SIXTH EDITION

Critical Care
Handbook of the
Massachusetts
General Hospital

Critical Care
Handbook of the
Massachusetts
General Hospital

Senior Editor

Jeanine P. Wiener-Kronish

Associate Editors

Aranya Bagchi

Jonathan E. Charnin

J. Perren Cobb

Matthias Eikermann

Sadeq A. Quraishi

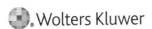 Wolters Kluwer

Philadelphia • Baltimore • New York • London
Buenos Aires • Hong Kong • Sydney • Tokyo

Acquisitions Editor: Keith Donnellan
Product Development Editor: Nicole Dernoski
Editorial Assistant: Kathryn Leyendecker
Marketing Manager: Dan Dressler
Production Project Manager: Priscilla Crater
Design Coordinator: Teresa Mallon
Manufacturing Coordinator: Beth Welsh
Prepress Vendor: S4Carlisle Publishing Services

6th edition

9 8 7 6 5 4 3 2

Printed in China

1-4511-9510-9
978-1-4511-9510-1
Library of Congress Cataloging-in-Publication Data available upon request

---

CCS0118

I would just thank the authors, the residents, the faculty, and above all, our patients who have given us the privilege of allowing us to care for them. We will engage in continuous learning to ensure that our care for our patients is optimal.

Jeanine P. Wiener-Kronish, MD

CONTRIBUTORS

Young Ahn, MD
Medical Director
Department of Anesthesiology
Perioperative Services—District of Columbia/Suburban Maryland
Kaiser Permanente: Mid-Atlantic Permanente Medical Group
Largo, Maryland

Aranya Bagchi, MBBS
Assistant in Anesthesia
Massachusetts General Hospital
Instructor in Anesthesia
Harvard Medical School
Boston, Massachusetts

Ednan K. Bajwa, MD, MPH
Medical ICU Director
Division of Pulmonary and Critical Care Medicine
Massachusetts General Hospital
Boston, Massachusetts

Peter L. Bekker, MD
Resident
Department of Anesthesia, Critical Care and Pain Medicine
Massachusetts General Hospital
Clinical Fellow
Harvard Medical School
Boston, Massachusetts

Lorenzo Berra, MD
Anesthesiologist and Critical Care Physician
Assistant Professor
Department of Anesthesia, Critical Care and Pain Medicine
Massachusetts General Hospital
Harvard Medical School
Boston, Massachusetts

Edward A. Bittner, MD, PhD, MS Ed, FCCP, FCCM
Program Director
Critical Care Medicine-Anesthesiology Fellowship
Associate Director, Surgical Intensive Care Unit
Assistant Professor of Anaesthesia
Harvard Medical School
Department of Anesthesia, Critical Care and Pain Medicine
Massachusetts General Hospital
Boston, Massachusetts

Kevin Blackney, MD
Resident in Anesthesiology
Department of Anesthesia, Critical Care and Pain Medicine
Massachusetts General Hospital
Harvard Medical School
Boston, Massachusetts

Sharon Brackett, RN, BS, CCRN
Attending Nurse, Surgical ICU
Massachusetts General Hospital
Boston, Massachusetts

Jeffrey Bruckel, MD, MPH, HMS
Fellow in Quality and Safety
Edward Lawrence Center for Quality and Safety
Massachusetts General Hospital
Boston, Massachusetts

Richard N. Channick, MD
Director, Pulmonary Hypertension and
    Thromboendarterectomy Program
Massachusetts General Hospital
Associate Professor of Medicine
Harvard Medical School
Boston, Massachusetts

Jonathan E. Charnin, MD
Instructor in Anesthesia
Harvard Medical School
Department of Anesthesia, Critical Care and Pain Medicine
Massachusetts General Hospital
Boston, Massachusetts

Sanjeev V. Chhangani, MD, MBA, FCCM
Assistant Professor of Anaesthesia
Harvard Medical School
Associate Anesthetist
Department of Anesthesia, Critical Care and Pain Medicine
Massachusetts General Hospital
Boston, Massachusetts

Hovig V. Chitilian, MD
Assistant Professor of Anesthesiology
Department of Anesthesia, Critical Care and Pain Medicine
Massachusetts General Hospital
Harvard Medical School
Boston, Massachusetts

Alexandra F. M. Cist, MD
Instructor
Harvard Medical School
Pulmonary and Critical Care Unit
Massachusetts General Hospital
Boston, Massachusetts

J. Perren Cobb, MD, FACS, FCCM
Vice-Chair for Critical Care
Department of Anesthesia, Critical Care and Pain Medicine
Massachusetts General Hospital
Associate Professor of Surgery and Anesthesiology
Harvard Medical School
Boston, Massachusetts

Gaston Cudemus, MD
Clinical Instructor
Department of Anesthesia, Critical Care and Pain Medicine
Massachusetts General Hospital
Harvard Medical School
Boston, Massachusetts

Brian M. Cummings, MD
Pediatric Critical Care, Assistant in Pediatrics
MassGeneral Hospital for Children
Instructor in Medicine
Harvard Medical School
Boston, Massachusetts

Marc A. de Moya, MD
Medical Director, Blake 12 ICU
Fellowship Director, Surgical Critical Care
Massachusetts General Hospital
Assistant Professor of Surgery
Harvard Medical School
Boston, Massachusetts

Matthias Eikermann, MD, PhD
Associate Professor of Anaesthesia
Harvard Medical School
Clinical Director, Critical Care Division
Massachusetts General Hospital
Boston, Massachusetts

Peter J. Fagenholz, MD
Attending Surgeon, Division of Trauma, Emergency
    Surgery, and Critical Care
Massachusetts General Hospital
Instructor in Surgery
Harvard Medical School
Boston, Massachusetts

David W. Fink, MD
Instructor
Trauma, Emergency Surgery, Surgical Critical Care
Massachusetts General Hospital
Boston, Massachusetts

Michael G. Fitzsimons, MD, FCCP
Director, Cardiac Anesthesia
Assistant Professor
Harvard Medical School
Department of Anesthesia, Critical Care and Pain Medicine
Massachusetts General Hospital
Boston, Massachusetts

Eugene Fukudome, MD
Clinical Fellow in Surgery
Department of Surgery
Brigham and Women's Hospital
Boston, Massachusetts

Jose P. Garcia, MD
Surgical Director, Cardiothoracic Transplantation
Artificial Heart and Lung Program
Massachusetts General Hospital
Harvard Medical School
Boston, Massachusetts

Klaus Goerlinger, MD
Department of Anesthesiology and Intensive Care Medicine
University Hospital Essen
Essen, Germany

Jessica Hahn, MD
Mass General Hospital for Children
Boston, Massachusetts

R. Scott Harris, MD
Associate Physician
Massachusetts General Hospital
Associate Professor of Medicine
Harvard Medical School
Boston, Massachusetts

Dean R. Hess, PhD, RRT
Assistant Director of Respiratory Care
Massachusetts General Hospital
Associate Professor of Anesthesia
Harvard Medical School
Boston, Massachusetts

Kathryn A. Hibbert, MD
Instructor in Medicine, Division of Pulmonary and Critical Care
Massachusetts General Hospital,
Harvard Medical School
Boston, Massachusetts

Ronald Hirschberg, MD
Massachusetts General Hospital
Department of Physical Medicine and Rehabilitation
Boston, Massachusetts

Craig S. Jabaley, MD
Clinical Fellow in Critical Care
Department of Anesthesia, Critical Care and Pain Medicine
Massachusetts General Hospital
Harvard Medical School
Boston, Massachusetts

Christina Jelly, MD, MSc
Clinical Fellow
Harvard Medical School
Department of Anesthesia, Critical Care and Pain Medicine
Massachusetts General Hospital
Boston, Massachusetts

Daniel W. Johnson, MD
Division Chief, Critical Care, Director
Critical Care Anesthesiology Fellowship
Assistant Professor
Department of Anesthesiology
University of Nebraska Medical Center
Omaha, Nebraska

Sameer S. Kadri, MD, MS
Physician-Scientist
Critical Care Medicine Department
Clinical Center
National Institutes of Health
Bethesda, Maryland

Rebecca I. Kalman, MD
Instructor of Anesthesia
Department of Anesthesia, Critical Care and Pain Medicine
Massachusetts General Hospital
Boston, Massachusetts

Corry "Jeb" Kucik, MD, MA, DMCC, FCCP, FUHM
Commander, Medical Corps, US Navy
Head, Healthcare Net Assessments
Navy Bureau of Medicine and Surgery
Falls Church, Virginia
Assistant Professor of Anesthesiology
Uniformed Services University
Bethesda, Maryland

Alexander S. Kuo, MD, MS
Fellow in Anesthesiology
Department of Anesthesia and Critical Care
Massachusetts General Hospital
Harvard Medical School
Boston, Massachusetts

Jean Kwo, MD
Assistant Professor of Anesthesia
Department of Anesthesia, Critical Care and Pain Medicine
Boston, Massachusetts

Yvonne Lai, MD
Department of Anesthesia, Critical Care and Pain Medicine
Massachusetts General Hospital
Boston, Massachusetts

Alice D. Lam, MD, PhD
Epilepsy Fellow
Department of Neurology
Massachusetts General Hospital
Boston, Massachusetts

Jarone Lee, MD, MPH
Instructor in Surgery
Harvard Medical School
Division of Trauma, Emergency Surgery, Surgical Critical Care
Massachusetts General Hospital
Boston, Massachusetts

Benjamin Levi, MD
Assistant Professor in Surgery
Division of Plastic and Reconstructive and Burn Surgery
University of Michigan
Director
Burn/Wound and Regenerative Medicine Laboratory
Ann Arbor, Michigan

Alexander R. Levine, PharmD
Critical Care Pharmacist
Department of Pharmacy
Massachusetts General Hospital
Boston, Massachusetts

Hsin Lin, PharmD
ICU Pharmacist
Pharmacy Department
Massachusetts General Hospital
Boston, Massachusetts

Andrew L. Lundquist, MD, PhD
Assistant Clinical Director
Division of Nephrology
Massachusetts General Hospital
Boston, Massachusetts

Laurie O. Mark, MD
Resident Physician
Department of Anesthesia, Critical Care and Pain Medicine
Massachusetts General Hospital
Boston, Massachusetts

Marcos Vidal Melo, MD, PhD
Associate Professor of Anesthesia
Department of Anesthesia, Critical Care and Pain Medicine
Massachusetts General Hospital
Harvard Medical School
Boston, Massachusetts

Sanjay Menon , MD
Clinical Fellow in Neurology
Department of Neurology
Massachusetts General Hospital
Boston, Massachusetts

Rebecca D. Minehart, MD
Assistant Professor
Massachusetts General Hospital
Harvard Medical School
Boston, Massachusetts

Jeremi R. Mountjoy, MSc, MD, FRCPC
Instructor in Anesthesia
Massachusetts General Hospital
Harvard Medical School
Boston, Massachusetts

Guido Musch, MD, MBA
Associate Professor of Anesthesia
Department of Anesthesia, Critical Care and Pain Medicine
Massachusetts General Hospital
Harvard Medical School
Boston, Massachusetts

Yasuko Nagasaka, MD, PhD
Fellow, Cardiothoracic Anesthesia
Department of Anesthesia, Critical Care and Pain Medicine
Massachusetts General Hospital
Boston, Massachusetts

John H. Nichols, MD
Resident in Anesthesiology
Department of Anesthesia and Critical Care
Massachusetts General Hospital
Boston, Massachusetts

Crystal M. North, MD
Clinical Research Fellow
Pulmonary and Critical Care Medicine
Massachusetts General Hospital
Boston, Massachusetts

Ala Nozari, MD, PhD
Department of Anesthesia, Critical Care and Pain Medicine
Massachusetts General Hospital
Harvard Medical School
Boston, Massachusetts

Madhukar S. Patel, MD, MBA, ScM
Resident in Surgery
Department of Surgery
Massachusetts General Hospital
Boston, Massachusetts

Pratik V. Patel, MD
Acting Assistant Professor
Department of Anesthesiology and Pain Medicine
University of Washington Hospital Harborview Medical Center
University of Washington
Seattle, Washington

Richard M. Pino, MD, PhD, FCCM
Associate Professor in Anesthesia
Harvard Medical School
Associate Anesthetist
Department of Anesthesia, Critical Care and Pain Medicine
Massachusetts General Hospital
Boston, Massachusetts

Justin M. Poltak, MD
Attending Physician
Department of Anesthesiology
Maine Medical Center
Portland, Maine

Kate Riddell, MD
Instructor in Anesthesia
Massachusetts General Hospital
Harvard Medical School
Boston, Massachusetts

Fiona D. Roberts, MA
Project Coordinator
Edward P. Lawrence Center for Quality and Safety
Massachusetts General Hospital
Boston, Massachusetts

Daniel Saddawi-Konefka, MD, MBA
Instructor
Department of Anesthesia, Critical Care and Pain Medicine
Massachusetts General Hospital
Harvard Medical School
Boston, Massachusetts

William J. Sauer, MD
Chief Resident
Department of Anesthesia, Critical Care and Pain Medicine
Massachusetts General Hospital
Boston, Massachusetts

Milad Sharifpour, MD, MS
Department of Anesthesia, Critical Care and Pain Medicine
Massachusetts General Hospital
Boston, Massachusetts

Kenneth Shelton, MD
Instructor in Anesthesia
Department of Anesthesia
Massachusetts General Hospital
Boston, Massachusetts

Robert Sheridan, MD, FACS
Department of Surgery
Massachusetts General Hospital
Boston, Massachusetts

Matthew J. G. Sigakis, MD
Clinical Fellow in Critical Care
Department of Anesthesia, Critical Care and Pain Medicine
Massachusetts General Hospital
Harvard Medical School
Boston, Massachusetts

Christopher R. Tainter, MD, RDMS
Assistant Clinical Professor
Department of Emergency Medicine
Department of Anesthesiology, Division of Critical Care
University of California, San Diego
San Diego, California

B. Taylor Thompson, MD
Division of Pulmonary and Critical Care
Massachusetts General Hospital
Harvard Medical School
Boston, Massachusetts

Andrea T. Tull, PhD
Director, Reporting and Analytics
Center for Quality and Safety
Massachusetts General Hospital
Boston, Massachusetts

Parsia A. Vagefi, MD, FACS
Associate Surgical Director, Liver Transplantation
Massachusetts General Hospital
Assistant Professor of Surgery
Harvard Medical School
Boston, Massachusetts

Olof Viktorsdottir, MD
Assistant in Anesthesia
Department of Anesthesia, Critical Care and Pain Medicine
Massachusetts General Hospital
Instructor in Anesthesia
Harvard Medical School
Boston, Massachusetts

Karen Waak, PT, DPT, CCS
Physical Therapy Clinical Specialist
Department of Physical Therapy
Massachusetts General Hospital
Boston, Massachusetts

Sarah Wahlster, MD
Acting Assistant Professor of Neurology
Harborview Medical Center
University of Washington
Seattle, Washington

M. Brandon Westover, MD, PhD
Harvard Medical School
Massachusetts General Hospital
Neurology Director
MGH Critical Care EEG Monitoring
Boston, Massachusetts

Jeanine P. Wiener-Kronish, MD
Anesthetist-in-Chief
Department of Anesthesia, Critical Care and Pain Medicine
Massachusetts General Hospital
Boston, Massachusetts

Stephen D. Wilkins, MD
Clinical Fellow in Cardiac Anesthesia
Department of Anesthesia, Critical Care and Pain Medicine
Massachusetts General Hospital
Harvard Medical School
Boston, Massachusetts

Elizabeth Cox Williams, MD
Instructor in Anesthesia
Department of Anesthesia, Critical Care and Pain Medicine
Massachusetts General Hospital
Boston, Massachusetts

Alison S. Witkin, MD
Division of Pulmonary and Critical Care Medicine
Massachusetts General Hospital
Boston, Massachusetts

Victor W. Wong, MD
Resident, Plastic and Reconstructive Surgery
Johns Hopkins Medical School
Baltimore, Maryland

Daniel Yagoda, MPH
Administrative Director
Center for Quality and Safety
Massachusetts General Hospital
Boston, Massachusetts

D. Dante Yeh, MD, FACS
Clinical Instructor in Surgery
Massachusetts General Hospital
Department of Surgery
Division of Trauma, Emergency Surgery, and Surgical Critical Care
Associate Director of Surgical Intensive Care Unit
Boston, Massachusetts

Kevin H. Zhao, MD
Critical Care Fellow
Department of Anesthesia, Critical Care and Pain Medicine
Massachusetts General Hospital
Boston, Massachusetts

PREFACE

The *Critical Care Handbook of the Massachusetts General Hospital* is meant to provide all health care providers with an overview of this enlarging and exciting field. Critical care now encompasses the care of all patients requiring intense physiologic monitoring. These patients include patients who now survive previously untreatable cancers, trauma victims of all ages, postoperative patients of all ages, patients whose age or comorbidities would have previously precluded anesthesia and surgery, and patients requiring mechanical support for prolonged periods.

The separation of ICUs is somewhat artificial since patients often have multiple problems requiring multiple medical specialties. Likewise, the skills of intensivists are expanding and include transthoracic echocardiography, transesophageal echocardiography, experience with ECMO and destination hearts as well as experience with liver, heart, face, and kidney transplants. In addition, intensivists must now learn to protect themselves from EBOLA and MERS as well as from influenza and antibiotic-resistant bacteria.

Some treatments have changed only slightly over the years, but the future of critical care will involve estimation of patient genetics and immunologic status as well as their microbiomes. Molecular techniques utilized only for research until recently will now come to the clinical arena. Critical care practitioners will need knowledge of these techniques, as well as an appreciation of epidemiology, disease states, and the economics of care. Communication skills need to be taught to improve patient care; patients need multiple providers when they have multiple organ dysfunction. Protocols and checklists improve aspects of care, as does optimal communication between practitioners and patients and their families.

The handbook has been heavily revised to reflect a multidisciplinary approach to care, the need to include all care providers to optimize treatment, and the need for ongoing education and learning. The challenges will continue, but so does the satisfaction in caring for our sickest patients and our goal of continually improving our patients' lives.

CONTENTS

Hemodynamic Monitoring

Christina Jelly and Daniel Saddawi-Konefka

I. **HEMODYNAMIC MONITORING** is one of the cornerstones of patient evaluation in the intensive care unit and provides diagnostic and prognostic value. The choice of monitoring depends on the diagnostic needs of the patient and the risk–benefit balance of monitor placement and maintenance. This chapter outlines an approach to assessment of hemodynamics and perfusion in critically ill patients and the technical principles of commonly used monitoring methods.

A. **Perfusion:** *The goal of hemodynamic monitoring is to ensure adequate tissue perfusion* for gas, nutrient, and waste exchange to ultimately decrease morbidity and mortality. To get from optimizing a single hemodynamic parameter to improving morbidity and mortality requires many assumptions (as shown in Fig. 1.1 for mean arterial pressure, MAP). For this reason, the intensivist should not rely solely on any one physical monitor and should look for other signs of adequate perfusion such as mental status, urine output, or laboratory findings (e.g., central venous oxygen saturation, base deficit, lactate).

B. **Optimizing Perfusion:** *Hemodynamic monitors by themselves are not therapeutic.* Hemodynamic data should be used to guide therapy. Optimizing perfusion may require fluid administration, diuresis, pharmacologic agents (e.g., vasoconstrictors, inotropic agents), or interventions (e.g., thrombectomy, intra-aortic balloon pump, ventricular assist devices, extracorporeal membrane oxygenation). With this in mind, any monitor must be used dynamically to ensure that employed therapies are optimizing perfusion over time.

1. **Fluid challenge:** The fluid challenge is a time-honored test that bears specific mention. Rapid administration of crystalloid (typically 500 cc–1 L) while monitoring hemodynamics is used to determine if a patient may benefit from fluid, as suggested by an increase in cardiac output or blood pressure, for example. A "passive leg raise" test provides similar information. To perform this test, a clinician passively elevates a supine patient's legs. Blood moves to the central veins from the elevated limbs, providing an "autotransfusion" of approximately 150 to 300 cc. An improvement in hemodynamics suggests fluid responsiveness, whereas deterioration in hemodynamics can be quickly reversed by lowering the legs.

II. **ARTERIAL BLOOD PRESSURE MONITORING**

A. **General Principles**

1. Blood pressure describes the pressure exerted by circulating blood within the blood vessels. Since this pressure drives flow, it is used as a

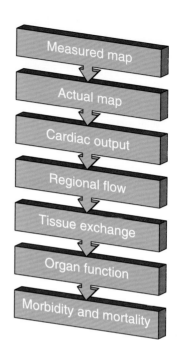

FIGURE 1.1 The assumptions when extrapolating MAP to a morbidity and mortality benefit.

surrogate measure of blood flow and, in turn, organ perfusion (Fig. 1.1). This simplified view has limitations and notably poor correlation with cardiac output in some situations, such as emergency resuscitation of the hypovolemic critically ill patient. Nonetheless, arterial blood pressure monitoring as a target for perfusion is used in almost all critical care settings and has been linked to morbidity and mortality outcomes.

2. Under normal circumstances, tissue perfusion is maintained across a range of pressures by autoregulation, which describes the intrinsic capacity of vascular beds to maintain flow by adjusting local vascular resistance. However, pathological conditions common in the intensive care unit such as chronic hypertension, trauma, and sepsis may impair autoregulation, resulting in blood flow that may depend directly on perfusion pressure.

3. The "gold standard" for blood pressure measurement is aortic root pressure, which is representative of the stresses faced by the major organs (e.g., heart, brain, kidneys). As the pressure wave travels distally from the aorta, the measured mean pressure decreases while the measured pulse pressure (systolic pressure minus diastolic pressure) is increased owing to pulse wave reflection from the high-resistant distal arterioles. In addition to being amplified, as one progresses distally, the arterial waveform is slightly delayed (Fig. 1.2). The difference in mean pressure is typically minimal given the low arterial resistance, but can be significant in some situations (e.g., high-dose vasoconstrictor administration).

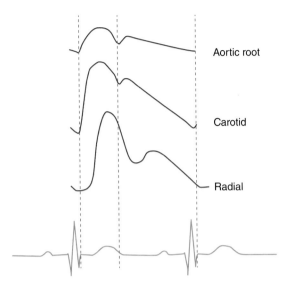

FIGURE 1.2 Arterial waveforms as one travels distally along the arterial tree.

B. **Noninvasive Blood Pressure Monitoring:** Various techniques can be used to measure blood pressure noninvasively including manual palpation, determination of Korotkoff sounds with a sphygmomanometer and stethoscope or Doppler ultrasound, and automated oscillometric methods, which are most common in the ICU.
   1. **Function:** The oscillometric method uses a pneumatic cuff with an electric pressure sensor, most commonly over the brachial artery. The cuff is inflated to a high pressure and then slowly deflated. Arterial pulsations are recorded as oscillations. The pressure that produces greatest oscillation recording is closely associated with mean arterial pressure. Systolic and diastolic pressures are then *calculated*, often using proprietary algorithms.
   2. **Technique:** Accurate noninvasive blood pressure measurement requires appropriate cuff sizing and placement. Most blood pressure cuffs display reference lines for an acceptable arm length, and the cuffs should be sized as recommended in relationship to arm circumference. Cuffs that are too small may overestimate blood pressure, whereas cuffs that are too large may underestimate blood pressure.
   3. **Limitations and risks:**
      a. The pressure measured by a noninvasive cuff is the pressure at the cuff site. When an extremity pressure is measured to estimate coronary perfusion, either the extremity should be elevated to the level of the heart, or the fluid column should be accounted for (e.g., a pressure measured at a site 10 cm below the heart will be 10 cmH_2O or approximately 7.4 mmHg greater than the pressure at the heart).
      b. Tissues, including vessels and nerves, can be damaged by cyclical compression of pneumatic cuffs with frequent cycling. Automatic methods may not be reliable in rapidly changing situations, such as

extremes of blood pressure, rapidly changing blood pressure, or patients with dysrhythmias.

C. Invasive Arterial Blood Pressure Monitoring provides beat-to-beat pressure transduction and allows convenient blood sampling.

1. **Indications** for placement of an arterial line include hemodynamic instability, need for tight blood pressure control, or need for frequent blood sampling.

2. **Site:** The radial artery is frequently selected given the existence of collateral circulation to distal tissues, convenient access for ongoing care, and patient comfort. Alternative sites in adults include the brachial, axillary, femoral, and dorsalis pedis arteries.

3. **Function:** Necessary equipment to monitor invasive arterial blood pressure includes an intra-arterial catheter, fluid-filled noncompliant tubing, transducer, continuous flush device, and electronic monitoring equipment. The flush device typically provides an infusion of plain or heparinized saline at a rate of 2 to 4 milliliters per hour through the tubing and catheter to prevent thrombus formation. Commonly employed arterial line pressure bag/transducer systems provide this slow flush by design. The transducing sensor is "connected" to arterial blood by a continuous line of fluid and measures a pressure deflection in response to the transmitted pressure wave of each heartbeat. The accuracy of intra-arterial blood pressure measurement depends on the proper positioning and calibration of the catheter–transducer monitoring system.

   a. **Positioning:** The arterial pressure transduced is at the level of the transducer, not at the level of the cannulation site. This is because of the fluid-filled tubing between the patient and transducer, which maintains energy by exchanging potential energy for pressure (Bernoulli's equation). For example, if the transducer is lowered, the fluid in the tubing exerts an additional pressure on the transducer and the measured pressure will be higher. Therefore, the arterial transducer should be placed at the level of interest. For example, positioning at the fourth intercostal space on the midaxillary line ("the phlebostatic axis") corresponds to the level of the aortic root, and positioning at the external acoustic meatus corresponds to the Circle of Willis.

   b. **Static calibration** zeroes the system to atmospheric pressure. The transducer is opened to air and the recorded pressure (the atmospheric pressure) is set to zero.

   c. **Dynamic calibration:** The two components of dynamic calibration of an oscillating system are resonance (which increases pulse pressure amplitude) and damping (which decreases pulse pressure amplitude).

      1. **Resonance:** When an arterial pulsation "hits" the elastic arterial wall, this vibrates and, just like a musical fork, generates an infinite series of sine waves of increasing frequency and decreasing amplitude. Typically, the natural frequencies of arterial pulse waveforms are in the 16-to-24-Hz range. The transducer system has its own natural frequency, commonly over 200 Hz. As the natural frequency of the arterial pulse approaches that of the transducer system, the system will resonate—pressure waveforms will be amplified versions of the intra-arterial waveform ("whipped" waveforms with erroneously wide pulse pressures). The resonant frequency of a system can be tested with a fast flush test. Displayed on a strip chart recorder, the resonant frequency of the

system can be calculated by measuring the distance between two subsequent peaks of the trace. Tachycardia or a steep systolic upstroke will increase the natural frequency of the arterial pulse and may contribute to resonance.

    2. Damping: The **damping coefficient** is a measure of how quickly an oscillating system comes to rest. A high damping coefficient indicates that the system absorbs mechanical energy well and will cause attenuation of the waveform. Factors that increase damping include loose connections, kinks, and large air bubbles. The ideal damping coefficient depends on the natural frequency of the system, though it is 0.6 to 0.7 for commonly used systems.

  4. Complications: Arterial cannulation is relatively safe. Risks depend on site of cannulation. For radial cannulation, reported serious risks include permanent ischemic damage (0.09%), local infection and sepsis (0.72% and 0.13%, respectively), and pseudoaneurysm (0.09%). Fastidious attention to the adequacy of distal perfusion is of great importance. Thrombotic sequelae are associated with larger catheters, smaller arterial size, administration of vasopressors, duration of cannulation, and multiple arterial cannulation attempts. With regard to infectious risk, aseptic technique was not standardized in the studies that yielded the aforementioned percentage of risk, and longer duration of cannulation increased risk. Less serious risks include temporary occlusion (19.7%) and hematoma (14.4%). Axillary and femoral sites are associated with higher risks of infection. Brachial cannulation has been associated with median nerve injury (0.2%–1.4%).

  5. Respiratory variation: Increased intrathoracic pressure decreases preload, arterial pressure, and pulse pressure. This effect is marked in hypovolemic patients who are more susceptible to increased intrathoracic pressures. Variation of more than 10% to 12% in systolic pressure or pulse pressure is suggestive of fluid responsiveness. Importantly, this is validated for patients with regular cardiac rhythm and breathing pattern, and it is dependent on the ventilatory pressure delivered.

  6. Arterial waveform analysis has been used to gauge stroke volume and is discussed later in this chapter.

D. Discrepancies between Noninvasive and Invasive Arterial Blood Pressure Measurements exist, with noninvasive measurements tending to yield higher measurements during hypotension and lower measurements during hypertension. These discrepancies persist even with appropriate cuff sizing in critically ill patients. Retrospective data suggests that the higher noninvasive systolic blood pressures during hypotension are overestimates of perfusion, since the incidence of acute kidney injury and mortality is higher with noninvasive versus invasive systolic blood pressures. There was no difference in acute kidney injury or mortality when mean pressures were compared. This suggests that mean pressures should be targeted when the hypotensive critically ill patient is treated with a noninvasive cuff.

III. CENTRAL VENOUS PRESSURE MONITORING

A. Indications for placement of a central venous catheter (CVC) include administration of certain drugs, concentrated vasopressors, or TPN; need for dialysis; need for long-term medication administration such as chemotherapy or intravenous antibiotics; need for IV access in patients with difficult peripheral access; or need for sampling central venous blood.

B. Site: Common central venous cannulations sites are the internal jugular, subclavian, and femoral veins. The ideal site of cannulation varies with

	Risks and Benefits of Different Central Line Access Approaches				
Site	Infection Risk	Bleeding Risk	Thrombotic Risk	Patient Comfort	Comments
Internal jugular	++	+	++	++	Compressible, low pneumothorax risk
Subclavian	+	+++	+	+++	Higher risk of pneumothorax, difficult to compress in case of bleeding
Femoral	+++	+	+++	+	Often easiest place in an emergency, high infection rate
PICC	+	−	++	+++	Good for long-term access, low flow rate

PICC, peripherally inserted central catheter.

the characteristics of the patient and the indications for insertion. For example, the subclavian site is relatively contraindicated in coagulopathic patients as it is not directly compressible, and the femoral vein may be ideal in emergency situations because of ease of cannulation. Table 1.1 summarizes the advantages and disadvantages of the most commonly used sites for venous access.

   C. **Central Venous Pressure Waveform**: Central venous pressure (CVP) provides an estimate of right ventricular preload and should be measured with the transducer positioned at the phlebostatic axis. The CVP tracing contains three positive deflections (Fig. 1.3). The *a*-wave corresponds with atrial contraction and correlates with the p wave on EKG. The *c*-wave corresponds with ventricular contraction (and bulging of tricuspid valve into the right atrium) and correlates with the end of the QRS complex on EKG. The *v*-wave corresponds to atrial filling against a closed tricuspid valve and occurs with the end of the T wave on EKG. The *x*-descent after the *c*-wave is thought to be due to the downward displacement of the atrium during ventricular systole and the *y*-descent by tricuspid valve opening during diastole.

      1. **Abnormal waveforms**: The loss of atrial contraction that occurs with atrial fibrillation results in loss of *a*-waves on CVP tracings. Large *a*-waves ("cannon a-waves") may occur when the atrium contracts against a closed valve as occurs during atrioventricular dissociation or ventricular pacing. Abnormally large *v*-waves may be associated with tricuspid regurgitation; they begin immediately after the QRS complex and often incorporate the *c*-wave. Abnormally large *v*-waves may also be observed during right ventricular failure or ischemia, constrictive pericarditis, or cardiac tamponade due to the volume and/or pressure overload seen by the right atrium. Tricuspid stenosis is a diastolic defect in atrial emptying and can elevate the CVP; the diastolic *y*-descent is attenuated the end diastolic *a*-wave is prominent.

   D. **Interpretation of CVP**:

      1. **Measurement**: CVP, when measured as a surrogate for end-diastolic filling, should be measured at the valley just before the *c*-wave (i.e., at the

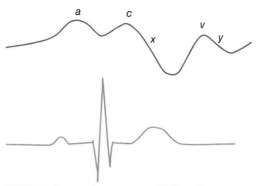

FIGURE 1.3 The central venous pressure (CVP) waveform.

end of diastole, just before ventricular contraction). As CVP changes with respiration (owing to changes in intrathoracic pressure), it should be measured at end expiration, when the lung is closest to functional residual capacity and confounding intrathoracic pressure influences are minimized.

2. **Utility and controversy**: In spite of recent evidence suggesting limited utility, CVP has been used clinically to assess fluid status for decades. The physiologic determinants of CVP include patient position, the circulating volume status, interactions between systemic and pulmonary circulations, and the dynamic changes in the respiratory system over the breathing cycle. Not surprisingly, the accurate interpretation of CVP can be difficult and a number of studies have challenged its use. Systematic review has suggested poor correlation of CVP with circulating blood volume as well as poor correlation of CVP (or trend in CVP) with fluid responsiveness.

3. **Clinical confounders**: When used clinically, CVP measurements are used to estimate end diastolic volume, given in the following relationship:

$$V_{RV} = C_{RV} \cdot \left(CVP - P_{extracardiac} \right)$$

where V_{RV} is end diastolic volume, C_{RV} is compliance of the right ventricle, CVP approximates the pressure inside the ventricle, and $P_{extracardiac}$ is extracardiac pressure. Given this relationship, the general categories of physiologic perturbation that alter the direct relation between CVP and volume are:

a. **Abnormal cardiac compliance**, as in concentric hypertrophy

b. **Altered extracardiac pressure**, as with high PEEP, abdominal compartment syndrome, or tamponade, for example

c. **Valvular abnormalities**, as with tricuspid insufficiency or stenosis (where CVP will no longer approximate right ventricular pressures)

d. **Ventricular interdependence**

E. **Complications**: Central venous cannulation complications vary based on selected anatomic site (see Table 1.1) and operator experience. Serious immediate complications include catheter malposition, pneumo- or hemothorax, arterial puncture, bleeding, air or wire embolism, arrhythmia, and thoracic duct injury (with left subclavian or left internal jugular approach). Delayed serious complications include infection, thrombosis and pulmonary emboli, catheter migration, catheter embolization, myocardial injury or perforation, and nerve injury. Recommendations for placement technique and avoidance of infection are described in *Clinical Anesthesia Procedures of the Massachusetts General Hospital, 7th Edition*, chapter 10.

IV. PULMONARY ARTERY CATHETERS

A. Indications for placement of a pulmonary artery (PA) catheter include need for monitoring pulmonary artery pressures, measuring cardiac output with thermodilution, assessing left ventricular filling pressures, and sampling true mixed venous blood. Additionally, some PA catheters have pacing ports and can be used for temporary transvenous pacing.

B. Technique: Pulmonary artery catheters are positioned by floating a distally inflated balloon through the right atrium and right ventricle into the pulmonary artery. Figure 1.4 shows the characteristic pressure waveforms seen as the pulmonary catheter is advanced. During placement, attention to the pressure tracing, electrocardiogram, systemic blood pressure, and oxygen saturation is essential to ensure proper placement of the catheter and to minimize known complications.

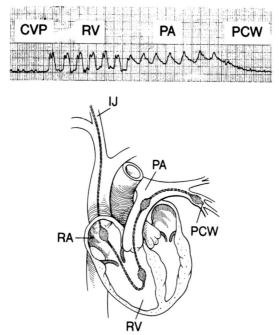

FIGURE 1.4 Characteristic pressure waves seen during insertion of a pulmonary artery catheter. CVP, central venous pressure; IJ, internal jugular; PA, pulmonary artery; PCW, pulmonary capillary wedge; RA, right atrium; RV, right ventricle.

1. Fluoroscopic guidance may be useful in certain situations, such as the presence of recently placed permanent pacemaker (generally within 6 weeks), the need for selective PA placement (e.g., following pneumonectomy) and the presence of significant structural or physiologic abnormality (e.g., severe RV dilation, large intracardiac shunts or severe pulmonary hypertension).

C. **Waveforms during Placement**: The right atrial pressure waveform is the same as the CVP waveform previously described. The pressure waveform in the right ventricle (RV) has a systolic upstroke (in phase with the systemic arterial upstroke) with low diastolic pressures that increase during diastole, owing to ventricular filling. The pulmonary artery pressure waveform will also be in phase with systemic pressures during systole, but will differ from the RV tracing as the pressure decreases during diastole. Often, the diastolic pressure will increase when the balloon enters the pulmonary artery, but the better marker of this advancement is the transition to a downward slope during diastole. The pulmonary artery occlusion pressure (PAOP) or wedge pressure waveform will resemble the CVP trace with *a*-, *c*-, and *v*-waves, though these are often difficult to distinguish clinically.

D. **Physiologic Data**

1. **Thermodilution cardiac output (CO)**

   a. **Method**: A rapid bolus of cold saline is injected proximal to the right heart, and temperature is monitored at the distal tip of the PA catheter. With higher cardiac output, more blood is mixed with the cold fluid bolus and the temperature recorded over time will be attenuated, as described by the Modified Stewart-Hamilton Equation:

   $$CO = \frac{T_{body} - T_{injectate}}{AUC}$$

   b. where CO is cardiac output, T_{body} is the temperature of the body, $T_{injectate}$ is the temperature of the saline bolus, V is the volume of the bolus, K reflects properties of the catheter system, and AUC is the area under the curve of temperature change.

   c. **Reliability**: Averaging of serial measurements is recommended for each CO determination as the calculated CO may vary by as much as 10% without a change in clinical condition. It is important to minimize variations in the rate and volume of injection, which also introduce error. Colder solutions (i.e., increased $T_{body} - T_{injectate}$) decrease error, though attention should be paid to potential tachy- or bradyarrhythmias. Tricuspid regurgitation may affect calculations as a result of recirculated blood between the right atrium and ventricle. Intracardiac shunt can likewise introduce error.

2. **PA occlusion pressure**: Occluding the PA recreates a static fluid column between the distal tip of the catheter and the left atrium, allowing equilibration of pressures between the two sites. In this manner, PAOP approximates left atrial pressure, a surrogate for left ventricular end-diastolic volume. For an accurate measure of PAOP, the proper atrial trace, similar to the "*a-c-v*" trace of the CVP waveform, should be visualized. As highlighted in the discussion of CVP measurements, volume is only one parameter that influences the PAOP measurements of other variables (e.g., cardiac compliance, intrathoracic pressures, valvular lesions, ventricular interdependence).

3. **Mixed venous oxygen saturation ($S\bar{v}o_2$)**: As cardiac output increases, tissue oxygen demand is met with less per-unit oxygen extraction and $S\bar{v}o_2$ increases. This is a loose correlation as $S\bar{v}o_2$ also depends on hemoglobin concentration and oxygen consumption, as outlined by the Fick Equation:

$$CO = \frac{\dot{V}o_2}{\left(Sao_2 - S\bar{v}o_2\right) \cdot hgb \cdot 1.34 \cdot 10}$$

where *CO* is cardiac output in liters per minute, $\dot{V}o_2$ is oxygen consumption in millimeters per minute, Sao_2 and $S\bar{v}o_2$ are arterial and mixed venous oxygen saturation, and hgb is hemoglobin in grams per deciliter.

In other words, $S\bar{v}o_2$ correlates with cardiac output, and a low $S\bar{v}o_2$ suggests low cardiac output (assuming adequate oxygen extraction by the tissues and an adequate hemoglobin). $S\bar{v}o_2$, an oxygen saturation drawn from a non-PA central line, can act as a surrogate for $S\bar{v}o_2$. It is typically higher than the $S\bar{v}o_2$ by about 5% as it does not include the oxygen-depleted blood from the heart itself (returned to the right atrium from the coronary sinus).

E. **Complications:** In addition to complications associated with central venous access, PA catheter placement is associated with increased risk of arrhythmia including right heart block (especially in patients with recent MI or pericarditis) and pulmonary artery rupture. Pulmonary artery rupture risk is increased with pulmonary hypertension, advanced age, mitral valve disease, hypothermia, and anticoagulant therapy and requires emergent thoracotomy. Catheter-related complications, including knotting or balloon rupture with subsequent air or balloon fragment emboli, have also been reported.

F. **Relative contraindications** to PA placement include left heart block (as a superimposed right heart block would lead to complete block), presence of a transvenous pacer or recently placed pacemaker or ICD leads, tricuspid or pulmonary stenosis or prosthetic tricuspid or pulmonary valves (given the associated difficulty in passing the catheter and balloon), patient predisposition for arrhythmia, coagulopathy, or severe pulmonary hypertension. Need for MRI is also a contraindication as most PA lines contain ferromagnetic material.

G. **Controversy on PA Catheters:** Although hemodynamic data derived from PA catheters enhances understanding of cardiopulmonary physiology, the risk-to-benefit profile has been questioned. Since the mid-1990s, several large outcome studies assessing the benefit of PA catheters have been conducted, and none shows clear evidence of benefit. Moreover, PA catheter-guided therapy has been associated with more complications than does central venous catheter-guided therapy. Although these results are not sufficiently convincing to completely discourage use of PA catheters, they underscore the importance of only using PA catheters when the benefit of management guidance derived from PA data are strongly believed to outweigh the associated risks.

V. **ALTERNATIVES TO BLOOD PRESSURE MONITORING**: Numerous alternative hemodynamic monitors have been developed to assess either cardiovascular function or tissue perfusion.
A. **Transthoracic Ultrasound:** The use of ultrasound for hemodynamic assessment of cardiac function and fluid status has been growing in critical care and is discussed further in **Chapter 3**.

B. Continuous Esophageal Doppler: Blood velocity in the descending aorta can be measured with a transesophageal Doppler ultrasound. The average velocity over one heartbeat is multiplied by the cross-sectional area of the aorta (either estimated on the basis of patient data or measured by the probe) to calculate stroke volume. Stroke volume is multiplied by heart rate to obtain cardiac output. Notably, as this is only the flow in a descending aorta, a certain percentage (typically around 30%) is added to determine total cardiac output. Modern probes are roughly the size of nasogastric tubes, much smaller than ordinary trans-esophageal echocardiography probes, and can provide "corrected flow time" and stroke volume variation in addition to cardiac output, which can be used to gauge fluid responsiveness.

   1. **Advantages:** Esophageal Doppler monitoring allows continuous measurement with minimal risk of infection, is simple to use with short set-up time, and has a low incidence of iatrogenic complications.
   2. **Disadvantages:** Esophageal Doppler monitoring can only be performed in intubated patients, requires frequent repositioning if the patient is moved, is operator dependent, and is not widely available.

C. Partial CO₂ Rebreathing Method: The partial CO_2 rebreathing method is based on the Fick principle:

$$CO = \frac{\dot{V}o_2}{Cao_2 - C\overline{v}o_2}$$

where CO is cardiac output, Cao_2 is the arterial blood oxygen content of oxygen $C\overline{v}o_2$ is the venous blood oxygen content, and $\dot{V}o_2$ is oxygen consumption.

   Clinical measurement of $\dot{V}o_2$ is challenging, so this technique is based on a restatement of the Fick equation for carbon dioxide elimination rather than oxygen consumption:

$$CO = \frac{\dot{V}o_2}{C\overline{v}co_2 - Caco_2}$$

Using an intermittent partial rebreathing circuit, the change in CO_2 production and end tidal CO_2 concentration in response to a brief, sudden change in minute ventilation is measured. The changes in end tidal CO_2 are used to calculate cardiac output.

   1. **Advantages:** This method is low risk, noninvasive, and can be performed every few minutes. The partial rebreathing CO_2 cardiac output method has also shown reasonably good agreement with gold standard thermodilution in clinical trials in some settings.
   2. **Disadvantages:** As currently designed, this method requires tracheal intubation for measurement of exhaled gases. Measurements can be affected by changing patterns of ventilation and intrapulmonary shunting. Furthermore, this technique has a relatively long response time.

D. Transpulmonary Thermodilution and Transpulmonary Indicator Dilution: With these techniques, the same principles for PAC thermodilution are employed, but only a CVC and arterial line are required. A bolus of either cold saline (with the PiCCO device) or lithium chloride (with the LiDCO device) is injected into the central line and the dilution over time in a peripheral artery is used to derive the cardiac output. These are commonly used in conjunction with pulse contour analysis (see next section) to provide continuous assessment of cardiac output.

1. **Advantages:** Both of these methods have been shown to correlate reasonably well with PA catheter thermodilution. Transpulmonary thermodilution has the added benefit of providing assessment of extravascular lung water and intrathoracic blood volume.

2. **Disadvantages:** Both methods require repetitive blood draws, and calibration may be affected by neuromuscular blocking agents. Notably, the PiCCO system typically requires placement of an axillary or femoral arterial catheter.

E. **Pulse Contour Analysis:** This modality for measuring cardiac output relies on the principle that stroke volume and cardiac output can be gauged from characteristics of the arterial waveform, using calculations that are based on estimates of compliance of the arterial tree. Commercially available devices require calibration, typically against thermodilution or indicator dilution methods.

1. **Advantages:** Pulse contour analysis devices are continuous and employ catheters (central venous catheters and arterial lines) that are commonly employed in ICU patients.

2. **Disadvantages:** This technique requires mechanically ventilated patients and has shown questionable accuracy in patients who are hemodynamically labile and patients on vasoactive medications. The altered arterial waveform of patients with aortic insufficiency may also decrease the accuracy of this technique.

F. **Impedance Cardiography (Also Known as Electrical Impedance Plethysmography):** With impedance cardiography, a high-frequency, low-magnitude current is applied to the chest, and impedance is measured. As the aorta fills with blood with each heartbeat, impedance decreases, and this change is used to determine stroke volume and cardiac output. Advances in phased-array and signal-processing technologies have improved impedance cardiography, largely overcoming artifact due to electrode placement, HR and rhythm disturbances, and differences in body habitus, though its use is still fairly limited in the ICU. Both electrical velocimetry and bioreactance employ similar principles. Electrical velocimetry relates the velocity of blood flow in the aorta to determine cardiac output, whereas bioreactance uses changes in electrical current frequency (rather than in impedance) to measure changes in blood flow during the cardiac cycle.

1. **Advantages:** This method is noninvasive and continuous.

2. **Disadvantages:** Impedance cardiography is difficult to set up, and its usefulness is limited with noisy environments, extravascular fluid accumulation, and arrhythmia.

G. **Tissue Perfusion Monitors:** Whereas most hemodynamic monitors are surrogates for adequate perfusion, a few aim to assess perfusion at the tissue level. Notably, these only assess tissue perfusion in the tissues where they are measured. Gastric tonometry measures gastric CO_2, which decreases with low perfusion states. Tissue oxygenation (Sto_2) measures percentage of oxygenated hemoglobin at the microcirculation/tissue level. While there are many others, most of these are still used primary for research and not for clinical applications at this time.

Respiratory Monitoring

Marcos Vidal Melo and Hovig V. Chitilian

I. **MONITORING**
   A. **Respiration** is the transport of oxygen from the environment to the cells of the body and the transport of carbon dioxide from those cells to the environment. Consequently, in its broadest sense, **respiratory monitoring** refers to the assessment of the processes involved with the exchange of respiratory gases between the environment and the subcellular pathways in which those gases are utilized and produced. Respiratory monitoring is performed to assure patient **safety**, maintain **homeostasis, and titrate treatment.**
   B. The main components of **respiratory physiology** are **gas exchange, respiratory mechanics, control of breathing,** and **pulmonary circulation.** This chapter will **address the monitoring of gas exchange** and **respiratory mechanics,** and comment on **control of breathing.** Monitoring of the circulation is addressed in Chapter 1.

II. **MONITORING GAS EXCHANGE**
   A. **Basic Concepts:**
   1. **Hypoxia** is the condition of deprived oxygen supply. It can apply to a region of the body (tissue hypoxia) or the whole body (generalized hypoxia). The complete deprivation of oxygen supply is denominated **anoxia.** These concepts are not equivalent to those of **hypoxemia,** which refers to the reduction of oxygen, i.e., low partial pressure of oxygen, in arterial blood. Reasons for **hypoxia** include the following:
      a. **Hypoxemia:** low partial pressure of O_2 in the blood
      b. **Ischemia:** a deficiency in oxygen supply due to insufficient blood flow
      c. **Hystotoxic:** inability of cells to use oxygen despite appropriate delivery (i.e., cyanide toxicity)
      d. **Anemia**
      e. **Inhibition of the function of hemoglobin** such as in carbon monoxide poisoning.
      f. As can be seen, in general, it is **easier to monitor hypoxemia** than hypoxia.
   2. Arterial blood gases and pH
      a. Arterial blood gas analysis is often considered the standard for assessment of pulmonary gas exchange.
   3. Arterial partial pressure of oxygen (PaO_2)
      a. The normal PaO_2 is 90 to 100 mmHg breathing room air at sea level.
   4. **Decreased PaO_2 (hypoxemia)** occurs with pulmonary diseases or conditions resulting in increased shunt ($\dot{Q}s/\dot{Q}T$), ventilation–perfusion ($\dot{V}/\dot{Q}$) mismatch, hypoventilation, and diffusion defect. A low mixed venous PO_2 (e.g., decreased cardiac output) will magnify the effect of shunt on PaO_2. The PaO_2 is also decreased with decreased inspired oxygen (e.g., at high altitude).

13

5. **Increased Pao$_2$ (hyperoxemia)** may occur when breathing supplemental oxygen. The Pao$_2$ also increases with hyperventilation.
6. Effect of Fio$_2$ (fraction of inspired oxygen)
   a. The Pao$_2$ should always be interpreted in relation to the level of supplemental oxygen. For example, a Pao$_2$ of 95 mmHg breathing 100% oxygen is quite different from a Pao$_2$ of 95 mmHg breathing air (21% oxygen).
7. Arterial partial pressure of CO$_2$ (Paco$_2$)
   a. The Paco$_2$ reflects the balance between carbon dioxide production ($\dot{V}co_2$) and alveolar ventilation ($\dot{V}A$):

$$Paco_2 = K \times \dot{V}co_2 / \dot{V}A$$

   where K is a constant.
8. Alveolar ventilation: the fraction of the minute ventilation that participates in gas exchange. Minute ventilation = tidal volume (VT) × respiratory rate.
   a. Paco$_2$ varies directly with **carbon dioxide production** and inversely with **alveolar ventilation.**
   b. Paco$_2$ is determined by **alveolar ventilation**, not **minute ventilation**. The difference between them is the **dead-space ventilation**, which is ventilation that does not participate in gas exchange. Dead-space ventilation is made up of ventilation of the portions of the airway that do not participate in gas exchange (anatomical dead space) and those alveolar regions that do not exchange gas optimally because of absence of (or insufficient) blood flow in relation to the corresponding ventilation (physiological dead space), e.g., embolized regions after a pulmonary embolism.
   c. Minute ventilation affects Paco$_2$ only to the extent that it affects the alveolar ventilation.
   d. Note that the **Pao$_2$** is predominantly related to $\dot{V}/\dot{Q}$ **mismatch and shunt**, while **Paco$_2$** is predominantly related to **alveolar ventilation.**
   e. The physiological dead space can be estimated using the Bohr equation:

$$\frac{\dot{V}DS}{\dot{V}T} = \left(\frac{Paco_2 - P\bar{E}co_2}{Paco_2} \right)$$

   where PĒco$_2$ is the mixed expired CO$_2$ partial pressure, as measured in exhaled air collected in a mixing bag or chamber, or computed from a volumetric capnogram. Very large $\dot{V}DS/\dot{V}T$ has been recently associated with poor prognosis in acute respiratory distress syndrome (ARDS).
9. **Arterial pH** is determined by bicarbonate (HCO$_3^-$) concentration and Paco$_2$, as predicted by the **Henderson–Hasselbalch equation:**

$$pH = 6.1 + \log\left[HCO_3^- / \left(0.03 \times Paco_2 \right) \right]$$

10. Blood gas errors
    a. Care must be taken to avoid sample contamination with air, as the Po$_2$ and Pco$_2$ of room air at sea level are approximately 155 and

0 mmHg, respectively. Care should also be taken to avoid contamination of the sample with saline or venous blood.

   b. A specimen stored in a plastic syringe at room temperature should be analyzed within 30 minutes.

   c. Leukocyte larceny (spurious hypoxemia, pseudohypoxemia). The Pao_2 in samples drawn from subjects with very high leukocyte counts can decrease rapidly. Immediate chilling and analysis are necessary.

11. Blood gases and pH

   a. Blood gases and pH are measured at 37°C. Once the results of blood gases are available, they are often used to adjust the patient's acid–base status through ventilation or medications. Two strategies for management exist. **α-stat** management is the acid–base adjustment method in which blood gas measurements (pH, $Paco_2$) obtained at 37°C from the blood gas machine are directly used to reach the targets ($Paco_2 = 40$ mmHg, pH = 7.4). Using empiric equations, the blood gas analyzer can adjust the measured values to the patient's body temperature. **pH-stat** management is an alternative method in which measurements obtained at 37°C are corrected to the patient's actual body temperature before use to achieve those same numerical targets. It may be necessary to enquire with your laboratory to determine whether the laboratory is reporting temperature-compensated values (that may facilitate the use of the pH-stat strategy).

   b. Most intensive care units (ICUs) utilize the **α-stat** strategy. The choice of ventilation strategy is becoming increasingly important with the use of induced hypothermia as a therapeutic tool. Because of increased gas solubility during hypothermia, the **α-stat** strategy results in relative hyperventilation. The pH-stat approach results in increased cerebral blood flow. There are different conditions in which each of these methods can be more or less advantageous.

B. Venous Blood Gases reflect Pco_2 and Po_2 at the tissue level.

   1. There is a large difference between **Pao_2** and **venous Po_2 (Pvo_2)**. Pvo_2 is affected by oxygen delivery and oxygen consumption, whereas Pao_2 is affected by lung function. Thus, Pvo_2 should not be used as a surrogate for Pao_2.

   2. Normally, **venous pH** is lower than arterial pH, and **venous Pco_2 ($Pvco_2$)** is higher than $Paco_2$. However, the difference between arterial and venous pH and Pco_2 is increased by hemodynamic instability. During cardiac arrest, for example, it has been shown that $Pvco_2$ can be very high even when $Paco_2$ is low, a consequence of low cardiac output for a similar CO_2 production.

   3. When venous blood gases are used to assess acid–base balance, **mixed venous** or **central venous** samples are preferable to peripheral venous samples. Mixed venous blood is the blood present in the pulmonary artery, a result of the mix of blood from the superior and inferior vena cavae, and coronary sinus.

   4. The partial pressure of mixed venous oxygen ($P\bar{v}o_2$) provides an indication of global tissue oxygen extraction. Normal mixed venous $P\bar{v}o_2$ is 35 to 45 mmHg, and normal mixed venous oxygen saturation ($S\bar{v}o_2$) is 65% to 75%. Factors affecting mixed venous oxygen level can be illustrated by the following equation, which is a rearrangement of the **Fick equation**:

$$S\bar{v}o_2 = Sao_2 - Vo_2/CO \times Hb \times 1.34$$

where $S\bar{v}O_2$ is the mixed venous oxygen saturation; SaO_2, arterial oxygen saturation; VO_2, oxygen uptake; CO, cardiac output; Hb, hemoglobin.

$S\bar{v}O_2$ is decreased if:

a. Oxygen consumption is increased in the absence of increased delivery, such as in hyperthermia or pain.

b. Cardiac output is decreased, such as in hypovolemia or shock.

c. The patient is anemic.

d. Oxygen saturation is decreased.

$S\bar{v}O_2$ is elevated under conditions of increased oxygen delivery such as increased inspired oxygen concentration or conditions of decreased oxygen utilization, such as hypothermia and sepsis.

C. **CO-oximetry**

  1. Spectrophotometric analysis of arterial blood is used to measure levels of oxyhemoglobin (oxygen saturation of hemoglobin), carboxyhemoglobin (carbon monoxide saturation of hemoglobin), and methemoglobin (amount of hemoglobin in the oxidized ferric form rather than the reduced ferrous form).

D. **Oxyhemoglobin** (HbO_2) measured by CO-oximetry is the gold standard for the determination of oxygen saturation. It is superior to other means of determining oxygen saturation, such as that calculated empirically by a blood gas analyzer or that measured by pulse oximetry. Normal HbO_2 is approximately 97%.

E. **Carboxyhemoglobin** (HbCO) levels should be measured whenever carbon monoxide inhalation is suspected. Endogenous HbCO levels are 1% to 2% and can be elevated in cigarette smokers and in those living in polluted environments. Because HbCO does not transport oxygen, the HbO_2 is effectively reduced by the HbCO level.

F. **Methemoglobin**

  1. The iron in the hemoglobin molecule can be oxidized to the ferric form in the presence of a number of oxidizing agents, the most notable being nitrates. Because methemoglobin (Hbmet) does not transport oxygen, the HbO_2 is effectively reduced by the Hbmet level.

G. **Point-of-care Blood Gas Analyzers** are available to measure blood gases, pH, electrolytes, glucose, lactate, urea nitrogen, hematocrit, and clotting studies (activated clotting time [ACT], prothrombin time [PT], and partial thromboplastin time [PTT]) at the patient's bedside.

  1. Advantages: Point-of-care analyzers are small and portable (some are handheld), they use very small blood volumes (several drops), and they provide rapid reporting of results (a few minutes). They are relatively easy to use (e.g., self-calibrating) and typically incorporate a disposable cartridge that contains the appropriate biosensors.

  2. Disadvantages: The cost/benefit of these devices need to be assessed on an individual basis. Accuracy and precision are variable in different systems and for different variables. Furthermore, appropriate quality control is necessary for compliance with the Clinical Laboratory Improvement Amendments or Joint Commission requirements.

H. **Pulse Oximetry**

  1. **Principles of operation**

     a. The commonly used pulse oximeter emits two wavelengths of light (e.g., infrared at 940 and red at 660 nm) from light-emitting diodes through a pulsating vascular bed to a photodetector. The ratio of absorption of red and infrared lights is used to determine the fraction of oxygenated hemoglobin. A variety of probes are available in disposable or reusable designs and include digital probes (finger or toe), ear probes, and nasal probes.

2. Accuracy

   a. Pulse oximeters use empiric calibration curves developed from studies of healthy volunteers. They are typically accurate within $\pm2\%$ for SpO_2 readings as low as 70%. Thus their accuracy may be reduced in the clinical setting (see Limitations later). As illustrated by the oxyhemoglobin dissociation curve (Fig. 2.1), if the pulse oximeter displays an oxygen saturation (SpO_2) of 95%, the true saturation could be as low as 93% or as high as 97%. This range of SpO_2 translates to a PaO_2 range from as low as about 60 mmHg to greater than 150 mmHg.

3. Multiple-wavelength pulse oximetry

   a. Multiple-wavelength pulse oximeters measure and report the concentrations of Hbco, Hbmet and total hemoglobin in addition to SpO_2.

4. **Limitations** of pulse oximetry should be recognized and understood by everyone who uses pulse oximetry data.

   a. **Saturation versus PO_2.** Because of the shape of the oxyhemoglobin dissociation curve, pulse oximetry is a poor indicator of hyperoxemia. It is also an insensitive indicator of hypoventilation. If the patient is breathing supplemental oxygen, significant hypoventilation can occur without HbO_2 desaturation.

   b. **Ventilation versus oxygenation.** Pulse oximetry provides little, if any, clinical information related to $PaCO_2$ and acid–base balance.

   c. **Differences between devices and probes.** Calibration curves vary from manufacturer to manufacturer. The output of the light-emitting diodes of pulse oximeters varies from probe to probe.

   d. **The penumbra effect** occurs when the pulse oximeter probe does not fit correctly and light is shunted from the light-emitting diodes

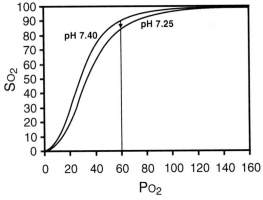

FIGURE 2.1 Oxyhemoglobin dissociation curve. Note that small changes in oxygen saturation relate to large changes in partial pressure of oxygen (PO_2) when the saturation is greater than 90%. Also note that the saturation can change without a change in PO_2 if there is a shift of the oxyhemoglobin dissociation curve.

directly to the photodetector. It leads to an SpO_2 reading that is erroneously lower than the actual value.

e. **Dyshemoglobinemia.** Traditional pulse oximeters use only two wavelengths of light and therefore evaluate only two forms of hemoglobin: HbO_2 and deoxyhemoglobin. **Carboxyhemoglobinemia** and **methemoglobinemia** result in significant inaccuracy in dual-wavelength pulse oximeters. Carboxyhemoglobinemia produces an SpO_2 greater than the true oxygen saturation. Methemoglobinemia causes the SpO_2 to move toward 85% regardless of the true oxygen saturation. Multiple-wavelength pulse oximeters address these issues by measuring HbCO and Hbmet. Fetal hemoglobin does not affect the accuracy of pulse oximeters.

f. **Endogenous and exogenous dyes and pigments** such as intravascular dyes (e.g., methylene blue) affect the accuracy of pulse oximetry. Nail polish can also affect the accuracy of pulse oximetry. Although this issue may be less problematic in newer generations of pulse oximeter, it is nonetheless prudent to remove nail polish before application of the pulse oximetry probe. Hyperbilirubinemia does not affect the accuracy of pulse oximetry.

g. **Skin pigmentation.** The accuracy and performance of pulse oximetry may be affected by deeply pigmented skin.

h. **Perfusion.** Pulse oximetry becomes unreliable during conditions of low flow such as low cardiac output or severe peripheral vasoconstriction. An ear probe may be more reliable than a digital probe under these conditions. A dampened plethysmographic waveform suggests poor signal quality. Newer technology uses signal processing software that improves the reliability of pulse oximetry with poor perfusion.

i. **Anemia.** Although pulse oximetry is generally reliable over a wide range of hematocrit, it becomes less accurate under conditions of severe anemia.

j. **Motion** of the oximeter probe can produce artifacts and inaccurate pulse oximetry readings. Newer-generation oximeters incorporate noise-canceling algorithms to lessen the effect of motion on signal interpretation. Newer technology uses signal processing software that improves the reliability of pulse oximetry with motion of the probe.

k. **High-intensity ambient light**, which can affect pulse oximeter performance, can be corrected by shielding the probe.

l. **Abnormal pulses.** Venous pulsations and a large dicrotic notch can affect the accuracy of pulse oximetry.

5. **Respiratory variation in the plethysmographic waveform.** Photoplethysmography of peripheral perfusion is displayed by some pulse oximeters. The beat-to-beat plethysmogram displayed on the pulse oximeter reflects beat-to-beat changes in local blood volume. The cyclic changes in the blood pressure and plethysmographic waveform baseline can be caused by changes in intrathoracic pressure relative to the intravascular volume (pulsus paradoxus).

a. Perfusion index is a measurement displayed on many pulse oximeters. It is the ratio of the pulsatile blood flow to the nonpulsatile and thus represents a noninvasive measure of peripheral perfusion.

b. Plethysmographic variability index is a measure of the dynamic changes in the perfusion index that occur during the respiratory cycle. The lower the number, the lesser the variability.

    c. Plethysmographic variability index may be increased in patients with severe airflow obstruction and in patients who are hypovolemic. It has been proposed as a predictor of fluid responsiveness in mechanically ventilated patients.

  6. Guidelines for use

    a. Pulse oximetry has become a standard of care in the ICU (particularly for mechanically ventilated patients). It is useful for titrating supplemental oxygen in mechanically ventilated patients. An SpO_2 of 92% or more reliably predicts a PaO_2 of 60 mmHg or more. SpO_2 should be periodically confirmed by blood gas analysis. Assessment of the plethysmographic waveform may be useful to monitor response to therapy in patients with severe airflow obstruction and those who are being volume resuscitated, although individual variability in waveform amplitude can indicate a limitation (Fig. 2.2).

I. Tissue Oxygenation
J. Near-Infrared Spectroscopy (NIRS)

  1. While arterial blood gases and $S\bar{v}O_2$ measurements provide insight into the global balance of oxygen supply and demand, tissue oxygen saturation (StO_2) provides information on the state of the microcirculation. NIRS utilizes reflectance of near-infrared wavelengths of light

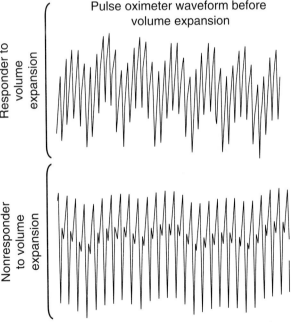

FIGURE 2.2 Pulse oximeter waveform from a patient who responded to volume expansion and from another who did not respond to volume expansion. From Cannesson M, Desebbe O, Rosamel P, et al. Pleth variability index to monitor the respiratory variations in the pulse oximeter plethysmographic waveform amplitude and predict fluid responsiveness in the operating theatre. *Br J Anaesth* 2008;101:200–206.

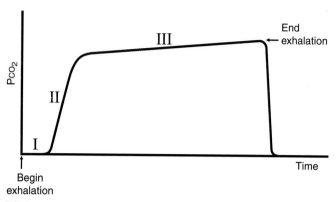

FIGURE 2.3 Normal capnogram. Phase I, anatomic dead space; phase II, transition from dead space to alveolar gas; phase III, alveolar plateau.

to determine the oxygen saturation in a volume of tissue at a depth of a couple of centimeters from the probe. NIRS of the thenar eminence has been investigated as a method of tracking Sto_2 and the state of the microcirculation. In trauma patients with hypovolemia, low Sto_2 at the thenar eminence has been shown to be predictive of poor outcome. Studies investigating the utility of this monitoring modality are ongoing and its role in the management of ICU patients remains to be determined.

K. Capnometry is the measurement of CO_2 at the airway. **Capnography** is the display of a CO_2 waveform called the **capnogram** (Fig. 2.3). The Pco_2 measured at end-exhalation is called the **end-tidal Pco_2** ($PETCO_2$).

   1. Principles of operation

   a. Quantitative capnometers measure CO_2 using the principles of infrared spectroscopy, Raman spectroscopy, or mass spectroscopy. Nonquantitative capnometers indicate CO_2 by a color change of an indicator material. Mainstream capnometers place the measurement chamber directly on the airway, whereas sidestream capnometers aspirate gas through tubing to a measurement chamber in the capnometer.

   2. The $PETCO_2$ represents alveolar Pco_2. It is a function of the rate at which CO_2 is added to the alveolus and the rate at which CO_2 is cleared from the alveolus. Thus, the $PETCO_2$ is a function of the ($\dot{V}/\dot{Q}$): with a normal and homogeneously distributed ($\dot{V}/\dot{Q}$), the $PETCO_2$ approximates the $Paco_2$. With a high $\dot{V}/\dot{Q}$ ratio (dead-space effect), the $PETCO_2$ is lower than the $Paco_2$. With a low $\dot{V}/\dot{Q}$ ratio (shunt effect), the $PETCO_2$ approximates the mixed venous Pco_2. Changes in $PETCO_2$ can be due to changes in CO_2 production, CO_2 delivery to the lungs, or changes in the magnitude and distribution of the alveolar ventilation.

   3. Abnormal capnogram. The shape of the capnogram can be abnormal with obstructive lung diseases (Fig. 2.4).

   4. Limitations

   a. There is considerable intra- and interpatient variability in the relationship between $Paco_2$ and $PETCO_2$. The P(a – et)co_2 is often too

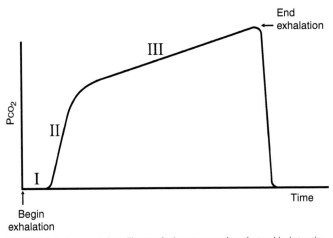

FIGURE 2.4 An increased phase III occurs in the capnogram in patients with obstructive lung disease.

variable in critically ill patients to allow precise prediction of $Paco_2$ from $Petco_2$.

5. Guidelines for clinical use
   a. The utility of $Petco_2$ to predict $Paco_2$ is limited in the ICU. Capnometry is useful for detecting esophageal intubation. $Petco_2$ monitoring to confirm tracheal intubation is generally regarded as the standard of care for clinically confirming the correct placement of the endotracheal tube. Low-cost, disposable devices that produce a color change in the presence of CO_2 are commercially available.
6. **Volumetric capnometry, also called volume-based capnometry,** displays exhaled CO_2 as a function of exhaled tidal volume (Fig. 2.5). Note that the area under the volume-based capnogram is the volume of CO_2 exhaled.

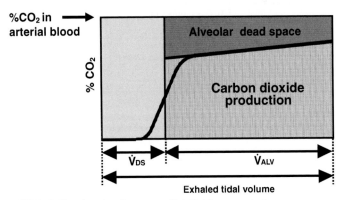

FIGURE 2.5 The volume-based capnogram. Note that the area under the curve represents carbon dioxide elimination, which equals carbon dioxide production during steady-state conditions.

Assuming steady-state conditions, this represents **carbon dioxide production** ($\dot{V}CO_2$). Because $\dot{V}CO_2$ is determined by metabolic rate, it can be used to estimate **resting energy expenditure** (REE):

$$REE = CO_2 \, (L/min) \times 5.52 \, kcal/L \times 1{,}440 \, min/d$$

Normal (co_2) is approximately 200 mL/min (2.6 mL/kg/min).

7. Using volume-based capnometry and a partial-rebreathing circuit, **pulmonary capillary blood flow** can be measured by applying a modification of the Fick equation (Fig. 2.6). With corrections for intrapulmonary shunt, this allows noninvasive estimation of cardiac output. There is significant variability in the clinical application of this method.

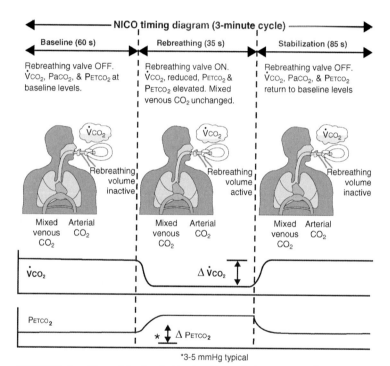

FIGURE 2.6 Use of the partial carbon dioxide rebreathing method to measure cardiac output using capnometry. Assuming that changes in pulmonary capillary carbon dioxide content (Cc'_{CO_2}) are proportional to changes in end-tidal CO_2 (P_{ETCO_2}), we can use the following equation to calculate pulmonary capillary blood flow (PCBF): $PCBF = \Delta CO_2/(S \times \Delta P_{ETCO_2})$, where ΔCO_2 is the change in CO_2 output and S is the slope of the CO_2 dissociation curve. Cardiac output is determined from PCBF and pulmonary shunt: $CO = PCBF/(1 - s/t)$. Noninvasive estimation of pulmonary shunt (s/t) is adapted from Nunn's isoshunt plots, which are a series of continuous curves for the relationship between partial pressure of oxygen (P_{aO_2}) and inspired oxygen (F_{IO_2}) for different levels of shunt. P_{aO_2} is estimated using a pulse oximeter. P_{aCO_2}, arterial partial pressure of CO_2. (Noninvasive cardiac output (NICO) timing diagram courtesy of Novametrix, Wallingford, CT.)

III. LUNG FUNCTION
A. Indices of Oxygenation
1. **Shunt fraction** is a measure of oxygenation inefficiency. It is calculated from the **shunt equation:**

$$\dot{Q}s/\dot{Q}T = (Cc'o_2 - Cao_2)/(Cc'o_2 - C\overline{v}o_2)$$

where $Cc'o_2$ is the pulmonary capillary oxygen content, Cao_2 is the arterial oxygen content, and $C\overline{v}o_2$ is the mixed venous oxygen content. Oxygen content is calculated from

$$Co_2 = (1.34 \times Hb \times Hbo_2) + (0.003 \times Pao_2)$$

To calculate $Cc'o_2$, we assume the pulmonary capillary Po_2 is equal to the alveolar Po_2 (Pao_2) and the pulmonary capillary hemoglobin is 100% saturated with oxygen. If measured when the patient is breathing 100% oxygen, the $\dot{Q}s/\dot{Q}T$ represents shunt (i.e., blood that flows from the right heart to the left heart without passing functional alveoli). If measured at Fio_2 less than 1.0, the $\dot{Q}s/\dot{Q}T$ represents shunt and $\dot{V}/\dot{Q}$ mismatch (i.e., venous admixture).

2. **Pao_2, $P(A - a)o_2$, Pao_2/Pao_2.** The Pao_2 is calculated from the alveolar gas equation:

$$Pao_2 = [Fio_2 \times (Pb - PH_2O)] - [Paco_2/R]$$

where Pb is the barometric pressure, PH_2O the water vapor pressure, and R the respiratory quotient. For calculation of Pao_2, an R of 0.8 is commonly used.

   a. An increased difference between Pao_2 and Pao_2, the **P(A – a)o₂ gradient**, is another measure of oxygen exchange inefficiency. It can be due to shunt, $\dot{V}/\dot{Q}$ mismatch, or diffusion defect. The $P(A - a)o_2$ is normally 10 mmHg or less breathing room air and 50 mmHg or less breathing 100% oxygen. The ratio of the Pao_2 to Pao_2 **(Pao₂/Pao₂)** can also be calculated as an index of oxygenation and is normally greater than 0.75 at any Fio_2.

3. **Pao₂/Fio₂** is the easiest of the indices of oxygenation to calculate, and another attempt to normalize the values of Pao_2 to the used Fio_2. It is used to classify the ARDS as mild ($200 \leq Pao_2/Fio_2 < 300$), moderate ($100 \leq Pao_2/Fio_2 < 200$), and severe ($Pao_2/Fio_2 < 100$).

B. Indices of Ventilation
1. **Dead space** ($\dot{V}Ds/\dot{V}T$) is calculated from the **Bohr equation**, which measures the ratio of dead space to total ventilation:

$$\dot{V}Ds/\dot{V}T = (Paco_2 - P\overline{E}co_2)/Paco_2$$

where Pco_2 is the mixed exhaled Pco_2. To determine Pco_2, exhaled gas is collected in a bag from the expiratory port of the ventilator and its CO_2 concentration is measured with a blood gas analyzer or capnometer. Alternatively, Pco_2 can be determined using volumetric capnometry:

$$Pco_2 = (Co_2 \times Pb)/E$$

where Pb is the barometric pressure. The normal $\dot{V}Ds/\dot{V}T$ is 0.3 to 0.4.

IV. LUNG MECHANICS

A. Plateau Pressure (Pplat) is the pressure measured during an inspiratory pause while on mechanical ventilation.

  1. Measurement

   a. Pplat is measured by applying an end-inspiratory breath-hold for 0.5 to 2.0 seconds. During the breath-hold, pressure equilibrates throughout the system so that the pressure measured at the proximal airway approximates the alveolar pressure (Fig. 2.7). For valid measurement of Pplat, the patient must be relaxed and breathing in synchrony with the ventilator.

  2. An increased Pplat indicates a greater risk of alveolar overdistention during mechanical ventilation. Many authorities recommend that Pplat be maintained at 30 cmH$_2$O or less in patients with acute respiratory failure. This assumes that chest wall compliance is normal. A higher Pplat may be necessary if chest wall compliance is decreased (e.g., abdominal distension).

  3. Occlusion pressure (P$_{0.1}$) is the negative airway pressure generated 100 ms after the onset of inhalation against an occluded airway.

   a. P$_{0.1}$ is an index of ventilatory drive. It can be measured manually and/or automatically on some ventilators.

   b. Normal P$_{0.1}$ is 3 to 4 cmH$_2$O.

   c. A P$_{0.1}$ greater than 6 cmH$_2$O has been associated with weaning failure.

  4. Maximum inspiratory pressure (P$_I$max or MIP), the most negative pressure generated during a maximal inspiratory effort against an occluded airway

   a. P$_I$max is an index of the strength of the inspiratory muscles.

   b. The off-ventilator manual measurement technique uses a one-way valve, allowing exhalation, but not inhalation, and an occlusion for approximately 15 to 20 seconds, provided no arrhythmias or desaturation occur. Some ventilators perform this measurement electronically by occluding both inspiratory and expiratory valves.

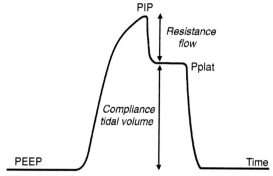

FIGURE 2.7 Peak alveolar pressure (Pplat) is determined by applying an end-inspiratory breath-hold. The peak inspiratory pressure (PIP)–Pplat difference is determined by resistance and end-inspiratory flow, and the Pplat–positive end-expiratory pressure (PEEP) difference is determined by compliance and tidal volume.

    c. Normal $P_{I}max$ is < -100 cmH$_2$O (varies with sex and age).

    d. Although $P_{I}max > -30$ cmH$_2$O has been associated with weaning failure, its predictive value is poor.

  5. Maximum expiratory pressure ($P_{E}max$ or MEP), the most positive pressure generated during a maximal inspiratory effort against an occluded airway

    a. $P_{E}max$ is an index of the strength of the expiratory muscles.

B. Esophageal Pressure

  1. Measurement. Esophageal pressure is measured by placing a thin-walled balloon containing a small volume of air (<1 mL) into the distal third of the esophagus. The measurement and display of esophageal pressure are facilitated by commercially available systems.

  2. Esophageal pressure changes reflect changes in pleural pressure, but the absolute esophageal pressure does not reflect absolute pleural pressure.

    a. Changes in esophageal pressure can be used to assess respiratory effort and the work of breathing during spontaneous breathing and patient-triggered modes of ventilation; to assess chest wall compliance during full ventilatory support; and to assess auto–positive end-expiratory pressure (PEEP) during spontaneous breathing and patient-triggered modes of ventilation.

    b. If exhalation is passive, the change in esophageal (i.e., pleural) pressure required to reverse flow at the proximal airway (i.e., trigger the ventilator) reflects the amount of auto-PEEP. Negative esophageal pressure changes that produce no flow at the airway indicate failed trigger efforts—in other words, the patient's inspiratory efforts are insufficient to overcome the level of auto-PEEP and trigger the ventilator (Fig. 2.8). Clinically, this is recognized as a patient respiratory rate (observed by inspecting chest wall movement) that is greater than the trigger rate on the ventilator.

    c. The increase in esophageal pressure (ΔPeso) during passive inflation of the lungs can be used to calculate chest wall compliance (Ccw): Ccw $= V_T/\Delta$Peso.

    d. Changes in esophageal pressure, relative to changes in alveolar pressure, can be used to calculate transpulmonary pressure (an indirect estimate of lung stress). This may allow more precise setting of tidal volume (and Pplat) in patients with reduced chest wall compliance. In this case, transpulmonary pressure (difference between Pplat and Peso) is targeted at <27 cmH$_2$O.

    e. Although esophageal pressure has been used to target the appropriate setting for PEEP, its clinical application is debated. The concept is that patients with a higher Peso require more PEEP to counterbalance the alveolar collapsing effect of the higher pleural pressure. Currently, our practice is to measure esophageal pressure for hypoxemic patients who weigh more than 120 kg.

    f. An alternative to esophageal pressure to assess changes in pleural pressure is respiratory variation in the central venous pressure waveform.

C. Gastric Pressure

  1. Gastric pressure is measured by a balloon-tipped catheter that is similar to that used to measure esophageal pressure. It reflects changes in intra-abdominal pressure. An alternative for measuring gastric pressure is measuring **bladder pressure**.

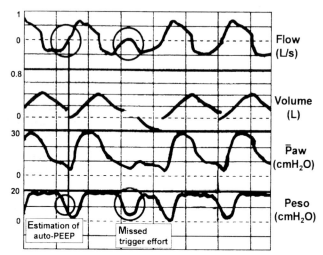

FIGURE 2.8 Use of esophageal pressure to determine auto–positive end-expiratory pressure (auto-PEEP). The change in esophageal pressure required to trigger the ventilator is the level of auto-PEEP. Also note the presence of missed trigger efforts in which the inspiratory effort of the patient is not sufficient to overcome the amount of auto-PEEP. P̄aw, mean airway pressure; Peso, esophageal pressure.

2. Clinical implications
   a. During a spontaneous inspiratory effort, gastric pressure normally increases because of contraction of the diaphragm. A decrease in gastric pressure with spontaneous inspiratory effort is consistent with diaphragmatic paralysis (Fig. 2.9). A high baseline gastric pressure reflects elevated intra-abdominal pressure, which may affect chest wall compliance and lung function.
3. Electrical activity of the diaphragm
   a. Neurally adjusted ventilatory assist (NAVA) is a ventilation mode that delivers ventilatory support synchronized with and proportional to the electrical activity of the patient's diaphragm (EAdi). EAdi is measured using esophageal electrodes positioned at the level of the diaphragm and provides a measure of respiratory drive. The ratio of tidal volume (Vt) to EAdi can be used as a measure of a patient's neuroventilatory efficiency.
D. **Compliance** (the inverse of elastance) is the change in volume (usually tidal volume) divided by the change in pressure required to produce that volume.
   1. Respiratory system, chest wall, and lung compliance
      a. **Respiratory system compliance** is most commonly calculated in the ICU: $C = \Delta V/\Delta P = Vt/(Pplat - PEEP)$ Respiratory system compliance is normally 100 mL/cmH$_2$O and is reduced to 50 to 100 mL/cmH$_2$O in mechanically ventilated patients, likely due to the supine or semirecumbent position and microatelectasis. It is determined by the compliance of the chest wall and the lungs. This measurement is often called *static compliance*, meaning that the measurement was

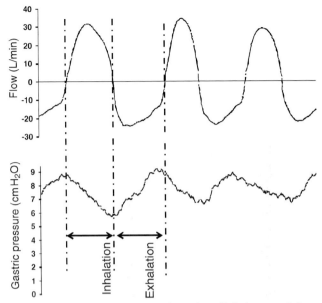

FIGURE 2.9 Gastric pressure measurement in a patient with diaphragm paralysis. Note that the gastric pressure decreases during the inspiratory phase.

performed in conditions of no flow or, more likely, a very low flow (quasistatic conditions) achieved by the end-inspiratory pause.

   b. **Chest wall compliance** is calculated from changes in esophageal pressure (pleural pressure) during passive inflation. It is normally 200 mL/cmH$_2$O and can be decreased because of abdominal distension, chest wall edema, chest wall burns, and thoracic deformities (e.g., kyphoscoliosis). It is also decreased with an increase in muscle tone (e.g., a patient who is bucking the ventilator) and increased with flail chest and paralysis.

   c. **Lung compliance** is calculated from changes in transpulmonary pressure. **Transpulmonary pressure** is the difference between alveolar pressure (Pplat) and pleural pressure (esophageal). Normal lung compliance is 100 mL/cmH$_2$O. Lung compliance is decreased with pulmonary edema (cardiogenic or noncardiogenic), pneumothorax, consolidation, atelectasis, pulmonary fibrosis, pneumonectomy, and mainstream intubation and is increased with emphysema.

2. Clinical implications

   a. When compliance is decreased, a larger transpulmonary pressure is required to deliver a given tidal volume into the lungs. Thus, a decreased compliance will result in a higher Pplat and peak inspiratory pressure (PIP). To avoid dangerous levels of airway pressure, lower tidal volumes are used to ventilate the lungs of patients with decreased compliance. Decreased lung compliance also increases the work of breathing, decreasing the likelihood of successful weaning from the ventilator.

E. **Mean Airway Pressure** ($\bar{P}$aw) is the average pressure applied to the lungs over the entire ventilatory cycle.
   1. Most current-generation microprocessor ventilators display $\bar{P}$aw by integrating the airway pressure waveform.
   2. Typical $\bar{P}$aw for passively ventilated patients are 5 to 10 cmH$_2$O (normal), 10 to 20 cmH$_2$O (airflow obstruction), and 15 to 30 cmH$_2$O (ALI (acute lung injury)/ARDS).
   3. Factors affecting $\bar{P}$aw are PIP (an increase in PIP increases aw), PEEP (an increase in PEEP increases aw), I:E ratio (inspiratory-to-expiratory ratio; the longer the inspiratory time, the higher the $\bar{P}$aw), inspiratory pressure waveform (a rectangular inspiratory pressure waveform produces a higher aw than does a triangular inspiratory pressure waveform).

F. **Airways Resistance** is determined by the driving pressure and the flow.
   1. **Inspiratory airways resistance** can be estimated during volume ventilation from the PIP–Pplat difference and the end-inspiratory flow:

$$R_I = (PIP \times Pplat)/r R_I = (PIP \times Pplat)/I$$

   where I is the end-inspiratory flow. A simple way to measure this is to set the ventilator for a constant inspiratory flow of 60 L/min (1 L/s). Using this approach, we have that the inspiratory airways resistance is the PIP – Pplat difference.
   2. Expiratory resistance can be estimated from the time constant (τ) of the lung (Fig. 2.10):

$$R_E = \tau/C$$

   3. **Common causes** of increased airways resistance are bronchospasm and secretions. Resistance is also increased with a small–inner-diameter endotracheal tube. For intubated and mechanically ventilated patients, airways resistance should be less than 10 cmH$_2$O/L/s at a flow of 1 L/s. Expiratory airways resistance is typically greater than inspiratory airways resistance.

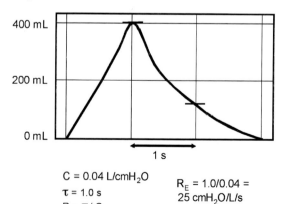

$$C = 0.04 \text{ L/cmH}_2\text{O}$$
$$\tau = 1.0 \text{ s}$$
$$R = \tau / C$$

$$R_E = 1.0/0.04 = 25 \text{ cmH}_2\text{O/L/s}$$

FIGURE 2.10 Use of the tidal volume waveform to measure time constant (τ) and calculate expiratory airways resistance.

G. Work of Breathing

1. **The Campbell diagram** (Fig. 2.11) is used to determine the work of breathing. This diagram includes the effects of chest wall compliance, lung compliance, and airway resistance on the work of breathing. Work of breathing is increased with decreased chest wall compliance, decreased lung compliance, or increased airways resistance.

2. Clinical implications

   a. Work of breathing requires special equipment and an esophageal balloon to quantify, and for this reason it is not frequently measured. Moreover, it is not clear that measuring work of breathing improves patient outcome. It may be useful for quantifying patient effort during mechanical ventilation, but this can often be achieved by simply observing the respiratory variation on a central venous pressure tracing. Large inspiratory efforts produce large negative deflections of the central venous pressure trace during inspiratory efforts. Increasing the level of ventilatory assistance should reduce these negative deflections.

H. The **static pressure–volume curve** measures the pressure–volume relationship of the respiratory system.

1. Measurement

   a. The manual method with a supersyringe is relatively simple but requires disconnecting the patient from the ventilator to perform

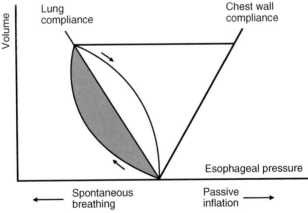

FIGURE 2.11 Campbell diagram. The chest wall compliance curve is determined by plotting volume as a function of esophageal pressure during positive-pressure breathing with the chest wall relaxed. The lung compliance curve is determined from the point of zero flow at end-exhalation to the point of zero flow at end-inhalation during spontaneous breathing. Because of airways resistance, the esophageal pressure is more negative than predicted from the lung compliance curve. The areas indicated on the curve represent elastic work of breathing and resistive work of breathing. Note that a decreased chest wall compliance will shift the compliance curve to the right, thus increasing the elastic work of breathing. A decrease in lung compliance shifts the curve to the left, also increasing the work of breathing. An increased airways resistance causes a more negative esophageal pressure during spontaneous breathing, increasing the resistive work of breathing.

the maneuver. Alternatively, a pressure–volume curve can be measured automatically in selected ventilators without disconnecting the patient from the ventilator. The multiple occlusion method performs repeated end-inspiratory breath occlusions at different lung volumes, and the constant flow technique measures the change in airway opening pressure with a constant slow flow (≤ 10 L/min). The best technique is unknown.

2. **Lower and upper inflection points** can be determined from the pressure–volume curve (Fig. 2.12). Some authors have suggested that the level of PEEP should be set above the lower inflection point to avoid alveolar collapse and that Pplat should be set below the upper inflection point to avoid alveolar overdistention. However, the clinical benefits of this approach are not clear, and setting the ventilator using the pressure–volume curve is not currently recommended because there are important limitations to the clinical use of pressure–volume curves. Accurate measurements require heavy sedation (and often paralysis); it is unclear whether the inflation or deflation curve should be assessed; it can be difficult to precisely determine the inflection points; the respiratory system pressure–volume curve can be affected by both the lungs and

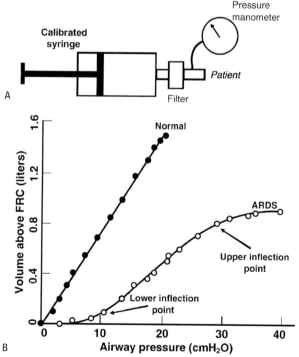

FIGURE 2.12 A: Supersyringe setup for measuring static compliance. **B:** Inspiratory pressure–volume curve for a patient with normal lung function and for a patient with acute respiratory distress syndrome (ARDS). FRC, functional residual capacity.

the chest wall; and the pressure–volume curve models the lungs as a single compartment.

I. **Functional Residual Capacity (FRC)** is the lung volume at the end of a normal exhalation.

 1. FRC is decreased in patients with ALI and increased in patients with obstructive lung disease.

 2. Some modern ventilators are able to measure FRC using a nitrogen washout procedure. The FRC procedure takes two measurements of approximately 20 breaths each. When an FRC measurement is started, the system first measures a baseline N_2 concentration. A constant FIO_2 is needed to accurately establish a baseline N_2 concentration for the nitrogen washout process. Once the baseline N_2 concentration is found, FIO_2 is changed by 10%. Because the only gases that are present are O_2, CO_2, and N_2, it is possible to determine the N_2 concentration indirectly by the measurement of O_2 and CO_2. FRC can be calculated from the washout of N_2 during the step change in FIO_2.

J. **Electrical Impedance Tomography (EIT)** is an imaging technique in which the conductivity is inferred from surface electrical measurements. EIT adhesive electrodes are applied to the skin and an electric current, typically a few milliamperes of alternating current at a frequency of 10 to 100 kHz, is applied across two or more electrodes. The resulting electrical potentials are measured, and the process is repeated for different configurations of applied current. The lungs become less conductive as the alveoli become filled with air and more conductive if alveoli become airless (collapsed, edematous, or consolidated).

Selected Readings

Albaiceta GM, Blanch L, Lucangelo U. Static pressure-volume curves of the respiratory system: were they just a passing fad? *Curr Opin Crit Care* 2008;14:80–86.

Batchelder PB, Raley DM. Maximizing the laboratory setting for testing devices and understanding statistical output in pulse oximetry. *Anesth Analg* 2007;105(6 suppl):S85–S94.

Bendjelid K. The pulse oximetry plethysmographic curve revisited. *Curr Opin Crit Care* 2008;14:348–353.

Bendjelid K, Schütz N, Stotz M, et al. Transcutaneous PCO_2 monitoring in critically ill adults: clinical evaluation of a new sensor. *Crit Care Med* 2005;33:2203–2206.

Cannesson M, Desebbe O, Rosamel P, et al. Pleth variability index to monitor the respiratory variations in the pulse oximeter plethysmographic waveform amplitude and predict fluid responsiveness in the operating theatre. *Br J Anaesth* 2008;101:200–206.

Cheifetz IM, Myers TR. Should every mechanically ventilated patient be monitored with capnography from intubation to extubation? *Respir Care* 2007;52:423–442.

Dhand R. Ventilator graphics and respiratory mechanics in the patient with obstructive lung disease. *Respir Care* 2005;50:246–261.

Fernández-Pérez ER, Hubmayr RD. Interpretation of airway pressure waveforms. *Intensive Care Med* 2006;32:658–659.

Gehring H, Nornberger C, Matz H, et al. The effects of motion artifact and low perfusion on the performance of a new generation of pulse oximeters in volunteers undergoing hypoxemia. *Respir Care* 2002;47:48–60.

Georgopoulos D, Prinianakis G, Kondili E. Bedside waveforms interpretation as a tool to identify patient-ventilator asynchronies. *Intensive Care Med* 2006;32:34–47.

Hess D. Detection and monitoring of hypoxemia and oxygen therapy. *Respir Care* 2000;45:65–80.

Hess DR, Bigatello LM. The chest wall in acute lung injury/acute respiratory distress syndrome. *Curr Opin Crit Care* 2008;14:94–102.

Hess DR, Medoff MD, Fessler MB. Pulmonary mechanics and graphics during positive pressure ventilation. *Int Anesthesiol Clin* 1999;37(3):15–34.

Jubran A. Advances in respiratory monitoring during mechanical ventilation. *Chest* 1999;116:1416–1425.

Krauss B, Hess DR. Capnography for procedural sedation and analgesia in the emergency department. *Ann Emerg Med* 2007;50:172–181.

Landsverk SA, Hoiseth LO, Kvandal P, et al. Poor agreement between respiratory variations in pulse oximetry photoplethysmographic waveform amplitude and pulse pressure in intensive care unit patients. *Anesthesiology* 2008;109:849–855.

Lucangelo U, Bernabé F, Blanch L. Respiratory mechanics derived from signals in the ventilator circuit. *Respir Care* 2005;50:55–67.

Lucangelo U, Bernabè F, Blanch L. Lung mechanics at the bedside: make it simple. *Curr Opin Crit Care* 2007;13:64–72.

Lucangelo U, Blanch L. Dead space. *Intensive Care Med* 2004;30:576–579.

McMorrow RC, Mythen MG. Pulse oximetry. *Curr Opin Crit Care* 2006;12:269–271.

Owens RL, Hess DR, Malhotra A, et al. Effect of the chest wall on pressure-volume curve analysis of acute respiratory distress syndrome lungs. *Crit Care Med* 2008;36:2980–2985.

Owens RL, Stigler WS, Hess DR. Do newer monitors of exhaled gases, mechanics, and esophageal pressure add value? *Clin Chest Med* 2008;29:297–312.

Shapiro BA. Point-of-care blood testing and cardiac output measurement in the intensive care unit. *New Horiz* 1999;7:244–252.

Talmor D, Sarge T, Malhotra A, et al. Mechanical ventilation guided by esophageal pressure in acute lung injury. *N Engl J Med* 2008;359:2095–2104.

Thompson JE, Jaffe MB. Capnographic waveforms in the mechanically ventilated patient. *Respir Care* 2005;50:100–109.

Yem JS, Tang Y, Turner MJ, et al. Sources of error in noninvasive pulmonary blood flow measurements by partial rebreathing: a computer model study. *Anesthesiology* 2003;98:881–887.

Use of Ultrasound in Critical Illness

Kenneth Shelton and Kate Riddell

Critical care ultrasonography (CCUS, or point-of-care ultrasound) has become increasingly popular in the management of critically ill patients as ultrasound technology has progressively become more portable, less expensive, and yet capable of high-quality imaging. Conceptually, CCUS functions as an extension of the physical examination. It is immediately available at the bedside, is noninvasive, and in skilled hands provides a wealth of information that can be used to narrow differential diagnoses and to initiate or modify treatment. CCUS is best used to complement results from other types of imaging, tests, and examinations and is not intended to replace them. Of the very broad range of techniques that comprise CCUS, in this chapter we will focus primarily on the use of ultrasound to evaluate cardiorespiratory status.

I. USE OF CRITICAL CARE ULTRASONOGRAPHY
   A. **Pros:** The use of ultrasound at the patient's bedside allows for rapid and noninvasive scanning. It can be used as an extension of the physical exam and be repeated often to monitor the progress of therapy or to evaluate an acute change in status. It does not involve risks associated with patient transport or radiation.
   B. **Cons:** Implementation of a high-quality point-of-care ultrasound program in any ICU requires an initial outlay of funding for equipment and time for training of personnel. Equipment must be maintained and quality assurance programs need to be established to ensure safety and accuracy. The critical care physician may encounter difficulty obtaining adequate scanning windows due to the patient's condition (pneumothorax, intra-abdominal free air, surgical dressings, and/or casts). Furthermore, the patient's hemodynamics may be too unstable to tolerate a change in position to facilitate appropriate ultrasound scanning.

II. ULTRASOUND PHYSICS
   A. The **wavelength** of a sound wave is the distance between two repetitive points along a single cycle. The wavelength helps to determine **spatial resolution**. The shorter the wavelength, the better the resolution. The frequency of a wave is the number of cycles per second. High-frequency waves provide excellent near-field resolution but poor tissue penetration, as they are subject to attenuation. Conversely, low-frequency waves offer improved tissue penetration, allowing visualization of deeper structures, but poor resolution. Thus we use a high-frequency probe for visualization of relatively superficial vascular structures, but a lower frequency probe for echocardiography of the heart.
   B. **Spatial resolution** differs from **temporal resolution**. Spatial resolution relates to the ability to determine the location of a structure in space. Temporal resolution relates to the ability to determine the position of a structure at a particular instant in time. Temporal resolution is determined by the pulse repetition frequency (PRF). The higher the PRF, the higher the temporal

resolution. A higher PRF increases the number of frames per second, and this allows for a smooth echo loop. This becomes important when assessing a fast-moving structure such as the heart.

C. **Doppler ultrasonography** is of great value in the assessment and quantification of blood flow through the heart (under both normal and pathologic conditions). Doppler techniques are divided into **pulse wave Doppler**, **continuous wave Doppler**, and **color Doppler**. Pulse wave Doppler (PWD) is used to measure flow velocities at a single defined location, such as at a point (defined by the sampling volume) in the left ventricular outflow tract. However, the maximum velocities that it can accurately measure is limited, beyond which PWD is susceptible to a form of sampling error called **aliasing**. **Continuous wave Doppler** (CWD) on the other hand, is not limited by aliasing and can be used to measure very high flow velocities (such as those from a stenotic aortic valve). However, the trade-off here is **range ambiguity**, that is, CWD cannot identify the precise location of the maximum velocity—it simply measures the maximum velocity anywhere in the path of the ultrasound beam. **Color Doppler** is a form of pulsed Doppler (and thus subject to aliasing) that measures flow at multiple sampling volumes on a two-dimensional grid rather than along a single line. One important caveat to the use of these techniques is that they are all **angle dependent**. In other words, they are accurate when the angle of the transducer beam is **<20°** to the direction of blood flow. Consequently, Doppler measurements may underestimate true flows, or provide inconsistent values on serial examination. Doppler examinations are not part of most basic critical care ultrasound protocols.

D. An important ultrasound feature for echocardiography that is frequently used in the ICU and the operating room is M-mode or motion mode. M-mode uses a single scan line of information and therefore provides the highest temporal resolution. This is useful for accurately measuring the size of structures such as the IVC or maximum aortic valve opening (see Figs. 3.1F and 3.2D).

III. **CARDIAC ULTRASOUND:** It is important to emphasize that intensivist-performed echocardiography is different from a formal cardiology echocardiographic exam. The critical care physician performs a **"goal-directed" examination**, designed to answer a specific question (most commonly, why is my patient hemodynamically unstable?), not a comprehensive examination. The primary skills involved in basic critical care ultrasound are **image acquisition** and **pattern recognition**. The critical care physician also uses the ultrasound as a monitoring tool, to evaluate the effect of his or her intervention. The **real-time acquisition and interpretation** of images in an acutely unstable patient that are then **interpreted in the context of the patients' physiology** is the hallmark of critical care echocardiography. ICU echocardiography can be broadly divided into **basic** and **advanced** categories. The scope of basic, **goal-directed critical care echocardiography** (GDE) has been defined by a number of authorities and will be the focus of this chapter. Practitioners should have an awareness of their limitations when it comes to echocardiography, and help from more experienced echocardiographers or cardiologists should be freely sought to resolve equivocal findings.

A. **Essential Views for Goal-Directed Echocardiography** (see Fig. 3.1): It is helpful to establish a sequence of images that are obtained in each patient to maximize efficiency. Many ICU physicians follow the following sequence: Parasternal long-axis (PLAX), parasternal short-axis (PSAX—midpapillary view), apical four chamber (A4C), subcostal four chamber (SC), and subcostal inferior vena cava (IVC) views. This sequence may be modified depending on the clinical situation—for example, during CPR it is most practical to begin with the subcostal four-chamber view (which will not interrupt chest compressions).

B. **Using Goal-Directed Echocardiography in the Hemodynamically Unstable Patient:** Acute hypotension is often caused by hypovolemia, left ventricular

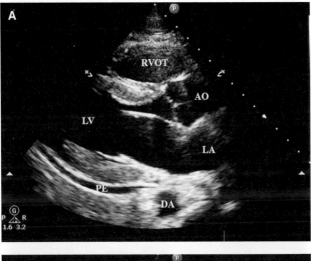

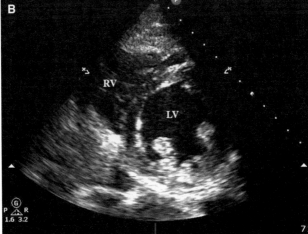

FIGURE 3.1 Transthoracic echocardiograms showing the views needed for a goal-directed echocardiographic examination in the ICU. Salient anatomic features are noted on the figures. **(A)** Parasternal long-axis view in diastole (mitral valve wide open; aortic valve closed). Note the small posterior pericardial effusion (PE); **(B)** Parasternal short-axis view. (*Continued*)

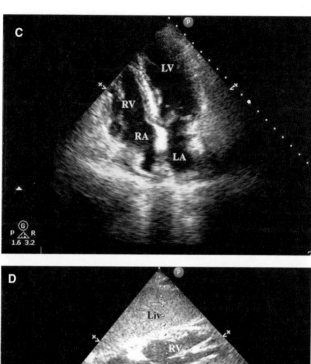

FIGURE 3.1 (C) Apical four-chamber view; **(D)** Subcostal four-chamber view; (*Continued*)

or right ventricular dysfunction, severe valvular disease (such as acute regurgitation), or pericardial tamponade. GDE can pick up all these findings, which are then integrated with the patient's history to categorize shock into one of the classic pathophysiologic mechanisms (hypovolemic, cardiogenic, obstructive, and distributive). **A finding should be confirmed in at least two orthogonal views** to reduce the risk of misinterpretation.

1. **Assessment of left ventricular (LV) function:** The left ventricle should be assessed in the PLAX, PSAX, A4C, and SC views. Is the LV dilated/ hypertrophied? What is the global function of the LV (hyperdynamic, normal, mildly, moderately, or severely depressed)? Research suggests

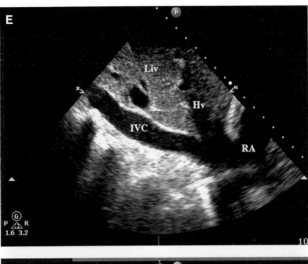

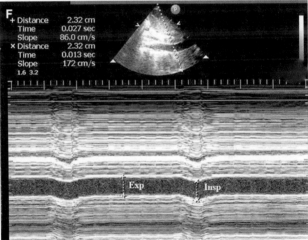

FIGURE 3.1 (E) Visualization of the inferior vena cava; **(F)** M-mode interrogation of the IVC—no change in diameter between inspiration and expiration. AO: Ascending Aorta; DA: Descending thoracic aorta; Hv: Hepatic vein; LA: Left atrium; LV: Left ventricle; Liv: Liver; PE: Pericardial effusion; RA: Right atrium; RV: Right ventricle; RVOT: Right ventricular outflow tract; Insp: Inspiration; Exp: Expiration (Images courtesy of Aranya Bagchi, MBBS).

that novice echocardiographers become proficient at "eyeballing" LV function after a short period of training. While the PSAX view allows assessment of regional wall motion abnormalities (RWMA) across all major coronary arterial territories, skill at detecting RWMA takes significant expertise and is typically out of the scope of a basic exam. More experienced echocardiographers can look for signs of **LV dynamic out-flow obstruction** or severe valvular stenosis/regurgitation.

2. **Assessment of right ventricular (RV) function:** The RV should be assessed using the A4C, PSAX, and SC views. Dilatation of the RVOT may be visible in the PLAX view. Basic assessment includes the size of the RV on A4C or SC views. A rule of the thumb is that if the RV is as large or larger than the LV, it is dilated. The interventricular septum is best

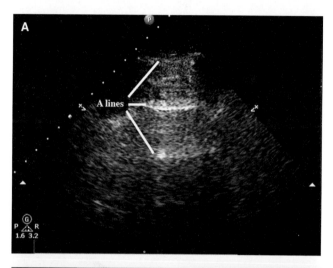

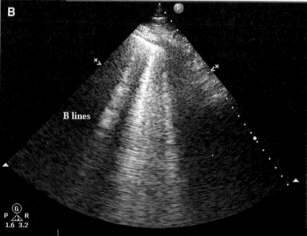

FIGURE 3.2 Ultrasound examination of the lung: **(A)** A-lines, which are consistent with normal aeration of the lung field under examination; **(B)** Multiple B lines seen in this sector, suggesting excess interstitial fluid. Note that A lines are not visible, since they are effaced by B lines; (*Continued*)

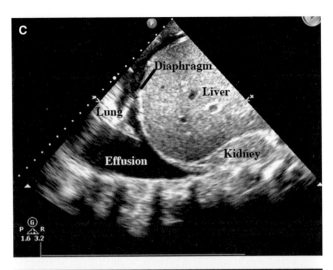

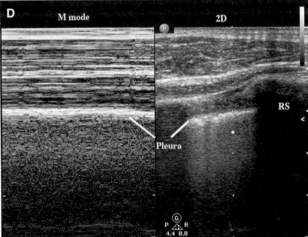

FIGURE 3.2 (C) An uncomplicated pleural effusion. It is important to use the anatomical landmarks (in this case, liver and diaphragm below and a portion of atelectatic lung above) to confirm the fluid being visualized is pleural fluid and not ascites; **(D)** M-mode interrogation of the pleural surface to show the "seashore sign" that is caused by the movement of the parietal and visceral pleura over each other. The 2D image being scanned by M-mode is shown to the right (RS: rib shadow) (Images courtesy of Aranya Bagchi, MBBS).

assessed in the PSAX view. It is flattened (the so-called "D sign") in the setting of RV volume (diastolic flattening) or pressure (systolic flattening) overload states. Assessment of the right ventricle can be critical in patients with ARDS on mechanical ventilators that are at risk of acute

RV failure. Once the RV septum has shifted, further fluid is not likely to improve cardiac output. RV dysfunction is almost always accompanied by a **dilated IVC**. More advanced measures of RV function include the **Tricuspid Annular Plane Systolic Excursion (TAPSE)** and measurement of RV systolic and pulmonary arterial pressures.

3. **Pericardial tamponade:** Pericardial tamponade is primarily a **clinical diagnosis**. However, the presence of pericardial fluid in a hemody-namically unstable patient should prompt a careful evaluation for the echocardiographic signs of tamponade. The best views to assess tam-ponade are the A4C and SC. Right atrial collapse during ventricular systole and right ventricular diastolic collapse are fairly sensitive and specific for tamponade, respectively. There is normally a small degree of respirophasic variation of flow across both the tricuspid and mitral valves. This variation is exaggerated with pericardial effusions that al-ter diastolic filling, both with spontaneous and mechanical ventilation. Initiation of positive pressure ventilation in a patient with suspected pericardial tamponade should be done very cautiously, as decreasing preload to the RV (from positive pressure ventilation) may precipitate cardiovascular collapse.

4. **Hypovolemia:** Assessment of intravascular volume status still remains a challenge in critically ill patients. While GDE can be extremely use-ful in helping to determine significant hypovolemia, it is important to use multiple methods to assess volume status since each method has drawbacks. Echocardiographic clues to significant hypovolemia include end-systolic ventricular effacement ("kissing papillary mus-cles") in PLAX/PSAX views, an IVC that is less than 1 cm in diameter (in spontaneously breathing patients), and an IVC diameter that varies by >12% to 18% on controlled ventilation (although assessing IVC vari-ation requires deep sedation/paralysis, and relatively large tidal vol-umes—in the 8–10 cc/kg range). The lung ultrasound exam (see below) can be a useful adjunct to the assessment of volume status. A patient with "A lines" over bilateral lung fields and a small IVC will likely be volume responsive, while a patient with "B lines" over the anterior lung fields (suggesting increased interstitial fluid; see Fig 3.2B) and a plump IVC will probably not benefit from more fluid (this technique has been called the **FALLS, or Fluid Administration Limited by Lung Ultrasound**). Ad-vanced practitioners can measure stroke volume (SV) variation with mechanical ventilation or after a small fluid challenge, but accurate SV measurement can be a technically challenging in ICU patients.

IV. THORACIC ULTRASOUND

A. For many years, the air-filled lungs were thought to be impossible to view in a meaningful way with ultrasound. However, taking advantage of artifacts produced by the air-filled lung interface with fluid and/or surrounding tissue can be quite useful. In fact, ultrasound has a higher sensitivity and specificity than auscultation and plain film X-ray for detection of pleural effusion, consolidation, and pneumothorax (PTX).

B. **The Normal Lung Point of Care (POC) Ultrasound Exam**

1. Using the linear or phased array probe in 2D mode (see Fig. 3.2), scan the chest in each of the four quadrants on both the left and right sides of a supine patient. The anterior border of the scanning area is defined by the parasternal line; the posterior border is defined by the posterior axillary line; and the midpoint of the scanning area is defined by the anterior axillary line. In the normal lung, the windows between each rib

should reveal the hyperechoic pleural line sliding along the chest wall with inspiration and expiration.

2. Ultrasound imaging of the normal lung in M-mode produces the characteristic "**seashore sign**" wherein a linear, laminar pattern appears in the tissue superficial to the hyperechoic pleural line and a granular, "sandy" pattern appears in the tissues deep to the pleural line (Fig. 3.2D). "Lung sliding" is produced by the movement of parietal pleura over the visceral pleura with inspiration and expiration and is seen in the 2D exam.

3. **A and B lines: A lines** are horizontal reverberation artifacts produced by the hyperechoic pleural line that repeat at regular intervals from the superficial to deep portion of the ultrasound image. These are present in normal lung, although patients with severe asthma/emphysema will also have an A-line pattern (Fig. 3.2A). **B lines** are vertical, discrete, laser-like reverberation artifacts that arise from the pleural line and extend to the bottom of the image without fading. B lines move synchronously with the pleural line during inspiration and expiration. A few B lines are normal in the dependent portions of the lung. However, multiple B lines in a lung field represent increased interstitial fluid. Patients with cardiogenic and noncardiogenic pulmonary edema will have an extensive B-line profile over their anterior lungs (Fig. 3.2B). B lines efface normal A lines.

4. **Pneumothorax**

   a. When the space between the parietal pleura and the visceral pleura becomes air-filled, normal pleural sliding is absent on POC ultrasound exam. Loss of lung sliding can be a sign of pleural pathology and pneumothorax. Loss of lung sliding is also seen in lung collapse and patients who have undergone pleurodesis.

   b. When visualized with M-mode, the "**stratosphere sign**" appears wherein horizontal, laminar artifact appears throughout the image—much like the thin, linear clouds in the stratosphere.

   c. Imaging of a lung point in pneumothorax can help define the physical limit of air in the space between the parietal and visceral pleura. "Lung point" refers to the absence of lung sliding at a physical point where this pattern transitions into an area of regular, consistent lung sliding. Finding a lung point using lung ultrasound is diagnostic of a pneumothorax.

5. **Effusion**

   a. Pleural effusion is best seen with the phased array probe and appears as a hypoechoic space between the chest wall and the consolidated lung tissue beneath. Often the lung itself appears as a hyperechoic tail of tissue floating in the effusion itself (Fig. 3.2C). It is important to delineate the boundaries of the effusion (the diaphragm below, visible lung tissue, and the chest wall) to avoid confusion with ascitic fluid.

V. OTHER USES OF POINT-OF-CARE ULTRASOUND IN THE ICU

A. The Focused Assessment with Sonography for Trauma (FAST) Exam

1. The FAST exam is a limited ultrasound scanning exam that allows for rapid diagnosis of fluid (hemorrhage) in the intraperitoneal or pericardial spaces. This exam can be completed with the curvilinear or phased array probes. The goal of the FAST exam is to identify significant bleeding, not to look for organ injury. A positive FAST examination in a hypotensive patient may suggest the need for emergent intervention (laparotomy or angio-embolization).

2. The FAST exam looks for free fluid in four areas: the perihepatic and hepatorenal space, the pelvis, the perisplenic space, and the pericardial space. The hepatorenal space is the most posterior portion of the upper abdominal cavity in a supine patient. The probe should be placed in the right posterior axillary line at the level of the 11th to 12th ribs. A perisplenic scan is accomplished by placing the probe in the left upper quadrant at the left posterior axillary line between the 10th and 11th ribs (Fig. 3.3). The pelvis is scanned by placing the probe midline and superior to the pubic symphysis. Finally, the pericardial space is

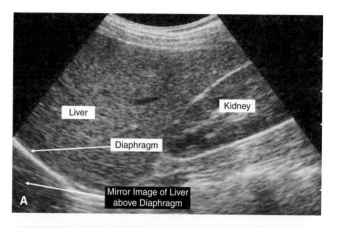

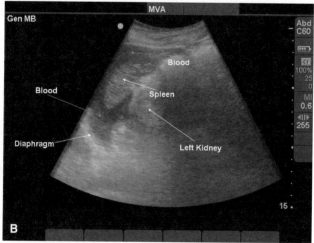

FIGURE 3.3 Selected images from a FAST exam. **(A)** Normal ultrasound view of Morrison's pouch. A mirror-image artifact of the liver is present above the hyperechoic diaphragm. **(B)** FAST exam of perisplenic space showing hemoperitoneum.

evaluated by pacing the probe inferior to the xiphoid process and an-
gling it upward and to the left toward the heart.

B. Detection of Deep Venous Thrombosis: Venous thrombosis and pulmonary
embolism are common in ICUs and add substantially to patient morbidity.
Studies have shown that intensivist-performed compression ultrasound is
sensitive and specific in the diagnosis of proximal lower-extremity DVT
compared with a formal vascular ultrasound (that included compression,
color augmentation, and spectral Doppler ultrasound). In addition,
using POC ultrasound resulted in significant time savings (diagnoses
were made >12 hours earlier when using POC ultrasound compared
with formal ultrasound). Compression ultrasound involves scanning
the lower extremity veins (common femoral, superficial femoral, and
popliteal veins) and compressing them enough to cause them to collapse
(the accompanying arteries should not be compressed during venous
compression). Lack of compressibility suggests the presence of a DVT.

C. Intracranial Pressure Measurement: Measurement of optic nerve sheath
diameter with POC ultrasound has been shown to correlate with
radiologic signs and symptoms of increased intracranial pressure (ICP). An
optic nerve sheath diameter of >5 mm correlates with an ICP >20 mmHg.
Measurement of optic nerve sheath diameter should be performed with
sterile ultrasound transmission gel and a sterile ultrasound probe sheath.
Using the linear 5 to 10 MHz probe, image the eye through closed eyelids.
Optic nerve sheath diameter measurements should be taken 3 mm behind
the globe where ultrasound contrast is the greatest and measurements
are therefore more reproducible. A contraindication to this technique is
ocular injury.

D. Airway Ultrasound: Occasionally, auscultation and end-tidal CO_2 fail to
provide anatomic proof that an endotracheal tube is in correct position.
This is especially true in situations of hemodynamic collapse. POC
ultrasound can provide visualization of the endotracheal tube and/or cuff.
Using the 7.5-to-10-MHz linear probe, begin above the thyroid cartilage
and scan down to the sternal notch. The frontal and lateral walls of the
trachea should be visible as well as portions of the endotracheal tube
provided it is in the correct location.

VI. ULTRASOUND-GUIDED PROCEDURES: Ultrasound-guided procedures (placement
of central venous and arterial catheters, peripheral IVs, thoracentesis,
paracentesis, etc.) have become commonplace, and the data support the
claim that many procedures can be performed faster and more safely under
ultrasound guidance. Space considerations preclude a detailed description of
ultrasound-guided procedures in this chapter.

Selected Readings

Cheung AT, Savino JS, Weiss SJ, et al. Echocardiography and hemodynamic indexes of left
    ventricular preload in patients with normal and abnormal ventricular function. *Anes-
    thesiology* 1994;81:376–387.

Kimberly HH, Shah H, Marill K, et al. Correlation of optic nerve sheath diameter with direct
    measurement of intracranial pressure. *Acad Emerg Med* 2008;15:201–204.

Koenig SJ, Narasimhan M, Mayo PH. Thoracic ultrasonography for the pulmonary special-
    ist. *Chest* 2011;140:1332–1341.

Kory PD, Pellecchia CM, Shiloh AL, et al. Accuracy of ultrasonography performed by critical
    care physicians for the diagnosis of DVT. *Chest* 2011;139:538–542.

Lichtenstein DA. Ultrasound in the management of thoracic disease. *Crit Care Med*
    2007;35:S250–S261.

Mayo PH, Beaulieu Y, Doelken P, et al. American College of Chest Physicians/La Société de Réanimation de Langue Francaise statement on competence in critical care ultrasonography. *Chest* 2009;135:1050–1060.

Raphael DT, Conrad FU. Ultrasound confirmation of endotracheal tube placement. *J Clin Ultrasound* 1987;15:459–462.

Via G, Hussein A, Wells M, et al. International evidence based recommendations for focused cardiac ultrasound. *J Am Soc Echocardiogr* 2014;27:683.e1–683.e33.

Volpicelli G, Elbarbary M, Blaivas M, et al. International evidence-based recommendations for point-of-care lung ultrasound. *Intensive Care Med* 2012;38(4):577–591.

Werner SL, Smith CE, Goldstein JR, et al. Pilot study to evaluate the accuracy of ultrasonography in confirming endotracheal tube placement. *Ann Emerg Med* 2007;49:75–80.

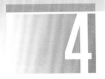

Airway Management

John H. Nichols and Jonathan E. Charnin

 Patient Positioning

 Direct Laryngoscopy

I. **INTRODUCTION:** Endotracheal intubation is indicated in the setting of acute respiratory failure (hypoxemic or hypercarbic) when noninvasive positive pressure ventilation (NIPPV) has failed or is contraindicated, obtundation (Glasgow Coma Score <8), airway obstruction, or anticipation of compromised airway patency due to trauma, edema, or other etiologies. This chapter will review airway evaluation, advanced airway placement/maintenance, and evaluation for withdrawal of advanced airway support.

II. **INDICATIONS FOR ADVANCED AIRWAY:** Intact respiratory function requires a central drive to breathe, appropriate respiratory neuromuscular function, a patent upper airway, the ability to protect the airway from aspiration, and effective ventilation and perfusion matching. Placement of an endotracheal tube (ETT) allows ventilation of a patient who lacks a respiratory drive, can support the work of breathing in a patient who is weak, provides an opening through an upper airway that may be prone to collapse, mitigates large volume aspiration, and, by using positive pressure, reexpands atelectatic lung regions that contribute to ventilation/perfusion mismatch.

III. **ASSESSMENT OF NEED FOR AN ADVANCED AIRWAY**
   A. **Cardiopulmonary Resuscitation:** Per ACLS guidelines, bag mask ventilation with 100% inspired oxygen is required. If bag-mask ventilation is inadequate, an advanced airway (ETT, supraglottic airway [SGA]) should be placed without interruption of chest compressions.
   B. **Decreased Level of Consciousness:** Intubation may be required due to airway obstruction, decreased respiratory drive, and risk of aspiration. Though GCS <8 is classically taught as an indication for intubation, significant risk of aspiration exists with GCS scores >8, and thus the presence of gastro-esophageal reflux disease (GERD), esophageal sphincter dysfunction, and full stomach may justify intubation in a stuporous patient.
   C. **Pulse Oximetry:** Continuous monitoring aids the assessment of patients with hypoxia. While more quantifiable and reliable than the appearance of cyanosis, there is no number that absolutely warrants intubation. Oxygen saturations below 88% usually require evaluation and may require intervention.
   D. **Respiratory Patterns:**
      1. **Respiratory rate (RR)/Tidal volume (TV):**
         a. ↓RR/↑TV: central cause (CNS disorder, opiate effect)
         b. ↑RR/↑TV: increased work of breathing to overcome changes in lung compliance (pulmonary edema, pneumothorax, alveolar

consolidation, ARDS) or need for greater levels of ventilation (CO_2 production, sepsis, increased dead space)

   c. ↑**RR/**⇔**TV:** other etiologies such as pain, bladder distention, and anxiety

2. **Symmetry:** The chest and abdomen should expand together with inspiration. Discordant movement may be seen during active exhalation, airway obstruction, and cervical spine paralysis with preserved diaphragm function. Pneumothorax, hemothorax, flail chest, splinting, and large bronchial obstructions can cause right/left asymmetry.

3. **Accessory muscle use:** Sternocleidomastoid and scalene muscle utilization suggests increased work of breathing and respiratory muscle fatigue/weakness. Firing of the external oblique muscles can signal active exhalation, a sensitive but not specific sign of respiratory distress.

4. **Inspiratory/expiratory timing:**
   a. Long inspiratory time: upper airway or extrathoracic obstruction
   b. Long expiratory time: intra-thoracic obstruction and/or bronchospasm
   c. Inspiratory/expiratory pauses: sustained apnea necessitates intubation, but periodic breathing does not usually require intubation, though the cause should be investigated.

5. **Auscultation/tactile exam:**
   a. Upper airway obstruction: Stridor, absent breath sounds, and lack of air movement from mouth/nose suggest upper airway obstruction (jaw thrust, chin lift, nasal airway may alleviate).
   b. Other: Wheezing, rales, and absent breath sounds may indicate bronchospasm, pulmonary edema/consolidation, or pneumothorax, respectively.

E. Ventilation/Oxygenation Data

1. **Arterial blood gas (ABG):** Oxygen and carbon dioxide tensions and pH should be used to assess severity of disease and the success/failure of clinical interventions. It should not substitute for clinical judgment or delay critical interventions, but remains the most reliable test for oxygenation and ventilation.

2. **Co-oximetry:** Evaluation of arterial blood, or via noninvasive multiwavelength oximeters, can assay methemoglobinemia, carboxyhemoglobinemia, and desaturated blood.

3. **Failed noninvasive positive pressure ventilation:** Bi-level positive pressure ventilation (BiPAP) and continuous positive airway pressure ventilation (CPAP) can help avoid endotracheal intubation in patients with respiratory failure secondary to chronic obstructive pulmonary disease (COPD) and acute cardiogenic pulmonary edema. Lack of improvement justifies endotracheal intubation.

IV. PREPARATION FOR PLACEMENT OF AN ADVANCED AIRWAY

A. Physical Exam/Patient History: A brief airway exam and history are necessary to minimize the chance of failing to ventilate/intubate, to predict the need for advanced intubation techniques, and to be aware of potential complications.

1. **Airway anatomy:** Less than three finger-breadths thyromental distance, small mouth opening, large incisors, limited ability to protrude the mandible, a large tongue, elevated Mallampati score, short neck, and limited cervical mobility may all contribute to difficult visualization of the glottis with laryngoscopy and should be checked.

2. **Potential difficulty with mask ventilation:** Facial hair, edentulousness, obesity, male gender, history of sleep apnea, and neck irradiation portend difficult mask ventilation.

3. **Data on prior intubation attempts:** If time permits, review old records for difficulty with prior intubation attempts and successful rescue techniques.
4. **Allergies:** Review for contraindications to the use of standard induction and maintenance drugs.
5. **Coagulation status:** Time permitting, a review of platelet count, PT/PTT, and current anticoagulation therapy is worthwhile, as profound anticoagulation may prohibit nasal airway manipulation given the risk of bleeding. The provider should be aware of potential for bleeding with multiple intubation attempts.
6. **Neuromuscular status:**
   a. Patients with burns, crush injuries, prolonged immobility ($>$1–2 weeks), extensive upper motor neuron injury (such as debilitating stroke), denervation injuries, and myopathies are at risk of hyperkalemic arrest with the use of succinylcholine. Rocuronium is a viable alternative for intubation.
   b. Cervical spine instability may require flexible fiberoptic or video laryngoscopic (e.g., GlideScope) intubation to minimize cervical manipulation.
   c. Increased intracranial pressure (ICP), presence of intracranial aneurysms, intracranial hemorrhage, and symptoms of cerebral ischemia/infarct should be noted and may affect choice of induction medications.
7. **Cardiovascular history:** Angina/ischemia, arrhythmias, congestive heart failure, hypertension, and aneurysms should be noted given risk of cardiovascular collapse with common induction agents.
8. **Aspiration risk:** Recent gastric feeding, GERD, hemoptysis, emesis, bowel obstruction, obesity, pregnancy, and depressed mental status increase aspiration risk and may require rapid sequence intubation (RSI).
9. **Hemodynamic stability:** Note vasopressor requirements, work of breathing, blood pressure, heart rate, and oxygen saturation. Instability may require judicious use of induction agents.

B. **Choice of Advanced Airway Placement Technique:** Options include direct laryngoscopy, video-assisted laryngoscopy, blind naso-tracheal intubation, flexible fiberoptic intubation (nasal/oral), and/or supraglottic airway placement.
1. **Direct laryngoscopy:** performed with a laryngoscope and direct visualization of the glottis
   a. **Advantages:** can be performed quickly with minimal equipment
   b. **Disadvantages:** uncomfortable for awake patients and difficult with unfavorable airway anatomy or cervical spine instability requiring cervical spine fixation
2. **Video-assisted laryngoscopy:** Modified laryngoscopy blades with an anteriorly angled camera at the blade tip are commonly used in the setting of predicted or encountered difficult direct laryngoscopy due to anterior/superior larynx, small mouth opening, obesity/redundant laryngeal soft tissue, or limited cervical mobility. Available devices include the C-Mac (Karl Storz) and the GlideScope (Verathon).
   a. **Advantages:** similar intubation mechanics to direct laryngoscopy with the advantage of an improved view of an anterior/superior glottis due to angled blade-tip camera
   b. **Disadvantages:** being not always available in critical care units, cost, fragility, need for power source, limited portability, and unfamiliarity with device compared with direct laryngoscopy
3. **Naso-tracheal Intubation:** performed when the oral opening is insufficient for direct glottis visualization, in neck instability, and when

access to a noninstrumented oral cavity is desired while maintaining an advanced airway

   a. **Advantages**: more easily tolerated by minimally sedated patients when compared with oro-tracheal intubation. It can be performed on patients with unfavorable airway anatomy, in the sitting position to improve spontaneous respiratory mechanics/minimize aspiration, and without general anesthesia or paralytic agents.

   b. **Disadvantages**: technically challenging, and spontaneous respiration must be present to guide blind placement via breath sounds. Placement under direct visualization with Magill forceps negates many advantages over oro-tracheal intubation. Contraindications include coagulopathy or planned anticoagulation/thrombolysis, nasal polyps, basilar skull fracture, and immunocompromise given increased risk of sinusitis. Endotracheal tube diameter may be limited given nasal passage size.

4. **Flexible fiberoptic intubation**: Insertion of an ETT over a flexible fiberscope with glottis visualization can be performed via the oral or nasal cavity.

   a. **Advantages:** can intubate patients with unfavorable airway anatomy with minimal cervical manipulation. Fiberoptic visualization of the ETT tip upon airway exit can confirm accurate placement depth.

   b. **Disadvantages**: technically difficult, equipment intensive, and visualization may be difficult with bleeding/excess secretions/distorted anatomy given decreased ability to suction or manipulate the airway

5. **Supra-glottic airway**: SGAs are the category of airway rescue devices that include the Laryngeal Mask Airway (LMA). As part of the ASA difficult airway algorithm, an SGA may be used as an emergency airway, especially as a bridge to endotracheal intubation. Some SGAs allow intubation through their lumens.

   a. **Advantages:** rapid/easy placement in majority of patients

   b. **Disadvantages**: not a long-term airway management strategy, decreased protection against aspiration, not tolerated by minimally sedated patients, risk of gastric insufflation with positive pressure ventilation if not placed appropriately

C. **Monitors/Equipment**: Essential monitors during acute airway management include pulse oximetry, blood pressure, and electrocardiography. All equipment must be ready for immediate use (a handy mnemonic is iSOAP).

1. **Intravenous (IV) access**: Adequate IV access should be available prior to intubation except in emergent cases such as cardiac arrest, which may necessitate intubation before IV access is obtained.

2. **Suction**: A functioning Yankauer or tonsil-tip suction device must be available.

3. **Oxygen**: An in-wall or tank oxygen (full) source and functioning bag-valve mask must be available for proper oxygenation.

4. **Airway**: A laryngoscope (Miller 2 or Macintosh 3 for adults, Miller 1 or Macintosh 2 for pediatrics), correctly sized endotracheal tube(s) (8.0 for men, 7.0 for women, see below for pediatrics) with stylet inserted and intact cuff must be available.

   a. **Pediatric ETT**: Recent literature supports the use of cuffed endotracheal tubes when ETT diameter is >3.5 mm, and inflating the cuff until a leak is present at 20 cmH$_2$O. If no cuff leak exists at 20 cmH$_2$O, downsize the ETT diameter by 0.5 mm, and repeat leak test (Table 4.1).

TABLE 4.1	Endotracheal Tube Sizes	
Age	**Size (ID, mm)—Un-cuffed**	**Size (ID, mm)—Cuffed**
Preterm	2.5	
1,000 g		
1,000–2,500 g		
Neonate to 6 mo	3.0	
6 mo to 1 y	3.0–3.5	3.0–3.5
1–2 y	3.5–4.0	3.0–4.0
>2 y	4.0–5.0	3.5–4.5
	(Age in y + 16) / 4	(Age in y / 4) + 3

TABLE 4.2	Contents of Emergency Airway Kit	
Airway Equipment	**Pharmacologic Agents**	
ETT with stylet (6.0, 7.0, 7.5 mm ID)	Propofol	
Laryngoscope handles (2—long, short)	Etomidate	
Laryngoscope blades (Mac 3, Miller 2)	Ketamine	
NPA	Midazolam	
OPA (No. 3, No. 5)	Fentanyl	
Bougie	Hydromorphone	
LMA (No. 4)	Rocuronium	
Syringes (3 cc, 5 cc, 10 cc, 30 cc)	Succinylcholine	
Tape	Phenylephrine	
End-tidal CO_2 detector	Ephedrine	
IV catheters (14–20 gauge)	Glycopyrrolate	
Surgical lubricant	Esmolol	

     5. **Pharmacology**: An induction agent, muscle relaxant, maintenance agent, vasopressor, vagolytic, and antihypertensive agent should be immediately available.
     6. Table 4.2: **Contents of Emergency Intubation Kit**

V. **INTUBATION TECHNIQUES**: Successful intubation requires optimal patient positioning, adequate preoxygenation (if possible), and proper intubation technique.
    A. **Patient Positioning**: Time to optimize position for intubation is well spent and should not be overlooked (Video 4.1: **Patient Positioning**).
      1. **Bed position in room**: Move the head of the bed away from any walls, remove headboard, and bring the head of the patient to the edge of bed. If the headboard cannot be removed, place the patient diagonally in the bed for improved airway access.
      2. **Bed height**: Elevate the bed so that the patient's pharynx is between the operator's umbilicus and xyphoid process. Consider slight reverse Trendelenberg position to minimize aspiration risk.
      3. **Align pharyngeal, laryngeal, and oral axes:** In the supine position, the laryngeal, pharyngeal, and oral axes are not parallel (Fig. 4.1a), inhibiting glottis visualization. Creating the "sniffing position" with neck flexion

via blankets under the occiput (Fig. 4.1b) and head extension on the at-lanto-axial joint (Fig. 4.1c) will align the three axes. Fig. 4.1c illustrates the ideal position where the laryngeal, pharyngeal, and oral axes are nearly parallel.

4. **Trauma patients:** All trauma patients who have not received definitive cervical spine clearance via NEXUS or Canadian C-spine rules, CT, or MRI (if obtunded), should be assumed to have a cervical spine injury. During airway management, the patient should remain in a c-collar or an assistant should hold the patient's neck/head in the neutral position. Awake fiberoptic intubation should be used for alert/awake patients in nonemergent cases, while direct orotracheal intubation with neck stabilization is appropriate in all other cases. Note that bag-mask ventilation is the time of greatest cervical manipulation.

B. **Pre-Oxygenation:** Replacement of functional residual capacity (FRC) nitrogen with oxygen is critical prior to intubation to maximize tolerated apnea time. This is especially relevant with obese patients, who should be preoxygenated to an end-tidal oxygen level >85%.

1. **Awake/alert patient:** Tightly seal bag-valve mask over nose and mouth, provide 100% oxygen at high flows >10 L/min, encourage tidal volume

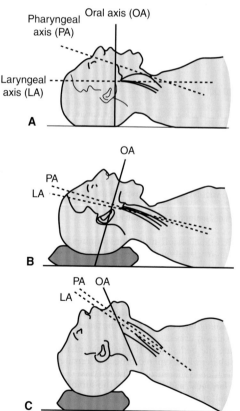

FIGURE 4.1 Optimal patient positioning

breathing for 3 minutes, or vital capacity breathing if time limited, and use gentle chin-lift/jaw thrust maneuvers as needed to ensure airway patency. Postinduction, maintain airway seal and patency during the time between induction and intubation, as apneic oxygenation can maintain oxygenation.

2. **Obtunded patient:** Without adequate respiratory effort, 8 to 10 breaths per minute of positive pressure ventilation/support with a bag-valve mask at 100% oxygen is required for preoxygenation. Airway adjuncts to ensure airway patency such as an oropharyngeal or nasopharyngeal airway may be required if bag-mask ventilation with head positioning and chin-lift/jaw thrust maneuvers is ineffective.

    a. **Oropharyngeal airway (OPA):** Provided in three adult sizes (Sizes 3, 4, 5–80, 90, 100 mm, respectively), which is the distance from the tip to flange. Proper size can be estimated by measuring distance from ear lobe to the ipsilateral corner of the lip. The distal tip is inserted facing upward against the hard palate and then rotated 180 degrees to advance into posterior pharynx. An OPA that is too short may cause obstruction by pressing the tongue into the posterior pharynx, while an OPA that is too long may push the epiglottis against the glottis opening. An OPA may cause laryngospasm or emesis in a conscious or semiconscious patient.

    b. **Nasopharyngeal airway (NPA):** Optimal for use in obstructed patients with intact oropharyngeal reflexes or minimal mouth opening when bag-mask ventilation is inadequate. NPAs are sized for adults by internal diameter (6–9 mm), should be inserted into the naris parallel to the hard palate after lubrication, and advanced until the flange rests on the outer naris. Use the largest diameter that will fit into the naris with minimal resistance. Bleeding tendency is a relative contraindication to NPA placement while basilar skull fractures are a more absolute contraindication to NPA placement. NPAs are less likely to induce vomiting and are better tolerated than OPAs in awake/minimally obtunded patients.

C. **Orotracheal Intubation:** Direct laryngoscopy, video-assisted laryngoscopy, and flexible fiberoptic intubation are common methods for oral ETT placement.

    1. **The laryngoscope:** Direct visualization of the glottis can be achieved using a laryngoscope with either a Macintosh or Miller blade. Some laryngoscopes have the light emitted from a bulb on the blade; some fiberoptic systems have the light source in the handle, with light carried to the blade tip. Non-fiberoptic handles and blades are not compatible with fiberobtic handles and blades. It is critical to ensure the system works (Fig. 4.2).

        a. **Laryngoscope handle:** provides a place to apply a firm grip with the left hand.

        b. **Macintosh blade:** a curved blade that is inserted into the vallecula (the space between the base of the tongue and the pharyngeal surface of the epiglottis). Upward pressure against the hyoepiglottic ligament elevates the epiglottis, exposing the glottis. Sizes range from No. 0 to No. 4, with No. 3 as the most commonly used blade in adults. Its deep flange provides more room for ETT passage when compared with a Miller blade (Video 4.2: **Direct Laryngoscopy**).

        c. **Miller blade:** A straight blade whose tip is inserted underneath the laryngeal surface of the epiglottis and lifted to expose the glottis. The smaller flange provides less space for ETT placement. Sizes range from No. 0 to No. 3, with No. 2 being the most common size for adults.

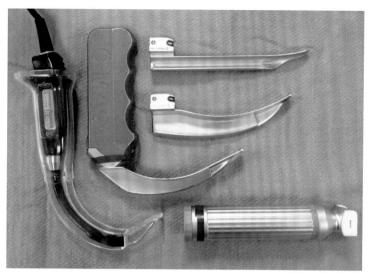

FIGURE 4.2 Laryngoscopes (Clockwise from bottom left: GlideScope, C-Mac, Miller 2, Macintosh 3, laryngoscope handle)

2. **Endotracheal tube:** Choose an appropriate-size ETT (7.5 for women, 8.0 for men) and insert a malleable stylet, making sure that the tip of the stylet does not extend past the tip of the ETT. Bending the tube/stylet 40 to 80 degrees anteriorly 2 to 3 inches from the tip of the ETT ("hockey stick") may aid in passage of the ETT along the posterior surface of the epiglottis if glottis visualization is suboptimal. Deflate the cuff prior to insertion.

3. **Direct laryngoscopy:** With the patient in optimal "sniffing" position and anesthetized, take the laryngoscope in your left hand near the meeting of the handle and blade and use your right hand to open the mouth via a scissoring maneuver during which you place your right thumb on the patient's right lower premolars and your right index finger on the right upper premolars, and press your thumb and index finger in opposing directions. With the mouth open, insert the laryngoscope blade in the right side of the mouth, and if using a Macintosh blade, use the curve of the blade to follow the tongue to its base while simultaneously using the flange to sweep the tongue to the left. Once the epiglottis is visualized, place the tip of the blade anteriorly into the vallecula. If using a Miller blade, advance the tip of the blade to the base of the epiglottis along its laryngeal surface, and note that tongue sweep will be much more difficult. Using either blade, following correct tip placement, lift the handle along its long axis to elevate the epiglottis for direct glottis visualization. Take care not to lever the laryngoscope handle with the maxilla as a fulcrum, as damage to the maxillary incisors may result.

   a. If the glottis cannot be visualized, attempt the following:
      1. Suction or manually extract any obstructing material.
      2. Utilize external laryngeal manipulation to move the larynx posteriorly or laterally into the field of view.

   3. Improve positioning with neck flexion and head extension.

   4. Change to a straight blade if the epiglottis is obstructing the view.

 b. If the glottis remains obscured, remove the laryngoscope, resume bag mask ventilation, and consider other approaches to securing the airway.

4. **ETT insertion:** While maintaining direct visualization of the glottis, hold the ETT in your right hand like a pencil and insert it into the right side of the mouth through the vocal cords. Following visualization of the cuff passing fully through the glottis, stop advancement, remove the stylet, and inflate the cuff with a volume of air that allows for no air leak with 20 cmH$_2$O of positive pressure ventilation. Tube depth should be measured at the upper incisors, with approximate proper depth of 21 cm for women and 23 cm for men.

5. **Video-assisted laryngoscopy:** The use of a GlideScope or other video laryngoscopy systems may be helpful with difficult airways as their anteriorly angled cameras facilitate glottis visualization unobtainable with direct laryngoscopy.

 a. **GlideScope:** Load the GlideScope handle/camera into a size 3 or 4 disposable GlideScope blade. Load a standard ETT onto the specialized GlideScope stylet. Without this stylet, passage of the ETT along the sharp curve of the GlideScope is nearly impossible. Following mouth opening as above, insert the GlideScope at the midline and advance the blade following the curvature of the tongue via rotation of the handle toward the nose until the base of the tongue is reached and the epiglottis can be seen. Continue advancement toward the epiglottis via rotation of the handle until visualization of the vocal cords. Keeping the vocal cords in the top one-third of the GlideScope screen, insert the styleted tube into the right side of the mouth and advance along the curvature of the blade until the tip of the ETT is visualized on the screen. Advance the tube between the vocal cords using small rotations as needed, and gradually begin to retract the stylet once the ETT tip is through the cords. Common errors are an inability to visualize the ETT tip by placing the camera too close to the glottis, excessively large rotations of the styleted ETT, and insertion of the Glidecope blade similar to direct laryngoscopy by not rotating the handle to follow the curvature of the blade and tongue.

 b. Many other rigid fiberoptic (Bullard, Upsher) or video laryngoscopy systems are available (C-mac, C-mac D, King Vision, McGrath). Each system will have unique operating requirements.

6. **ETT placement confirmation:** The most common mistake during endotracheal intubation is esophageal intubation, which must be recognized quickly via the following confirmatory techniques. None alone will guarantee proper ETT placement, and if any doubt exists regarding proper ETT placement, remove the ETT, initiate bag mask ventilation, and attempt intubation a second time.

 a. **Direct visualization:** Watch the ETT pass through the glottis.

 b. **Chest rise:** Observe symmetric bilateral chest rise with positive pressure ventilation.

 c. **Water vapor:** Observe condensation in the ETT on expiration and its disappearance on inspiration.

 d. **Auscultation:** Listen for clear bilateral inspiratory breath sounds in the upper thorax and their absence in the stomach. Lack of breath sounds in the left thorax may suggest right main-stem intubation, and the ETT should be retracted until bilateral breath sounds are confirmed.

      e. **CO_2 measurement**: A capnometer on the mechanical ventilator or a disposable calorimetric CO_2 detector should be used to confirm persistent end-tidal CO_2 on expiration. End-tidal CO_2 may be absent despite endotracheal placement without adequate cardiopulmonary circulation. Conversely, end-tidal CO_2 may be transiently be present following esophageal intubation due to residual CO_2 in the stomach from mask ventilation and will gradually disappear.

      f. **Ventilation and oxygenation**: Only leave the patient under the care of others once several minutes of adequate oxygenation and ventilation have been observed.

  7. **Secure the ETT**: Tape the ETT to bony structures of the maxilla. Take care to avoid pinching the lip against the ETT with tape, and note the depth of the ETT at the upper incisors in the chart while also summarizing the procedure and noting any complications.

  8. **Chest radiograph**: Obtain a chest plain radiograph to confirm ETT placement. The tip of the ETT should be approximately 2 to 4 cm above the carina.

D. Nasotracheal Intubation: Endotracheal intubation via the nares is a technique to be used when an orotracheal tube is not feasible, such as the inability to open the mouth or predicted oral surgery. The technique is as follows:

  1. **Nasal vasoconstriction**: To avoid excessive bleeding, nasal application of 0.25% to 1% phenylephrine solution or 0.05% Oxymetazoline several minutes prior to nasal instrumentation is recommended.

  2. **Antisialogogue**: 0.2 mg Glycopyrrolate IV

  3. **Anesthesia**: Apply cotton-tipped nasal swabs dipped in 4% Lidocaine solution to both nares. Nebulized 2% Lidocaine via facemask and gargling of 2% Lidocaine for more distal airway anesthesia may be considered.

  4. **ETT**: A standard ETT or Nasal Rae Tube can be used. Sizes are 7.0 to 7.5 mm for men and 6.0 to 6.5 mm for women. Standard depth measured at the nares is 26 cm for women and 28 cm for men. A flexible-tipped ETT may minimize airway trauma. Generously lubricate the endotracheal tube cuff, but avoid lubrication in the lumen of the ETT (Fig. 4.3).

  5. **Nare dilation**: To dilate the nares and ensure patency, insert a well-lubricated, nasopharyngeal airway of the largest diameter that does not meet resistance. The inner diameter of the NPA should be no smaller than that of the ETT. Remove the NPA prior to intubating.

  6. **Nasal ETT insertion basics**: Insert the ETT perpendicular to the plane of the face and parallel to the hard palate. If resistance is met in the pharynx, the ETT may be impacting the posterior pharyngeal wall, and the ETT should be retracted, the neck extended, and the ETT readvanced. Do not advance against resistance.

  7. **Blind nasal ETT placement**: When intubating a spontaneously breathing patient, the operator can advance the ETT while listening for breath sounds at the proximal end of the ETT, which should become louder as the glottis nears. Sudden loss of breath sounds suggests placement in the esophagus, piriform recess, or vallecula, whereas a cough, condensation on the interior of the ETT, and loss of voice suggests endotracheal intubation. Common maneuvers to correct placement errors are the following:

      a. Neck extension and/or cricoid pressure can move the larynx posteriorly and direct the ETT away from the esophagus.

      b. Neck flexion can direct the ETT away from the vallecula.

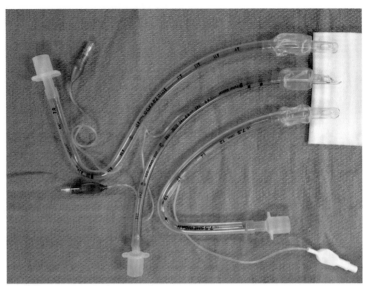

FIGURE 4.3 Endotracheal tubes (Top to bottom: Nasal Rae, standard ETT with Parker flex tip, oral Rae)

   c. Tilting (not rotating) the head toward the nare chosen for intuba-
      tion and rotating the ETT toward the midline directs the tube away
      from the piriform recess.
   d. Inflate the cuff to move the tip of the ETT off the posterior pharyn-
      geal wall in a patient with an anterior larynx, making sure to deflate
      the cuff prior to passage through the cords.
8. **Direct visualization:** In an anesthetized patient, following insertion of
   the ETT into the oropharynx via the nare, direct laryngoscopy is performed, and Magill forceps are used to guide the ETT through the vocal
   cords under direct visualization. The ETT should be grasped proxi-
   mally to the cuff to prevent cuff damage.
9. **Fiberoptic intubation:** A flexible fiberoptic bronchoscope can be inserted
   into the lumen of the ETT and used to guide the ETT through the glottis
   (technique described later).
E. **Fiberoptic Intubation (FOI):** Intubation with a flexible fiberoptic bronchoscope
   is recommended in cases of predicted difficult airways (body habitus, airway
   anatomy, neck/head flexibility limitations) and can be performed awake or
   asleep via the nasal or oral routes with similar technique.
   1. **Preparation:**
      a. Consider preprocedure low dose anticholinergic treatment to mini-
         mize oral secretions.
      b. Connect the bronchoscope to a video screen or eye piece and ensure
         proper white balance/focus. (Adult size will have greater resolution
         than pediatric size.)
      c. Lubricate the fiberoptic bronchoscope.
      d. Remove the stylet from an ETT with an inner diameter larger than
         the bronchoscope diameter, advance the bronchoscope through the

ETT, and lightly tape the proximal end of the ETT to the proximal end of the bronchoscope.

 e. Connect suction tubing to the suction port of the bronchoscope.

 f. Minimize bronchoscope tip condensation by touching the tip of the bronchoscope to the patient's tongue or using a defogging solution.

2. **Anesthesia**: Proper local anesthesia is critical for an FOI performed with an awake patient. Nasal anesthesia is described above, and for oral anesthesia, the operator may consider nebulized lidocaine via facemask, lidocaine liquid gargling, and gradual advancement of an OPA coated with 4% lidocaine paste (as patient tolerates). Glossopharyngeal, superior laryngeal, and transtracheal blocks are more advanced techniques (out of the scope of this book). Care must always be taken to avoid local anesthetic toxicity.

3. **Oral insertion**: While holding the proximal end of the bronchoscope with the dominant hand and the distal end with the nondominant hand, an assistant should insert an Ovassapian airway or pull the tongue out of the mouth to maximize space in the oropharynx. Keeping the bronchoscope straight at all times, insert the tip into the mouth and feed it slowly forward with the nondominant hand. Upon reaching the base of the tongue, the tip should be flexed anteriorly and advanced toward the epiglottis. Slide the tip underneath the epiglottis, advance through the glottis after visualization, and advance distally in the trachea until 3 to 4 cm above the carina. If visualization becomes unclear at any point, retract the bronchoscope until landmarks are recognized, and reattempt placement. Once the bronchoscope is intratracheal, an assistant should advance the ETT over the bronchoscope to the standard depth. If resistance is met, rotate the ETT 90 degrees to place the bevel in a more favorable position. After ETT advancement, firmly hold the ETT and retract the bronchoscope making sure to visualize that the tip of the ETT is intratracheal at the appropriate depth.

4. **Nasal insertion**: The technique/preparation is identical to oral insertion, except entry is via the nare. Insert the bronchoscope perpendicular to the face, and advance only when the lumen of the nare is clearly visualized. Lubricating the ETT cuff prior to insertion is advised.

F. **Supraglottic Airway**: There are many SGAs, each with its own system of utilization. Because the laryngeal mask airway (LMA) is most commonly used, it is described here. The LMA does not protect against aspiration and should not be placed in a patient with intact airway reflexes.

1. **Sizes**: LMAs come in sizes 1 to 5 based on patient size, with the most common adult sizes being No. 3 through No. 5.

2. **Insertion**: Generously lubricate the LMA cuff, place your index finger in the angle between the cuff and connecting tube, and using pressure with the index finger, advance along the hard palate until the cuff lodges into the pharynx. Inflate or deflate the cuff such that a leak begins to appear with positive pressure of 20 cmH$_2$O.

3. **Common errors**:
 a. Forcing the tip of the LMA superiorly into the nasopharynx
 b. Folding the epiglottis over the trachea
 c. Folding the tip of the cuff upon itself
 d. Lateral rotation of the cuff within the oropharynx

4. **Specialized supraglottic airways**:
 a. **Intubating SGA (Air Q, Mercury Medical)**: lumen large enough for passing ETT blindly or with fiberoptic visualization after SGA placement (Fig. 4.4).

    b. Blind Insertion Airway Device (BIAD) (Combitube): A single lumen tube with esophageal and pharyngeal balloons which, when inflated, allows ventilation from a port between the balloon sites. Used in emergency settings.

G. Cricothyrotomy: When endotracheal intubation, LMA placement, and mask ventilation fail to provide adequate ventilation, cricothyrotomy should be performed emergently.

    1. Needle cricothyrotomy: Puncture the cricothyroid membrane with a 14G intravenous catheter attached to a syringe, and advance until air is aspirated from the trachea. Remove the needle, secure the catheter with your hand, and attach the catheter via tubing to either a jet ventilator or wall oxygen supply. Cyclically deliver oxygen, anticipating that exhalation may not be able to occur, but oxygenation may be possible. Avoid elevated intrathoracic pressures. Call for help!

    2. Surgical cricothyrotomy: Using a scalpel, incise the skin and subcutaneous tissue at the cricothyroid notch until piercing the cricothyroid membrane. Expand the membrane bluntly or with the scalpel, and insert either a small tracheostomy tube (No. 4–6) or a No. 6–6.5 ETT cut near its distal end into the trachea.

    3. Complications: Bleeding, subcutaneous/mediastinal emphysema, tracheal mucosal trauma, and barotrauma from inadequate expiration can all occur from cricothyrotomy and jet ventilation. The above

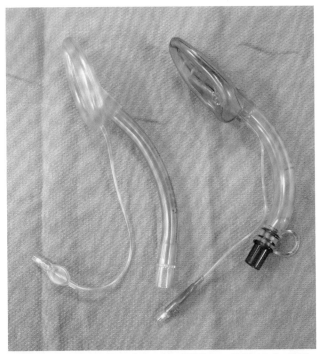

FIGURE 4.4 Supraglottic airways (Left to right: LMA Unique, Air-Q intubating LMA)

techniques should only be used temporarily while a more definitive surgical airway is achieved.

H. Emergent Tracheostomy: Requires time and surgical equipment and may take longer for placement. Its use as an emergent procedure depends on the operator and the equipment available.

VI. INTUBATION PHARMACOLOGY: Hypnotics, neuromuscular blockers, analgesics, and local anesthetics are the primary agents used during endotracheal intubation.

A. Hypnotics/Amnestics: Used to prevent consciousness and recall.

1. **Propofol (GABA-A agonist):** 1 to 2 mg/kg IV for induction, though care must be taken in hemodynamically unstable patients given its ability to decrease systemic vascular resistance and inotropy.
2. **Midazolam (Benzodiazepine):** titrated via 0.5 to 1-mg IV incremental doses to achieve sedation/anterograde amnesia without major hemodynamic effects. Onset is within 60 to 90 seconds and duration is 20 to 60 minutes.
3. **Dexmedetomidine (Alpha-2 agonist):** 1 mcg/kg IV over 10 minutes, followed by an infusion of 0.4 mcg/kg/h. Side effects include hypotension and bradycardia, and induction is much more prolonged than the above agents.
4. **Ketamine (NMDA antagonist):** 2 mg/kg IV for induction, and common side-effects include nystagmus, tonic-clonic movements, hypertension, and vivid nightmares. It produces a dissociative anesthesia, often with eyes open, and benzodiazepines are commonly administered concomitantly to avoid nightmares.
5. **Etomidate (GABA-A agonist):** 0.5 mg/kg IV for induction, and primarily only used in hemodynamically unstable patients given side effects, which include adrenal suppression, myotonic movements, and pain on injection.

B. Neuromuscular Blockers (NMBD): All drugs in this class induce paralysis, respiratory arrest, abolishment of airway reflexes, and vocal cord relaxation. Concomitant sedation is required, and intubation must be achieved in a timely manner as the patient will remain in respiratory arrest.

1. **Depolarizing NMBDs (Succinylcholine):** Following a 1-mg/kg IV intubating dose, fasciculations will appear within 30 seconds, at which point the patient is ready for intubation. Succinylcholine is the drug of choice for rapid sequence intubation, but the operator must be aware of the contraindications (history of malignant hyperthermia, neuromuscular disease, upper motor neuron injury, burns, or immobility), given risk of hyperkalemia.
2. **Nondepolarizing NMBDs:** For emergent intubation without succinylcholine, 1.2 mg/kg IV of Rocuronium is recommended.

C. Analgesics: Intubation is painful. Opioids and local anesthetics can blunt the sympathetic response to intubation.

1. **Opioids:** Fentanyl 50 to 500 mcg IV provides rapid analgesia (peak within 3–5 minutes) and cough suppression during intubation with a brief duration of action (30–60 minutes). Morphine 2 to 10 mg IV has a much slower onset (peak >30 minutes) and longer duration of action (3–4 hours). Hydromorphone 0.5 to 2 mg IV has an intermediate onset (peak 10–20 minutes) and duration (2–3 hours).
2. **Local anesthetics:** Topical local anesthetics (gargled Lidocaine, nebulized Lidocaine, and Benzocaine spray may all provide analgesia for endotracheal intubation, though care must be taken to avoid accidental local anesthetic overdose/toxicity with unmetered use.

3. **Nerve blocks**: Glossopharyngeal, superior laryngeal, and transtracheal nerve blocks can be used for analgesia, but should be avoided in patients with coagulopathies.

D. **Cardiovascular Drugs:**
   1. β-**Blockers**: Esmolol 10 to 100 mg IV may be titrated to minimize tachycardia from sympathetic surge following endotracheal intubation.

E. **Vasopressors**: Phenylephrine (80–160 mcg IV), ephedrine (5–10 mg IV), and epinephrine (10–20 mcg) can be titrated to minimize blood pressure and heart rate lability during induction.

VII. SPECIAL INTUBATING CIRCUMSTANCES

A. **Rapid Sequence Intubation (RSI)**: In patients with full stomachs or high risk of gastric aspiration, an RSI is indicated to minimize the time between airway reflex inhibition and endotracheal intubation. In quick succession, an analgesic (fentanyl), hypnotic (propofol, ketamine, etomidate), and NMBD (succinylcholine, rocuronium) are provided in sequence, and intubation is achieved as rapidly as possible. Cricoid pressure has been considered a standard of care, but given a lack of evidence of its value, and potential to complicate laryngoscopy, many clinicians are abandoning the use of cricoid pressure. Bag-mask ventilation is generally avoided to minimize gastric insufflation and the risk of regurgitation, though should be used if intubation is not immediately successful, or if rapid/severe oxygen desaturation occurs. If an NGT is in place, suction is indicated prior to induction to minimize gastric contents.

B. **Difficult Intubation**: defined as the inability to place an ETT after three attempts by an experienced laryngoscopist. The American Society of Anesthesiologists (ASA) difficult airway algorithm provides a framework for predicted and unpredicted difficult airways (Fig. 4.5). In all cases of difficult intubation, backup personnel should be summoned immediately, including those with surgical airway expertise.
   1. **Predicted**: Based on airway exam, body habitus, lack of neck mobility, and many other clinical factors, a difficult airway may be predicted prior to any attempt at laryngoscopy. The safest approach is to maintain spontaneous respiration and to perform an awake fiberoptic intubation (described above), blind nasal intubation, or elective surgical airway under sedation. If induction of general anesthesia is needed, personnel capable of performing an emergent surgical airway should be present in the event that endotracheal intubation is not achieved rapidly.
   2. **Unpredicted**: When intubation attempts have failed and spontaneous/assisted respirations are absent, an airway emergency is in progress and the next step is placement of an SGA. If ventilation is successful, the SGA can be used as a bridge to endotracheal intubation. If ventilation via SGA is unsuccessful, a surgical cricothyrotomy should be performed by trained personnel. If no persons with surgical expertise are available, needle cricothyrotomy should be performed, followed by jet ventilation. Subcutaneous emphysema and bleeding after needle cricothyrotomy may make subsequent surgical cricothyrotomy impossible.

C. **Increased Intracranial Pressure (ICP)**: Airway management in patients with elevated ICP should be achieved with minimal stimulation to avoid transient ICP increases. Induction with propofol, thiopental, or etomidate is appropriate, followed by muscle relaxation with a nondepolarizing NMBD. Ketamine and succinylcholine should be avoided given their propensity to increase ICP. Adjunctive opioids and β-blockade should be considered to minimize sympathetic stimulation with intubation.

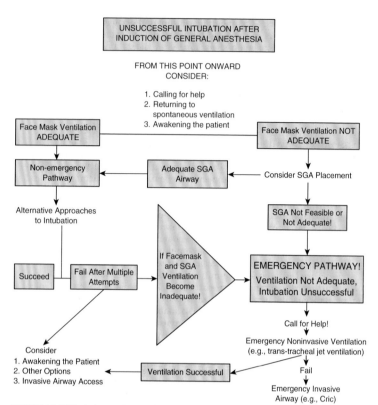

UNSUCCESSFUL INTUBATION AFTER
INDUCTION OF GENERAL ANESTHESIA

FROM THIS POINT ONWARD
CONSIDER:

1. Calling for help
2. Returning to
   spontaneous ventilation
3. Awakening the patient

Face Mask Ventilation
ADEQUATE

Face Mask Ventilation NOT
ADEQUATE

Non-emergency
Pathway

Adequate SGA
Airway

Consider SGA Placement

Alternative Approaches
to Intubation

SGA Not Feasible or
Not Adequate!

If Facemask
and SGA
Ventilation
Become
Inadequate!

Succeed

Fail After Multiple
Attempts

EMERGENCY PATHWAY!
Ventilation Not Adequate,
Intubation Unsuccessful

Call for Help!

Emergency Noninvasive Ventilation
(e.g., trans-tracheal jet ventilation)

Consider
1. Awakening the Patient
2. Other Options
3. Invasive Airway Access

Ventilation Successful

Fail

Emergency Invasive
Airway (e.g., Cric)

FIGURE 4.5 Difficult airway algorithm (Redrawn and simplified from "Practice guidelines for management of the difficult airway." *Anesthesiology* 2013;118:251–270).

D. Myocardial Ischemia/Recent Infarction: Avoidance of hypo/hypertension and tachycardia during intubation is critical to avoid ischemic injury. Etomidate or midazolam in conjunction with deep opioid analgesia may provide optimum conditions. Aggressive β-blockade with esmolol should be used to minimize tachycardia, and vasopressors (e.g., phenylephrine) and vasodilators (e.g., nitroglycerin) should be immediately available to maintain blood pressure at the patient's baseline.

E. Neck Injury: Unstable cervical vertebrae present a risk of spinal cord injury with intubation, and the head, neck, and thorax should remain in the neutral position throughout any intubation attempts. A second individual should provide bi-manual stabilization of the head, neck, and thorax ("in-line stabilization") if the patient is not wearing a protective collar. If intubation is nonemergent, awake fiberoptic intubation (oral or nasal) is advised. In an emergent scenario, direct laryngoscopy should be performed with minimal neck/head extension, and if glottis visualization is not readily achieved, asleep fiberoptic intubation or surgical cricothyrotomy should be performed. A video laryngoscope (GlideScope or C-Mac) may be a useful for laryngoscopy with minimal head/neck manipulation.

F. **Oropharyngeal/Facial Trauma**: Cranial base fractures are a relative contraindication to nasal intubation given the risk of penetrating the cranial vault with a fiberoptic bronchoscope or ETT. Emergent oral intubation is preferred, and with severe facial/neck trauma, an emergent cricothyrotomy or tracheostomy may be preferable. One should always consider the possibility of elevated ICP when presented with facial trauma.

G. **Emergency Pediatric/Neonatal Intubations**: Direct laryngoscopy is the method of choice for intubation of pediatric patients given lack of cooperation for awake intubation and potential for rapid oxygen desaturation (increased oxygen consumption). A low-pressure high-volume cuffed tube (size as previously discussed) is preferable, and the cuff should be inflated such that leak occurs at ~20 cmH$_2$O to prevent mucosal ischemia and to reduce the risk of tracheomalacia and tracheal stenosis as the tracheal cartilage in prepubertal children is not fully developed.

H. **Common Complications of Intubation**:

1. **Hypertension/tachycardia**: Stimulation from laryngoscopy and ETT insertion can produce profound tachycardia and hypertension.

2. **Hypotension**: Severe hypotension can occur following induction of a patient in respiratory distress. In addition to the SVR lowering and negative inotropic effects of many induction agents, the removal of the drive to breathe and its sympathetic stimulation, combined with hyperinflation from aggressive mask ventilation and the resultant preload reduction, can cause profound hypotension.

3. **Bradycardia**: Vagal responses to laryngoscopy can be seen.

I. **Gastric Aspiration**: At highest risk are patients with a full stomach or who are not completely paralyzed prior to laryngoscopy.

VIII. ENDOTRACHEAL AND TRACHEOSTOMY TUBES

A. **ETT Materials**: Most endotracheal tubes are made from polyvinylchloride. Specialized tubes designed to resist infection, resist airway fires, or resist mechanical obstruction due to kinking are available.

B. **Cuff Designs**:

1. **Low pressure/high volume (Hi-Lo)**: Found on standard disposable ETTs, these cuffs are highly compliant, conform to the irregular tracheal wall, and are less likely to cause tracheal mucosal ischemia at cuff pressures <30 cmH$_2$O.

2. **High pressure/low volume**: Found on specialty ETTs, the small area of contact with the tracheal wall, the high pressure required to achieve appropriate cuff inflation, and the required deformation of the tracheal wall to achieve an effective seal all place the trachea at risk for mucosal ischemia.

3. **Low profile (Lo-Pro)**: Often used in pediatrics, these low-pressure/high-volume tubes have cuffs that lie closer to the ETT for ease of visualization during intubation.

C. **Preformed ETT**: designed to move the ETT away from surgical field

1. **Oral RAE**: ETT with an acute curvature at the proximal end for placement inferiorly along the chin

2. **Nasal Rae**: ETT with less acute curvature closer to the proximal end and exits the nare superiorly

D. **Supra-Glottic Suction Tubes**: marketed to reduce ventilator associated pneumonia by facilitating removal of secretions that pool above the endotracheal tube cuff

E. **Tracheostomy Tubes**: available in many sizes, designs, and brands. Key design differences include cuffed/noncuffed, inner cannula/single lumen, fenestrated/nonfenestrated, metal/PVC/silicone.

1. **Sizes**: vary depending on manufacturer and style of tube
2. **Obturator**: a relatively rigid stylet used to aid insertion of a tracheostomy tube. It fits in the lumen of the tracheostomy tube and is removed following insertion.
3. **Inner cannula**: a disposable or reusable cannula that reduces the inner diameter of the tracheostomy tube, but allows for cleaning by removal/replacement of the cannula, thus minimizing risk of obstruction
4. **Key features**:
   a. **Cuffed**: used for patients requiring mechanical ventilation. Phonation can be achieved with fenestration.
   b. **Uncuffed**: mostly used in nonventilated patients at low aspiration risk and allows coughing/phonation around the tube. Often worn over a long period of time. Should not be used if mechanical ventilation is needed.

IX. ENDOTRACHEAL AND TRACHEOSTOMY TUBE MAINTENANCE
A. General Care
1. **Suctioning**: The pharynx and trachea of intubated patients may need periodic suctioning to clear secretions.
2. **Cuff pressure**: Pressure should be less than 25 to 30 cmH$_2$O to avoid mucosal damage and should be monitored routinely. A dedicated ETT cuff monitor (Posey® Cufflator Endotracheal Tube Manometer) or a CVP transducer can be used.
3. **Securing the ETT**: Tape or a dedicated holder can be used to secure the ETT and should be reapplied/adjusted as needed. With oral tubes, lip impingement should be avoided. With nasal tubes, the patient should routinely be assessed for sinusitis, otitis media, and nare ischemia/necrosis.
B. Common Endotracheal and Tracheostomy Tube Problems
1. **Cuff leak**: noted via audible flow of air around the anterior portion of the ETT cuff during positive pressure ventilation while the patient is supine, often with delivered tidal volumes less than expected. Leaks can often be repaired via reinflation with a small volume of air, but large leaks generally require urgent reintubation. Common causes of persistent large volume cuff leak are supraglottic cuff position, cuff damage, and tracheal dilatation.
   a. **Supraglottic cuff position**: A cuff that is above the vocal cords can be seen on chest radiograph or laryngoscopy and is fixed via cuff deflation and ETT advancement.
   b. **Damaged cuff system**: The cuff or its inflation system may slowly or quickly leak air. In either case, ETT replacement is needed, and the level of urgency depends on the speed of the leak.
   c. **Tracheal dilatation**: An ETT with a cuff that is unable to seal a widened tracheal lumen will need to be replaced with an ETT with a larger volume air-filled cuff or a foam cuff tube (Bivona Fome-Cuff). This scenario is seen as a leak with a widened trachea on chest radiograph.
2. **Main-stem intubation**: Following initial intubation or subsequent position changes, the ETT may migrate such that the tip is in the left or right main-stem bronchus. High airway pressures and desaturation may occur. Confirmation is via unilateral breath sounds and chest radiograph, and the problem can be fixed via cuff deflation and retracting the ETT to the appropriate depth.

3. **Airway obstruction**: Triggering of the high airway pressure or low-volume alarm in the absence of obvious changes in pulmonary compliance/ bronchial obstruction suggests ETT obstruction. Common causes are ETT kinking and secretions. Head/neck manipulation may relieve positional ETT kinks, while suctioning via soft suction catheter may relieve obstructing secretions. A kinked ETT will not let a soft suction catheter pass. In either case, if manual ventilation is not possible, immediate ETT replacement is required.

4. **Mal-positioned tracheostomy tubes**: Pressure from the tracheostomy tube on the anterior or posterior tracheal walls can damage the tracheal mucosa, cause obstruction, and predispose to decannulation.

5. **Airway bleeding**: Return of blood during airway suctioning requires prompt evaluation. The primary etiologies are repeated trauma from suctioning and mucosal erosion, both of which must be evaluated. Fiberoptic bronchoscopy can be used to examine the airway for trauma. If bleeding is persistent or without clear source, evaluation by an otolaryngologist is advised. If bleeding is minimal, the airway will require time to heal, and the irritant should be removed, either from less frequent suctioning or replacement of the tracheostomy tube or ETT distal to the lesion. Bleeding from a tracheostomy tube can be particularly dangerous with the risk of erosion into mediastinal vessels causing exsanguination and/or clotting with ETT obstruction, or trachea-esophageal fistula causing aspiration and/or airway obstruction. In cases of persistent obstruction/bleeding from a tracheostomy, urgent laryngotracheal intubation followed by surgical evaluation/exploration is indicated.

C. **ETT Replacement**: often required in the setting of mechanical ETT failure, size inadequacy, and location (oral vs. nasal) changes. Techniques for tube exchange include direct laryngoscopy, bronchoscopy, and use of a tube exchanger.

1. **Direct laryngoscopy**: reintubation as previously described. Useful in patients without a prior difficult airway and minimal airway trauma/ edema.

2. **Bronchoscopy**: After loading a fresh ETT on a flexible bronchoscope, the bronchoscope is advanced via the nasal or oral route until the glottis is visualized, all while maintaining ventilation by the intact old ETT. With glottis visualization, the old ETT cuff is deflated, and the bronchoscope tip is passed around the deflated cuff into the trachea. Maintaining tracheal visualization, an assistant will remove the old ETT followed by advancement of the fresh ETT into the trachea over the bronchoscope.

D. **Tube exchanger**: A long, malleable stylet can be inserted blindly into the existing ETT and advanced to the appropriate tracheal depth using the depth markers. Once advanced to the appropriate depth, the old ETT can be removed over the stylet and the new ETT, blindly or under direct laryngoscopy, can be advanced into the trachea over the exchange stylet. Some specialized tube exchangers have a small lumen through which the patient can be oxygenated or jet ventilated.

X. **TRACHEOSTOMY**: can be performed safely at the bedside as a percutaneous procedure or in the operating room as an open surgical procedure. Most bedside tracheostomies are performed using a modified Ciaglia technique, which utilizes sequential wire-guided plastic or balloon tracheal dilators prior to tracheostomy tube placement.

A. Advantages Over Oral ETT:
1. Improved patient comfort
2. Decreased risk of laryngeal damage/dysfunction
3. Improved oral/pharyngeal hygiene
4. Potential for phonation when cuff is deflated

B. Disadvantages:
1. Potential for tracheal stenosis at stoma site
2. Stoma infection
3. Erosion of neighboring vascular tissue leading to hemorrhage
4. Scarring and/or granulation tissue formation at stoma site
5. Operative complications

C. Timing of Placement: Given the risk of laryngeal damage with prolonged trans-laryngeal intubation, a tracheostomy should be considered after 2 to 3 weeks of oral intubation.

D. Tracheostomy Tube Change: Replacing a tracheostomy tube may be required due to improper size, malposition, or failure. Given difficulty with recannulation of a fresh tracheostomy tract and the risk of false tract creation, it is advisable to wait until the tract is 7 to 10 days old before attempting a tracheostomy tube exchange. If it is necessary to change within 7 to 10 days of initial cannulation, exchange should be made over a malleable stylet, equipment for laryngotracheal intubation should be readily available, and preferably the surgeon who initially placed the tracheostomy tube should present in case surgical reexploration is necessary.

1. **Technique**:
   a. Be fully prepared for emergent laryngotracheal intubation.
   b. Preoxygenate with 100% oxygen.
   c. Clean the tracheostomy site with chlorhexidine and suction the trachea with a soft suction catheter.
   d. Check that the new tracheostomy tube is mechanically intact and that the cuff inflates appropriately. Insert the obturator within the lumen to ensure a smooth distal surface for cannulation.
   e. Deflate the cuff on the existing tube and remove the tube using the natural angulation of the tube. Slight resistance may be felt as the deflated cuff passes through the anterior tracheal wall.
   f. Insert the new tracheostomy tube/obturator smoothly into the existing stoma along the curvature of the tube, being careful to avoid excessive resistance, which is suggestive of a new tract.

E. Manually ventilate with 100% oxygen and ensure proper placement as described previously.

XI. EXTUBATION: Removal of a laryngotracheal ETT or tracheostomy tube in the ICU is indicated once the patient is able to ventilate, oxygenate, clear secretions, and protect the airway without support.

A. Criteria:
1. **Subjective criteria**
   a. Underlying disease process improving
   b. Appropriate cough/gag with airway suctioning
2. **Objective criteria**
   a. GCS >13, minimal sedation
   b. Hemodynamically stable
   c. Sao_2 >90%, Pao_2 >60 mmHg, Pao_2/Fio_2 >150
   d. PEEP <5 to 8 cmH_2O

        e. F_{IO_2} <0.4 to 0.5

        f. $Paco_2$ <60 mmHg

        g. pH >7.25

   3. Ventilator criteria (during SBT)

        a. Rapid shallow breathing index (RSBI: RR/VT) <100

        b. Negative inspiratory force (NIF) >20 cmH$_2$O

        c. Tidal volumes >5 mL/kg

        d. Vital capacity >10 mL/kg

        e. RR <30

B. Devices that may aid in transition to decannulation of a tracheostomy tube:

   1. Fenestrated cuffed tracheostomy tube: With the balloon down, inner cannula removed, and speaking valve in place, the airway is not protected, but the patient can be tested for tolerance to decannulation.

   2. Small/Cuffless tracheostomy tube: A No. 4 Shiley CFS has insignificant airway resistance and performs as a guard against ventilatory failure and as a conduit for tracheal suctioning while the patient is evaluated for decannulation tolerance.

C. Speech and Swallow Evaluation: A modified barium swallow exam can elucidate potential causes of aspiration, and a speech therapist can provide recommendations for aspiration risk minimization following extubation.

Selected Readings

Adnet F, Baud F. Relation between Glasgow coma scale and aspiration pneumonia. *Lancet* 1996;348(9020):123–124.

Cote CJ, Lerman J, Anderson B, eds. *A practice of anesthesia for infants and children.* 5th ed. Philadelphia: Elsevier/Saunders, 2013:251.

Fine GF, Borland LM. The future of the cuffed endotracheal tube. *Paediatr Anaesth* 2004;14(1):38–42.

Frumin MJ, Epstein RM, Cohen G. Apneic oxygenation in man. *Anesthesiology* 1959;20:789–798.

Ghafoor AU, Martin TW, Gopalakrishnan S, et al. Caring for the patients with cervical spine injuries: what have we learned? *Clin Anesth* 2005;17(8):640–649.

Longnecker DE, Brown DL, Newman MF, et al. *Anesthesiology.* 2nd ed. New York: McGraw-Hill, 2012:709.

MacIntyre NR, et al. Evidence-based guidelines for weaning and discontinuing ventilatory support: a collective task force facilitated by the ACCP, AARC, and the ACCCM. *Chest* 2001;120(6 suppl):375S–395S.

Roberts JR, Spadafora M, Cone DC. Proper depth placement of oral endotracheal tubes in adults prior to radiographic confirmation. *Acad Emerg Med* 1995;2(1):20–24.

Sinz E, Navarro K, Soderberg ES, et al. *Advanced cardiovascular life support provider manual.* Dallas: American Heart Association, 2011.

Smith KJ, Dobranowski J, Yip G, et al. Cricoid pressure displaces the esophagus: an observational study using magnetic resonance imaging. *Anesthesiology* 2003;99(1):60–64.

Tournadre J, Chassard D, Berrada K, et al. Cricoid cartilage pressure decreases lower esophageal sphincter tone. *Anesthesiology* 1997;86(1):7–9.

Walkey AJ, Wiener RS. Use of noninvasive ventilation in patients with acute respiratory failure, 2000–2009: a population-based study. *Ann Am Thorac Soc* 2013;10(1):10–17.

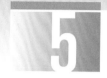

Mechanical Ventilation

Kathryn A. Hibbert and Dean R. Hess

I. **MECHANICAL VENTILATION** provides artificial support of gas exchange.
   A. **Indications**
      1. **Hypoventilation**
         a. **Evaluation: arterial pH** should be evaluated for evidence of hypoventilation. Chronic compensated hypercapnia is a stable condition that usually does not require mechanical ventilatory support and therefore arterial partial pressure of carbon dioxide ($PaCO_2$) is not useful in isolation.
         b. **Hypoventilation resulting in an arterial pH of less than 7.30** is often considered an indication for mechanical ventilation, but patient fatigue and associated morbidity must be considered and may prompt initiation of mechanical ventilation at a higher or lower pH.
         c. **Noninvasive ventilation (NIV)** may be considered for hypoventilation due to chronic obstructive lung disease (COPD).
      2. **Hypoxemia**
         a. **Supplemental oxygen** should be administered to all hypoxemic patients to attain arterial oxygen saturation by pulse oximetry (SpO_2) >90% regardless of diagnosis (e.g., appropriate oxygen therapy should not be withheld from hypercapneic patients with chronic obstructive pulmonary disease [COPD]).
         b. Patients with **hypoxemic respiratory failure** due to atelectasis and/or pulmonary edema may benefit from **continuous positive airway pressure (CPAP)** administered by face mask.
         c. **Endotracheal intubation and mechanical ventilation** should be considered for severe hypoxemia (SpO_2 <90% at a fraction of inspired oxygen [FIO_2] equal to 1.0) unresponsive to more conservative measures and can be considered earlier for lung protection if ARDS is suspected.
      3. **Respiratory fatigue**
         a. Tachypnea, dyspnea, use of accessory muscles, nasal flaring, diaphoresis, and tachycardia may be an indication for mechanical ventilation before abnormalities of gas exchange occur.
      4. **Airway protection**
         a. Mechanical ventilation may be initiated in patients who require endotracheal **intubation for airway protection**, even in the absence of respiratory abnormalities (e.g., increased aspiration risk due to decreased mental status or massive upper GI bleed).
         b. **The presence of an artificial airway** is not an absolute indication for mechanical ventilation (e.g., many long-term tracheostomy patients do not require mechanical ventilation).
   B. **Goals of Mechanical Ventilation**
      1. Provide adequate oxygenation and alveolar ventilation.
      2. Avoid alveolar overdistension.
      3. Maintain alveolar recruitment.
      4. Promote patient–ventilator synchrony.

5. Avoid auto-PEEP.
6. Use the lowest possible F_{IO_2}.

II. THE VENTILATOR SYSTEM

A. **The ventilator** is powered by gas pressure and electricity. Gas pressure provides the energy required to inflate the lungs (Fig. 5.1).
   1. Gas flow is controlled by **inspiratory and expiratory valves.** The electronics (microprocessor) of the ventilator controls these valves so that gas flow is determined by ventilator settings.
      a. **Inspiratory phase:** The inspiratory valve controls gas flow and/or pressure, and the expiratory valve is closed.
      b. **Expiratory phase:** The expiratory valve controls positive end-expiratory pressure (PEEP), and the inspiratory valve is closed.

B. **The Ventilator Circuit** delivers flow between the ventilator and the patient.
   1. Due to gas compression and the elasticity of the circuit, part of the gas volume delivered from the ventilator is not received by the patient. This **compression volume** is typically about 3 to 4 mL for every cmH_2O inspiratory pressure—some ventilators compensate for the compression volume while others do not.
   2. The volume of the circuit containing gas that the patient rebreathes during the respiratory cycle is **mechanical dead space.** Mechanical dead space should be as low as possible. This is particularly an issue when low tidal volumes are used.

C. **Gas Conditioning**
   1. **Filters** may be placed in the inspiratory and expiratory limbs of the circuit.
   2. **The inspired gas** is actively or passively humidified.
      a. **Active humidifiers** pass the inspired gas over a heated water chamber for humidification. Some also use a **heated circuit** to decrease condensate within the circuit.
      b. **Passive humidifiers** (artificial noses or heat and moisture exchangers) are inserted between the ventilator circuit and the patient. They trap heat and humidity in the exhaled gas and return that on the subsequent inspiration. Passive humidification is satisfactory for many patients, but it is less effective than active humidification, increases the resistance to inspiration and expiration, and increases mechanical dead space.

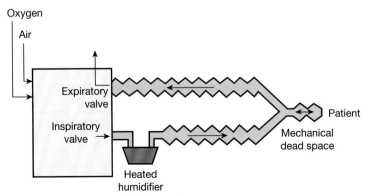

FIGURE 5.1 Simplified block diagram of a mechanical ventilator system.

    c. The presence of **water droplets** in the inspiratory circuit near the patient (or in the proximal endotracheal tube if a passive humidifier is used) suggests that the inspired gas is adequately humidified.

D. Delivery of Inhaled Medications and Gases during Mechanical Ventilation

    1. Inhaled medications can be delivered by **metered-dose inhaler** or **nebulizer** during mechanical ventilation. Dry-powder inhalers cannot be adapted to the ventilator circuit. Inhaled gases (e.g., inhaled NO) can be added directly to the inhaled gas mixture.

    2. A variety of factors influence aerosol delivery during mechanical ventilation (Fig. 5.2).

    3. With careful attention to technique, either inhalers or nebulizers can be used effectively during mechanical ventilation.

    4. The mesh nebulizer is commonly used because it overcomes issues with the use of jet nebulizers (mostly related to additional gas flow into the circuit) and is cost-effective compared with HFA metered-dose inhalers.

    5. Inhaled nitric oxide (NO) can be injected into the ventilator circuit. Mixtures of helium and oxygen (heliox) can also be delivered. However, gases with physical characteristics different from oxygen and air have the potential to interfere with ventilator function.

III. CLASSIFICATION OF MECHANICAL VENTILATION

A. Negative- versus Positive-Pressure Ventilation

    1. The **iron lung** and **chest cuirass** create negative pressure around the thorax during the inspiratory phase. Although useful for some patients with neuromuscular disease requiring long-term ventilation, these devices are almost never used in the intensive care unit (ICU).

    2. **Positive-pressure ventilation** applies pressure to the airway during the inspiratory phase.

    3. **Exhalation** occurs passively with both positive-pressure ventilation and negative-pressure ventilation.

Ventilator related
- Ventilation mode
- Tidal volume
- Respiratory rate
- Duty cycle
- Inspiratory waveform
- Breath-triggering mechanism

Device related - MDI
- Type of spacer or adapter
- Position of spacer in circuit
- Timing of MDI actuation
- Type of MDI

Drug related
- Dose
- Formulation
- Aerosol particle size
- Targeted site for delivery
- Duration of action

Device related-Nebulizer
- Type of nebulizer
- Fill volume
- Gas flow
- Cycling inspiration vs. continuous
- Duration of nebulization
- Position in the circuit

Patient related
- Severity of airway obstruction
- Mechanism of airway obstruction
- Presence of dynamic hyperinfiation
- Patient-ventilator synchrony

Circuit related
- Endotracheal tube size
- Humidity of inhaled gas
- Density of inhaled gas

FIGURE 5.2 Factors affecting aerosol delivery during mechanical ventilation. MDI, metered-dose inhaler. (Modified from Dhand R. Basic techniques for aerosol delivery during mechanical ventilation. *Respir Care* 2004;49:611–622, with permission.)

B. Invasive versus Noninvasive Ventilation

1. **Invasive ventilation** is delivered through an endotracheal tube (orotracheal or nasotracheal) or a tracheostomy tube.

2. Although mechanical ventilation through an artificial airway remains the standard in the most acutely ill patients, **NIV** is preferred in some patients such as those with an exacerbation of COPD, those with acute cardiogenic pulmonary edema, or immunocompromised patients with acute respiratory failure. NIV is also useful to prevent postextubation respiratory failure. There are many patients, however, in whom NIV is not appropriate.

   a. NIV can be applied with a nasal mask, oronasal mask, nasal pillows, total face mask, or helmet. Oronasal masks and total face masks are preferred in acutely ill dyspneic patients, in whom mouth leak is often problematic.

   b. Although bilevel ventilators are most commonly used for NIV, any ventilator can be used to provide this therapy. Current generation ventilators designed for critical care have both invasive and noninvasive modes, and some have good leak-compensation algorithms.

   c. **Pressure support** is most commonly used for NIV. For bilevel ventilators, this is achieved by setting inspiratory positive airway pressure **(IPAP)** and expiratory positive airway pressure **(EPAP)**. The difference between IPAP and EPAP is the level of pressure support.

   d. An algorithm for use of NIV (including evaluation of contraindications) in the critical care setting is provided in Figure 5.3.

C. Full versus Partial Ventilatory Support

1. **Full ventilatory support** provides the entire minute ventilation, with little interaction between the patient and the ventilator. This usually requires sedation and sometimes neuromuscular blockade. Full ventilatory support is indicated for patients with severe respiratory failure, patients who are hemodynamically unstable, patients with complex acute injuries while they are being stabilized, and all patients receiving paralysis.

2. **Partial ventilatory support** provides a variable portion of the minute ventilation, with the remainder provided by the patient's inspiratory effort. The patient–ventilator interaction is important during partial ventilatory support.

   a. Partial ventilatory support is indicated for patients with moderately acute respiratory failure or patients who are recovering from respiratory failure.

      1. **Advantages** of partial ventilatory support include avoidance of muscle weakness during long periods of mechanical ventilation, preservation of the ventilatory drive and breathing pattern, decreased requirement for sedation and neuromuscular blockade, a better hemodynamic response to positive-pressure ventilation, and better ventilation of dependent lung regions.

      2. **Disadvantages** of partial ventilatory support include a higher work of breathing for the patient and difficulty achieving lung protective ventilation if the patient has a strong respiratory drive.

IV. THE EQUATION OF MOTION

   A. Delivery of gas into the lungs is determined by the interaction between the ventilator, respiratory mechanics, and respiratory muscle activity, which is described by the **equation of motion** of the respiratory system:

$$\text{Pvent} + \text{Pmus} = V_T/C + \dot{V} \times R$$

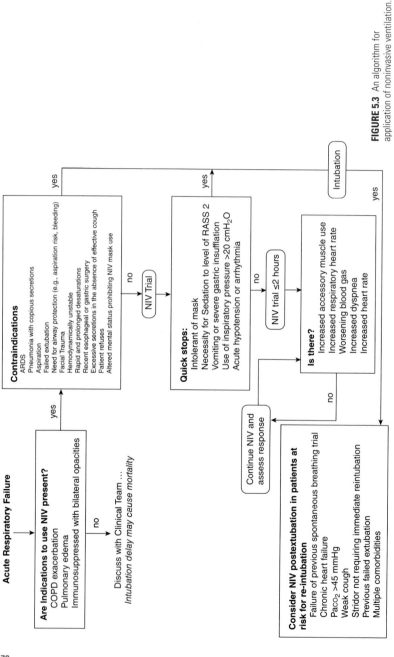

FIGURE 5.3 An algorithm for application of noninvasive ventilation.

Acute Respiratory Failure

Are Indications to use NIV present?
COPD exacerbation
Pulmonary edema
Immunosuppressed with bilateral opacities

no → Discuss with Clinical Team ...
Intubation delay may cause mortality

yes →

Contraindications
ARDS
Pneumonia with copious secretions
Aspiration
Failed extubation
Need for airway protection (e.g., aspiration risk, bleeding)
Facial Trauma
Hemodynamically unstable
Rapid and prolonged desaturations
Recent esophageal or gastric surgery
Excessive secretions in the absence of effective cough
Patient refuses
Altered mental status prohibiting NIV mask use

yes → Intubation

no → NIV Trial

Quick stops:
Intolerant of mask
Necessity for Sedation to level of RASS 2
Vomiting or severe gastric insufflation
Use of inspiratory pressure >20 cmH$_2$O
Acute hypotension or arrhythmia

yes → Intubation

no → NIV trial ≤2 hours →

Is there?
Increased accessory muscle use
Increased respiratory heart rate
Worsening blood gas
Increased dyspnea
Increased heart rate

yes → Intubation

no → Continue NIV and assess response

Consider NIV postextubation in patients at risk for re-intubation
Failure of previous spontaneous breathing trial
Chronic heart failure
Paco$_2$ >45 mmHg
Weak cough
Stridor not requiring immediate reintubation
Previous failed extubation
Multiple comorbidities

where Pvent is the pressure applied by the ventilator, Pmus is the pressure generated by the respiratory muscles, VT is tidal volume, C is compliance, $\dot{V}$ is gas flow, and R is airway resistance.

1. Pressure generated from either the respiratory muscles (spontaneous breathing), the ventilator (full ventilatory support), or both (partial ventilatory support) applied to the respiratory system results in gas flow into the lungs.

2. For a given pressure, gas flow is opposed by airways resistance and the elastance (inverse of compliance) of the lungs and chest wall.

3. Larger tidal volumes, lower compliance, higher flow, and higher resistance all require a higher pressure.

V. PHASE AND CONTROL VARIABLES

A. The **trigger variable** starts the inspiratory phase.

   1. The trigger variable determines when the ventilator initiates a breath.

   2. The ventilator detects patient inspiratory effort by either a pressure change **(pressure trigger)** or a flow change **(flow trigger).**

   3. The **trigger sensitivity** is set to both prevent excessive patient effort and avoid autotriggering. Pressure trigger sensitivity is commonly set at 0.5 to 2 cmH$_2$O, and flow trigger sensitivity is set at 2 to 3 L/min.

      a. Autotrigger can be caused by artifacts such as cardiac oscillations and leaks. This is corrected by making the trigger less sensitive.

      b. Ineffective trigger can be due to neuromuscular disease or auto-PEEP. Switching the trigger variable is rarely effective to deal with failed triggers.

   4. Pressure triggering and flow triggering are equally effective if sensitivity is optimized and closely monitored.

B. The **control variable** remains constant throughout inspiration. Most common of these are volume control, pressure control, and adaptive control (Table 5.1).

   1. **Volume control.** Despite the name, the ventilator actually controls flow (the time derivative of volume) to maintain a **constant delivered tidal volume** regardless of airways resistance or respiratory system compliance.

      a. A decrease in respiratory system compliance or an increase in airways resistance results in an increased peak inspiratory pressure during volume control. Decreased compliance also results in an increased plateau pressure (the pressure during an inspiratory pause when flow is zero).

      b. With volume control, the **inspiratory flow is fixed** regardless of patient effort. This unvarying flow may induce patient–ventilator dyssynchrony.

         1. Inspiratory flow patterns during volume control include **constant flow** (rectangular wave) (Fig. 5.4) or **descending-ramp flow** (Fig. 5.5).

         2. Use of the constant-flow waveform results in a higher peak pressure, which is largely borne by the airways and not the alveoli.

         3. Use of a descending-ramp waveform results in maximal flow early in the breath when lung volume is minimal. This reduces peak pressures but decreases expiratory time, which may increase the risk of auto-PEEP and dynamic hyperinflation.

      c. The **inspiratory time** during volume control is determined by inspiratory flow, the inspiratory flow pattern, and tidal volume.

      d. Volume control is preferred when an assured minute ventilation or tidal volume is desirable (e.g., avoiding hypercarbia in patients with intracranial hypertension or preventing overdistention in acute respiratory distress syndrome [ARDS]).

TABLE 5.1 Comparison of Several Breath Types during Mechanical Ventilation

	Pressure Control Ventilation	Volume Control Ventilation	Adaptive Control Ventilation	Pressure Support Ventilation	Proportional Assist Ventilation
Tidal volume	Variable	Set	Minimum set	Variable	Variable
Peak inspiratory pressure	Limited by pressure control setting	Variable	Variable	Limited by pressure support setting	Variable
Plateau pressure	Limited by pressure control setting	Variable	Variable	Limited by pressure support setting	Variable
Inspiratory flow	Descending; variable	Set; constant or descending ramp	Descending; variable	Variable	Variable
Inspiratory time	Set	Set (flow and volume settings)	Set for adaptive pressure control; variable for adaptive pressure support	Variable	Variable
Respiratory rate	Minimum set (patient can trigger)	Minimum set (patient can trigger)	Minimum set for adaptive pressure control; not set for adaptive pressure support	Variable; rate not set	Variable; rate not set

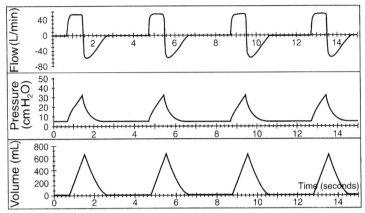

FIGURE 5.4 Constant-flow volume ventilation.

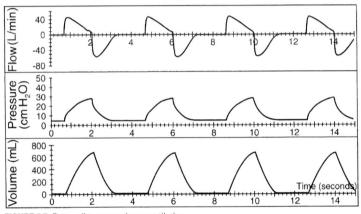

FIGURE 5.5 Descending-ramp volume ventilation.

2. **Pressure control**
   a. With pressure control (Fig. 5.6), **the pressure applied to the airway is constant** regardless of the airways resistance or respiratory system compliance.
   b. **The inspiratory flow** during pressure control is exponentially descending and determined by the pressure-control setting, airways resistance, and respiratory system compliance. With low respiratory system compliance (e.g., ARDS), flow decreases rapidly. With high airways resistance (e.g., COPD), flow decreases slowly.
   c. Some ventilators allow the adjustment of the **rise time,** which is the pressurization rate of the ventilator at the beginning of the inspiratory phase (Fig. 5.7). The rise time is the amount of time required

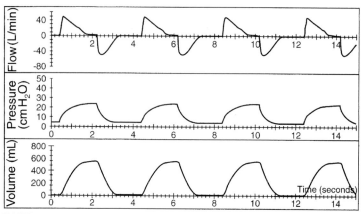

FIGURE 5.6 Pressure-controlled ventilation.

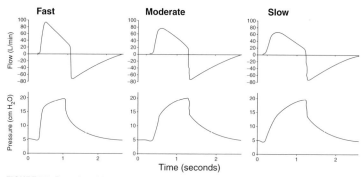

FIGURE 5.7 Examples of fast, moderate, and slow rise times during pressure ventilation.

for the pressure-control level to be reached after the ventilator is triggered.

A rapid rise time delivers more flow at the initiation of inhalation, which may be useful for patients with a high respiratory drive.

d. **Factors that affect tidal volume** during pressure control are respiratory system compliance, airways resistance, pressure setting, rise time setting, and the inspiratory effort of the patient. Increasing the inspiratory time will affect tidal volume during pressure-controlled ventilation only if the end-inspiratory flow is not zero. Once the flow decreases to zero, no additional volume is delivered.

e. Unlike volume control, **inspiratory flow is affected by patient effort**—increased patient effort will increase the flow from the ventilator and therefore delivered tidal volume. This may improve patient–ventilator synchrony, but results in unpredictable tidal volumes and the potential for overdistention.

    f. With pressure control, **the inspiratory time is set** on the ventilator.

        1. If the inspiratory time is set to be longer than the expiratory time, pressure-controlled inverse ratio ventilation (PCIRV) results. This strategy has been used to improve oxygenation in patients with ARDS, but has generally fallen out of favor in recent years because it has not been shown to improve patient outcomes and can adversely affect hemodynamics.

        2. Pressure control can be desirable for improving patient–ventilator synchrony, but this is controversial. It is also used as an alternative to pressure support when a fixed inspiratory time or rate is desired.

3. Adaptive control

    a. With adaptive control, the breath is ventilator- or patient-triggered, pressure-limited, and ventilator- or patient-cycled. With adaptive pressure control, the pressure limit is not constant, but varies breath to breath on the basis of a comparison of the set and delivered tidal volume.

    b. Although the ventilator is capable of controlling only pressure or volume at any time, adaptive control combines features of pressure control (variable flow) and volume control (constant tidal volume) (Table 5.1).

    c. **Pressure-regulated volume control (PRVC on Servo, Viasys), AutoFlow (Draeger), and VC+ (Puritan-Bennett)** are trade names that function in a similar manner. With this form of adaptive pressure control, the pressure control level increases or decreases in an attempt to deliver the desired tidal volume.

    d. With **Volume support (VS)**, the pressure support level varies on a breath-to-breath basis to maintain a desired tidal volume. If the patient's effort increases (increased tidal volume for the set level of PSV), the ventilator decreases the support of the next breath. If the compliance or patient effort decreases, the ventilator increases the support to maintain the set volume. This combines the attributes of PSV with the guaranteed minimum tidal volume.

    e. The clinical utility of adaptive control is yet to be determined and has potential drawbacks:

        1. Tidal volumes may exceed the desired tidal volume if the patient makes vigorous inspiratory efforts, which could result in overdistention lung injury.

        2. If the tidal volume exceeds the target volume, the ventilator will decrease the level of pressure support. This may increase the patient's work of breathing in the setting of increased respiratory demand.

        3. If the lungs become stiffer (i.e., compliance decreases) and the tidal volume does not meet the target, the ventilator will increase the pressure, which could result in overdistention lung injury.

4. The choice of volume control, pressure control, or adaptive control usually is the result of clinician familiarity, institutional preferences, and personal bias.

C. **Cycle** is the variable that terminates inspiration, which is commonly time (volume control or pressure control) or flow (pressure support ventilation).

VI. BREATH TYPES DURING MECHANICAL VENTILATION

  A. **Spontaneous Breaths** are triggered and cycled by the patient.

  B. **Mandatory Breaths** are either triggered by the ventilator or the patient and cycled by the ventilator.

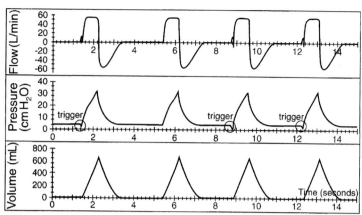

FIGURE 5.8 Continuous mandatory ventilation (assist-control ventilation).

VII. **MODES OF VENTILATION.** The combination of the various possible breath types and phase variables determines the mode of ventilation (Table 5.1). There are many modes of ventilation, and their nomenclature can be confusing as manufacturers will often use different names for similar ventilation modes. Only a few of the more commonly used modes are discussed in the following section.

   A. **Continuous Mandatory Ventilation (CMV) or Assist-Control (A/C) Ventilation**
      1. Every breath is a mandatory breath type (Fig. 5.8). Although CMV is more descriptive, the terms CMV and A/C are used interchangeably.
      2. **The patient can trigger** additional breaths but always receives at least the set respiratory rate.
      3. All breaths, whether ventilator triggered or patient triggered, are either volume control, pressure control, or adaptive control (i.e., all breaths are the same).
      4. Triggering at a rapid rate may result in hyperventilation, hypotension, and dynamic hyperinflation (auto-PEEP).

   B. **Continuous Spontaneous Ventilation.** With continuous spontaneous ventilation modes, all breaths are triggered and cycled by the patient. There is no set rate, inspiratory time, or expiratory time.
      1. **Continuous positive airway pressure (CPAP).** During CPAP, the ventilator provides no inspiratory assist.
         a. Strictly speaking, CPAP applies a positive pressure to the airway. However, current ventilators allow the patient to breath spontaneously without applying positive pressure to the airway (CPAP = 0).
         b. CPAP can be applied to an endotracheal tube (invasive) or to a face mask (noninvasive).
      2. **Pressure support (PS)**
         a. **The patient's inspiratory effort is assisted** by the ventilator at a preset pressure with PS. All breaths are spontaneous breath types (Fig. 5.9).
         b. A pressure **rise time** can be set during pressure support, similar to pressure control ventilation.
         c. Because the ventilator delivers only patient-triggered breaths, appropriate apnea alarms must be set on the ventilator. The lack of a backup rate may result in apnea and sleep-disordered breathing in some patients.

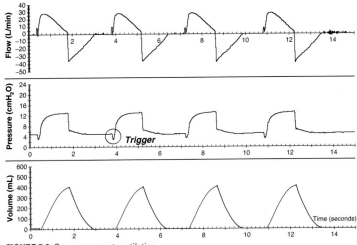

FIGURE 5.9 Pressure support ventilation.

    d. The ventilator cycles to the expiratory phase when the flow decreases to a predetermined value (e.g., 5 L/min or 25% of the peak inspiratory flow). **If the patient actively exhales,** the ventilator may pressure cycle to the expiratory phase. The ventilator may not cycle correctly **in the presence of a leak** (e.g., bronchopleural fistula or mask leak with NIV). A secondary time cycle will terminate inspiration at 3 to 5 seconds (depending on the ventilator, sometimes adjustable).

    e. Some ventilators allow the clinician to **adjust the flow cycle** criteria during PS (Fig. 5.10). This allows adjustment of the inspiratory time to better coincide with the patient's neural inspiration (thus avoiding active exhalation or double triggering). If the ventilator is set to cycle at a greater percentage of peak flow, the inspiratory time is decreased. Conversely, if the ventilator is set to cycle at a lower percentage of the peak flow, the inspiratory time is increased. As a general rule, a higher flow cycle is necessary for obstructive lung disease and a lower flow cycle is necessary for restrictive lung disease (e.g., patients recovering from acute lung injury).

    f. The tidal volume, inspiratory flow, inspiratory time, and respiratory rate may vary from breath to breath with PS.

    g. **Tidal volume** is determined by the level of pressure support, rise time, lung mechanics, and the inspiratory effort of the patient.

    h. With a strong respiratory drive, the resultant tidal volume and transpulmonary pressure may not be lung protective.

3. Proportional assist ventilation (PAV)

    a. PAV provides ventilatory support as a proportion of the patient's calculated work of breathing.

    b. The ventilator monitors the inspiratory flow of the patient, integrates flow to volume, measures elastance and resistance, and then calculates the pressure required from the equation of motion.

    c. This mode is only available on the Puritan-Bennett 840 and 980 ventilators for invasive ventilation, and the Philips Respironics V60 for NIV.

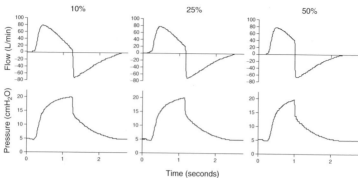

Time (seconds)

FIGURE 5.10 Examples of pressure support ventilation with termination flows of 10%, 25%, and 50% of peak flow.

    d. Using the pressure calculated from the equation of motion and the tidal volume, the Puritan Bennett 849 and 980 ventilators calculate work of breathing (WoB): WoB = $\int P \times V$. These calculations occur every 5 minutes during breath delivery.
        1. The ventilator estimates resistance and elastance (compliance) by applying end-inspiratory and end-expiratory pause maneuvers of 300 minutes. These maneuvers are randomly applied every 4 to 10 seconds.
        2. The clinician adjusts the percentage of support (from 5% to 95%), which allows the work to be partitioned between the ventilator and the patient.
        3. Typically, the percentage of support is set so that the WoB is in the range of 0.5 to 1.0 joules/L.
    e. If the percentage of support is high, patient WoB may be inappropriately low and excessive volume and pressure may be applied (runaway).
    f. If the percentage of support is too low, patient WoB may be excessive.
    g. PAV applies a pressure that varies from breath to breath due to changes in patient's elastance, resistance, and flow demand. This differs from PS, in which the level of support is constant regardless of demand, and VC, in which the level of support decreases when demand increases.
    h. The cycle criteria for PAV is flow, similar to pressure support.
    i. PAV requires the presence of an intact ventilatory drive and a functional neuromuscular system.
C. Synchronized Intermittent Mandatory Ventilation (SIMV)
    1. With SIMV (Fig. 5.11), the ventilator is set to deliver both mandatory and spontaneous breath types.
    2. The mandatory breaths can be either volume-control, pressure-control, or adaptive-control breaths.
    3. There is a set respiratory rate for the mandatory breaths, and the mandatory breaths are synchronized with patient effort.
    4. Between the mandatory breaths, the patient may breathe spontaneously and the spontaneous breaths may be pressure supported (Fig. 5.12).

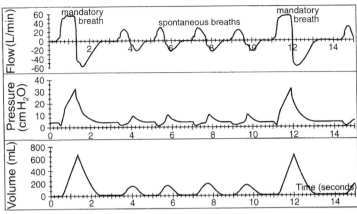

FIGURE 5.11 Synchronized intermittent mandatory ventilation.

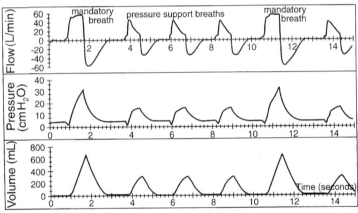

FIGURE 5.12 Synchronized intermittent mandatory ventilation with pressure support.

5. The patient's inspiratory efforts may be as great during the mandatory breaths as the spontaneous breaths. It is therefore a myth that SIMV rests the patient during the mandatory breaths and allows patient work only during spontaneous breaths.

6. The different breath types during SIMV may induce patient–ventilator asynchrony.

7. Note that CMV and SIMV become synonymous if the patient is not triggering the ventilator (e.g., with neuromuscular blockade).

D. **Airway Pressure Release Ventilation (APRV)** allows spontaneous breathing at alternating high and low CPAP levels (Fig. 5.13). On some ventilators, APRV is achieved using modes called BiLevel (Puritan-Bennett) or BiVent (Maquet).

1. High and low airway pressures are set and tidal breathing occurs at both levels, though the time at the high-pressure level is greater than

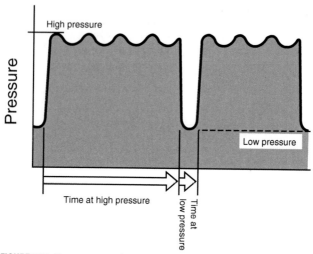

FIGURE 5.13 Airway pressure release ventilation (APRV).

the time at the low-pressure level, which is reached during a transient release.

2. Minute ventilation is determined by lung compliance, airways resistance, the magnitude of the pressure release, the duration of the pressure release, and the magnitude of the patient's spontaneous breathing efforts.

3. Oxygenation is largely determined by the high-pressure setting. Spontaneous breathing by the patient may also provide recruitment of dependent lung regions.

4. Because the patient is allowed to breathe spontaneously at both levels of pressure (due to an active exhalation valve), the need for sedation may be decreased.

5. A proposed advantage of APRV is to provide lung recruitment at lower overall airway pressures than with traditional positive pressure ventilation by taking advantage of the spontaneous breathing efforts. This may increase PaO_2 while minimizing barotrauma, hemodynamic instability, and the need for sedation. However, it may be an uncomfortable breathing pattern for some patients and can lead to tidal recruitment–derecruitment (atelectrauma).

6. Of concern is the potential for overdistention during tidal breathing at the high-pressure level.

7. Depending on the ventilator brand, APRV may be applied using BiLevel, BIPAP, BiVent, BiPhasic, PCV+, or DuoPAP.

8. Evidence is lacking for improved outcomes with the use of APRV.

E. The choice of the mode of ventilation depends on the capability of the ventilator, the experience and preference of the clinician, and, most important, the needs of the patient. Rather than relying on a single best mode of ventilation, one should determine the mode that is most appropriate for each individual situation. However, the more complex and adaptive modes of ventilation have not consistently shown to improve outcomes.

VIII. HIGH-FREQUENCY VENTILATION (HFV)

A. With HFV, the patient is ventilated with higher-than-normal rates (i.e., >60/min) and smaller tidal volumes (<5 mL/kg).

B. Theoretical advantages include a lower risk of alveolar overdistension due to smaller tidal volumes (thereby limiting peak alveolar pressure), better alveolar recruitment, and improved gas exchange.

C. High-Frequency Oscillatory Ventilation (HFOV) delivers small tidal volumes by oscillating a bias gas flow in the airway. The oscillator has an active inspiratory and expiratory phase.

1. The determinants of CO_2 elimination are the pressure amplitude (ΔP) and frequency. HFOV tidal volume and CO_2 elimination varies directly with ΔP. In contrast to conventional ventilation, CO_2 elimination varies inversely with frequency.

   a. ΔP is initially set at about 20 cmH_2O above the $Paco_2$ or to induce wiggling that is visible to the patient's mid-thigh.

   b. The rate is adjustable from 3 to 15 Hz (180–900/min). Higher rates (12–15 Hz) are used in neonates and lower rates (3–6 Hz) are used in adults.

2. The primary determinant of oxygenation during HFOV is mean airway pressure, which is essentially the level of PEEP. The ventilator oscillates the gas to pressures above and below (ΔP) the mean airway pressure.

3. Initial evidence suggested that arterial oxygenation was improved in some patients with ARDS, but subsequent studies in adults showed either no benefit or increased mortality, and HFOV has therefore largely fallen out of favor.

D. High-Frequency Jet Ventilation delivers gas from a high-pressure source through a jet directed into the airway. Viscous shearing drags gas into the airway.

1. Tidal volume is determined by the driving pressure, inspiratory time, catheter size, and respiratory system mechanics.

2. Mean airway pressure is controlled by driving pressure, I:E ratio, and PEEP.

3. High-frequency jet ventilation uses rates of 240 to 660 breaths/min.

4. In the United States, jet ventilators are occasionally used in operating rooms but are not available for use in ICUs.

E. High-Frequency Percussive Ventilation, also called volumetric diffusive respiration, uses a sliding nongated venturi to separate inspired and expired gases and provide PEEP. It is commercially available only on the Percussionaire VDR ventilator.

1. Minute ventilation is controlled by respiratory rate and peak inspiratory pressure.

2. Respiratory rates of 180 to 600 breaths/min are used.

3. Oxygenation is determined by peak inspiratory pressure, I:E ratio, and PEEP.

4. High-frequency percussive ventilation has popularity in the care of patients with burn injury despite lack of high-level evidence reporting better outcomes.

IX. SPECIFIC VENTILATOR SETTINGS

A. A Tidal Volume target of 4 to 8 mL/kg predicted body weight is used. Ideal body weight is determined by the height and the sex of the patient.

$$\text{Male patients: PBW} = 50 + 2.3 \times [\text{height (inches)} - 60]$$

$$\text{Female patients: PBW} = 45.5 + 2.3 \times [\text{height (inches)} - 60]$$

1. Lower tidal volumes decrease the risk and extent of alveolar overdistention and **ventilator-induced lung injury (VILI)**.
2. Use a tidal volume of 6 mL/kg (4–8 mL/kg) for patients with **ARDS**.
3. Accumulating evidence supports the use of tidal volumes of <8 mL/kg for all mechanically ventilated patients.
4. Monitor the **plateau pressure (Pplat)** and consider tidal volume reduction if the Pplat is greater than 30 cmH$_2$O.
   a. Because lung injury is a function of transalveolar pressure, a higher plateau pressure may be acceptable if pleural pressure is increased (e.g., obesity or abdominal hypertension).
   b. Lower Pplat is desirable and may be associated with improved outcomes.
   c. With a strong inspiratory effort, transalveolar pressure may be injurious despite that airway pressure is acceptable (e.g., during PC or PS).
5. Tidal volume may also be adjusted to minimize **driving pressure** (Pplat – PEEP). A recent individual subject meta-analysis suggests that tidal volume and PEEP should be selected such that the driving pressure is <15 cmH$_2$O; higher driving pressure increases the mortality risk.

B. Respiratory Rate

1. The respiratory rate and tidal volume determine **minute ventilation.**
2. Set the rate at 15 to 25/min to achieve a minute ventilation of 8 to 12 L/min.
   a. With low tidal volumes and a low pH, a higher respiratory rate may be necessary.
   b. A lower respiratory rate (and longer expiratory phase) may be necessary to avoid air trapping and dynamic hyperinflation.
   c. In the recovery phase, spontaneous modes (e.g., PS, PAV) can be used to allow the patient to choose his or her own respiratory rate.
3. Adjust the rate to achieve the desired pH and Paco$_2$.
4. **A high-minute-ventilation** (>10 L/min) requirement may be required for increased carbon dioxide production or high dead space.

C. Inspiratory:Expiratory (I:E) Ratio

1. **Inspiratory time** can be determined by flow, tidal volume, and flow pattern; it is not directly set with all modes of ventilation.
2. **Expiratory time** is determined by the inspiratory time and respiratory rate and is not directly set in any mode of ventilation.
3. The expiratory time generally should be longer than the inspiratory time (e.g., I:E of 1:2).
4. **The expiratory time should be lengthened** (e.g., higher inspiratory flow, lower tidal volume, lower respiratory rate) positive-pressure ventilation causes a blood pressure drop or if auto-PEEP is present. If air trapping is significant and accompanied by an acute drop in blood pressure, the patient may be temporarily disconnected from the ventilator (about 30 seconds) to allow exhalation and then reconnected.
5. **Inspiratory time can be lengthened** to increase mean airway pressure and may thus improve oxygenation in some patients by limiting derecruitment.
   a. With other options to increase mean airway pressure (e.g., increased PEEP), there is little role for an inverse I:E (i.e., inspiratory time longer than expiratory time).
   b. When long inspiratory times are used, hemodynamics and auto-PEEP must be closely monitored.

D. Oxygen Concentration (FIO_2)

1. Initiate mechanical ventilation with an FIO_2 of 1.0.
2. Titrate the FIO_2 using pulse oximetry. A target SpO_2 of 88% to 95% is usually acceptable.
3. Severe, persistent hypoxemia (requiring FIO_2 >0.60) usually indicates the presence of shunt (intrapulmonary or intracardiac).

E. Positive End-Expiratory Pressure

1. **Appropriate levels of PEEP** increase the functional respiratory capacity, decrease intrapulmonary shunt, and improve lung compliance (by preventing derecruitment).
   a. Because lung volumes are typically decreased with acute respiratory failure, it is reasonable to use a PEEP of at least 5 cmH_2O with the initiation of mechanical ventilation for most patients.
   b. **Maintaining alveolar recruitment** in disease processes like ARDS may decrease the likelihood of ventilator-associated lung injury.
   c. Although higher levels of PEEP often increase PaO_2, evidence has not shown that higher levels of PEEP (compared with modest levels of PEEP) decrease mortality.
2. A number of methods have been used to titrate the best level of PEEP in patients with acute lung injury.
   a. PEEP can be titrated with a goal to allow a decrease in FIO_2 to 0.6 or less.
   b. PEEP can be set according to a table of FIO_2/PEEP combinations to achieve an SpO_2 of 88% to 95%, as was done in the ARDSnet trials.
   c. PEEP can be set 2 to 3 cmH_2O above the lower inflexion point of the pressure–volume curve to prevent end-tidal derecruitment. However, this is difficult to measure reliably in critically ill patients.
   d. PEEP can be set to achieve the best respiratory system compliance. The best compliance can be determined from either an incremental or a decremental PEEP trial. A decremental PEEP trial may theoretically achieve a greater lung volume for a given level of PEEP but may result in progressive derecruitment over time if adequate time for equilibration is not spent at each PEEP level.
   e. PEEP can be adjusted to the best stress index, as assessed from the slope of the pressure–time curve during constant flow volume ventilation. This may require special software and can be difficult to estimate at the bedside.
   f. PEEP can be titrated with an esophageal balloon in place to measure esophageal pressure (Pes) as a proxy for pleural pressure. The goal with this method is to set PEEP $\geq$ Pes to prevent end tidal derecruitment.
   g. There is little evidence that any approach to setting PEEP is superior to another in terms of patient outcomes.
   h. Modest levels of PEEP (8–12 cmH_2O) should be used for mild ARDS and higher levels of PEEP (12–20 cmH_2O) should be used for moderate and severe ARDS.
3. In patients with COPD, PEEP may be used to counterbalance auto-PEEP, thereby decreasing work of breathing and improving the patient's ability to trigger the ventilator.
4. In patients with left ventricular failure, PEEP may improve cardiac performance by decreasing venous return and left ventricular afterload.
5. **Adverse effects of PEEP**
   a. PEEP may **decrease cardiac output** by decreasing venous return. Hemodynamics should be monitored during PEEP titration.

   b. High levels of PEEP may result in **alveolar overdistention** during the inspiratory phase. It may be necessary to decrease the tidal volume with high PEEP.
   c. PEEP may **worsen oxygenation with focal lung disease** because it results in a redistribution of pulmonary blood flow from overdistended lung units to the unventilated lung units. PEEP may also worsen oxygenation with cardiac shunt (e.g., patent foramen ovale).

X. COMPLICATIONS OF MECHANICAL VENTILATION
A. Ventilator-Induced Lung Injury
   1. Overdistension injury (volutrauma) occurs if the lung parenchyma is subjected to an abnormally high transpulmonary pressure.
   a. Overdistension injury produces inflammation and increased alveolar–capillary membrane permeability.
   b. Tidal volume should be limited (e.g., 6 mL/kg in patients with ALI/ARDS) and Pplat limited to 30 cmH$_2$O (or lower) to prevent overdistension injury.
   c. Because the risk of overdistension lung injury is related to transpulmonary pressure, higher plateau pressures may be acceptable if pleural pressure is increased (e.g., abdominal distention, chest wall burns, chest wall edema, obesity).
   2. Pressure-related injury (barotrauma) occurs when the airways and alveoli are subjected to high transmural pressures, resulting in extravasation of gas through the bronchovascular sheath into the pulmonary interstitium, mediastinum, pericardium, peritoneum, pleural space, and subcutaneous tissue.
   a. Manifestations of barotrauma include **tension pneumothorax**, which should be suspected if there is a sudden increase in peak inspiratory pressure or sudden hemodynamic instability in a mechanically ventilated patient.
   b. Barotrauma can occur with spontaneous breathing (e.g., spontaneous pneumothorax in status asthmaticus) but is classically associated with high airway pressures in a mechanically ventilated patient.
   c. High transpulmonary pressures may promote alveolar injury **in the absence of high airway pressures** (e.g., strong inspiratory effort on PC or PS).
   3. Derecruitment injury (Atelectrauma) occurs if there is cyclic alveolar opening and closing with tidal breathing.
   a. This injury may be avoided by use of appropriate levels of PEEP to maintain alveolar recruitment. In ARDS, this may require 8 to 20 cmH$_2$O, and sometimes more depending on pleural pressure.
4. Oxygen toxicity
   a. High concentrations of oxygen for long periods may cause lung damage, worsen $\dot{V}/\dot{Q}$ matching, and promote atelectasis.
   b. Although the precise role of oxygen toxicity in patients with respiratory failure is unclear, it is prudent to reduce the F$_{IO_2}$ to the minimum necessary to maintain adequate arterial oxygenation (usually SpO$_2$ 88%–95%), although some patients tolerate lower SpO$_2$.
   c. Appropriate levels of inspired oxygen should never be withheld for fear of oxygen toxicity.

B. Patient–Ventilator Asynchrony

1. **Trigger asynchrony** refers to the inability of the patient to trigger the ventilator.

   a. Trigger asynchrony may be due to an **insensitive trigger setting** on the ventilator, which is corrected by adjusting the trigger sensitivity.

   b. Flow trigger instead of pressure trigger can be tried, though this rarely solves the problem.

   c. A common cause of trigger asynchrony is the presence **of auto-PEEP**. If auto-PEEP is present, the patient must generate enough inspiratory effort to overcome the auto-PEEP before triggering can occur. This can be addressed by reducing auto-PEEP (e.g., administer bronchodilators, increase expiratory time). Setting the extrinsic PEEP to equal auto-PEEP can improve trigger synchrony.

   d. Autotrigger is another form of asynchrony. In this case, the ventilator is triggered by an artifact other than the patient's inspiratory effort. Examples include oscillations in the flow or pressure at the proximal airway due to the heart beating against the lungs or a leak causing the airway flow or pressure to change.

2. **Flow asynchrony**

   a. During volume control, flow is fixed and may not meet the patient's inspiratory flow demands. The inspiratory pressure waveform will demonstrate a characteristic scalloped pattern if patient makes additional inspiratory effort.

   b. Flow asynchrony may be improved during volume control ventilation by increasing the inspiratory flow or changing the inspiratory flow pattern.

   c. Changing volume control to pressure control or pressure support, in which flows are variable, may also be helpful. However, this runs the risk of overdistention due to high tidal volumes if the patient generates a strong inspiratory effort.

3. **Cycle asynchrony** occurs when the patient's expiratory effort begins before or after the end of the inspiratory phase set on the ventilator. Cycle asynchrony can occur if the inspiratory time is inappropriately short or long. This is corrected by adjusting the inspiratory time.

   a. If the inspiratory flow is too high or the inspiratory time setting is too short, the patient may double trigger the ventilator.

      1. This can be addressed during VC by reducing the flow setting or adding an inspiratory pause.

      2. During PC, this can be addressed by setting a longer inspiratory time.

   b. If the inspiratory flow is too low or the inspiratory time setting is too long, the patient may actively exhale.

      1. This can be addressed during VC by using a higher inspiratory flow.

      2. On PC, this is addressed by setting a shorter inspiratory time.

   c. When PSV is used in patients with high airways resistance and high lung compliance (e.g., COPD), it may take a long time for inspiratory flow to decrease to the flow cycle criteria set in the ventilator. The patient may therefore actively exhale to terminate the inspiratory phase.

      1. This can be corrected by using pressure-control rather than pressure-support setting. The inspiratory time is then set so that inspiratory flow does not reach zero.

      2. Most ventilators allow the clinician to adjust the termination flow during pressure support to improve synchrony.

   3. This problem may improve with the use of a lower pressure-support setting.
   4. Reducing airways resistance (e.g., with bronchodilators, secretion clearance) can resolve this problem.
 4. Asynchrony can be the result of acidosis, pain, and anxiety. These non-ventilator factors should also be considered when asynchrony is present. Sedation and paralysis may be required in some patients.
C. Auto-PEEP
  1. **Auto-PEEP** is the result of gas trapping (dynamic hyperinflation) due to insufficient expiratory time and/or increased expiratory airflow resistance. The pressure exerted by this trapped gas is called auto-PEEP or intrinsic PEEP.
  2. The increase in alveolar pressure due to auto-PEEP may adversely affect hemodynamics by reducing venous return.
  3. The presence of auto-PEEP can produce trigger dyssynchrony as discussed above.
  4. **Detection of auto-PEEP**
     a. Some ventilators allow auto-PEEP to be measured directly.
     b. In spontaneously breathing patients, auto-PEEP can be measured using an **esophageal balloon.**
     c. The **patient's breathing pattern** can be observed. If exhalation is still occurring when the next breath is delivered, auto-PEEP is present.
     d. If flow graphics is available on the ventilator, it can be observed that **expiratory flow** does not return to zero before the subsequent breath is delivered.
     e. Inspiratory efforts **that do not trigger the ventilator** suggest the presence of auto-PEEP.
  5. **Factors affecting auto-PEEP**
     a. **Physiologic factors.** A high airways resistance increases the likelihood of auto-PEEP.
     b. **Ventilator factors.** A high tidal volume, high respiratory rate, or prolonged inspiratory time increases the likelihood of auto-PEEP. Reducing minute ventilation and increasing expiratory time decreases the likelihood of auto-PEEP.
D. Hemodynamic Perturbations
  1. Positive-pressure ventilation increases intrathoracic pressure and **decreases venous return.** Right ventricular filling is limited by the reduced venous return, and cardiac output therefore decreases.
  2. When alveolar pressure exceeds pulmonary venous pressure, pulmonary blood flow is affected by alveolar pressure rather than left atrial pressure, producing an **increase in pulmonary vascular resistance.** Consequently, right ventricular afterload increases and right ventricular ejection fraction falls.
  3. **Left ventricular filling is limited** by reduced right ventricular output and decreased left ventricular diastolic compliance.
  4. Increased right ventricular size affects left ventricular performance by shifting the interventricular septum to the left.
  5. **Intravascular volume resuscitation** counteracts the negative hemodynamic effects of PEEP.
  6. Increased intrathoracic pressure may **improve left ventricular ejection fraction and stroke volume, reducing afterload.** This beneficial effect may be significant in patients with poor ventricular function.
E. Infection-Related Ventilator-Associated Complications: Please see Chapter 27.

Selected Readings

Amato MBP, Meade MO, Slutsky AS, et al. Driving pressure and survival in the acute respiratory distress syndrome. *N Engl J Med* 2015;372:747–755.

Branson RD, Johannigman JA. What is the evidence base for the newer ventilation modes? *Respir Care* 2004;49:742–760.

Brower RG, Lanken PN, MacIntyre N, et al. Higher versus lower positive end-expiratory pressures in patients with the acute respiratory distress syndrome. *N Engl J Med* 2004;351:327–336.

Chatburn RL. Classification of ventilator modes: update and proposal for implementation. *Respir Care* 2007;52:301–323.

Dhand R. Inhalation therapy in invasive and noninvasive mechanical ventilation. *Curr Opin Crit Care* 2007;13:27–38.

Fan E, Needham DM, Stewart TE. Ventilatory management of acute lung injury and acute respiratory distress syndrome. *JAMA* 2005;294:2889–2896.

Ferguson ND, Cook DJ, Guyatt GH, et al. High-frequency oscillation in early acute respiratory distress syndrome. *N Engl J Med* 2013;368:795–805.

Habashi NM. Other approaches to open-lung ventilation: airway pressure release ventilation. *Crit Care Med* 2005;33(3 suppl):S228–S240.

Hess DR. Ventilator waveforms and the physiology of pressure support ventilation. *Respir Care* 2005;50:166–186.

Hess DR, Thompson BT. Patient-ventilator dyssynchrony during lung protective ventilation: what's a clinician to do? *Crit Care Med* 2006;34:231–233.

Lellouche F, Mancebo J, Jolliet P, et al. A multicenter randomized trial of computer-driven protocolized weaning from mechanical ventilation. *Am J Respir Crit Care Med* 2006;174:894–900.

MacIntyre NR. Is there a best way to set positive expiratory-end pressure for mechanical ventilatory support in acute lung injury? *Clin Chest Med* 2008;29:233–239.

Meade MO, Cook DJ, Guyatt GH, et al. Ventilation strategy using low tidal volumes, recruitment maneuvers, and high positive end-expiratory pressure for acute lung injury and acute respiratory distress syndrome: a randomized controlled trial. *JAMA* 2008;299:637–645.

Mercat A, Richard JC, Vielle B, et al. Positive end-expiratory pressure setting in adults with acute lung injury and acute respiratory distress syndrome: a randomized controlled trial. *JAMA* 2008;299:646–655.

Myers TR, MacIntyre NR. Respiratory controversies in the critical care setting. Does airway pressure release ventilation offer important new advantages in mechanical ventilator support? *Respir Care* 2007;52:452–460.

NIH/NHLBI ARDS Network. Ventilation with lower tidal volumes as compared with traditional tidal volumes for acute lung injury and the acute respiratory distress syndrome. *N Engl J Med* 2000;342:1301–1308.

Nilsestuen JO, Hargett KD. Using ventilator graphics to identify patient-ventilator asynchrony. *Respir Care* 2005;50:202–234.

Ramnath VR, Hess DR, Thompson BT. Conventional mechanical ventilation in acute lung injury and acute respiratory distress syndrome. *Clin Chest Med* 2006;27:601–613.

Hemodynamic Management

Milad Sharifpour and Edward A. Bittner

I. **HEMODYNAMIC PERTURBATIONS** are common during intensive care unit admission. Both hypotensive and hypertensive emergencies threaten cardiovascular system's ability to provide sufficient oxygen and metabolic substrates to meet the demands of the body's tissues. In the event that supply is insufficient to meet demand, pathophysiologic alterations lead to the clinical manifestations of progressive end-organ damage, be it neurologic, cardiovascular, pulmonary, renal, gastrointestinal, hematologic, or musculocutaneous. The goal of the hemodynamic management of such patients is to maintain end-organ oxygenation and perfusion in order to preserve function.

II. **SHOCK** is a state of inadequate tissue perfusion, leading to tissue hypoxia and organ dysfunction. In its early stages, shock may be *compensated*: potent neurohumoral reflexes, including activation of the sympathetic nervous system and the renin–angiotensin–aldosterone system, act to maintain a supply of oxygen sufficient to meet cellular demands. With the failure of these reflexes, however, shock becomes *progressive* and, ultimately, *irreversible*: as demand for intracellular energy outstrips supply, anaerobic metabolism predominates and lactic acid production rises, membrane-associated ion transport pumps fail, the integrity of cell membranes is compromised, and cell death ensues. Shock is classified according to one of four mechanisms: hypovolemic, cardiogenic, obstructive, or distributive. The first three mechanisms may be categorized as states of *hypodynamic* shock, while the last may be categorized as a state of *hyperdynamic* shock.

A. **Types of Shock**

1. **Hypovolemic shock** occurs with the depletion of effective intravascular volume, due to insufficient intake, excessive loss, or both. Common causes include dehydration, acute hemorrhage, gastrointestinal and renal losses, and interstitial fluid redistribution occurring in the context of severe tissue trauma, burn injuries, or pancreatitis. Hemorrhage is the most common cause of shock in trauma patients and has been categorized by the American College of Surgeons into four classes, providing a correlation between the percentage of total blood volume lost and the expected attendant physiologic changes in mental status, blood pressure, heart rate, respiratory rate, and urine output (Table 6.1). Hemodynamically, hypovolemic shock is characterized by **decreased cardiac output, decreased filling pressures** (see Chapter 1), and increased systemic vascular resistance (SVR).

2. **Cardiogenic shock** is defined as persistent hypotension and inadequate tissue perfusion due to primary cardiac dysfunction occurring in the context of adequate intravascular volume and adequate or elevated left ventricular filling pressures. It may be caused by abnormalities of heart rate, rhythm, or contractility, although it occurs most commonly after extensive acute myocardial infarction (AMI) or ischemia leading to left or right ventricular failure. Other etiologies of cardiogenic

TABLE 6.1	American College of Surgeons Hemorrhage Classification[a]			
	Class			
	I	**II**	**III**	**IV**
Blood loss (mL)	<750	750–1,500	1,500–2,000	>2,000
Blood loss (%)	<15	15–30	30–40	>40
SBP	Normal	Normal	Decreased	Decreased
HR (beats/min)	<100	100–120	120–140	>140
RR (breaths/min)	14–20	20–30	30–40	>35
UOP (mL/h)	>30	20–30	5–15	Negligible
Mental status	Slightly anxious	Mildly anxious	Anxious, confused	Confused, lethargic

[a] Based on 70-kg individual.
SBP, systolic blood pressure; HR, heart rate; RR, respiratory rate; UOP, urine output.

shock include acute (e.g., tako-tsubo) and chronic cardiomyopathies, myocarditis, and **myocardial contusion.** The hemodynamic profile of cardiogenic shock is characterized by **decreased cardiac output, increased filling pressures,** and increased SVR.

3. **Obstructive shock** occurs as a result of an impediment to the normal flow of blood either to or from the heart, producing impairment of venous return or arterial outflow. Common causes include **tension pneumothorax, abdominal compartment syndrome, pulmonary embolism, pericardial tamponade,** auto-PEEP, severe aortic stenosis, dissecting aortic aneurysm, and severe aortic coarctation. Hemodynamically, obstructive shock is characterized by **decreased cardiac output, increased filling pressures,** and increased SVR.

4. **Distributive shock** is characterized by **normal or high cardiac output** and a low SVR. In the critical care setting, it is most commonly caused by sepsis. Other etiologies include neurogenic shock, anaphylaxis, adrenal insufficiency, hepatic failure, and high-output arteriovenous fistulae. The hemodynamic and metabolic profiles of the various types of shock are summarized in Tables 6.2 and 6.3.

B. **Clinical Presentation of Shock** reflects the macro- and microvascular consequences of inadequate tissue perfusion and oxygenation.

1. **Neurologic:** altered mental status manifested as anxiety, disorientation, delirium, and frank obtundation

2. **Cardiac:** chest pain, hypotension, electrocardiographic and enzymatic evidence of myocardial damage, echocardiographic wall motion abnormalities, vasoconstriction, cool limbs, poor capillary refill, weak pulses

TABLE 6.2	Hemodynamic Parameters in Shock			
Type of Shock	**MAP**	**CO**	**PAOP**	**SVR**
Hypovolemic	↓	↓	↓	↑
Cardiogenic	↓	↓	↑	↑
Obstructive	↓	↓	↓/↑	↑
Distributive	↓	↔/↑	↔/↓	↓

MAP, mean arterial blood pressure; CO, cardiac output; PAOP, pulmonary artery occlusion pressure; SVR, systemic vascular resistance.

TABLE 6.3	Metabolic Parameters in Shock	
Type of Shock	$S\bar{v}o_2$, $Sc\bar{v}o_2$	**Lactate**
Hypovolemic	↓	↑
Cardiogenic	↓	↑
Obstructive	↓	↑
Distributive	↔/↑	↑

$S\bar{v}o_2$, mixed venous oxygen saturation; $Sc\bar{v}o_2$, central venous oxygen saturation.

3. **Respiratory:** increased respiratory rate and minute ventilation, respiratory muscle failure
4. **Renal:** decreased urine output, renal ischemia, acute tubular necrosis, uremia
5. **Gastrointestinal:** hepatic centrilobar necrosis and elevated transaminases, stress ulceration, bacterial translocation
6. **Hematologic:** coagulopathy, thrombosis, thrombocytopenia, disseminated intravascular coagulation
7. **Musculocutaneous:** weakness, fatigue

C. **Monitoring** in shock should be directed toward detecting, if not preventing, the progression of tissue hypoperfusion as well as toward assessing the adequacy of resuscitation.

1. **Standard monitors** (continuous electrocardiography, pulse oximetry, noninvasive blood pressure, urinary output, temperature) should not preclude the vigilance of the clinician in performing a comprehensive history and serial physical examinations.

2. **Monitors of tissue perfusion** include both hemodynamic and metabolic indices, the utility of which are likely greater when followed over time rather than when examined at discrete time points.

   a. **Hemodynamic indices.** Measurement of systemic blood pressure allows for a global rather than a regional assessment of the adequacy of tissue perfusion. Given the desire for continuous arterial pressure monitoring and the need for frequent blood draws to track trends in arterial blood gases and serum lactate levels (see later), most patients in shock will have an **indwelling arterial cannula** placed for systemic blood pressure measurement (see Chapter 1). The need to infuse potent vasoactive medications, measure central venous oxygen saturation, and establish large-volume access frequently requires placement of a **central venous catheter.** Placement of a **pulmonary artery (PA) catheter (PAC)** may further assist in the differential diagnosis of shock when the hemodynamic profile is not clear from peripheral assessment and may aid in monitoring cardiac responses (e.g., PA occlusion pressure, cardiac output) to therapeutic interventions. However, clinical trials have demonstrated that placement of PACs does not improve patient outcomes. This should not be a surprise given that PACs are monitoring devices and not therapeutic interventions. Additional monitors (e.g., esophageal Doppler monitors, echocardiography, arterial pulse waveform analysis) are now available to allow less-invasive assessment of cardiac output, stroke volume, and SVR (see Chapter 1).

   b. **Metabolic indices**

      1. **Serum pH.** Metabolic acidemia may reflect a state of increased anaerobic metabolism and endogenous acid production occurring

with progressive tissue hypoperfusion. It may also signal worsening renal and hepatic function and an inability to metabolize and clear the increasing endogenous acid load.

2. **Serum lactate.** In the absence of sufficient cellular levels of oxygen, demand for energy sources such as ATP exceeds supply, the citric acid cycle and oxidative phosphorylation fail, and pyruvate generated by glycolysis is increasingly reduced to lactate.

3. **Mixed venous ($S\bar{v}o_2$) and central venous ($Sc\bar{v}o_2$) oxygen saturations** reflect the balance between systemic oxygen delivery (Do_2) and systemic oxygen consumption ($\dot{V}o_2$). When supply is insufficient to meet demand or demand exceeds supply, $S\bar{v}o_2$ falls below the normal range of 65% to 75%. Given that $S\bar{v}o_2$ reflects the balance between Do_2 and $\dot{V}o_2$, it is affected by the variables that determine them, including body temperature, metabolic rate, hemoglobin concentration, arterial oxygen partial pressure, and cardiac output (Fig. 6.1). It is important to note that $S\bar{v}o_2$ can be falsely elevated in septic shock secondary to mitochondrial dysfunction (cytopathic dysoxia).

D. Management of Shock
1. **General principles.** If shock is defined as a state of inadequate tissue perfusion and oxygenation, it makes sense that treatment should be aimed at increasing Do_2 while minimizing $\dot{V}o_2$.
   a. **Supplemental oxygen.** Supplemental oxygen should be supplied and the institution of endotracheal intubation with controlled mechanical ventilation should be considered early.
   b. **Circulation.** Delivery of well-oxygenated blood to the tissues depends on an adequate cardiac output and driving pressure. Thus, fluid resuscitation plays an integral role in the treatment of shock. In the event that infusion of crystalloid, colloid, or blood products is insufficient to establish and maintain adequate systemic oxygen delivery, pharmacologic therapy with inotropes and/or vasopressors may be required.

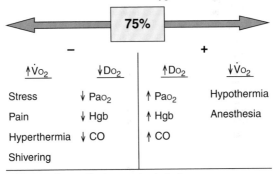

FIGURE 6.1 Factors affecting central and mixed venous oxygen saturation. After Rivers EP, Ander DS, Powell D. Central venous oxygen saturation monitoring in the critically ill patient. *Curr Opin Crit Care* 2001;7(3):204–211. $\dot{V}o_2$, systemic oxygen consumption; Do_2, systemic oxygen delivery; Pao_2, arterial oxygen partial pressure; Hgb, hemoglobin concentration; CO, cardiac output.

2. **Fluid resuscitation** is the cornerstone of the treatment of hypotension and shock. Its aim is both to increase effective circulating intravascular volume and, through the Frank-Starling mechanism, to increase cardiac ventricular preload and therefore cardiac output. Unfortunately, it is often difficult to predict whether, and by how much, the **cardiac output will increase in response to volume loading.** While inadequate fluid replacement may result in continued tissue hypoperfusion and the progression of shock, **overly aggressive resuscitation may result in heart failure** and pulmonary and tissue edema, which in turn will further compromise tissue perfusion. The fluids available for resuscitation include crystalloids, colloids, and blood products; however, the optimal choice of fluid remains controversial.

   a. **Crystalloids.** The most commonly used crystalloid solutions are **lactated Ringer's** and 0.9% **normal saline solutions,** which are inexpensive, easily stored, and readily available. Because these fluids readily leave the intravascular space, however, they require a volume equal at least to three to five times the intravascular deficit to restore circulating volume. In addition, by expanding the interstitial volume, they have the potential to create tissue edema and worsen tissue perfusion, thus providing an at least theoretical argument for the use of colloids in fluid resuscitation instead.

   b. **Colloids** include both natural and synthetic solutions. Because of their high molecular weight and increased osmotic activity, colloids remain in the intravascular space longer than crystalloids and thus require less volume to achieve the same hemodynamic goals.

      1. **Human albumin** is derived from pooled human plasma and is available as 5% and 25% solutions in normal saline. Heat treatment eliminates the risk of transmission of viral infections. Although there is no evidence of harm from the use of albumin as a resuscitation fluid (except perhaps in head injury victims), no clear benefit has been shown either and its relatively high cost limits its widespread use.

      2. **Synthetic colloids** include **dextran** and **hydroxyethyl starch (HES).** Because of their antigenicity and high incidence of anaphylactic and anaphylactoid reactions, the dextrans have largely been replaced by starch-based compounds. **Hydroxyethyl starches** are high-polymeric glucose compounds available with a variety of mean molecular weights and molar substitution patterns and dissolved in normal saline or sodium lactate. Fluid resuscitation with HES has been associated with increased need for renal replacement therapy. Based on these results, the use of HES in patients with severe sepsis and septic shock is discouraged.

   c. **Blood products.** While not recommended for pure volume expansion due to their potential for disease transmission, immunosuppression, transfusion reaction, and transfusion-related acute lung injury, as well as their limited availability and high cost, administration of packed red blood cells may be indicated to improve systemic oxygen delivery when infusion of crystalloid or colloid and institution of vasoactive agents have proven insufficient to halt the progression of shock. The choice of a transfusion trigger for any given patient in any given situation remains unclear. However, general agreement exists that the hemoglobin level in stable anemic patients does not need to be increased above a concentration of 10 mg/dL.

3. **Specific considerations**
   a. **Hypovolemic shock.** Since hypovolemic shock entails a reduction in effective intravascular volume, it would seem logical that its treatment would involve rapid and early volume resuscitation. However, in the case of hemorrhagic shock with ongoing blood loss, aggressive fluid administration prior to definitive hemostasis may increase bleeding from disrupted vessels and promote the progression of tissue hypoperfusion. As such, delayed and initially limited, rather than immediate and vigorous, fluid resuscitation may be beneficial. It must also be kept in mind that massive hemorrhage also involves loss of platelets and coagulation factors, such that balanced infusions of packed red blood cells and fresh frozen plasma may be required. As is the case with any massive transfusion, care must be taken to guard against development of the lethal triad of cold, coagulopathy, and acidemia.
   b. **Cardiogenic shock.** The abnormalities in rate, rhythm, contractility, and valvular mechanics associated with cardiogenic shock may require a host of specialized interventions, ranging from pacemaker and defibrillator placements to antithrombotic therapy, percutaneous coronary intervention with angioplasty, stenting, open coronary revascularization, mechanical support with intra-aortic balloon counter pulsation devices, and even left ventricular assist devices (see Chapter 18). Despite such sophisticated treatments, the initial approach to the management of patients in cardiogenic shock adheres to the same basic principles of rectifying the imbalance between systemic oxygen delivery and systemic oxygen consumption until definitive treatment can be obtained.
   c. **Obstructive shock** requires specific interventions targeted to the cause of blood flow impairment. Tension pneumothorax is treated with needle decompression followed by tube thoracostomy, abdominal compartment syndrome is treated with surgical decompression, pulmonary embolism is treated with supportive care and may involve the use of thrombolysis or surgical embolectomy, cardiac tamponade is treated with pericardiocentesis, auto-PEEP requires temporary suspension of mechanical ventilation and adjustment of ventilator settings.
   d. **Distributive shock.** In the critical care setting, distributive shock is most commonly caused by *systemic inflammatory response syndrome* (inflammation) or *sepsis*. Guidelines for the management of **severe sepsis** and **septic shock** are reviewed in **Chapter 30.** In brief, appropriate initial management rests upon the triad of early broad-spectrum antimicrobial antimicrobial therapy, hemodynamic resuscitation, and source control. **Anaphylactic shock** is another form of distributive shock resulting from an acute, immunoglobulin E (IgE)–mediated reaction involving the release of multiple inflammatory mediators from mast cells and basophils. Initial management requires immediate identification and discontinuation of the suspected antigen, prompt provision of ventilatory and cardiovascular support, and pharmacologic therapy directed at the immune mediators of the symptomatology, including epinephrine, the histamine H_1- and H_2-receptor blockers diphenhydramine and ranitidine, respectively, and corticosteroids.

III. **PHARMACOLOGIC THERAPIES OF HYPOTENSION AND SHOCK.** When appropriate fluid replacement fails to restore adequate blood pressure and tissue perfusion, pharmacologic therapy with vasopressors and/or inotropes is required. Even with the return of physiologic systemic filling and perfusion pressures (e.g., CVP 8–12 mmHg, MAP 65–90 mmHg), regional perfusion abnormalities may cause refractory tissue hypoperfusion. Persistent metabolic acidemia, elevated serum lactate levels, and depressed S$\bar{v}o_2$ suggest the need for further pharmacologic intervention, although the choice of a specific agent will depend on the clinical context. Tables 6.4 and 6.5 summarize the common vasopressor and inotropic agents, including their receptor-binding affinity and major hemodynamic effects and side effects.

TABLE 6.4	Commonly Used Vasopressor and Inotropic Agents: Receptor Selectivity					
Drug	α_1	α_2	β_1	β_2	**DA**	**Other**
Phenylephrine	+++++	0	0	0	0	
Ephedrine	+++	0	+++	++	0	
Vasopressin	0	0	0	0	0	V_1/V_2
Dopamine[a]	+++	0	++++	++	+++++	
Norepinephrine	++++	0	+++	+	0	
Epinephrine	+++++	+++	++++	+++	0	
Isoproterenol	0	0	+++++	+++++	0	
Dobutamine	+	0	+++++	+++	0	
Milrinone						

[a] Effects of dopamine vary with dose, from predominantly DA agonism at low doses to predominantly α agonism at high doses.

α_1, α_1 receptor; α_2, α_2 receptor; β_1, β_1 receptor; β_2, β_2 receptor; DA, dopamine receptors; V_1/V_2, vasopressin receptors; 0, zero receptor affinity; + through +++++, minimal to marked receptor affinity.

TABLE 6.5	Commonly Used Vasopressor and Inotropic Agents: Hemodynamic Effects and Major Clinical Side Effects					
Drug	**HR**	**MAP**	**CO**	**SVR**	**Renal Blood Flow**	**Side Effects**
Phenylephrine	↓	↑↑↑	↓	↑↑↑	↓↓↓	Reflex bradycardia, HTN, peripheral and visceral vasoconstriction
Ephedrine	↑↑	↑↑	↑↑	↑	↓↓	Tachycardia
Vasopressin	0	0	0	↑	↑	Peripheral and visceral vasoconstriction
Dopamine[a]	↑↑	↑	↑↑↑	↑	↑↑↑	Arrhythmias
Norepinephrine	↓	↑↑↑	↑/↓	↑↑↑	↓↓↓	Arrhythmias
Epinephrine	↑↑	↑	↑↑	↓/↑	↓↓	HTN, arrhythmias, cardiac ischemia
Isoproterenol	↑↑↑	↓	↑↑↑	↓↓	↓/↑	Arrhythmias
Dobutamine	↑	↑	↑↑↑	↓	↑	Tachycardia, arrhythmias
Milrinone	0	↓	↑↑	↓↓↓	↓	Arrhythmias, hypotension
Levosimendan	0	↓	↑↑	↓↓↓	↓	Tachycardia, hypotension

[a] Effects of dopamine vary with dose, from predominantly DA agonism at low doses to predominantly α agonism at high doses.

HR, heart rate; MAP, mean arterial pressure; CO, cardiac output; SVR, systemic vascular resistance; 0, zero receptor affinity; ↓↓↓ through ↑↑↑, decrease through increase in effect; HTN, hypertension.

A. **Non–Catecholamine Sympathomimetic Agents** are synthetic drugs used primarily as vasopressors. They are classified according to their affinity for activation of α- and/or β-adrenergic receptors.

   1. **Phenylephrine** is a selective α_1 adrenergic agonist that causes arterial vasoconstriction. By increasing SVR, it rapidly raises mean arterial pressure, although reflex bradycardia may cause a reduction in cardiac output. Because of its rapid onset, its ease of titration, and its ability to be administered through a peripheral intravenous (IV) line, phenylephrine is often used as a first-line, temporizing agent to treat hypotension. Its indications include hypotension secondary to peripheral vasodilatation, such as following the administration of potent hypnotic medications or epidural local anesthetics. Because of its pure vasoconstrictive effect, phenylephrine may be poorly tolerated in patients with compromised left ventricular function.

   2. **Ephedrine** is a direct and indirect α- and β-adrenergic agonist that causes an increase in heart rate and cardiac output with modest vasoconstriction. As such, its hemodynamic profile is similar to that of epinephrine, although much less potent.

   3. **Arginine vasopressin (AVP)** (antidiuretic hormone, ADH) is a nonapeptide hormone endogenously synthesized in the hypothalamus and stored in the posterior pituitary. In addition to its roles in osmoregulation and volume regulation, which are mediated through the V_2 **receptors,** AVP also acts through V_1 **receptors** to increase arteriolar smooth muscle tone and thus SVR. While vasopressin levels in hypovolemic (hemorrhagic) and cardiogenic shock are appropriately elevated, serum levels in patients with septic shock have been found to be inappropriately low. Given this relative vasopressin deficiency in septic shock, **low-dose infusions in the range of 0.01 to 0.04 U/min** may produce V_1-mediated vasoconstriction while potentiating the effects of other vasoactive and inotropic agents. While pharmacologic doses (>0.1 U/min) may cause potentially deleterious vasoconstriction of splanchnic, renal, pulmonary, and coronary vascular beds, physiologic infusions (0.01–0.04 U/min) do not.

B. **Catecholamines** include endogenous compounds **dopamine, norepinephrine,** and **epinephrine** and synthetic compounds such as **isoproterenol** and **dobutamine.**

   1. **Endogenous**

      a. **Dopamine** is the immediate precursor to norepinephrine and epinephrine. Its actions vary with its dosing. At low doses, it affects primarily dopaminergic receptors in splanchnic, renal, coronary, and cerebral vascular beds, leading to vasodilatation and increased blood flow. At intermediate doses, dopamine increasingly stimulates β_1-adrenergic receptors producing positive inotropic and chronotropic effects. At high doses, α_1-adrenergic effects predominate, causing an increase in SVR. However, its use in patients in shock is limited by its arrhythmogenicity. Furthermore, in a subset of patients with cardiogenic shock, dopamine use has been associated with higher mortality.

      b. **Norepinephrine** is an endogenous catecholamine with both α- and β-adrenergic activity. Its potent vasoconstrictive and inotropic effects frequently make it the drug of choice to treat hemodynamically unstable patients who require the support of both vascular tone and myocardial contractility. Compared with epinephrine, it lacks β_2 activity. Based on its hemodynamic properties, norepinephrine is the first-line vasopressor in treatment of septic shock.

  c. **Epinephrine** is the primary endogenous catecholamine produced by the adrenal medulla. As mentioned earlier, epinephrine has potent α_1, β_1, and β_2 activities, which together act to increase heart rate and contractility. It is the mainstay of cardiopulmonary resuscitation and second-line vasopressor in treatment of septic shock when an additional agent is needed to achieve hemodynamic goals. Its effect on BP is due to positive inotropic and chronotropic effects and to vasoconstriction in vascular beds, especially the skin, mucosae, and kidney. Its strong β_2 effect promotes bronchodilation and blocks mast cell degranulation, making it the drug of choice for **anaphylaxis**.

 2. **Synthetic**

  a. **Isoproterenol** is a pure β-adrenergic agonist whose β_1 effects increase heart rate, contractility, and cardiac output. Because of its β_2 activation, both diastolic and mean arterial pressures may slightly decrease. The combination of increased cardiac work and decreased diastolic pressures may compromise coronary perfusion and lead to myocardial ischemia, particularly in patients with preexisting coronary artery disease. Despite these limitations, isoproterenol may be useful in cases of cardiogenic shock in heart transplant recipients, where the donor organ is denervated and will only respond to direct-acting sympathomimetic agents.

  b. **Dobutamine** is another synthetic catecholamine with predominantly β activity. With its high affinity for β_1 receptors, dobutamine is a potent inotrope with moderate chronotropic effects. The β_2 effects of dobutamine produce a modest decrease in SVR. Taken together, dobutamine's potent inotropic and slight vasodilatory effects make it a suitable agent for patients with cardiogenic shock with depressed left ventricular function, elevated filling pressures, and increased SVR.

 C. **Phosphodiesterase-III (PDE-III) Inhibitors. Amrinone** and **milrinone** exert their effects by inhibiting PDE-III, an enzyme especially abundant in vascular smooth muscle and cardiac tissues, where it increases cAMP levels, which in turn leads to increased chronotropy and inotropy. Amrinone has been largely replaced by milrinone due to its shorter duration of action, easier titratability, and decreased risk of thrombocytopenia. Milrinone is indicated for IV administration in patients with acute heart failure and may be of some benefit to patients with right heart failure secondary to elevated PA pressures. Milrinone is administered with a loading dose of 50 μg/kg followed by a continuous infusion of 0.25 to 1.0 μg/kg/min. Its elimination half-life is 30 to 60 minutes. Hypotension and tachycardia are the main side effects that limit its use.

 D. **Calcium Sensitizers.** The calcium sensitizer **levosimendan** stabilizes the conformational change in troponin C as it binds to calcium, thus facilitating myocardial cross-bridging and augmenting contractility. Given its ability to increase cardiac output while lowering central filling pressures, levosimendan has been approved in Europe for treatment of acute heart failure. Levosimendan is not available in the United States.

IV. **HYPERTENSION.** As was the case with shock, hypertensive crises may also compromise blood flow and the delivery of oxygen to tissues, complicating the care of patients and necessitating treatment in a higher acuity critical care setting. According to the seventh report of the Joint National Committee on Prevention, Detection, Evaluation, and Treatment of High Blood Pressure, patients with blood **pressures higher than 180/120 mmHg** and with evidence of acute or progressive end-organ damage are classified as having a **"hypertensive emergency"** and require immediate blood pressure reduction, albeit not necessarily to normal ranges, to limit end-organ damage.

A. The **clinical presentation** of hypertensive emergencies largely reflects the macro- and microvascular consequences of compromised tissue perfusion and oxygenation.

1. **Neurologic:** encephalopathy with the symptoms and signs of increased intracranial pressure secondary to cerebral hyperperfusion, including headache, nausea, vomiting, visual disturbances, papilledema, altered mental status, confusion, obtundation, localized or generalized seizure activity, and stroke

2. **Cardiovascular:** angina, acute coronary syndrome with electrocardiographic and enzymatic evidence of ischemia and/or AMI, acute heart failure, and acute aortic dissection

3. **Respiratory:** dyspnea, acute pulmonary edema, respiratory failure

4. **Renal:** oliguria, acute renal failure

5. **Obstetric:** severe preeclampsia, HELLP (**h**emolysis, **e**levated **l**iver enzymes and **l**ow **p**latelets) syndrome, eclampsia

6. **Hematologic:** hemolytic anemia, coagulopathy

B. **Management:** The goal of therapy is to limit end-organ damage and restore the balance between tissue oxygen supply and demand. Rapid and excessive reduction in blood pressure may compromise organ blood flow and precipitate cerebral, coronary, or renal ischemia. Therefore, it is best to manage patients with hypertensive emergencies with continuous intravenous infusions of easily titratable, short-acting agents, such as esmolol, clevidipine, nitroglycerine, and sodium nitroprusside. In the case of hypertensive emergencies not complicated by recent ischemic stroke or acute aortic dissection, a general goal is to reduce blood pressure by 15% to 20% within 30 to 60 minutes, provided the patient remains clinically stable. If these changes are well tolerated, further reduction toward a normal blood pressure can be made over the course of the next 24 to 48 hours.

1. **Acute ischemic stroke.** In patients who have suffered an acute ischemic stroke, higher pressures may be tolerated in an attempt to improve perfusion to metabolically compromised tissues. For patients not eligible for thrombolytic therapy (see Chapter 31) and lacking evidence of other end-organ involvement, the American Stroke Association recommends pharmacologic intervention for systolic blood pressure (SBP) >220 mmHg and/or diastolic blood pressure (DBP) >140 mmHg, aiming for a 10% to 15% reduction in blood pressure. Patients eligible for thrombolytic therapy require intervention for SBP >185 mmHg and DBP >110 mmHg.

2. **Acute aortic dissection.** For patients with acute aortic dissections, various consensus guidelines published in 2001 recommend achieving an SBP between 100 and 120 mmHg, provided that symptoms and signs of neurological and/or renal compromise do not develop. In general, the goals of pharmacologic intervention are to reduce the force of left ventricular contraction and to decrease the rate of rise of the aortic pulse pressure wave (i.e., the "dP/dT") while maintaining the blood pressure as low as possible without compromising organ function. If the strength of left ventricular contraction can be reduced and the rate

of rise of arterial pressure as function of time mitigated, the risk of dissection extension and rupture may be minimized.

C. Pharmacologic Therapies

  1. Vasodilators

    a. Sodium nitroprusside is a potent arterial and (to a lesser extent) venous vasodilator. Its rapid onset and short duration of action make it ideal for continuous infusion. **Central administration** is preferred. The normal dose range is 20 to 200 µg/min. Because sodium nitroprusside is photodegradable, protection with foil wrapping is necessary. **Adverse effects** include **cyanide toxicity**–free cyanide ions (CN^-) bind to cytochrome oxidase and uncouple oxidative metabolism, causing tissue hypoxia. At low infusion rates, cyanide can be converted to thiocyanate (by thiosulfate and rhodanase), which is less toxic than CN^-. The risk of cyanide and thiocyanate toxicity is dose dependent and increases with renal impairment. **Signs of cyanide toxicity** include tachyphylaxis, increased mixed venous Pao_2, and metabolic acidosis. Pharmacologic treatment depends on facilitating cyanide metabolism through two nontoxic pathways by providing **sodium nitrite** to increase production of methemoglobin, or **sodium thiosulfate** to provide additional sulfur donors. In addition, **hydroxocobalamin** may be given, which combines with cyanide to form cyanocobalamin (vitamin B_{12}), which is excreted by the kidneys. Other potentially adverse effects of nitroprusside infusion include increased intracranial pressure with cerebral vasodilation, intracoronary steal with coronary vasodilatation, and impairment of hypoxic pulmonary vasoconstriction. **Rebound hypertension** may occur when SNP is abruptly discontinued.

    b. Nitroglycerine is a venous and (to a lesser extent) arterial vasodilator. By dilating venous capacitance vessels, nitroglycerine reduces preload and offloads the heart, decreasing ventricular end-diastolic pressure, myocardial work, and myocardial oxygen demand. At the same time, nitroglycerine dilates large coronary vessels and relieves coronary artery vasospasm, promotes the redistribution of coronary blood flow to ischemic regions, and decreases platelet aggregation, all of which serve to improve myocardial oxygen supply. Nitroglycerine's salutary effects on the balance between supply and demand of myocardial oxygen render it of particular use in hypertensive emergencies associated with acute coronary syndromes or acute cardiogenic pulmonary edema. **IV administration** of NTG is easy to titrate to effect and is the preferred route for critically ill patients. Common rates of infusion range from 25 to 1,000 µg/min. Because NTG is absorbed by polyvinyl chloride IV tubing, its dose may decrease after 30 to 60 minutes, once the IV tubing is fully saturated. **Hypotension, reflex tachycardia,** and **headache** are common side effects. Nitroglycerine administration may **worsen hypoxemia** during acute respiratory failure by increasing pulmonary blood flow to poorly ventilated areas of the lung, which can worsen ventilation–perfusion mismatch and shunt. **Tachyphylaxis** is common with continuous exposure to the drug.

    c. Nicardipine is a second-generation dihydropyridine calcium-channel blocker that causes vascular and coronary vasodilation through relaxation of vascular smooth muscle. The reduction in afterload and cardiac work accompanied by coronary vasodilatation and increased coronary blood flow make nicardipine useful in hypertensive crises associated with angina and coronary artery disease. The normal dose range is 5 to 15 mg/h. The development of reflex tachycardia may limit its benefit in some patients. A newer, third-generation dihydropyridine, **clevidipine,** has recently received FDA approval for treatment of perioperative hypertension. An ultra-short-acting and selective arteriolar vasodilator, clevidipine reduces afterload and increases cardiac output without causing reflex tachycardia. It is metabolized by erythrocyte esterases so that its clearance is not prolonged in cases of renal or hepatic dysfunction.

   d. Fenoldopam is an arteriolar vasodilator acting primarily as a δ_1 dopamine receptor agonist. At low doses (up to 0.04 μg/min), it results in renal vasodilation and natriuresis without systemic hemodynamic effects. At higher doses, it is a potent antihypertensive. Its onset is within 5 minutes and its duration of action is 30 to 60 minutes. In addition to its antihypertensive effects, fenoldopam has been shown to improve creatinine clearance in severely hypertensive patients with and without impaired renal function. Its administration may lead to increased intraocular pressure and so should proceed with caution in patients with glaucoma.

   e. Hydralazine is an arteriolar vasodilator with a not well-understood mechanism of action. Its delayed onset of action (5–15 minutes) makes it difficult to titrate in most hypertensive emergencies. It is often used on an as-needed basis (10–20 mg IV) as an additional means of controlling BP high points. High doses may be accompanied by immunologic reactions, including a lupus-like syndrome with arthralgias, myalgias, rashes, and fever.

2. Adrenergic inhibitors

   a. Labetalol is a selective β_1- and nonselective α-antagonist with an α- **to β-blocking ratio of 1:7** following IV administration. With this receptor profile, labetalol reduces arterial pressure and SVR while largely maintaining heart rate, cardiac output, and coronary and cerebral blood flow. Initial IV doses of 5 to 10 mg can be increased to 15 to 20 mg in 5-minute intervals and followed by a continuous infusion of 1 to 5 mg/min.

   b. Esmolol is short-acting β_1-selective antagonist with a rapid onset of action lending to its ease of titratability. As is the case with clevidipine, it contains an ester linkage that is rapidly hydrolyzed by erythrocyte esterases. In cases of hypertensive emergencies complicating and complicated by acute aortic dissection, esmolol is frequently the α-blocker of choice to combine with a vasodilator such as nitroprusside to achieve hemodynamic control.

Selected Readings

Binanay C, Califf RM, Hasselblad V, et al. Evaluation study of congestive heart failure and pulmonary artery catheterization effectiveness: the ESCAPE trial. *JAMA* 2005;294:1625–1633.

Bickell WH, Wall MJ Jr, Pepe PE, et al. Immediate versus delayed fluid resuscitation for hypotensive patients with penetrating torso injuries. *NEJM* 1994;331:1105–1109.

Chobanian AV, Bakris GL, Black HR, et al. Seventh report of the Joint National Committee on prevention, detection, evaluation, and treatment of high blood pressure. *Hypertension* 2003;42(6):1206–1252.

De Backer D, Biston P, Devriendt J, et al. Comparison of dopamine and norepinephrine in the treatment of shock. *NEJM* 2010;362:779–789.

Dellinger RP, Levy MM, Rhodes A, et al. Surviving sepsis campaign: international guidelines for management of severe sepsis and septic shock: 2012. *Crit Care Med* 2013;41:580–637.

Finfer S, Bellomo R, Boyce N, et al. A comparison of albumin and saline for fluid resuscitation in the intensive care unit. *NEJM* 2004;350:2247–2256.

Marik PE, Varon J. Hypertensive crises: challenges and management. *Chest* 2007;131:1949–1962.

Marik PE, Rivera R. Hypertensive emergencies: an update. *Curr Opinion Crit Care* 2011;17:569–580.

Myburgh JA, Finfer S, Bellomo R, et al. Hydroxyethyl starch or saline for fluid resuscitation in intensive care. *NEJM* 2012;367:1901–1911.

Perner A, Haase N, Guttormsen AB, et al. Hydroxyethyl starch 130/0.42 versus Ringer's acetate in severe sepsis. *NEJM* 2012;367:124–134.

Russell JA, Walley KR, Singer J, et al. Vasopressin versus norepinephrine infusion in patients with septic shock. *NEJM* 2008;358:877–887.

Sandham JD, Hull RD, Brant RF, et al. A randomized, controlled trial of the use of pulmonary artery catheters in high-risk surgical patients. *NEJM* 2003;348:5–14.

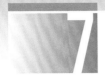

Sedation and Analgesia

Hsin Lin and Matthias Eikermann

I. INTRODUCTION

A. The management of pain, sedation, and delirium has a significant impact on patients' clinical and functional long-term outcome. Many patients are admitted to intensive care unit (ICU) for respiratory distress requiring mechanical ventilation. Traditionally, these patients often receive continuous infusions of sedatives and analgesics to improve tolerance of mechanical ventilation and to reduce anxiety, but not all patients who are endotracheally intubated need continuous sedation and analgesia. Sedation for mechanically ventilated patients aims to reduce distress, ease adaption to the ventilator, reduce oxygen consumption and carbon dioxide production, and protect patients with brain injury from development of edema or ischemia. However, clinical observations, clinical effectiveness research as well as interventional trials have suggested that sedation is often overused and leads to delayed ambulation.

B. There is a complex relationship among wakefulness, pain, and agitation that need to be addressed in an individualized fashion. Curley et al suggested pain and anxiety management should be driven by the goal of optimizing patient's comfort while minimizing the risk of adverse drug effects. Protocolized sedation does not always reduce the duration of mechanical ventilation. We have therefore systematized the parallel assessment of sedation, pain, and agitation (Fig. 7.1), such that sedation, pain, and agitation can be treated in an integrative fashion with an aim to maximize the benefit of pharmacological management across these symptoms and to minimize the undesired adverse effects.

C. Goal of a protocolized approach is to use just enough sedative and analgesic for the shortest possible time to avoid deleterious cardiopulmonary effects and minimize the later neurological and muscular effects. The requirement of sedation and analgesia varies among patients, and we will in this chapter focus the discussion on the principles and goals of sedation and analgesia in the ICU.

D. Some patients with acute refractory respiratory failure require deep sedation and/or even neuromuscular transmission block in order to prevent ventilator–patient asynchrony and to avoid the risk of barotrauma due to uncontrolled and excessive spontaneous breathing. In these patients, respiratory depressant side effects of propofol and opioid infusions can be utilized to control respiratory drive and achieve patient–ventilator synchrony until gas exchange improves. In addition, deep sedation may be required temporarily when controlling elevated intracranial pressure in head injury and status epileptics or to achieve anxiolysis during pharmacological paralysis.

In contrast, some long-term ventilated patients without severe critical illness might require very little or no sedation. Accordingly, sedation strategies must recognize and respond to this problem. Daily interruption of sedative-drug infusions (if indicated) decreases the duration of

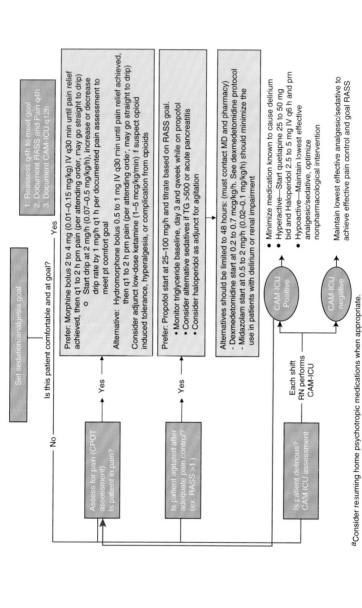

Set sedation/analgesia goal

Is this patient comfortable and at goal? ——— Yes

No

Assess for pain (CPOT assessment)
Is patient in pain?

——— Yes

Prefer: Morphine bolus 2 to 4 mg (0.01–0.15 mg/kg) IV q30 min until pain relief achieved, then q1 to 2 h prn pain (per attending order, may go straight to drip)
  o Start drip at 2 mg/h (0.07–0.5 mg/kg/h), increase or decrease drip rate by 1 mg/h q1 h per documented pain assessment to meet pt comfort goal
Alternative: Hydromorphone bolus 0.5 to 1 mg IV q30 min until pain relief achieved, then q1 to 2 h prn pain (per attending order, may go straight to drip)
Consider adjunct low-dose ketamine (1–5 mcg/kg/min) f suspect opioid induced tolerance, hyperalgesia, or complication from opioids

Is patient agitated after adequate pain control?
(ex. RASS >1)

——— Yes

Prefer: Propofol start at 25–100 mg/h and titrate based on RASS goal.
• Monitor triglyceride baseline, day 3 and qweek while on propofol
• Consider alternative sedatives if TG >500 or acute pancreatitis
• Consider haloperidol as adjunct for agitation

Alternatives should be limited to 48 hours: (must contact MD and pharmacy)
- Dexmedetomidine start at 0.2 to 0.7 mcg/kg/h. See dexmedetomidine protocol
- Midazolam start at 0.5 to 2 mg/h (0.02–0.1 mg/kg/h) should minimize the use in patients with delirium or renal impairment

Is patient delirious?
CAM ICU assessment

Each shift
RN performs
CAM-ICU

CAM-ICU Positive

CAM-ICU negative

• Minimize medication known to cause delirium
• Hyperactive—Start quetiapine 25 to 50 mg bid and Haloperidol 2.5 to 5 mg IV q6 h and prn
• Hypoactive—Maintain lowest effective analgesic/sedative, optimize nonpharmacological intervention

Maintain lowest effective analgesic/sedative to achieve effective pain control and goal RASS

1. Reassess q4h to meet goal
2. Document RASS and Pain q4h
3. Document CAM-ICU q12h

aConsider resuming home psychotropic medications when appropriate.

FIGURE 7.1 SICU pain, agitation, delirium guideline for intubated patients not receiving NMBAs.

mechanical ventilation and the length of stay in the ICU. In addition, the incidence of toxic-metabolic coma, delirium, drug-induced respiratory depression, immobility-induced muscle wasting, and constipation can be minimized. The goal of sedation should be established daily with the multidisciplinary team, and the goal should change as the patient's status evolves. Nonparalyzed patients should receive sufficient sedatives to be comfortable and awake enough to communicate their needs. Anxiety is reported by up to 85% of the critically ill patients as assessed by the Anxiety Faces Scale and persisted at a year after discharge in 62% of survivors. Note that non-pharmacologic measures may reduce anxiety and pain.

E. Over the last decade, numerous studies have reported on the benefits of lighter sedation of patients undergoing mechanical ventilation. ICU patients who are able to interact with ICU staff are more likely to participate in early mobility activities, which will likely shorten their duration on mechanical ventilation as well as their ICU length of stay. The early mobilization is clearly not feasible when patients are deeply sedated. It should be noted that neuromuscular blocking agents do not have amnesic properties and sedation to the point of amnesia is required to avoid awake and paralyzed patients. In the extreme cases, patients in a vegetative state and coma, sedation is not required.

F. Low sedation levels may also help prevent delirium in the ICU. Delirium is a cognitive disturbance with an acute onset or fluctuating clinical course. The reported incidence of delirium in the ICU ranges from 11% to 87%. Most commonly recognized risk factors are age >65 years, male sex, dementia, history of delirium, immobility, dehydration, coexisting medical conditions, treatment with psychoactive and anticholinergic drugs, and malnutrition. Other modifiable risk factors are sedative hypnotics, narcotics, infection, surgery, pain, and prolonged sleep deprivation.

G. Early mobilization has been shown to decrease delirium in the ICU. In addition, judicious use of medications known to potentiate delirium may reduce ICU delirium.

II. **SEDATION TITRATION:** Poorly monitored and/or coordinated sedation may predispose patients to delirium, posttraumatic stress disorder (PTSD), prolonged ventilator time, and mortality. If sedation is required, the coordination of a daily awakening and breathing trial has been shown to be an effective procedure to reduce mortality in ICU patients. The best strategy is to avoid excessive sedation and use of sedation scales and protocol, including targeted sedation and daily interruption of all sedative medications. Richmond Agitation Sedation Scale (RASS) is one of the most commonly used scales in the United States. With established daily RASS goal, nurses can titrate the sedation to a targeted goal. In addition to use of an objective sedation scale, daily interruption of all sedative medications can facilitate recognition of the time when sedatives are no longer needed and have been shown to decrease amount of sedative used and improve outcomes. We have noticed a tendency that clinicians aggressively sedate patients early in their ICU course and keep the same level of deep sedation indefinitely. Daily cessation of sedation allows the opportunity to test sedative needs for each patient everyday.

A. Continuous Infusion versus Intermittent Administration of Sedatives and Opioids

1. Continuous infusion of opioids can provide a constant level of analgesia; however, context sensitive half-live needs to be taken into account since clinical duration of action of some frequently used drugs (fentanyl, midazolam) markedly increases with duration of infusion compared with single-dose intermittent administration. The context-sensitive half-time describes the time required for the plasma drug concentration to decline by 50% after terminating an infusion. In general, context-sensitive half-time increases with duration of infusion. Context refers to the infusion duration. The context-sensitive half-times can be markedly different from elimination half-lives.

2. Given the concern of oversedation associated with continuous infusions, strategies such as intermittent bolus administration of lorazepam was compared with the continuous administration of propofol with daily interruption. Intermittent boluses of lorazepam were associated with longer ventilator days compared with daily interruption of propofol infusion. This was due to lorazepam's long half-life, persistent sedative effects, and an increased risk of delirium.

B. Sedative Medications: Sedatives and opioids increase the risk of respiratory complications. When given in high doses, the clinician needs to expect a decrease in respiratory arousal, leading to a diminished drive to respiratory pump muscles and—even more importantly, upper airway dilator muscles, which increase the vulnerability of airway collapse.

1. **Propofol**

   a. Propofol is one of the most commonly used sedative in the ICUs. It is a GABAergic agent that quickly crosses the blood–brain barrier due to its lipophilicity. Propofol has an immediate onset of action of seconds and the duration of action of 10 to 15 minutes. These pharmacokinetic characteristics are particularly useful for patients who require frequent neurological assessment. However, long-term infusions can result in accumulation within lipid stores and prolong the duration of action. Multiple studies showed propofol use is associated with shorter time to mental status recovery, liberation from ventilator, and cost effectiveness when compared to benzodiazepine sedation regimens in the ICU.

   b. Propofol causes vasodilation and myocardial suppression; hypotension is common with propofol use especially at high doses. Propofol is formulated in lipid emulsion, and thus triglycerides should be monitored every 3 to 7 days while the patient receives a continuous infusion. The phospholipid emulsion provides 1.1 kcal/mL and should be counted as a caloric source when formulating nutrition plans.

   c. Propofol infusion syndrome (PRIS) is a rare but possibly fatal complication of prolonged propofol infusion, characterized by myocardial depression and shock, profound metabolic acidosis, rhabdomyolysis, and renal failure. PRIS is mostly reported among critically ill children, particularly those with traumatic brain injury, receiving high doses of propofol. However, PRIS has been reported in adults as well. The clinician should have a high suspicion to recognize this complication, which includes monitoring pH, lactate, and creatinine kinase, especially when prolonged high-dose propofol infusion is required.

2. **Dexmedetomidine**

   a. Dexmedetomidine is a selective α2-receptor agonist. Stimulation of the 2A receptor will produce sedation, anxiolysis, and partial analgesia effects; stimulation of the 2B receptor induces peripheral vasoconstriction, produces analgesia, and suppresses shivering. Unlike other sedatives, it does not suppress the respiratory center, and arousal may occur during its administration. It allows for a more awake, interactive, and mobilized patient and is associated with fewer days on the ventilator and a decrease in length of stay in the ICU. Dexmedetomidine is approved for short-term sedation (<24 hours); however, it has been studied in long-term sedation at dosages that exceeds the proprietary upper limit of 0.7 mcg/kg/h. In recent controlled trials where higher doses were allowed, dexmedetomidine was safe and at least as effective as lorazepam and midazolam in providing targeted sedation and was associated with fewer days on the ventilator and in the ICU.

b. The most common indication for use of dexmedetomidine is to provide short-term sedation to patients who are otherwise ready to be extubated but cannot safely be weaned off other sedative-hypnotics. A reasonable opportunity to initiate the transition to dexmedetomidine is when a patient qualifies for daily awakenings with traditional sedative therapies. A bolus dose of 0.5 to 1 mcg/kg can expedite the target concentration achievement of dexmedetomidine. A reasonable alternative to a bolus dose of dexmedetomidine is to initiate an infusion at 0.6 to 0.7 mcg/kg/h and adjust the infusion rate by 0.1 to 0.2 mcg/kg/h, at intervals no more frequent than every 30 minutes. This should minimize hemodynamic fluctuations. Figure 7.2 is an example of transitioning from propofol-based sedation to dexmedetomidine. This approach should optimize comfort while dexmedetomidine achieves target sedation. Due to frequent dosage adjustments during this transition, a protocalized approach can help to guide bedside nurses.

c. Dexmedetomidine doses exceeding 1.5 mcg/kg/h offers minimal benefits. Traditional agents, antipsychotics, should be incorporated into the regimen to augment dexmedetomidine if this rate is reached. Dexmedetomidine may be discontinued abruptly in most patients. Withdrawal syndromes characterized by agitation and tachycardia can result in discontinuation of long-term infusion, and dexmedetomidine weaning may be required. Dexmedetomidine use is limited by its inability to produce deep sedation and hypotension and bradycardia. The most common intervention is to interrupt the infusion, administer atropine or glycopyrrolate. Of note, high-dose dexmedetomidine has dose-dependent respiratory side effects: It affects hypoxic ventilatory control and can induce upper airway obstruction.

3. Benzodiazepines

a. Benzodiazepines are potent anxiolytic and sedative medications. They act on GABA receptors and have a dose-dependent pharmacodynamic and toxicological profiles. These drugs have antiepileptic properties and are useful for seizures and alcohol withdrawal. Although benzodiazepines were used as first-line sedatives in the past, recent studies show when used for ICU sedation, these agents are associated with excessive sedation, slow awakening, delayed tracheal extubation, and acute brain dysfunction. Furthermore, benzodiazepines can cause paradoxical agitation and confusion, particularly in the elderly, and have been repeatedly associated with the development of delirium in the ICU. Patients who received prolonged infusions of benzodiazepines are at risk for withdrawal on discontinuation, and slow weaning is required. There is also an association with increased mortality.

- Do not initiate infusion if patient is bradycardia (sustained HR <50 bpm), hypotensive (sustained SBP <90 mmHg)
- Assess and document patient's blood pressure, heart rate at baseline
- **Obtain baseline QTc prior to the initiation and daily QTc when patient is on dex**
- Monitor vital signs continuously during the administration of dex
  o If patient becomes hypotensive (SBP <90 mmHg) or bradycardia (HR <50 bpm with hemodynamic instability), 2nd- and 3rd-degree heart block, stop the infusion for 30 minutes and restart at half of previous rate.
  o Call MD for sustained SBP <90 mmHg, HR <40 bpm and stop dex infusion.
- Dex infusion should be increased no more frequently than q30 minute interval (range 0.2–1.5 mcg/kg/h) unless authorized by the ICU fellow or attending but can be decreased more rapidly if necessary. Consider increasing dex at a slower rate when patient is hypotensive or bradycadia.
- Option of dex load –0.25 to 1 mcg/kg over 30 minutes to quick achieve target RASS[a] (1)

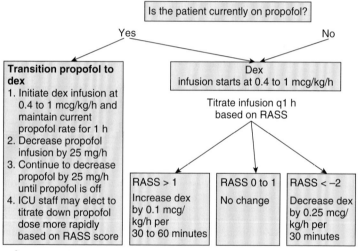

1. [a]Attending physician or fellow must be present in the ICU unit when the dexmedetomidine loading dose is given.
2. If the patient becomes hemodynamically unstable, consider eliminating any concommitent negative inotropic agents.
3. For selected patient population (e.g., substance abuse, alcohol withdrawal, delirious), higher maintainance dose may be required temporarily when refractory to other pharmacological options.

FIGURE 7.2 SICU dexmedetomidine (Dex) guideline.

b. The two most commonly used drugs for ICU sedation are midazolam and lorazepam. Midazolam is a potent short-acting benzodiazepine with an onset of action of 2 to 3 minutes. Midazolam is lipophilic and can accumulate in adipose tissues, where the drug is not readily metabolized; therefore, accumulation occurs during prolonged infusions, particularly in obese patients. In addition, midazolam is broken down into active metabolites that can accumulate in the renal failure. Midazolam also seems to develop tachyphylaxis more rapidly than other benzodiazepines. Because of concerns for unpredictable awakening after prolonged infusion, midazolam is recommended only for short-term (<48 hours) sedation. Lorazepam is less lipophilic compared with midazolam; therefore, it has slower onset of action. It does not have active metabolites and is the preferred benzodiazepine in patients with renal failure.

III. **PAIN ASSESSMENT:** Pain is frequently the root cause of distress in many ICU patients, and most critically ill patients will experience pain during their ICU stay. The etiology of pain may include underlying medical condition (such as postoperative wound and incision discomfort, trauma, burn, bone fracture, etc.) as well as routine ICU-related care such as mechanical ventilation, indwelling catheters, physical therapy, repositioning, and ICU noise from monitoring devices. It is estimated that as many as 70% of patients experience at least moderate-intensity pain during their ICU stay. Patients with inadequate pain control are prone to development of PTSD. Accordingly, pain should be addressed to ensure patient comfort and reduce adverse events. Furthermore, the management of preexisting chronic pain must be optimized to prevent the patient from experiencing additional stress and pain while staying in the ICU.

Pain assessment and management in ICU is challenging because of patient's inability to communicate effectively due to cognitive impairment from injury, sedation, or chemical paralysis. Therefore, several scales have been developed to facilitate pain assessment. For patients who are unable to self-report but who have intact motor function and observable behaviors, the Critical Care Pain Observation Tool (CPOT) is a validated and one of the most reliable behavioral pain scales for multiple ICU patient populations. CPOT includes four behavioral categories: (1) facial expression (2) body movements (3) muscle tension, and (4) ventilator compliance in ventilated patients. Each of these four indicators is scored from 1 (*no response*) to 4 (*full response*), assuming that a relationship exists between each score and the intensity of pain. Therefore, the possible range score of CPOT is 3 to 12. For patients able to communicate, a multidimensional scale that measures pain and quality of analgesia has been proposed.

When an enteral route is available, enteral opioids offer several theoretical advantaged over parenteral opioids, including greater convenience, decreased infectious complication, and improved maintenance of mucosal structure and function, which could possibly prevent gut atrophy and bacterial translocation.

A. **Opioids:** the most effective commonly used analgesics in the ICU. The primary mechanism of action is to stimulate the opioid receptor and inhibit the central nervous system pain response. The activation of opioid receptors is also associated with respiratory depression and hypercapnia. Patients with sleep apnea or chronic apnea are particularly prone to respiratory depression from opioids.

In addition to their effects on regulating pain transmission in the brain, opioid receptors are also distributed in the peripheral nervous system and the gastrointestinal tract, such as in the myenteric plexus. Opioids therefore decrease GI motility, increase transit time, and cause constipation and ileus. Opioid-induced bowel hypomotility can promote reflux of enteral tube feeds and aspiration. Other consequences include delay in resuming enteral nutrition and prolonged hospitalization. Increasingly, neurotoxicity is reported as a complication associated with opioid use particularly older ages with larger doses of opioids. The reported symptoms include rigidity, myclonus, and hyperalgesia.

An understanding of drug pharmacology should guide the specific type of opioid. Prolonged continuous infusions of opioids lead to tolerance, resulting in dose escalation to achieve the same analgesic effects.

1. Morphine has an onset of 5 minutes and a peak effect between 10 and 40 minutes after intravenous (IV) administration, with a variable duration of action of 2 to 5 hours. Intermittent IV doses of 2 to 10 mg or 1 to 3 mg/h by constant infusion are usually adequate for relief of moderate pain in the average adult. The dose required depends on factors such as tolerance and metabolic and excretory abilities. Morphine is metabolized through the liver to morphine-3-glucuronide and morphine-6-glucoronide (a potent analgesic, 20–40 times the potency of morphine). Both metabolites are eliminated by the kidney and may accumulate in patients with renal impairment; for this reason, alternative opioids are preferred.

2. Hydromorphone is five- to sevenfold more potent than morphine, with a peak onset time of 10 to 20 minutes and duration of action of 4 to 6 hours. Hydromorphone does not significantly accumulate in fat tissues and does not have active metabolites. Therefore, it is well suited for continuous infusions even in patients with moderate renal insufficiency.

3. Fentanyl is approximately hundredfold more potent than morphine. It is a highly lipid-soluble, synthetic opioid with very quick onset and short duration of action when used as an intermittent bolus. With repeated injections or given as continuous infusion, large stores of drug may accumulate in lipophilic tissues that then must be metabolized to terminate the drug action. This leads to prolonged effects after discontinuation. However, fentanyl does not have any renally excreted metabolites, which make it an ideal drug for patients with renal impairment.

4. Remifentanil has a short onset of action and is metabolized into inactive metabolites by unspecific esterases that are widespread throughout the plasma, red blood cells, and interstitial tissue, so it is not affected by hepatic or renal failure. Context-sensitive half-time of remifentanil is consistently short even after an infusion of long duration. However, hyperalgesia, a paradoxical increased sensitivity to pain, can occur with remifentanil due to its short half-life. This limits its use in the ICU.

5. Methadone is approximately equipotent to morphine when administered parenterally (IV or IM) and one-half as potent when given orally. It has duration of 15 to 40 hours, although it often seems to wear off earlier in ICU patients. Methadone is used primarily in patients who are chronic users of IV opioids.

6. Meperidine should be avoided because it is associated with myocardial depression and has vagolytic properties, which cause tachycardia and hypotension. It is rarely used in the ICU other than for the treatment of shivering. Meperidine's major metabolite, normeperidine, can accumulate in renal failure and cause seizures in high concentration.

B. Nonopioid Analgesics

1. **Ketamine:** Ketamine induces rapid sedation and analgesia through a dual mechanism of antagonizing central nervous system NMDA receptors and activating opioid u and k receptors. Ketamine administration results in inhibition of central desensitization, also known as the "wind-up phenomenon" and may lead to improved efficacy of other opioids and reduced likelihood of dependency. Most notably, ketamine preserves spontaneous respiratory reflexes, stimulates central nervous

system outflow, and decreases catecholamine reuptake. It has been shown to reduce opioid consumption after surgery. By blocking NMDA receptors, ketamine can prevent the development of opioid tolerance. In addition, unlike other anesthetics, ketamine activates respiratory effort and promotes bronchodilation. At subanesthetic plasma concentration, ketamine reduces both opioid and propofol requirements. Patients are not required to be intubated while on low-dose ketamine infusion; the doses range from 1 to 5 mcg/kg/min and can increase infusions up to 10 mcg/kg/min.

There are also several downsides to ketamine that may limit its use. Ketamine is associated with hypersalivation and emergence phenomenon, which may result in severe confusion, dreaming, nightmares, and hallucinations. Ketamine is also reported to cause hypertension and tachycardia and acts as a negative inotrope in patients with heart failure and cardiogenic shock. Although known to produce hallucinations and nightmares, the occurrence at low-dose ketamine ($<$5 mcg/kg/min) infusions is rarely reported. Ketamine can be an effective analgesic for procedures such as debridement and dressing changes and can also be used as an opioid-sparing analgesic adjunct (Fig. 7.3).

2. **Acetaminophen:** Acetaminophen is an analgesic used to treat mild to moderate pain. When combined with an opioid, acetaminophen produces a greater analgesic effect than higher doses of the opioid alone. The maximum total daily dose should not exceed 4 g per day and should be used carefully in patients with hepatic dysfunction. Ketorolac is the most potent parenteral NSAID currently available. The dose of ketorolac is 15 to 30 mg every 6 to 8 hours. The analgesic effect of 30 mg is similar to 10 mg of morphine. The use of ketorolac is associated with an increased risk of gastrointestinal bleeding, renal failure, and platelet dysfunction. Elderly patients and those with a tenuous volume status are particularly susceptible to its renal toxicity. To minimize adverse effects, ketorolac should be given for 3 days or less. Ibuprofen is the most commonly used enteral NSAID in the United States. Although effective, it seems less potent than ketorolac. The analgesic dose is 200 to 600 mg every 6 to 8 hours. Ibuprofen has a similar toxicological profile as ketorolac.

C. **Regional Analgesia:** Regional analgesia with local anesthetics can provide immediate success in otherwise "intractable" pain when relief cannot be achieved by orally and intravenously administered analgesics. It is accepted that epidural analgesia compared with IV opioid therapy provides superior pain control and potentially other benefits, including early mobility, improved cardiopulmonary function, and reduced risk of venous thromboembolism. These benefits are countered by increased risks of hypotension, motor block, urinary retention, and rare but catastrophic neurologic injury in the presence of anticoagulants. Strongest evidence in favor of epidural analgesia supports the use of epidural analgesia in patients with traumatic or surgical chest pain. Epidural analgesia is associated with reduction in mortality for patients with multiple rib fractures, but is underused, in part due to potential risks of epidural hematomas. Thoracic paravertebral catheters have improved pain and pulmonary function for patients with rib fractures. Interpleural catheters have also demonstrated effectiveness, although the insertion site can be a significant source of discomfort, and, especially with bilateral catheters, the risk of local anesthetic toxicity must be weighed. Similarly, rib blocks can be considered, but multiple, repeated blocks carry concern for local anesthetic toxicity.

Titration of opioids and propofol following start of ketamine

- RNs should use their experience and clinical judgment when using this guideline.
- Titration of analgesics and anesthetics should be started 1 hour after initiation of ketamine.
- Titration priority (sedation or analgesia) should be based on the goal of therapy.
    o E.g., if patient develops opioid tolerance, opioid induced constipation or opioid associated hypercarbia → consider to titrate down continuous opioid
- If patient becomes agitated /delirious during the titration, may consider haloperidol 2.5 to 5 mg IV or a GABA ergic drugs such as propofol

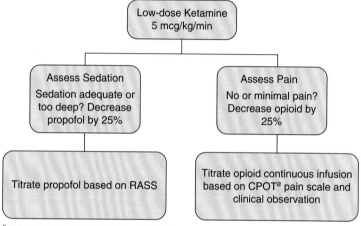

^aCPOT—The Critical-Care Pain Observation Tool

FIGURE 7.3 Low (subanesthetic)-dose ketamine for analgesia.

IV. **NEUROMUSCULAR BLOCKADE:** If patient–ventilator synchrony cannot be achieved with medications that cause respiratory depression, paralysis may be considered in patients with refractory respiratory failure (P/F ratio <150) receiving >60% oxygen and a PEEP >10 cmH$_2$O.

   During neuromuscular blockade, it is imperative to achieve deep sedation in order to decrease the risk of PTSD. It is reasonable to add EEG monitoring (e.g., the BIS/Sedline monitor) to achieve a high likelihood of adequate sedation during paralysis. Steroidal neuromuscular blocking agent infusions should not be used. The infusion rate of the neuromuscular blocking agent cisatracurium should be based on objective monitoring (TOF-ratio or PTC). Typically, a moderate neuromuscular block where the infusion is titrated to one-three visible twitches in response to train-of-four stimulation is sufficient. If patient–ventilator synchrony cannot be achieved by using the above-defined *moderate* depth of neuromuscular blockade, it may be useful to intensify the neuromuscular blockade to achieve "deep" neuromuscular blockade, characterized as absence of the response to train-of-four stimulation while a posttetanic count of 1 or 2 can be demonstrated. The need for continuous paralysis should be *reevaluated every 12 hours on patient rounds.* If the P/F ratio increases and hemodynamic stability has been achieved (stable vasopressor dose), an attempt should be made to discontinue the cisatracurium infusion. In case of reoccurrence of patient–ventilator asynchrony, neuromuscular blockade should be reestablished for a period of up to 48 hours.

Selected Readings

Balachundhar A, Brett SA. Epidural analgesia–the jury is in. *Ann Surg* 2014;259:1068–1069.

Block BM, Liu SS, Rowlingson AJ, et al. Efficacy of postoperative epidural analgesia: a meta-analysis. *JAMA* 2003;290:2455–2463.

Brochard L. Less sedation in intensive care: the pendulum swings back. *Lancet* 2010;375(9713):436–438.

Carson SS, Kress JP, Rodgers JE, et al. A randomized trial of intermittent lorazepam versus propofol with daily interruption in mechanically ventilated patients. *Crit Care Med* 2006;34(5):1326–1332.

Curley MA, Wypij D, Watson RS, et al. Protocolized sedation vs usual care in pediatric patients mechanically ventilated for acute respiratory failure: a randomized clinical trial. *JAMA* 2015;313(4):379–389.

Danielson Å, Ebberyd A, Cedborg AH, et al. Sedation with dexmedetomidine or propofol impairs control of breathing in healthy male volunteers. A randomized cross-over study [Abstract LBC07]. American Society of Anesthesiologists Annual Meeting 2014; New Orleans, USA.

Ebert TJ, Hall JE, Barney JA, et al. The effects of increasing plasma concentrations of dexmedetomidine in humans. *Anesthesiology* 2000;93(2):382–394.

Eikermann M, Vidal Melo MF. Therapeutic range of spontaneous breathing during mechanical ventilation. *Anesthesiology* 2014;120(3):536–539.

Flagel BT, Luchette FA, Reed RL, et al. Half-a-dozen ribs: the breakpoint for mortality. *Surgery* 2005;138:717–725.

Girard TD, Kress JP, Fuchs BD, et al. Efficacy and safety of a paired sedation and ventilator weaning protocol for mechanically ventilated patients in intensive care (awakening and breathing controlled trial): a randomized controlled trial. *Lancet* 2008;371: 126–134.

Himmelseher S, Durieux ME. Ketamine for perioperative pain management. *Anesthesiology* 2005;102:211–220.

Hughes MA, Glass PS, Jacobs JR. Context-sensitive half-time in multicompartment pharmacokinetic models for intravenous anesthetic drugs. *Anesthesiology* 1992;76:334–341.

Kam PCA, Cardone D. Propofol infusion syndrome. *Anaesthesia* 2007;62:690–671.

Kress JP, Pohlman AS, O'Connor M, et al. Daily interruption of sedative infusions in critically ill patients undergoing mechanical ventilation. *New Eng J Med* 2000;342:1471–1477.

Lehmann N, Joshi GP, Dirkmann D, et al. Development and longitudinal validation of the overall benefit of analgesia score: a simple multi-dimensional quality assessment instrument. *Br J Anaesth* 2010;105(4):511–518.

Lonardo NW, Mone MC, Nirula R, et al. Propofol is associated with favorable outcomes compared with benzodiazepines in ventilated intensive care unit patients. *Am J Respir Crit Care Med* 2014;189(11):1383–1394.

McKinley S, Stein-Parbury J, Chehelnabi A, et al. Assessment of anxiety in intensive care patients by using the Faces Anxiety Scale. *Am J Crit Care* 2004;13(2):146–152.

Mehta S, Cook D, Devlin JW, et al. Prevalence, risk factors, and outcomes of delirium in mechanically ventilated adults. *Crit Care Med* 2015;43(3):557–566.

Mikkelsen ME, Christie JD, Lanken PN, et al. The adult respiratory distress syndrome cognitive outcomes study: long-term neuropsychological function in survivors of acute lung injury. *Am J Respir Crit Care Med* 2012;185(12):1307–1315.

Pandharipande PP, Pun BT, Herr DL, et al. Effect of sedation with dexmedetomidine vs lorazepam on acute brain dysfunction in mechanically ventilated patients: the MENDS randomized controlled trial. *JAMA* 2007;298:2644–2653.

Payen JF, Chanques G, Mantz J, et al. Current practices in sedation and analgesia for mechanically ventilated critically ill patients: a prospective multicenter patient-based study. *Anesthesiology* 2007;106(4):687–695.

Riker RR, Shehabi Y, Bokesh PM, et al. Dexmedetomidine vs. midazolam for sedation of critically ill patients. *JAMA* 2009;301:489–499.

Sasaki N, Meyer MJ, Eikermann M. Postoperative respiratory muscle dysfunction: pathophysiology and preventive strategies. *Anesthesiology* 2013;118(4):961–978.

Schweickert WD, Pohlman MC, Pohlman AS, et al. Early physical and occupational therapy in mechanically ventilated, critically ill patients: a randomized controlled trial. *Lancet* 2009;373(9678):1874–1882.

Segredo V, Caldwell JE, Matthay MA, et al. Persistent paralysis in critically ill patients after long-term administration of vecuronium. *N Engl J Med* 1992;327(8):524–528.

Sessler CN, Gosnell MS, Grap MJ, et al. The Richmond agitation-sedation scale: validity and reliability in adult intensive care unit patients. *Am J Respir Crit Care Med* 2002;166:1338–1344.

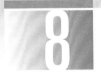

Fluids, Electrolytes, and Acid–Base Management

Yvonne Lai and Aranya Bagchi

Optimal management of fluids, electrolytes, and acid–base status in critically ill patients requires a general understanding of their normal composition and regulation. Disease processes, trauma, and surgery can all affect the manner by which the body controls its fluid balance and electrolytes.

I. FLUID COMPARTMENTS
A. The Total Body Water (TBW) ranges from 50% to 70% of the body mass and is determined by lean body mass, gender, and age (Table 8.1). There is an inverse relationship between TBW and percentage body fat due to the low water content of adipose tissues.

B. Compartments of TBW
1. The **intracellular** compartment is approximately 66% of TBW (approximately 40% of body mass).
2. The **extracellular** compartment is approximately 34% of TBW (approximately 20% of body mass) and can be further divided into the following:
   a. the **intravascular** compartment, composed of plasma. It is approximately 5% of total body mass.
   b. the **extravascular** compartment, composed of interstitial fluid, lymph, bone fluid, fluids of the various body cavities, and mucosal/secretory fluids. The extravascular compartment represents approximately 15% of total body mass.
   c. the **third space,** an ill-defined space invoked to account for otherwise inexplicable fluid losses in the perioperative period or in critically ill patients. It may be considered "nonfunctional" interstitial fluid that cannot equilibrate with the circulating blood volume. However, many experts doubt the existence of a discrete third space.

C. Ionic Composition of the Fluid Compartments. Various physiologic terms describe the concentrations of ions in a solution:
1. **Molarity:** Moles of solute per liter of solution

	Total Body Water as a Percentage of Body Weight (%)	
	Male	**Female**
Thin	65	55
Average	60	50
Obese	55	45
Neonate	75–80	
First year	65–75	
Ages 1–10 y	60–65	
Ages 10 y to adult	50–60	

2. **Molality:** Moles of solute per kilogram of solvent
3. **Osmolarity:** Osmoles per liter of solution. The number of osmoles is determined by multiplying the number of moles of solute by the number of freely dissociated particles from one molecule of solute. For example, 1 mole of NaCl will yield 2 osmoles (Osm) in solution.
4. **Osmolality:** Osmoles per kilogram of solvent
5. Electrolytes in physiology are generally described in terms of milliequivalents per liter (mEq/L). The fluids of each compartment are electrically neutral. Average concentrations of each electrolyte in various compartments are given in Table 8.2.

D. Movement of Water in the Body

1. Water is generally readily permeable through cell membranes and moves freely throughout the different fluid compartments. Movement of water is largely determined by **osmotic pressure** and **hydrostatic pressure**. The osmotic pressure depends on the number of osmotically active molecules in solution.
2. The movement of water between extracellular interstitial and intravascular compartments is described by **Starling's equation:**

$$Q_f = K_f \left[\left(P_c - P_i \right) - \sigma \left(pi_c - pi_i \right) \right]$$

where Q_f is the fluid flux across the capillary membrane; K_f is a constant reflecting the permeability of capillaries to water and their surface area; P_c and P_i are the hydrostatic pressures in the capillary and the interstitium, respectively; σ is the *reflection coefficient* (see below); and pi_c and pi_i are the colloid osmotic pressures in the capillary and interstitium, respectively.

a. Large, negatively charged intravascular proteins to which vascular membranes are impermeable are responsible for the osmotic pressure gradient between intravascular and interstitial compartments. This component of osmotic pressure, known as the **oncotic pressure** or **colloid osmotic pressure**, contributes a small amount to the total osmotic pressure of the fluids. The positive ions that are associated with the negatively charged proteins also contribute to the osmotic pressure. **Albumin** is the predominant type of protein

 TABLE 8.2   Fluid Electrolyte Composition of Body Compartments

	Plasma (mEq/L)	Interstitial (mEq/L H_2O)	Intracellular[a] (mEq/L H_2O)
Cations			
Na	142	145	10
K	4	4	159
Ca	5	5	<1
Mg	2	2	40
Anions			
Cl	104	117	3
HCO_3	24	27	7
Proteins	16	<0.1	45
Others	9	9	154

[a]Intracellular electrolytes are difficult to measure, and most of the measurements are from myocytes, which might or might not be applicable to other cell types.

responsible for the oncotic pressure, accounting for approximately two-thirds of the total oncotic pressure. Cells do not contribute to the oncotic pressure.

b. The **reflection coefficient** (σ) describes the permeability of plasma proteins for a specific capillary membrane. Its value ranges from 0 (completely permeable) to 1 (impermeable) and varies in different disease states; it is approximately 0.7 in healthy tissues.

c. **Edema** occurs when the rate of interstitial fluid accumulation is greater than the rate of removal of interstitial fluids by the lymphatic system.

II. FLUID DEFICITS AND REPLACEMENT THERAPY

A. **Fluid Volume Deficits** and appropriate fluid therapy are dependent on the source and type of fluid loss. Because all membranes are permeable to water, fluid deficits in one compartment will affect all other compartments. Fluid losses can be broadly classified on the basis of the initial source of loss. Fluid losses also lead to electrolyte abnormalities.

1. **Intracellular fluid (ICF) compartment** deficits arise from **free water loss.**

   a. **Sources of free water loss** include the following:
      1. **Insensible losses** through skin and respiratory tract
      2. **Renal losses** secondary to inability to recollect water, such as in neurogenic or nephrogenic diabetes insipidus (DI; see **Section III.C**)

   b. With free water loss, both intracellular and extracellular volumes decrease in proportion to their volumes in the body; therefore, two-thirds of the loss will be intracellular. Similarly, **free water replacement** will be distributed in proportion to their volumes in the body, and only one-third of the administered free water will end up in the extracellular space and even less in the intravascular space.

   c. **Therapy** includes replacement of water with either **hypotonic saline** (5% dextrose in water with 0.45% sodium chloride solution) or **free water** (5% dextrose in water). Electrolytes (especially sodium) must be monitored with therapy.

2. **Extracellular fluid (ECF) compartment deficit**

   a. In general, ECF losses are isotonic. Losses may occur in each compartment, and fluid losses from one compartment are rapidly reflected in others.

   b. Clinical manifestations of ECF losses are notoriously variable. Although textbooks routinely refer to clinical findings associated with quantified losses (3%–5% losses leading to dry mucous membranes and oliguria to >20% losses leading to circulatory collapse), these signs are frequently unreliable. See the discussion on intravascular fluid deficit below.

   c. Causes of ECF losses include blood loss, vomiting, diarrhea, and "third spacing."
      1. Replacement of ECF volume loss usually requires isotonic salt solutions. Volumes required to replace ECF deficits can vary considerably among patients on the basis of the inciting event and comorbid processes.

3. **Intravascular fluid (plasma volume) deficit**

   a. Intravascular volume deficits will lead to interstitial fluid depletion as the two compartments equilibrate. It should be noted that with acute blood loss, laboratory values such as hemoglobin levels are not accurate indices of the severity of blood loss till equilibration with the ECF has taken place.

   b. The clinical utility of classifications based on percentage volume loss and clinical manifestations (such as the ATLS classification of hemorrhage) is questionable, as signs of bleeding, including tachycardia, diaphoresis, and so forth, are extremely variable. Perhaps the most relevant clinical feature associated with intravascular volume loss is **orthostatic hypotension** (or **orthostatic tachycardia**) in a relatively stable patient. In an unstable patient, clinicians should use a combination of **noninvasive** or **invasive methods** to assess blood volume and **"fluid responsiveness,"** the ability of volume administration to increase cardiac output significantly. For a discussion of static and dynamic parameters predicting fluid responsiveness, see **Chapters 1** and **3.** Patients should be resuscitated early and aggressively—however, reliance on static numbers (e.g., 30 mL/kg crystalloid) or goals (e.g., give fluids till CVP is 8–12 mmHg) should be avoided in favor of frequent reassessment of both parameters of fluid responsiveness and global/regional perfusion indices.

B. Fluid Replacement Therapy (see **Chapter 33**)

   1. Crystalloid solutions (see Table 8.3 **for the composition of commonly used crystalloids**)

      a. Maintenance fluids are used to replace constitutive losses of fluids and electrolytes via urine, sweat, respiration, and gastrointestinal (GI) tract.

         1. Insensible water losses include normal losses by skin and lungs, and total approximately 600 to 800 mL/d. **Sensible losses** of water include losses from the kidneys and GI tract. The obligate minimal urine output is 0.3 mL/kg/h and the average urine output is 1 mL/kg/h in an average 70-kg person (approximately 1,700 mL/d).

         2. General guidelines for hourly maintenance fluid replacement based on body weight (note that these guidelines should be tempered by frequent assessment of the patient's volume status):

           a. 0 to 10 kg: 4 mL/kg/h

           b. 11 to 20 kg: 40 mL + 2 mL/kg/h for each kilogram above 10 kg

           c. >20 kg: 60 mL + 1 mL/kg/h for each kilogram above 20 kg

         3. Maintenance fluid composition. In general, **hypotonic maintenance fluids** are used to replace insensible losses. Additional losses from other sources are often present in critically ill patients (e.g., through drains, fistulas, etc.) and require **isotonic fluid repletion.**

   b. For ECF repletion and intravascular fluid deficit (blood loss), isotonic solutions are used. The goal of **replacement fluid therapy** is

TABLE 8.3   Composition of Crystalloid Solutions

	Na	Cl	K	Ca	Buffer	Dextrose	pH	Osmolarity
D5W	0	0	0	0	0	5	4.5	252
D5 0.45% NaCl	77	77	0	0	0	5	4.0	406
0.9% NaCl	154	154	0	0	0	0	5.0	308
7.5% NaCl	1283	1283	0	0	0	0	5.0	2567
Lactated Ringer's	130	109	4	3	28[a]	0	6.5	273

[a] Lactate.

Na, Cl, K, Ca, and buffer concentrations are in milliequivalent per liter; dextrose is in grams per 100 mL.
D_5W, 5% dextrose in water; D_5 0.45% NaCl, 5% dextrose in water with 0.45% sodium chloride solution.

to correct abnormalities in volume status or serum electrolytes. Because electrolytes are permeable through capillary membranes, crystalloids will rapidly redistribute from the intravascular compartment throughout the entire ECF, in the normal distribution of 75% extravascular to 25% intravascular.

2. **Colloid solutions (see** Table 8.4 **for the composition of commonly used colloids).** Colloid solutions are most commonly used for intravascular volume expansion. Unlike crystalloid solutions, the colloid elements do not freely cross-intact capillary membranes and therefore do not redistribute as readily into the entire ECF compartment in the absence of a severe capillary leak state. Colloids have been thought to have a number of important **potential advantages** over crystalloids, although clinical evidence for these advantages is weak.

   a. More effective volume expansion and less edema formation

   b. Better at maintaining endothelial integrity

   c. Improved microcirculation

   d. Less immunomodulation

   e. The chief disadvantage of colloids is their **significantly higher cost compared** with crystalloids (see below for the harmful effects specific to the hydroxyethyl starches).

3. **Transfusions** of blood and blood components are important for maintaining the oxygen-carrying capacity of blood and for coagulation. A detailed discussion of transfusions as a part of fluid management can be found in **Chapter 33**.

   a. Transfusion should be restricted in critically ill patients who are not actively bleeding and do not have evidence of ongoing myocardial ischemia.

   b. Patients needing massive transfusion should be transfused early with a 1:1:1 ratio of PRBCs to FFP to platelets for the best outcomes (see **Chapter 33**).

4. **Clinical use: Crystalloids versus Colloids.** The controversy over the ideal resuscitation fluid is an old one and is unlikely to be definitively answered in the near future. Nonetheless, in the last 3 to 4 years a number of large, well-designed trials have provided some guidelines for evidence-based fluid resuscitation—the recommendations below are based on our interpretation of these trials.

   a. The initial choice of resuscitation fluid should almost always be a crystalloid. In spite of the expected advantages of colloids at volume expansion, the data shows only a 30% to 40% decrease in total volumes infused with colloid-based resuscitation compared with crystalloids (rather than the expected threefold difference), over days to weeks.

| T A B L E **8.4** | Physiologic and Chemical Characteristics of Colloid Solutions |

Fluid	Weight–Average Molecular Weight (kd)	Oncotic Pressure (mmHg)	Serum Half-Life (h)
5% albumin	69	20	16
25% albumin	69	70	16
6% hetastarch	450	30	2–17

   b. Lactated ringer's (LR, or a balanced crystalloid) may be preferred in most instances to normal saline, even in the presence of renal dysfunction. With large-volume resuscitation, NaCl is associated with greater hyperchloremic acidosis, which may actually cause more hyperkalemia in patients with renal dysfunction than LR. In addition, accumulating evidence suggests that excessive chloride administration may be associated with worse renal outcomes, and perhaps worse mortality. One exception to this occurs in patients with neurologic injury, where resuscitation with relatively hypotonic fluids like LR is not recommended.
   c. **Hydroxyethyl starches (HES) are contraindicated in patients with severe sepsis** and septic shock. There is high-quality evidence linking HES solutions and worse renal injury and mortality in patients with sepsis. It is probably prudent to avoid HES solutions in critically ill patients altogether.
   d. Albumin is safe in most critically ill patients (**with the exception of those with head injury, in whom it worsens mortality**). The administration of albumin is not associated with improved outcomes in the broad population of critically ill patients. However, there are some groups of patients in whom albumin should be considered:
      1. Patients with liver disease and cirrhosis undergoing large-volume paracentesis
      2. Patients with septic shock and hypoalbuminemia. A recent study showed that keeping serum albumin levels >3 g/dL was associated with a mortality benefit in patients with septic shock (subgroup analysis of the ALBIOS trial).

III. ELECTROLYTES AND ELECTROLYTE ABNORMALITIES: SODIUM
   A. The normal range of serum (plasma) sodium concentration is 136 to 145 mEq/L. Abnormalities in serum sodium suggest abnormalities in both water and sodium balance.
   B. **Hyponatremia** is defined by a serum sodium of <136 mEq/L. Severe hyponatremia can cause central nervous system (CNS) and cardiac abnormalities, such as seizures and dysrhythmias. Hyponatremia can be classified on the basis of concomitant plasma tonicity.
      1. **Isotonic hyponatremia** (approximately 290 mOsm/kg H_2O) occurs when there are elevated levels of other ECF constituents such as protein and lipids. This form of hyponatremia is also known as **pseudohyponatremia** and is an artifact of measurement due to lipid and protein displacement of volume for a given volume of plasma. Therapy for this hyponatremia is not required.
      2. **Hypertonic hyponatremia** is due to the movement of intracellular water into the ECF compartment under the influence of **osmotically active substances** (e.g., glucose, mannitol) with consequent dilution of ECF sodium. A common example of hypertonic hyponatremia is seen with **hyperglycemia,** which can decrease serum sodium concentration by approximately 1.6 mEq/L for each 100 mg/dL of blood glucose. Removal of the osmotically active etiologic substance and restoration of volume are goals of therapy.
      3. **Hypotonic hyponatremia** is the most common form of hyponatremia. This type of hyponatremia is due to higher TBW relative to total body sodium. Hypotonic hyponatremia is further classified on the basis of the ECF volume status (hypovolemic, hypervolemic, and isovolemic). In all three scenarios, the extracellular compartment volume status

does not always correlate with the intravascular or effective arterial volume status.

a. **Hypovolemic hypotonic hyponatremia** can result from renal or nonrenal sources. In either case, water and salt are lost, but the loss of sodium is greater than the loss of water.

   1. **Renal causes** include the use of diuretics (particularly thiazide diuretics), osmotic diuresis, mineral corticoid deficiency/hypoaldosteronism, hypothyroidism, and, rarely, renal salt-wasting nephropathy, cerebral salt wasting, and certain types of renal tubular acidosis (RTA).

   2. **Nonrenal causes** include fluid losses from the GI tract, skin (burns), cerebral salt wasting syndrome, and intravascular volume depletion via third spacing.

   3. Renal and nonrenal causes can be distinguished by urine electrolytes. A urine sodium of >20 mEq/L suggests a renal source, while a urine sodium of <10 mEq/L suggests a nonrenal etiology.

   4. **The goal of therapy is to replace extracellular volume with isotonic sodium solutions** and to allow for appropriate renal-free water excretion.

b. **Hypervolemic hypotonic hyponatremia** is associated with congestive heart failure (CHF), renal failure with nephritic/nephrotic syndrome, and cirrhosis.

   1. **Mechanism:** In these disease processes, the effective arterial intravascular volume is low even if the total intravascular volume is normal or increased. The activation of the renin–angiotensin–aldosterone system and the sympathetic nervous system and the release of ADH lead to oliguria and salt retention. The result is expansion of ECF volume.

   2. **Manifestations** include edema, elevated jugular venous pressures, pleural effusions, and ascites.

   3. The **goal of therapy** is to control the primary disease process. Fluid and salt restriction and the use of proximal and loop diuretics may also be appropriate.

c. **Isovolemic hypotonic hyponatremia**

   1. **Causes:** Syndrome of inappropriate ADH secretion (SIADH), psychogenic polydipsia, medications (e.g., oxytocin), physiologic nonosmotic stimulus for ADH release (e.g., nausea, anxiety, pain), hypothyroidism, and adrenal insufficiency.

   2. Causes of SIADH include neurologic (head injury, subarachnoid hemorrhage, intracranial surgery), pulmonary (pneumonia, COPD, tuberculosis), malignancies, major surgeries (postoperative pain and nausea stimulate ADH secretion), and medications (desmopressin, cyclophosphamides, TCA, SSRI). It is important to **contrast SIADH** from **cerebral salt wasting syndrome**, a form of hypovolemic hyponatremia associated with head injury. **The volume status is the only way to distinguish between SIADH and cerebral salt wasting** in traumatic brain injury patients who are hyponatremic.

4. **Therapy for hyponatremia**

   a. **General guidelines:** Most patients with hyponatremia have a chronic electrolyte abnormality and will be mostly asymptomatic. Thus, if these patients require treatment, it would be a slow correction through fluid restriction (euvolemic or hypervolemic etiology) or isotonic saline/oral salt tablets (hypovolemic or diuretic etiology).

More aggressive therapy would be instituted in patients with symptomatic or severe hyponatremia, which would include hypertonic saline and potentially vasopressin receptor antagonists.

b. **Treatment of underlying disease:** If the patient is hyponatremic from adrenal insufficiency, administer glucocorticoids that will directly suppress the release of ADH. If the patient were hyponatremic due to reversible causes of SIADH (e.g., nausea, pain, anxiety), treat the underlying cause first. Iatrogenic/drug causes of hyponatremia should be approached by stopping the medication first.

c. Fluid restriction is an appropriate intervention for euvolemic and hypervolemic hyponatremia. The amount of fluid restriction is dependent on the level of urine output, but, in general, restriction to 50% to 60% of daily fluid requirements may be the treatment.

d. **Urgent intervention** is required in patients with symptomatic hyponatremia (nausea, vomiting, lethargy, altered level of consciousness, and seizures). The sodium deficit can be calculated as follows:

$$\text{Sodium deficit} = \text{TBW} \times 140 - [\text{Na}]_{\text{serum}}$$

The rate of correction of the serum sodium is important and must be tailored to the individual patient. Both delayed and rapid correction can be associated with neurologic injury. Safe correction can be achieved with **hypertonic saline (3% NaCl)** in euvolemic patients and with infusion of NS in hypovolemic patients. The rate of infusion should result in a correction of serum sodium of 1 to 2 mEq/L per hour for the first 24 hours or until serum sodium reaches a level of 120 mEq/L and then be reduced to a correction rate of 0.5 to 1 mEq/L/h.

e. The **vaptans** are active nonpeptide vasopressin receptor antagonists that are used in the treatment of euvolemic and hypervolemic hyponatremia including patients with chronic heart failure, cirrhosis, SIADH, or hyponatremia from other causes. Experience with these agents is limited, particularly in ICU patients.

C. Hypernatremia is defined by serum sodium of >145 mEq/L. Hypernatremia is also a description of total body sodium content relative to TBW and can exist in hypovolemic, euvolemic, and hypervolemic states. Hypernatremia could be due to water loss (more common) or increased salt intake without water. In all cases, the serum is hypertonic. Clinical manifestations of hypernatremia include tremulousness, irritability, spasticity, confusion, seizures, and coma. Symptoms are more likely to occur when the rate of change is rapid. When the change is gradual and chronic, cells in the CNS will increase the cellular osmolality, thereby preventing cellular water loss and dehydration. This process starts approximately 4 hours after the onset and stabilizes in 4 to 7 days. This change in CNS cellular osmolality is an important concept when considering therapy.

1. Hypovolemic hypernatremia

a. Caused by the loss of hypotonic fluids through extrarenal (e.g., skin or GI losses) or renal (e.g., osmotic diuresis and drug-induced) sources. There is loss of water and salt, with a greater proportion of water loss, which results in a decrease in the ECF volume and the effective arterial intravascular volume. Osmotic diuresis renally can be due to glucose, mannitol, or urea. GI losses include vomiting or osmotic diarrhea while skin losses include burns or perspiration.

   b. It is recommended that isotonic saline be used for initial volume re-pletion, followed by hypotonic crystalloid solutions, such as 0.45% NS.
 2. Euvolemic hypernatremia
   a. Caused by the loss of free water through extrarenal (e.g., excessive insensible loss through skin or respiration) or renal (e.g., osmotic di-uresis and drug-induced) sources.
   b. Measuring urine osmolality (Uosm) is important. Extrarenal pro-cesses cause a high Uosm (>800 mOsm/kg H_2O), whereas renal processes cause a low Uosm (approximately 100 mOsm/kg H_2O).
   c. In most cases of hypernatremia from free water loss, the intravascu-lar and extracellular fluid volumes appear normal. Therapy involves replacement of free water.
   d. Central and nephrogenic DI (see **Chapter 26**) are among the renal causes of euvolemic hypernatremia. Evaluation of urinary osmolal-ity (usually urine osmolality is less than the plasma osmolality) and the response to ADH may help to determine the site of the lesion.
     1. Central (neurogenic) DI can be caused by pituitary damage from tumor, trauma, surgery, granulomatous disease, and idiopathic causes. Central DI is treated with desmopressin (intranasal, 5–10 µg daily or twice daily).
     2. Nephrogenic DI can be caused by severe hypokalemia with renal tubular injury, hypercalcemia, chronic renal failure, interstitial kidney disease, and drugs (e.g., lithium, amphotericin, demeclo-cycline). Therapy includes correcting the primary cause if feasi-ble and possibly free water repletion.
 3. Hypervolemic hypernatremia is caused by addition of excess sodium and usually results from the infusion or intake of solutions with high sodium concentration. The acute salt load leads to intracellular de-hydration with ECF expansion, which can cause edema or CHF. The goal of therapy is to remove the excess sodium; this can be accom-plished by using nonmedullary gradient disrupting diuretics (e.g., thiazides).
 4. Free water deficit and correction of hypernatremia

$$\text{Free water deficit} = \text{TBW} * \left\{1 - \left(140 / \left[\text{Na}\right]\right)\right\}$$

   The correction of hypernatremia should occur at approximately 1 mEq/L/h. Approximately one-half of the calculated water deficit is adminis-tered during the first 24 hours and the rest over the following 1 to 2 days. Aggressive correction is dangerous, especially in chronic hypernatremia, where rapid correction can cause cerebral edema. Rapid correction is reasonable if the hypernatremia is acute (<12 hours). Neurologic status should be carefully monitored while correcting hypernatremia, and the rate of correction should be decreased if there is any change in neuro-logic function.

IV. POTASSIUM
 A. In an average adult, the total body potassium is approximately 40 to 50 mEq/kg. Most of the potassium is in the ICF compartment. In general, intake and excretion of potassium are matched. The electrocardiogram (**ECG**) is useful in diagnosing true potassium imbalance because the level of polarization of an excitable cell and the ability for repolarization are determined by the extracellular and intracellular potassium concentrations.

B. Hypokalemia: serum potassium concentration of <3.5 mEq/L. A general rule is that a 1 mEq/L decrease in serum potassium represents approximately a total body potassium deficit of 200 to 350 mEq.
1. **Causes of hypokalemia**
   a. Transcellular redistribution (increased entry into cells mostly through increased Na/K/ATPase pump)
      1. **Alkalemia** (a 0.1–0.7 mEq/L change per 0.1 U change in pH).
      2. Increased circulating **catecholamines** via β_2 adrenergic receptors
      3. Increased **insulin**.
   b. **Renal-associated causes**
      1. Without hypertension
         a. With **acidosis**
            i. Diabetic ketoacidosis (DKA) and renal tubular acidosis (RTA) types 1 and 2.
         b. With **alkalosis**
            i. Diuretics
            ii. Vomiting
            iii. Nasogastric suction (leading to hyperaldosteronism)
            iv. Transport defects—thick ascending limb: Bartter's syndrome; cortical collecting duct: Gitelman's syndrome
      2. With hypertension
         a. Renal artery stenosis
         b. **Hyperaldosteronism due to tumor (Conn's syndrome, adrenal adenoma)**
         c. **Glucocorticoid-mediated hyperadrenalism**
         d. **Pseudo-hyperadrenalism**
            i. Licorice ingestion
            ii. Cushing's syndrome
            iii. Liddle's syndrome
   c. Hypomagnesemia
   d. Acute leukemia
   e. Excessive GI losses
   f. Dietary
   g. Lithium toxicity
   h. Hypothermia
2. **Manifestations** of hypokalemia include myalgias, cramps, weakness, paralysis, urinary retention, ileus, and orthostatic hypotension. **ECG manifestations,** in order of progression of worsening hypokalemia, are decreased T-wave amplitude, prolonged QT interval, U wave, dragging of ST segment, and increased QRS duration. **Arrhythmias** are common, including atrial fibrillation, premature ventricular beats, supraventricular and junctional tachycardia, and Mobitz-I second-degree atrioventricular block (see **Chapter 17**).
3. **Therapy: IV potassium replacement** is appropriate in patients who have severe hypokalemia or who cannot take oral preparations. The rate of replacement should be governed by the clinical signs. The recommended maximal rate of infusion is 0.5 to 0.7 mEq/kg/h, with continuous ECG monitoring. **Hypomagnesemia** should be corrected prior to potassium repletion (see **Section IV.C**).
C. Hyperkalemia: serum potassium of >5.5 mEq/L.
1. **Causes** of hyperkalemia
   a. Hemolysis of sample
   b. Leukocytosis (white blood cell count >50,000/mm^3)
   c. Thrombocytosis (platelet count >1,000,000/mm^3)

      d. Transcellular redistribution:
         1. Acidemia
         2. Insulin deficiency, hyperglycemia, hyperosmolality
         3. Drugs (digitalis, β-blockers, succinylcholine)
      e. Malignant hyperthermia
      f. Cell necrosis (rhabdomyolysis, hemolysis, burns)
      g. Increased intake via replacement therapy and transfusions
      h. Decreased renal potassium secretion
         1. Renal failure
         2. Hypoaldosteronism
         3. Drugs: Heparin, angiotensin-converting enzyme inhibitors, and potassium-sparing diuretics
  2. **Manifestations** of hyperkalemia include muscle weakness and cardiac conduction disturbances. **ECG changes** include atrial and ventricular ectopy (serum potassium of 6–7 mEq/L), shortened QT interval, and peaked T waves. Worsening hyperkalemia will lead to widening of the QRS and eventually **ventricular fibrillation.**
  3. Therapy for hyperkalemia is emergent in the presence of ECG changes, particularly when serum potassium is >6.5 mEq/L. Continuous ECG monitoring is recommended. Therapy should begin in an ICU if the potassium levels show an increasing trend, even in the absence of ECG changes (see **Chapter 23, Section VII.C**).

V. ELECTROLYTE ABNORMALITIES: CALCIUM, PHOSPHORUS, AND MAGNESIUM

  A. **Calcium** acts as a key signaling element for many cellular functions and is the most abundant electrolyte in the body. Normal values of total serum calcium range from 8.5 to 10.5 mg/dL (4.5–5.5 mEq/L). However, because calcium is bound to protein (approximately 40%), the appropriate range of total serum calcium that can provide for adequate ionized calcium is dependent on the total serum calcium and the amount of serum protein (particularly albumin). The **ionized calcium** provides a better functional assessment, with **normal values ranging from 4 to 5 mg/dL (2.1–2.6 mEq/L, 1.05–1.3 mmol/L)**. Direct measurement of ionized calcium is commonly available and is superior to "corrected" calcium values based on albumin levels. Ionized calcium can be affected by the pH of the serum, with acidemia leading to higher ionized calcium and alkalemia to lower ionized calcium. Modulators of calcium homeostasis include PTH and 1,25-vitamin D, which increase calcium levels, and calcitonin, which decreases calcium levels.
  1. **Hypercalcemia (see Chapter 26):** A total serum calcium >10.5 mg/dL or ionized calcium >5.0 mg/dL (2.6 mEq/L or 1.29 mmol/L)
      a. **Causes** of hypercalcemia:
         1. Primary hyperparathyroidism
         2. Immobilization
         3. Malignancy (bone destruction from metastases or hormone secretion)
         4. Granulomatous diseases (tuberculosis, sarcoidosis), secondary to increased 1,25-vitamin D production by the granulomatous tissue
         5. Thyrotoxicosis
         6. Primary bone reabsorption abnormalities (Paget's disease)
         7. Adrenal insufficiency
         8. Pheochromocytoma
         9. Milk-alkali syndrome: High intake of calcium (>5 g/d)
        10. Drugs (thiazides, vitamin D, lithium, estrogens)

   b. Diagnosis
   1. **PTH levels**: low in malignancy-associated hypercalcemia, high in primary, secondary, and tertiary hyperparathyroidism
   2. **1,25-Vitamin D levels**: elevated in granulomatous disease
   3. **PTH-related protein**: elevated in malignancy-associated hypercalcemia (breast, lung, thyroid, renal cells)
   4. **Protein electrophoresis**: monoclonal band associated with myeloma
   5. Thyroid-stimulating hormone (TSH)
   6. **Chest radiographs**: evaluate for malignancy and granulomatous disease

   c. Manifestations: Hypercalcemia will affect multiple organ systems, including renal, GI, musculoskeletal, neurologic, and cardiovascular. Polyuria, nephrolithiasis, and nephrogenic DI are the renal effects. GI manifestations include nausea/vomiting, constipation, and pancreatitis. The patient will also exhibit muscle weakness, lethargy, and possibly coma. EKG abnormalities will include bradycardia, shortened QT interval, increased PR and QRS intervals, and atrioventricular block.

   d. Treatment is described in detail in **Chapter 26**. Here we summarize the main considerations. Treatment should be initiated if neurologic symptoms are present, total serum calcium is >12 to 13 mg/dL, or calcium/phosphate product is >75.
   1. **Immediate hydration** with NS to restore volume status and decrease serum calcium concentration by dilution
   2. After establishing euvolemia, a loop diuretic can be added to NS with the goal of generating a urine output of 3 to 5 mL/kg/h.
   3. Other electrolytes should be repleted.
   4. Hemodialysis, if the above therapy is ineffective
   5. The use of pamidronate, calcitonin, and glucocorticoids is described in detail in **Chapter 26**. Calcium-channel blockers can also be used to treat the cardiotoxic effects of hypercalcemia.

2. Hypocalcemia (see **Chapter 26**): an ionized calcium of <4 mg/dL
   a. Causes of hypocalcemia:
   1. **Sequestration of calcium** can be caused by hyperphosphatemia (from renal failure), pancreatitis, intravascular citrate (from packed red blood cells), and alkalemia.
   2. **PTH deficiency:** PTH deficiency can be caused by surgical excision of parathyroid gland, autoimmune parathyroid disease, amyloid infiltration of parathyroid gland, severe hypermagnesemia, hypomagnesemia, HIV infection, and hemochromatosis.
   3. **PTH resistance:** PTH resistance is due to congenital abnormality or secondary to hypomagnesemia.
   4. **Vitamin D deficiency** is caused by malabsorption, poor nutritional intake, liver disease, anticonvulsants (phenytoin), inadequate sunlight, and renal failure.
   5. **Inappropriate calcium deposition** can be due to formation of complex with phosphorus in hyperphosphatemic states (rhabdomyolysis), acute pancreatitis, and postparathyroidectomy.
   6. **Sepsis** and **toxic shock syndrome**

   b. Manifestations of hypocalcemia include generalized excitable membrane irritability leading to paresthesias and progressing to tetany and seizures. The classic physical examination findings include **Trousseau's sign** (spasm of the upper extremity muscles that causes flexion of the wrist and thumb with the extension of the fingers and can be elicited by occluding the circulation to the arm) and **Chvostek's sign** (contraction of ipsilateral facial muscles elicited by tapping over the facial nerve at the jaw). **ECG changes** include prolonged QT and heart block. Respiratory manifestations will include apnea, bronchospasm, and laryngeal spasm (typically seen after thyroidectomy or parathyroidectomy surgery). Anxiety and depression may also be noted as some neurologic indications of hypocalcemia.

   c. **Diagnosis**
   1. Confirm true hypocalcemia by checking ionized calcium and pH.
   2. Rule out hypomagnesemia.
   3. Check PTH level; if low or normal, hypoparathyroidism may be involved; if high, check for phosphorus level. A low phosphorus level is indicative of pancreatitis or vitamin D deficiency, while a high phosphorus level suggests rhabdomyolysis and renal failure.

   d. **Therapy of hypocalcemia:** Infusion of calcium at 4 mg/kg of elemental calcium with either **10% calcium gluconate** (93 mg of calcium/10 mL) or **10% calcium chloride** (272 mg of calcium/10 mL). A bolus should be followed by an infusion because the bolus will increase the ionized form of calcium for 1 to 2 hours. To avoid precipitation of calcium salts, **IV calcium solutions should not be mixed with IV bicarbonate solutions.** Calcium chloride is caustic to peripheral veins and should be given via central venous access if possible. Suspected vitamin D or PTH deficiency is treated with calcitriol (0.25 µg, up to 1.5 µg PO once a day). Oral calcium repletion with at least 1 g of elemental calcium a day should be given together with vitamin D therapy.

B. **Phosphorus** exists mainly as a free ion in the body. Approximately 0.8 g to 1 g of phosphorus is excreted in the urine per day. Phosphorus excretion is affected by PTH (which inhibits proximal and distal nephron phosphorus reabsorption), vitamin D, high dietary phosphorus intake, cortisol, and growth hormone.

   1. **Hypophosphatemia** occurs in 10% to 15% of hospitalized patients.
      a. **Causes**
      1. **GI:** malnutrition, malabsorption, vitamin D deficiency, diarrhea, and use of aluminum-containing antacids
      2. **Renal losses:** primary hyperparathyroidism, renal transplantation, ECF expansion, diuretics (acetazolamide), Fanconi's syndrome, post–obstructive and post–acute tubular necrosis (ATN), glycosuria, DKA
      3. **Redistribution:** alkalosis, postalcohol withdrawal, parenteral hyperalimentation, burns, and continuous venovenous hemofiltration
      b. **Clinical symptoms** usually occur when phosphorus is <1.0 mg/dL.
      1. **Neurologic:** metabolic encephalopathy
      2. **Muscular:** myopathy, respiratory failure, cardiomyopathy
      3. **Hematologic:** hemolysis, white blood cell dysfunction
      c. **Diagnosis**
      1. Urinary phosphorus <100 mg/d implies GI losses.
      2. Urinary phosphorus >100 mg/d suggests renal wasting.
      3. Elevated serum calcium suggests hyperparathyroidism.
      4. Elevated PTH suggests primary or secondary hyperparathyroidism or vitamin D–resistant rickets.
      d. **Treatment**
      1. Increase oral intake to 1,000 mg/d.
      2. Elemental phosphorus, 450 mg per 1,000 kcal of hyperalimentation

3. Dose of IV phosphorus should not exceed 2 mg/kg (0.15 mmol/kg) of elemental phosphorus.

2. Hyperphosphatemia
a. Causes
1. **Renal:** decreased glomerular filtration rate (GFR), increased tubular reabsorption, hypoparathyroidism, pseudohypoparathyroidism, acromegaly, thyrotoxicosis
2. **Endogenous:** tumor lysis, rhabdomyolysis
3. **Exogenous:** vitamin D administration, phosphate enemas

b. Clinical symptoms are related to hypocalcemia due to calcium phosphate deposition and decreased renal production of 1,25-vitamin D.

c. Treatment
1. Phosphate binders to reduce GI absorption
2. Volume expansion and dextrose 10% in water with insulin may reduce acutely elevated phosphorus levels.
3. Hemodialysis and peritoneal dialysis

C. Magnesium: Serum magnesium is maintained between 1.8 and 2.3 mg/dL (1.7–2.1 mEq/L); 15% is protein bound.

1. Hypermagnesemia is rare in patients with normal renal function. It is defined as >2.5 mg/dL.
a. Causes
1. Acute and chronic renal failure
2. Magnesium administration for toxemia of pregnancy, magnesium-containing antacids and laxatives
3. Hypothyroidism
4. Lithium toxicity

b. Signs and symptoms
1. Cardiac dysrhythmias
2. Decreased neuromuscular transmission
3. CNS dysfunction: confusion, lethargy
4. Hypotension
5. Respiratory depression

c. Treatment
1. IV calcium
2. Hemodialysis to remove magnesium in renal failure

2. Hypomagnesemia is defined as serum magnesium <1.8 mg/dL.
a. Causes
1. **GI**
   a. Decreased intake (chronic alcoholism)
   b. Starvation
   c. Magnesium-free enteral feedings
   d. Decreased GI intake due to nasogastric suction and malabsorption
2. **Renal losses**
   a. Diuretic therapy
   b. Postobstructive diuresis
   c. Recovery (polyuric phase) from ATN
   d. DKA versus hypercalcemia
   e. Primary hyperaldosteronism
   f. Barter's syndrome
   g. Aminoglycoside, cisplatin, and cyclosporine nephrotoxicity

b. Manifestations
1. Hypokalemia and hypocalcemia; hypokalemia is the result of excess urine losses, which can only be corrected with magnesium repletion.

        2. ECG changes mimic hypokalemia.

        3. Digoxin toxicity is magnified by hypomagnesemia.

        4. Neuromuscular fasciculations with Chvostek's and Trousseau's signs may be present.

     c. Treatment for hypomagnesemia should be initiated when ECG changes and/or signs of tetany are present.

        1. IV: with $MgSO_4$, 6 g in 1 L of 5% dextrose in water over 6 hours.

        2. Oral: with magnesium oxide, 250 to 500 mg four times a day.

VI. ACID–BASE PHYSIOLOGY: Acid–base homeostasis is essential for maintaining life. Significant acid–base derangements have major physiologic consequences that can be life threatening. However, it is the primary cause of the derangement that largely determines prognosis. Patients in the ICU often have important acid–base disturbances that require prompt diagnosis and treatment of the underlying condition and occasionally require symptomatic treatment of the acid–base disturbance itself. There are three major methods for quantifying acid–base disorders: the **physiological** approach, the **base-excess** approach, and the **physicochemical** (or **Stewart**) approach. In this section, we present a systematic approach to acid–base disorders relying primarily on the physiological approach.

A. Physiological Approach to Acid–Base Disturbances: The physiological approach uses the carbonic acid–bicarbonate system:

$$H^+ + HCO_3^- \leftrightarrow H_2CO_3 \leftrightarrow H_2O + CO_2$$

A primary change in $Paco_2$ causes a secondary (adaptive) response in the HCO_3 concentration and vice versa. Since the concentration of hydrogen ions in plasma is very low (approximately 40 nEq/l), the pH (the negative logarithm of the hydrogen ion concentration) is used clinically. H_2CO_3 is in equilibrium with the dissolved CO_2. The **Henderson–Hasselbach equation** describes the relationship between the pH, $Paco_2$, and HCO_3:

$$pH = 6.1 + \log \left\{ \left[HCO_3^- \right] / \left(0.03 \times Paco_2 \right) \right\}$$

Because pH = –log[H], the equation can be rearranged (this form is also known as the **Henderson equation**):

$$\left[H^+ \right] = 24 \times \left(Paco_2 / \left[HCO_3^- \right] \right)$$

The above equation can be used to verify the reliability of a blood gas value, using the $Paco_2$ from the blood gas result, and a HCO_3 from a simultaneously drawn metabolic panel (the HCO_3 value reported in a blood gas is calculated, not measured). The $[H^+]$ is roughly estimated by adding or subtracting 10 nEq/L per change in 0.1 pH units from 40 nEq/L. The four primary acid–base disorders comprise two metabolic disorders (acidosis and alkalosis) and two respiratory disorders (acidosis and alkalosis).

B. A Systematic Approach to the Diagnosis of Acid–Base Disorders: All steps listed below are often not necessary. However, this approach enables an efficient and thorough evaluation for patients with complex acid–base abnormalities.

     1. History and physical examination: A thorough clinical evaluation often provides important diagnostic clues. The medical history, including medications being taken, may predispose a patient toward specific acid–base disturbances. Vital signs, the presence of fever, neurological, pulmonary, and gastrointestinal signs and symptoms may indicate the severity of the disturbance as well as point to the type of acid–base disorder.

2. Determine the **primary acid–base disorder**: The pH defines whether the patient is **acidemic** (pH <7.38) or **alkalemic** (pH >7.42). The serum [HCO_3^-] (measured separately on a metabolic panel) determines whether there is a **metabolic acidosis** ([HCO_3^-] <22 mEq/L), or a **metabolic alkalosis** ([HCO_3^-] >26 mEq/L). The $Paco_2$ defines the presence of a **respiratory acidosis** ($Paco_2$ >42 mmHg) or **respiratory alkalosis** ($Paco_2$ <38 mmHg).

3. Define the **secondary** (or **compensatory**) **response**: The **predicted** $Paco_2$ for a given [HCO_3^-] or vice versa can be calculated (Table 8.5). The presence of a **mixed acid–base disorder** (i.e., two or even three coexisting acid–base disturbances) is suggested if the measured value is greater or less than predicted. For example, a patient with a pH of 7.16 with a [HCO_3^-] of 12 mEq/L has a primary metabolic acidosis. The predicted $Paco_2$ for this patient would be 26 mmHg. If the actual $Paco_2$ is 40 mmHg, the patient has a superimposed respiratory acidosis (even though the $Paco_2$ is "normal").

4. Calculate the **corrected anion gap** (**AG_{corr}**): For a metabolic acidosis, the AG is calculated ([Na^+] − [Cl^-] − [HCO_3^-]). The normal value is typically between 5 to 12 mEq/L, depending on the laboratory. Since albumin accounts for up to 75% of the anion gap, the AG should **always** be corrected for hypoalbuminemia (common in critically ill patients) to give the **corrected anion gap** (**AG_{corr} = AG + 2.5 × (4.0 − Pt Albumin (in g/dL))**).

TABLE 8.5	Simple Acid–Base Disorders and Compensatory Changes

Disorder	Mechanism	Primary Disturbance	Compensation	Compensatory Change
Metabolic acidosis, pH <7.37	H^+ retention or production; HCO_3^- loss	↓ HCO_3^- from 24 mEq/L	↓ $Paco_2$	$\Delta Paco_2 = 1.2 \times \Delta HCO_3^-$
Metabolic alkalosis, pH >7.43	HCO_3^- retention or production; H^+ loss	↑ HCO_3^- from 24 mEq/L	↑ $Paco_2$	$\Delta HCO_3^- = 0.7 \times \Delta Paco_2$
Respiratory acidosis, pH <7.37	$Paco_2$ retention	↑ $Paco_2$ from 40 mmHg	↑ HCO_3^-	Acute: $\Delta HCO_3^- = 0.1 \times \Delta Paco_2$; $\Delta pH = 0.08/10$ mmHg $\Delta Paco_2$ Chronic: $\Delta HCO_3^- = 0.4 \times \Delta Paco_2$; $\Delta pH = 0.03/10$ mmHg $\Delta Paco_2$
Respiratory alkalosis, pH >7.43	Excessive $Paco_2$ reduction	↓ $Paco_2$ from 40 mmHg	↓ HCO_3^-	Acute: $\Delta HCO_3^- = 0.2 \times \Delta Paco_2$; $\Delta pH = 0.08/10$ mmHg $\Delta Paco_2$ Chronic: $\Delta HCO_3^- = 0.5 \times \Delta Paco_2$; $\Delta pH = 0.03/10$ mmHg $\Delta Paco_2$

5. Calculate the **delta–delta (Δ–Δ) or delta gap**: In patients with a high AG metabolic acidosis, calculating the delta gap may help to diagnose a concomitant metabolic acidosis or a normal anion-gap acidosis. The delta gap is the comparison between the increase in AG_{corr} above the upper reference value (above 12 mEq/L) and the decrease in $[HCO_3^-]$ below the lower reference value (24 mEq/L). In theory, high AG acidosis is characterized by an increase in the AG_{corr} that is closely matched by a decrease in $[HCO_3^-]$. Thus the delta gap is close to zero (0 ± 5 mEq/L) in a pure AG acidosis. If the gap is **>5 mEq/L,** it suggests the presence of a **concomitant metabolic alkalosis**; if the gap **is <–5 mEq/L,** a **superimposed normal anion-gap acidosis** is diagnosed.

6. Calculate the **urinary anion gap (UAG)**: The UAG ($[Na^+] + [K^+] - [Cl^-]$) is a convenient surrogate for the excretion of urinary ammonium. The UAG is negative in extrarenal causes of normal anion-gap acidosis (e.g., diarrhea or ureteral diversion), whereas it is positive in conditions where urinary excretion of ammonium (as ammonium chloride) is impaired, such as renal failure, distal renal tubular acidosis (RTA), or hypoaldosteronism. In certain cases (urine pH >6.5, urinary $[Na^+]$ <20 mEq/L, polyuria), the **urine osmolal gap** may be more reliable.

7. Calculate the **serum osmolal gap**: In any patient with an unexplained, high AG acidosis, a serum osmolal gap should be calculated since laboratory confirmation of toxic alcohol (or propylene glycol) intoxication is often not rapidly available and may require immediate treatment. The serum osmolal gap is the difference between the measured and calculated serum osmolality (calculated serum osmolality = $2 \times [Na^+]$ (in mEq/L) + (Glucose in mg/dL ÷ 18) + (BUN in mg/dL ÷ 2.8)). Normal values are <10 mOsm/kg.

8. Measurement of **urinary [Cl⁻]**: History and clinical examination are often sufficient to determine the causes of metabolic alkalosis. In case of ambiguity, urinary $[Cl^-]$ may be measured. Urinary $[Cl^-]$ <25 mEq/L is typically associated with gastric fluid losses (**chloride-responsive alkalosis**), while values >40 mEq/L suggest inappropriate renal excretion of NaCl (hyperaldosteronism or severe hypokalemia; **chloride-resistant alkalosis**).

C. Metabolic Acidosis is caused by a primary decrease in $[HCO_3^-]$ due to one of three mechanisms: (a) buffering of a strong acid (endogenous or exogenous) by bicarbonate, (b) GI or renal bicarbonate losses, and (c) dilution of the ECF by large volumes of non–bicarbonate-containing fluids (such as normal saline). Note that lactated ringer's solution typically does not cause a hyperchloremic acidosis since the administered lactate is rapidly metabolized by the liver to bicarbonate. Metabolic acidosis is classified as high anion gap or normal anion gap (Table 8.6).

D. High Anion-Gap Acidosis

1. **Lactic acidosis** is common in critically ill patients. Conventionally, lactic acidosis has been classified as type A (associated with evidence of tissue hypoxia) and type B, or nonhypoxic (thiamine deficiency, medications [e.g., metformin, propofol, iron, etc.], intoxications [methanol, ethylene glycol, etc.]). However, it has become clear in recent years that in patients with septic shock, a significant fraction of the lactate is generated aerobically, via catecholamine-driven accelerated glycolysis and increased activity of the Na^+, K^+-ATPase pump. Some clinically relevant points regarding lactic acidosis in critically ill patients are mentioned below:

   a. Although the pathophysiology of hyperlactatemia is complicated, the evidence strongly suggests an **association between elevated**

| **8.6** | Classification of Metabolic Acidoses |

Anion-gap metabolic acidosis
Endogenous
  Diabetic ketoacidosis; severe ketoacidosis (alcohol, starvation); uremia; lactate
Exogenous
  Toxins
    Ethylene glycol, methanol, salicylate
Non–anion-gap metabolic acidosis
Gastrointestinal losses
  Diarrhea; pancreatic, biliary, and enterocutaneous fistulas; ostomies
Ureterosigmoidostomy
    Infusion and ingestion of chloride-containing salts: total parenteral nutrition;
      cholestyramine
RTA
  Distal RTA
  Proximal RTA
  Type IV RTA
Metabolic acidosis of renal failure

RTA, renal tubular necrosis.

      lactate and a poor outcome. This is true even in the presence of "high-normal" lactates (2–4 mmol/L) and even in the **absence of associated hypotension.**

    b. The AG_{corr} and **base deficit do not reliably predict** increased lactate levels—they are sensitive but not specific. The advantage of the AG and base deficit is that they are routinely reported and can alert the clinician to the possibility of metabolic acidosis, but if lactic acidosis is suspected, the lactate level should be measured.

    c. Some studies support using lactate clearance as a marker of adequate resuscitation. Given the complexity of lactate generation, however, it would be wise to consider the lactate levels in the context of the whole patient and not continue to administer fluids only because the lactate has not been normalized.

  2. Diabetic ketoacidosis (DKA, see **Chapter 26):** Insulin deficiency leads to excess hepatic ketone production and is treated by insulin administration. DKA is treated with intravenous insulin infusion and crystalloids to replace fluid losses form glycosuria-driven osmotic diuresis. Bicarbonate therapy is not recommended in children with DKA unless pH falls below 6.9 because of the association between bicarbonate treatment and cerebral edema. However, in adults, it is reasonable to individualize therapy (see below) rather than treat using arbitrary numbers. **Patients with a substantial hyperchloremic (normal anion-gap) acidosis** can benefit from bicarbonate at higher pH values.

  3. Starvation ketoacidosis: Ketones are present in serum and urine. Treatment includes refeeding and correction of associated metabolic and electrolyte abnormalities such as hypophosphatemia and hypokalemia.

  4. Alcoholic ketoacidosis: Seen in patients with chronic alcoholism and binge drinking. **A high AG and a normal lactate level** in such a patient may be a clue to alcoholic ketoacidosis since the test widely used to detect ketonuria (the nitroprusside test) **detects only acetoacetate and not**

β-**hydroxybutyrate,** the primary keto acid seen in alcoholic ketoacidosis. Treatment includes IV hydration, along with intravenous thiamine, glucose, and phosphorus administration.

   5. Intoxications and ingestions: Please see **Chapter 31.**

E. Normal Anion-Gap Acidosis

  1. Nonrenal causes:

    a. GI losses: Often seen with severe diarrhea, ileus, enterocutaneous fistulas, ostomies, laxative abuse, and villous adenoma of the rectum. Therapy includes bicarbonate replacement. Volume replacement is also essential as avid sodium retention by the kidney decreases its ability to excrete hydrogen ions.

    b. Ureterosigmoidostomy: Urinary diversion through the intestine can cause a normal gap acidosis, hypokalemia, and sometimes hypocalcemia and hypomagnesemia. These abnormalities are less severe when urinary diversion is done with ileal conduits.

  2. Renal causes:

    a. Renal Tubular Acidosis (RTA)

      1. Type 1 RTA:

        a. Mechanisms: impairment of the apical membrane H^+/ATPase and decreased ability to acidify urine

        b. Diagnosis: positive UAG, urine pH >5.5, low serum potassium, possible nephrocalcinosis and nephrolithiasis, filtered bicarbonate excreted <10

        c. Therapy: bicarbonate replacement (1–2 mEq/kg/24h) and potassium replacement

      2. Type 2 (proximal) RTA:

        a. Mechanisms: impaired proximal bicarbonate absorption with bicarbonaturia

        b. Diagnosis: UAG unreliable due to the presence of an additional anion–bicarbonate in the urine; urine pH <5.5, low serum potassium; filtered bicarbonate >15

        c. Therapy: high doses of bicarbonate (10–25 mEq/kg/24h), potassium, calcium, and vitamin D supplementation

      3. Type 4 (hyperkalemic) RTA:

        a. Mechanisms: selective aldosterone deficiency (common in types 1 and 2 diabetic nephropathy) and hyporeninemic hypoaldosteronism

        b. Diagnosis: positive UAG, urine pH <5.5, high serum potassium, percentage of filtered bicarbonate <10

        c. Therapy: treat hyperkalemia with exchange resins (as long as there is no ileus) and loop diuretics

      4. Renal failure: Renal failure can cause both a high anion-gap acidosis and a normal anion-gap acidosis. As the GFR falls below 30 to 40 mL/min, ammonium production falls below the level required to secrete the daily acid load, which is buffered by bicarbonate in the ECF, causing bicarbonate levels to fall. Normal-gap acidosis due to chronic renal insufficiency may be treated by oral bicarbonate supplementation to reduce the adverse effects of prolonged acidosis—muscle wasting and bone demineralization.

F. Physiologic Effects of Severe Acidemia: Irrespective of the cause, accumulation of H^+ ions can have important consequences, most prominently affecting the cardiovascular system. These include decreased cardiac contractility, arteriolar dilatation, sensitization to ventricular arrhythmias, and decreased responsiveness to catecholamines. The result is often severe hemodynamic instability. Other adverse effects include hyperventilation (Kussmaul breathing), respiratory muscle fatigue, increased pulmonary vascular resistance, hyperkalemia, insulin resistance, obtundation, and coma.

G. **Symptomatic Management of Severe Acidemia:** While the primary treatment of severe acidemia is the amelioration of the underlying condition causing the acidemia, on occasion it is necessary to provide symptomatic treatment and improve extracellular and intracellular pH to avoid hemodynamic collapse and to buy time for the treatment of the underlying condition to take effect. Symptomatic treatment is often required when the pH <7.15, and rarely if it is >7.20. However, decisions must be individualized, as certain comorbidities (e.g., severe pulmonary hypertension with right ventricular dysfunction) may require symptomatic treatment at higher pH values.

  a. **Bicarbonate administration** is often the initial buffer used to treat severe acidemia. The dose of bicarbonate is titrated to effect. Some have recommended the following formula to calculate the bicarbonate dose: Wt (kg) × BD (base deficit) × 0.3, provided as an infusion. In cases with identifiable bicarbonate losses, bicarbonate is therapeutic as well as symptomatic. However, bicarbonate administration has a number **of potential drawbacks:**

1. Some patients cannot eliminate the excess CO_2 generated by bicarbonate administration (either because of respiratory fatigue or because of the limits of lung protective ventilation), and in them bicarbonate may exacerbate intracellular acidosis.

2. Bicarbonate can stimulate glycolysis (by inducing phosphofructokinase) and increase lactate production.

3. It may cause hypernatremia, hypervolemia, and hyperosmolality.

  b. **Nonbicarbonate buffers** have been under investigation for many years, but only one—**THAM** (Tris-Hydroxymethyl-Amino-Methane)—is in clinical use. THAM is a more effective buffer than bicarbonate (its pK is 7.8, compared with 6.3 for bicarbonate), and it does not generate CO_2; it buffers H^+ by generating NH_3^+ that is eliminated by the kidneys. Thus, **preserved renal function** (or renal replacement therapy) is required for its effect. It also avoids a sodium load. The initial dose of THAM in mls (of a 0.3 molar solution) is weight × base deficit. The maximum dose is 15 mmol/kg, although the maximum dose is seldom required. Side effects of THAM include respiratory depression (not an issue in mechanically ventilated patients), hypoglycemia, and venous irritation. Hyperkalemia has been documented with THAM, and it should not be used in the setting of renal failure (unless on replacement therapy) and hyperkalemia.

  c. It should be noted that the data for the symptomatic treatment of acidemia are poor and no high-quality trials exist. Management is governed largely by physiologic principles.

H. **Metabolic Alkalosis**

  1. **Causes:**

    a. **GI Losses:** proton losses from the upper GI tract due to vomiting or nasogastric suctioning

    b. **Diuretics** cause a **contraction alkalosis** (reduction of the ECF volume around existing bicarbonate concentrations due to the excretion of bicarbonate-free urine) along with chloride and potassium wasting, which alter normal renal handling of protons and bicarbonate.

    c. Hyperaldosteronism causes metabolic alkalosis by increasing $[H^+]$ losses at the distal nephron.

    d. Other causes:

        1. Posthypercapneic alkalosis

        2. Hypokalemia

        3. Bicarbonate or citrate infusion. **Massive transfusion** can cause metabolic alkalosis (provided that the patient has been adequately resuscitated and has normal hepatic function) due to the citrate transfused with blood products.

   2. Management: Chloride-responsive metabolic alkalosis (see **Section VI.B.8**) responds to volume repletion with NaCl. Potassium repletion often ameliorates chloride-resistant alkalosis. Although treatment of symptomatic alkalosis with 0.1 N hydrochloric acid has been reported, it is extremely unusual in clinical practice.

I. Respiratory Acidosis is due to decreased CO_2 excretion resulting in a rising $Paco_2$ and a compensatory decrease in $[HCO_3^-]$. Hypoventilation results from decreased ventilating capacity, either in patients who **can't breathe** (neuromuscular disease, respiratory fatigue, severe obstructive lung disease, etc.) or in patients who **won't breathe** (altered responsiveness of the respiratory center to $Paco_2$ as in narcotized patients). Treatment centers on the underlying disorder. Occasionally patients with severe respiratory acidosis may require symptomatic therapy (see above). A fascinating recent approach to symptomatic hypercapnea is the **partial extracorporeal removal of CO_2**, allowing the use of very low tidal volumes (approximately 4 cc/kg) in ARDS.

J. Respiratory Alkalosis is due to alveolar hyperventilation. Hyperventilation may be due to a metabolic cause (fever), pain, anxiety, or neurogenic (head injuries or strokes) in patients with normal pulmonary function. Patients with intrinsic lung disease (pneumonia or pulmonary embolism) may also present with hyperventilation. Management is directed at the underlying cause.

K. The Physicochemical (Stewart) Approach to Acid–Base Physiology: Critics of the physiologic approach argue that the bicarbonate buffer system is only one of numerous buffers in the body and that changes in the bicarbonate buffers is reflective of the cumulative effect of multiple metabolic and respiratory processes. The Stewart physicochemical approach defines mathematically the determinants of acid–base balance in aqueous solutions on the basis of the laws of mass action, conservation of mass, and conservation of charge. The Stewart approach defines **three independent variables**, namely, **$Paco_2$, SID (strong ion difference),** and **A_{tot} (total weak acids),** that completely describe the acid–base status of a closed system. Other changes, including changes in $[H^+]$ and $[HCO_3^-]$ are secondary to changes in the independent variables. The details of the Stewart system are beyond the scope of this chapter. Its proponents believe that complex acid–base disorders are easier to understand and explain by the Stewart method and that it is mathematically sound. However, critics of the Stewart method contend that there is no evidence that patient management using the Stewart approach produces superior results compared with the physiological approach and that the Stewart approach introduces greater complexity without improving understanding. Using the stepwise approach to the diagnoses of acid–base disturbance outlined above (**Section VI.B**) provides a thorough description of complex acid–base disorders using the physiologic approach. For these reasons, the physiologic approach continues to be the preferred method of diagnosing acid–base disturbances at the authors' institution.

Acknowledgements

The authors of the current chapter gratefully acknowledge the contributions of Dr. Gauran and Dr. Steele, the authors of this chapter in the earlier (5th) edition.

Selected Readings

Berend K, de Vries APJ, Gans ROB. Physiological approach to the assessment of acid–base disturbances. *N Engl J Med* 2014;371:432–445.

Caironi P, Tognoni G, Masson S, et al. Albumin replacement in patients with severe sepsis or septic shock. *N Engl J Med* 2014;370:1412–1421.

Cerda J, Tolwani AJ, Warnock DG. Critical care nephrology: management of acid–base disorders with CRRT. *Kidney Int* 2012;82:9–18.

Finfer S, Bellomo R, Boyce N, et al. A comparison of albumin and saline for fluid resuscitation in the intensive care unit. *N Engl J Med* 2004;350:2247–2256.

Holmdahl MH, Wiklund L, Wetterberg T, et al. The place of THAM in the management of acidemia in clinical practice. *Acta Anesth Scand* 2000;44:524–527.

Kraut JA, Madias NE. Differential diagnosis of nongap metabolic acidosis: value of a systematic approach. *Clin J Am Soc Nephrol* 2012;7:671–679.

Kraut JA, Madias NE. Lactic acidosis. *N Engl J Med* 2014;371:2309–2319.

Kurtz I, Kraut J, Ornekian V, et al. Acid–base analysis: a critique of the Stewart and bicarbonate-centered approaches. *Am J Physiol Renal Physiol* 2008;294:F1009–F1031.

Perner A, Haase N, Guttormsen AB, et al. Hydroxyethyl starch 130/0.42 versus Ringer's acetate in severe sepsis. *N Engl J Med* 2012;367:124–134.

Rastegar A. Use of the $\Delta AG/\Delta HCO_3$ ratio in the diagnosis of mixed acid–base disorders. *J Am Soc Nephrol* 2007;18:2429–2431.

Yunos NM, Bellomo R, Hegarty C, et al. Association between a chloride-liberal vs chloride-restrictive intravenous fluid administration strategy and kidney injury in critically ill adults. *JAMA* 2012;308:1566–1572.

9

Trauma

David W. Fink and Peter J. Fagenholz

I. **INTRODUCTION**: Trauma remains a major cause of morbidity and mortality in the United States, as well as a major source of patients requiring intensive care unit (ICU) admission. The most recent data from the Centers for Disease Control lists "unintentional injury" as the leading cause of death for patients aged 1 to 44. Suicide and homicide are in the top five causes of death for patients between the ages of 10 and 44. The bulk of the critical care of trauma patients is similar to the care of other critically ill patients, but a few aspects are unique. This chapter will explain the initial evaluation of trauma patients, highlight some aspects of critical care unique to trauma patients, and address the care of specific commonly encountered injuries.

II. **INITIAL EVALUATION AND PRIMARY SURVEY, THE ABCS**: The initial evaluation of the trauma patient begins in the emergency department and should be complete by the time of transfer to the ICU, but the ICU provider should have some familiarity with this evaluation process. This standardized evaluation, promulgated through courses such as the American College of Surgeons' Advanced Trauma Life Support, is remarkably similar at different institutions. Hemorrhage and respiratory compromise are the most common causes of preventable trauma deaths, and the initial evaluation is aimed at rapid identification of these entities. Clinical evaluation is based on history, physical exam, and portable diagnostic adjuncts such as x-ray or ultrasound, which are immediately available in the trauma bay.

A. **Airway.** An awake, talking patient has a stable airway, unless there are other reasons to worry about the durability of that airway (e.g., bleeding, expanding neck hematoma, subcutaneous emphysema). Please see Chapter 4 for an excellent review and details of airway management, including rapid sequence intubation. Specific indications for securing the airway and considerations for managing the airway in trauma patients are described below:

1. **Indications for endotracheal intubation**
   a. **Glasgow Coma Scale (GCS)** ≤8.
   b. Respiratory distress with signs of potential impending airway collapse such as stridor or crepitus, expanding neck hematoma, or severe facial injury.

2. **Special situations**
   a. **Head injury**—In these cases, it is important to minimize the intracranial hypertension associated with laryngeal stimulation, the hypotension sometimes associated with induction regimens, and hypoxemia, as all of these can worsen outcome in head injury. No specific pharmacologic adjuncts have been proven effective.
   b. **Basilar skull fracture**—Nasotracheal intubation should be avoided to prevent inadvertent passage of foreign bodies into the cranial vault.
   c. **Suspected laryngotracheal injury**—Consider awake fiber-optic intubation in the operating room for awake patients who are controlling

their airway. Paralysis and direct laryngoscopy can precipitate an emergency. Whenever possible, surgical assistance should be available in case tracheostomy is required.

  d. **Maxillofacial injury**—In cases of severe maxillofacial injury, consider early placement of a surgical airway if orotracheal intubation fails.

B. **Breathing**. Victims of trauma can present with varied pathology that will affect their breathing including pneumothorax, hemothorax, aspiration, flail chest, and diaphragmatic rupture. Initial evaluation begins with a physical exam including auscultation of breath sounds bilaterally and palpation of the thorax to feel for crepitus or flail segments. Additional adjuncts include portable chest x-ray and chest ultrasonography. The most common initial interventions affecting breathing are tube thoracostomy and endotracheal intubation. In unstable patients with absent breath sounds, radiographic confirmation of pneumothorax or hemothorax is not necessary and only delays treatment; place a chest tube immediately. In cases of suspected pneumothorax or hemothorax without obvious signs on physical exam, either ultrasound or chest x-ray performed in the trauma bay can be used for immediate further evaluation. See the sections on pneumothorax, hemothorax, and pulmonary contusion below regarding further management of these injuries.

C. **Circulation**. Hemorrhage is the most common cause of circulatory compromise in trauma. Hemodynamically significant bleeding can occur in five locations, which are evaluated as noted below:

  1. **External**—physical exam
  2. **Thoracic cavity**—chest x-ray, ultrasound, empiric chest tube placement
  3. **Abdominal cavity**—ultrasound (focused abdominal sonography for trauma [FAST exam]), diagnostic peritoneal aspiration
  4. **Extraperitoneal pelvis**—physical exam, pelvic x-ray
  5. **Thighs**—physical exam, x-ray

D. Other less common but important causes of circulatory compromise in trauma include tension pneumothorax, pericardial tamponade, and neurogenic shock. Pericardial tamponade is most frequently diagnosed by ultrasound. Neurogenic shock from spinal cord injury is identified by the combination of bradycardia and hypotension and findings of lower body paralysis.

E. Once the "ABCs" have been reviewed, the patient should undergo a complete history and physical exam (the secondary survey) and will typically either travel for a therapeutic procedure (e.g., to the operating room or angiography suite) or to undergo further diagnostic imaging (usually computed tomography [CT]).

III. TRAUMA RESUSCITATION

A. **Goals of Resuscitation**. These are determined by the patient and the suspected injuries. Young healthy patients with suspected bleeding can undergo "permissive hypotension" while en route to definitive control of the bleeding source. If they are awake and mentating, they have an acceptable blood pressure. If they are sedated, we select an arbitrary but relatively low systolic pressure goal of 90 mmHg. Patients with suspected head injury or older patients who are more likely to have a higher baseline systolic pressure may not be candidates for this type of resuscitation strategy and have more standard resuscitation goals.

B. **Choice of Resuscitation Fluid**. Hypovolemia secondary to bleeding should be treated with blood products. The optimum ratio of packed red cells, plasma, and platelets remains an area of controversy. We favor a ratio of one unit of FFP for every two units of PRBC given, and consider platelets after the fourth unit of PRBC. We never consider colloid (albumin) in patients with head injuries or burns and rarely use it in the initial resuscitation of any patient.

IV. SPECIFIC INJURIES:

A. Head Injuries—For the critically ill head injured patient, a checklist approach to physiologic management goals may improve outcomes. Invasive intracranial pressure monitoring is typically utilized when the GCS is ≤8. Standard parameters include the following:

1. SBP >90—control with fluid boluses and/or vasopressor use
2. $PaCO_2$ 35 to 40—control with mechanical ventilation
3. PaO_2 >60, SaO_2 >90%—control with supplemental oxygen
4. Glucose between 90 and 150—control with dextrose infusions and insulin
5. Temperature 36.5° to 37.5°C—control with external warming or cooling, acetaminophen
6. ICP <20—control by mechanical or medical means
   a. mechanical (elevate head of bed, loosen c-collar)
   b. medical (analgesia/sedation, hyperosmolar therapy)
7. Seven days of antiepileptic therapy is also standard for patients with traumatic intracranial hemorrhage.
8. Presence of a head injury may impact the management of other concurrent injuries. Specific instances where head injuries shift management paradigms include solid organ injuries (splenic and liver lacerations) where the potential for continued bleeding and resulting hypotension and impaired cerebral perfusion may lower the threshold for intervention on the bleeding organ. Similarly, there may need to be a lower threshold for intervening on aortic pathology (dissection or contained rupture) with coincident head injury in order to liberalize blood pressure parameters and improve cerebral perfusion. Anticoagulation for blunt cerebrovascular injuries may need to be avoided when there is concomitant head injury.

B. Blunt Cerebrovascular Injury (BCVI)—Severe acceleration/deceleration or flexion/extension forces can injure the intima of the carotid or vertebral vessels, resulting in thrombus formation and risk of emboli/stroke. Finding this injury requires a high index of suspicion as there are usually no clinical signs or symptoms until an often catastrophic stroke has occurred. Screening CT angiography of the neck vessels should be utilized in accordance with the guidelines set forth by the Eastern Association for the Surgery of Trauma (EAST):

1. Patients presenting with any neurologic abnormality that is unexplained by a diagnosed injury
2. Blunt trauma patients presenting with epistaxis from a suspected arterial source after trauma
3. Asymptomatic patients with significant blunt head trauma and
   a. Glasgow Coma Scale score ≤8
   b. Petrous bone fracture
   c. Diffuse axonal injury
   d. Cervical spine fracture particularly those with (i) fracture of C1 to C3 and (ii) fracture through the foramen transversarium
   e. Cervical spine fracture with subluxation or rotational component
   f. Lefort II or III facial fractures

4. The standard treatment is full anticoagulation with unfractionated or low-molecular-weight heparin. While no head-to-head trial of efficacy of heparin versus aspirin has been conducted, aspirin 325 mg has been used as an alternative treatment for BCVI and is thought to be safer in patients with other risks for bleeding (head injury, liver laceration, etc.). Even when other injuries may preclude immediate anticoagulation (intracranial hemorrhage, solid organ injury), it is still important to know the full extent of injuries and competing interests to allow the care team to weigh the risks and benefits of interventions like antiplatelet agents or anticoagulation.

C. Pneumothorax

1. As previously stated, a patient with absent breath sounds and hypotension or respiratory distress should have a chest tube placed without waiting for imaging.

2. **Occult pneumothorax.** An "occult" pneumothorax is one that is found on CT but not seen on plain radiography. Previously, it was thought that any patient requiring positive pressure ventilation with a pneumothorax required tube thoracostomy. Randomized controlled trials have shown that positive pressure ventilation does not influence the progression of occult pneumothoraces. We no longer routinely place chest tubes for stable patients with occult pneumothoraces who will undergo positive pressure ventilation, but caregivers must be alert for progression, and we typically monitor these patients with serial chest x-rays.

D. Hemothorax. Posttraumatic hemothorax comes from the chest wall, lung, or intrathoracic vessels. Drainage allows for lung reexpansion and assessment of bleeding severity. Surgical intervention should be considered when the initial output is >1,500 mL, is >200 mL/h over the first 4 hours, or there is hemodynamic stability, as this degree of bleeding is less likely to stop spontaneously. If bleeding stops, and chest X-ray shows persistent effusion, chest computed tomography is useful to evaluate for retained hemothorax, which may be treated with intrapleural thrombolytics or thoracoscopic evacuation.

E. Rib Fracture. The presence of rib fractures should alert the intensivist to the potential for associated injuries including pneumothorax, hemothorax, pulmonary contusion, liver or spleen laceration, and diaphragmatic injury. Adequate pain control and pulmonary toilet are the cornerstones of rib fracture management. This can be accomplished with epidural, paravertebral, or intercostal nerve blocks, opioids, nonsteroidal anti-inflammatory medication, or combinations of these and other adjuncts. The goals should be normal tidal volumes, normal mobility, an effective cough, and secretion clearance. Patients with flail chest (two or more consecutive ribs fractured in two or more places) and respiratory failure or severe chest wall deformity may benefit from open reduction and internal fixation of rib fractures.

F. Pulmonary Contusion. Reticular opacities related to membrane thickening were first noted in World War II victims of overpressure "blast" injury. This is more commonly seen associated with blunt traumatic injury to the chest wall. Unlike most sequelae of trauma, pulmonary contusions usually take 24 to 48 hours to "bloom" and fully manifest. Management includes minimizing fluid resuscitation but even with careful fluid management, many patients will require intubation. Colloid resuscitation does not improve outcomes compared with crystalloid. Pulmonary contusion rarely presents as an isolated injury and is often associated with rib, diaphragm, and extrathoracic injuries.

G. Aortic Injury. This is usually related to a significant deceleration injury (fall from height or motor vehicle collision) resulting in a contained rupture of the aorta, most commonly immediately distal to the origin of the left subclavian artery. It is most often diagnosed by chest computed tomography with intravenous contrast. Surgical control of a contained rupture is nonemergent, but close control of heart rate and blood pressure should be maintained until repair, which can usually be accomplished with an endovascular stent.

H. Blunt Cardiac Injury. This injury is associated with significant chest wall trauma and manifests as hypotension and/or new arrhythmias. More significant, time-sensitive injuries like cardiac tamponade or tension pneumothorax must be ruled out before hypotension is attributed to blunt cardiac injury. Suspected blunt cardiac injury should be evaluated with an EKG and a serum troponin measurement. If both are normal, no blunt cardiac injury exists. If either an elevated troponin or a new arrhythymia are found, the patient should be admitted to a monitored bed for 24 hours. If either exists with hypotension or significant arrhythmias, the patient should be admitted to the ICU and undergo a trans-thoracic echocardiogram to look for a traumatic valvular lesion, tamponade, or segmental wall motion abnormality. Occasionally, inotropic support is required until the myocardium recovers.

I. Abdominal Solid Organ Injury. The spleen, liver, and kidneys are susceptible to injury (laceration, contusion, hematoma), particularly in blunt trauma. In the absence of hemodynamic instability or peritonitis, these injuries can be managed with serial abdominal exams and serial measurement of hematocrit. Large bore intravenous lines and reversal of coagulopathy are important in managing these injuries. If there are signs of continued bleeding, these injuries can be managed by angio-embolization or by surgery. There are no absolute values for minimum hematocrit, or number of units of transfused blood, or hemodynamic parameters to guide the decision to intervene on these injuries. Rather the clinician must evaluate the entire patient and how the solid organ injury affects management.

J. Pelvic Fracture. These can cause significant bleeding and rapid decompensation, and management should focus on large-bore intravenous access and reversal of any coagulopathy. There are three modalities for managing severe bleeding from pelvic fractures: pelvic fixation, extraperitoneal pelvic packing, and bilateral internal iliac artery angioembolization. In unstable patients, they are often employed simultaneously. Patients with extraperitoneal packing will require reoperation for pack removal. Since angioembolization is typically done with absorbable gelatin foam, a small percentage of patients with recurrent bleeding will require repeat angioembolization.

K. Extremity Compartment Syndrome. This secondary injury is related to swelling, crush injury, or periods of ischemia with reperfusion (tourniquet application, vascular injury, long bone fracture with or without vascular injury). Clinically, compartment syndrome will present as a tense compartment with the following:
1. Pain out of proportion to injury
2. Paresthesias
3. Pallor
4. Pulselessness
5. Poikilothermia (cooler than other extremities)
6. Paralysis (late finding)

7. This diagnosis is easiest to make in an awake, sober, cooperative patient. The level of suspicion must be high. Splints or plasters need to be removed for evaluation in at-risk patients. Typically, pain and paresthesia are the earliest symptoms. If there is any doubt about the diagnosis, compartment pressures can be measured directly with commercially available devices or with a transducer and large-bore needle. Although different thresholds have been proposed, surgical decompression is usually required when compartment pressures reach 25 to 30 mmHg and should be performed urgently.

L. **Cervical Spine Injury.** Most blunt trauma patients requiring ICU admission will have had a high energy mechanism of injury, such that the possibility of cervical spine injury must be considered. Many patients will arrive to the ICU with a hard cervical collar in place to provide in-line stabilization. For patients who are clinically evaluable (not intoxicated, no distracting injury), the cervical spine can be cleared by physical exam alone. If there is no posterior midline tenderness or no pain or paresthesia with axial loading, flex, extension, or rotation, there is no need for further evaluation. Patients who cannot be clinically cleared by exam should undergo CT of the cervical spine. When injuries are found, they can be treated appropriately (either with immobilization or surgery). When no injuries are found on CT, in-line stabilization is typically maintained until a clinical evaluation can be performed to assess for possible ligamentous injury. If patients are likely to be clinically evaluable shortly after CT is performed, it is appropriate to wait for the opportunity to examine them. If not, or if the physical exam is abnormal despite a normal CT scan, cervical spine MRI should be performed to evaluate for ligamentous injury. It should be performed as soon as feasible since prolonged cervical collar application is associated with a number of complications from pressure ulceration to ventilator-associated pneumonia.

V. OTHER CONSIDERATIONS

A. **Thromboprophylaxis.** Trauma patients are at high risk for deep venous thrombosis and pulmonary embolism. Because trauma can be associated with bleeding and significant tissue damage, there is occasionally confusion or reluctance about how or when to initiate thromboprophylaxis and what agents to use.

1. Mechanical prophylaxis is safe for virtually all patients and reduces the risk of DVT compared with no prophylaxis.
2. Pharmacologic prophylaxis is more effective than mechanical prophylaxis.
3. LMWH is more effective than unfractionated heparin.
4. Combined mechanical and pharmacologic prophylaxis is more effective than either alone.
5. Prophylactic IVC filter placement has not been proven to be effective in trauma patients. IVC filters should only be routinely used in patients with thromboembolism and absolute contraindications to therapeutic anticoagulation, and failure of anticoagulation when there is acute proximal venous thrombosis.
6. Immediate pharmacologic prophylaxis is safe in patients without a major hemorrhagic injury or intracranial hemorrhage.
7. Pharmacologic prophylaxis should generally be considered safe 48 hours after bleeding control in patients with hemorrhagic injuries or 48 hours after stable intracranial imaging in patients with intracranial hemorrhage.

B. **Damage Control.** Damage control surgery refers to the tactic of controlling bleeding and limiting contamination without necessarily performing definitive reconstruction at the time of initial operation in unstable trauma patients. This may involve using temporary packs to control bleeding, performing intestinal resection without anastomosis, or placing temporary intravascular shunts rather than performing bypass grafts. The ICU physician needs to understand the state of the incomplete anatomy (e.g., cannot provide enteral feeding to a patient whose GI tract is out of continuity) and the physiologic derangements (e.g., hypothermia, coagulopathy) that need to be corrected to allow for definitive treatment of the patient's injuries.

C. **Open Abdomen.** After laparotomy for trauma, the abdominal cavity may be left open for one of two reasons: (1) closure results in intraabdominal hypertension or abdominal compartment syndrome, or (2) a damage control operation was performed and early reoperation is anticipated to remove packs or definitively address injuries. The open abdomen is usually managed with a closed suction dressing. An open abdomen per se does not require neuromuscular blockade or cessation of enteral feeding. If the abdomen was left open due to concerns for compartment syndrome, multiple procedures may be required to achieve primary fascial closure. The key is to begin the closure process early before abdominal domain is lost. If physiologically tolerated, a negative fluid balance may also increase the rate of fascial closure.

D. **Tertiary Survey.** Patients undergo primary and secondary survey as above. Since these occur in the heat of the moment in the trauma bay, it is possible to miss non–life-threatening, but nonetheless significant, injuries. A repeated head-to-toe physical exam and review of systems (the "tertiary survey") has been shown to reduce the rate of missed injuries. Patients undergoing urgent interventions shortly after presentation who may have never had a complete secondary survey are at particularly high risk for missed injuries.

E. **Antibiotic Prophylaxis.** Trauma patients do not require antibiotic prophylaxis exceeding that of other critically ill or surgical patients. Penetrating injuries should undergo appropriate wound care and/or closure, but do not require prophylaxis per se. Periprocedural prophylaxis is appropriate for patients undergoing laparotomy or emergency tube thoracostomy, but even in the presence of hollow viscus injury, antibiotic administration should not be routinely extended beyond 24 hours.

VI. **SUMMARY:** The greatest immediate risks to trauma patients are hemorrhage and respiratory compromise, and the initial evaluation focuses on identifying and addressing these without the luxury of axial imaging. Once patients have been stabilized, further imaging and a tertiary survey are performed to identify all injuries. The bulk of critical care for trauma is identical to the care for any critically ill patient, but there are key differences in certain aspects of care (thromboprophylaxis, resuscitation strategies). Commonly, different injuries present competing management priorities, requiring the intensivist to actively evaluate and manage the entire patient and entire injury burden.

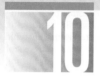

Critical Care of the Neurological Patient

Sarah Wahlster and Ala Nozari

I. INTRODUCTION

A. Common Problems and Diagnoses Requiring Neurocritical Care

1. Increased intracranial pressure (ICP) → requiring close monitoring, hyperosmolar therapy, and/or surgical intervention: related to edema (traumatic brain injury, strokes: posterior fossa or large strokes affecting the middle cerebral artery), lesions with mass effect (intracranial tumors, bleeding, and abscesses), hydrocephalus (mass or blood obstructing ventricles, disturbances in CSF homeostasis), CNS infections
2. Subarachnoid hemorrhage (SAH) → requiring close neurological and hemodynamic monitoring
3. Refractory seizures and status epilepticus → requiring intubation due to poor mental status, in the setting of sedating medications, or burst suppression
4. Infections of the CNS (meningitis, encephalitis) → requiring intubation due to poor mental status, ICP monitoring, seizure control
5. Neuromuscular disease presenting with respiratory failure (Guillain-Barré syndrome/acute inflammatory demyelinating polyneuropathy [AIDP], myasthenia gravis, amyotrophic lateral sclerosis) → requiring mechanical ventilation
6. Toxidromes: serotonin syndrome, neuroleptic malignant syndrome, benzodiazepine or alcohol withdrawal → requiring seizure control, close hemodynamic and cardiac monitoring, thermoregulation and intubation
7. Spinal cord injury → requiring close hemodynamic monitoring and management of autonomic dysregulation
8. Cardiac or pulmonary failure in the context of neurological injury
9. Impaired arousal with inability to maintain patent airways or need for mechanical ventilation

B. General Principles of Neurocritical Care: multimodal neuromonitoring (see Section II), neuroprotection, intracerebral hemodynamics

II. MONITORING

A. Neurological Examination: In general, minimize sedation and follow serial bedside exams, monitoring relevant parameters such as cortical, brainstem, and spinal cord function. In patients with status epilepticus or patients requiring sedation for elevated ICPs or pharmacological paralysis, the exam may be limited to checking brainstem reflexes.

1. **Red Flags:** *Pupillary asymmetries* (make sure patient has not been exposed to pharmacological stimuli such as atropine drops or nebulizers)—concerning for increasing ICP, ruptured posterior cerebral artery (PCA) or posterior communicating artery aneurysm; *Cushing triad* (combination of elevated blood pressure, bradycardia, and irregular respiration)—concerning for increasing ICP; *impaired upgaze*—concerning for hydrocephalus; *decreasing NIFs/vital capacity or decreasing strength affecting the neck and bulbar muscles*—concerning for worsening neuromuscular

failure; *meningismus*—concerning for SAH or CNS infection; *acute loss of reflexes and ascending paralysis*—concerning for progressive AIDP

2. **Document the exam** in a simple and easily reproducible manner, and report findings in the following order: cognition (level of alertness, orientation, attention, language: ability to express and comprehend), cranial nerves, strength, sensation, deep tendon reflexes.

3. **Start with a minimal stimulus** and then escalate as needed (whisper before yelling, give verbal commands before pinching).

4. If the patient has a gaze preference or neglect, stand on the side that the patient's gaze is turned towards.

5. **Cortical function:** In essentially all right-handed individuals and 70% of left-handed individuals, **language is processed in the left hemisphere** and **attention in the right hemisphere.** The **motor cortex** (precentral gyrus) controls the **contralateral limbs. Sensation** is processed in the postcentral gyrus of the **contralateral hemisphere.** The frontal eye fields direct gaze to the contralateral side, therefore a stroke (lack of stimulation on affected side) drives gaze toward the side of the injury (e.g., L-gaze deviation in a L-sided stroke) while a seizure (excessive stimulation on affected side) drives gaze toward the unaffected side (R-gaze deviation with L-sided seizure).

6. **Brainstem function:** The brainstem controls involuntary eye movements, pupillary function, facial sensation, and vital functions. Knowledge of its functions is critical in the evaluation of the comatose patient and the posterior circulation acute stroke syndromes (see Table 10.1).

7. **Spinal cord function:** In contrast to brainstem and cortical injuries, spinal cord injury often produces bilateral, symmetric impairment of the limbs but never facial weakness. Always distinguish anterior column function (strength, sensation of pin/temperature) from posterior column function (sensation of vibration, proprioception), document reflexes and sacral functions (anal sphincter tone, bulbocavernosus reflex). The aim of localization is to identify the highest level of injury.

   a. **Brown-Séquard syndrome** of hemicord dysfunction is characterized by ipsilateral loss of motor and proprioceptive functions and contralateral loss of pain and temperature (fibers carried in the spinothalamic tract decussate at the spinal cord level).

 Common Findings in Brainstem Lesions

Lesion Level	Common Findings	Anatomic Pathway
Midbrain	Midposition fixed pupils	Light reflex pathways
	Ophthalmoplegia	Oculomotor nuclei
	Hemiparesis, Babinski sign	Cerebral peduncles
High pons	Pinpoint, reactive pupils	Sympathetic fibers
	Internuclear ophthalmoplegia	Medial longitudinal fasciculus
	Facial weakness	Facial nerve
	Reduced corneal sensation	Trigeminal nerve
Low pons	Horizontal reflex gaze paralysis	Abducens nerve, horizontal gaze center
	Hemiparesis, Babinski sign	Corticospinal, corticobulbar tracts
Medulla	Disordered breathing	Respiratory center
	Hypotension, hypertension, dysrhythmias	Vasomotor center

b. **Anterior spinal artery syndrome** is characterized by bilateral symmetric motor weakness and dissociated sensory loss, with impairments in pain and temperature sensation and preservation of proprioception and vibration (fibers for the latter are carried in the posterior column, which is supplied by the posterior spinal arteries).

c. **Central cord syndrome** is common in cervical spinal cord injuries and characterized by motor and sensory impairment predominantly affecting the upper extremities.

d. **Cauda equina syndrome** is characterized by variable degrees of bilateral lower motor neuron weakness in the legs (sparing the arms), sensory loss of the lower extremities and sacrum, and dysfunction of bowel and bladder.

B. ICP Monitoring

1. **Intracranial compliance:** The skull is a rigid box filled with incompressible brain parenchyma. When the volume inside the skull increases, there is evacuation of cerebrospinal fluid (CSF) into the extracranial subarachnoid space followed by a rapid rise in **ICP** (Fig. 10.1). **ICP** is normally less than 10 mmHg (5–15 mmHg); transient elevations up to 30 mmHg are usually tolerated. When ICP rises above 20 mmHg (or **cerebral perfusion pressure [CPP]** falls below 60 mmHg), **cerebral blood flow (CBF)** may be inadequate. Pressure gradients may exist between different compartments of the brain and can lead to clinical herniation even though measured or global ICP may not be significantly elevated.

2. **ICP-monitoring devices and potential complications**

a. The most common device is an **external ventricular drain (EVD)**, usually placed in the right lateral ventricle. The ventricular catheter is connected to a transducer. The risks of complications include intracranial hemorrhage upon insertion and infection (the latter increases with duration of catheter presence). The great advantage

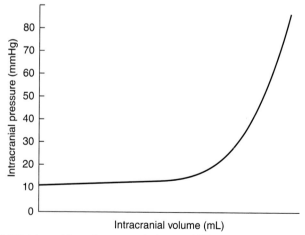

Intracranial volume (mL)

FIGURE 10.1 Intracranial compliance curve. In the normal ICP range; increases in intracranial volume produce minimal changes in ICP initially. Further small increases in intracranial volume at the "elbow" of the curve, however, can produce an abrupt increase in ICP. ICP, intracranial pressure.

is that this allows for drainage of CSF and can be recalibrated. Compared with other ICP-monitoring devices, EVDs are least susceptible to false readings over time.

b. Less invasive than EVDs are the transducer-tipped **fiberoptic intraparenchymal catheters,** which can be placed through a minicraniotomy. The device is placed several millimeters into the cortex but cannot be recalibrated once it has been placed. This requires special signal transducing monitors and may not be compatible with the available monitoring systems if patients are transferred between institutions. External transducers require periodic recalibration to remain accurate, sometimes called "zeroing" because of the task of zero calibrating to the level of the foramen of Monro.

c. In patients with temporal lesions, high ICPs at the level of injury might not be accurately measured by the monitoring device (which mostly capture ICPs in higher regions), so clinical judgment should be used when assessing the risk of herniation.

3. **ICP waveforms:**
   a. There are three components to an ICP wave: P1 (percussion wave) represents arterial pulsation, P2 (tidal wave) represents intracranial compliance, and P3 (dicrotic wave) represents aortic valve closure. Normally, P1 has the highest peak; if P2 > P1, there should be concern for impaired intracranial compliance and increased ICP in the appropriate clinical context (Fig. 10.2).
   b. Lundberg A waves ("plateaus") are characterized by increased ICP lasting >5 min, at times up to hours. They are pathological and strongly concerning for intracranial hypertension with the risk of herniation. Lundberg B waves are oscillations of ICP at a frequency of 0.5 to 2 waves/min. They have been noted in cerebral vasospasm and in the right clinical context can be associated with high ICP;

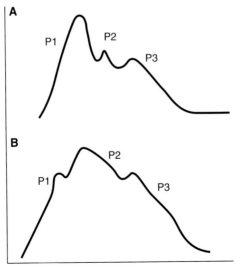

FIGURE 10.2 Intracranial pressure wave.

at times they can progress to Lundberg A waves. Lundberg C waves are oscillations with a frequency of 4 to 8 waves/min. They have been noted in healthy individuals and are of unclear clinical significance.

C. **Electroencephalogram (EEG):** Long-term monitoring (LTM) EEG is frequently used in the ICU with the goal to capture paroxysmal events, monitor patients with fluctuating or poor mental status (to evaluate the background and rhythm and assess for nonconvulsive status epilepticus), ongoing seizures, status epilepticus requiring burst suppression, or patients requiring titration of AEDs under EEG surveillance. Quantitative EEG may also aid in detecting small changes in the EEG that can correlate with changes in ICP or impending ischemia. New modalities are emerging, such as the compressed spectral array, which transforms the EEG into a succinct graphic display of changes in frequency and amplitude, allowing a simplified yet efficient screening of LTM data.

D. **CSF Microdialysis:** Microdialysis probes can be inserted into brain tissue and allow for serial sampling of physiological markers such as glucose, lactate, pyruvate, amino acids as well as drug concentrations. These measurements may provide information regarding impending cerebral ischemia and also allow for more precise adjustments in medications such as antibiotic or insulin therapy. These probes are gradually making their way from the bench to the bedside as research studies begin to explore their benefits.

E. **Brain Tissue Oxygenation:** Oxygen partial pressure measurements can be made using fiberoptic catheters placed within the brain tissue, usually as part of ICP-monitoring catheters. This type of monitoring provides information about local brain tissue oxygen levels. Additional probes can measure temperature and pH. Adjustments in cerebral perfusion, systemic oxygenation, temperature management, and transfusion strategies can be made to optimize tissue oxygenation, as indicated.

F. **Jugular Bulb Oxygen Tension:** Continuous monitoring of the jugular bulb oxygen saturation may provide information regarding global brain tissue oxygen extraction. Patients with jugular saturations below 50% (indicating a supply–demand mismatch) tend to have poor outcomes.

III. NEUROIMAGING

A. **Computed Tomography (CT):** used routinely, in many ICUs as a portable scanner, to evaluate for gross pathology (such as ICH, evolving strokes, mass lesion, edema, hydrocephalus) or perform an interval screening (to assess evolution of an ICH, large stroke, or midline shift). CT-angiogram is used to assess for clots and stenoses in the intracranial and neck vasculature as well as aneurysms. Given the relatively large contrast load, it is prudent to assess renal function before ordering CT-angiogram. CT spine can help rule out fractures and misalignments.

   Edema and ischemia tend to be hypodense, whereas **blood and calcifications** (the latter being brighter based on Hounsfield units) appear as hyperdense structures on CT.

B. **Magnetic Resonance Imaging (MRI):** allows for evaluation of the brain in greater detail compared to CT, but takes longer time to complete (challenging in agitated patients as well as patients with high ICPs who cannot tolerate being in a flat position for the duration of the study) and requires careful screening for contraindications prior to the study. Indications include characterization of masses (extent of spread, extra vs. intracranial location, pattern and degree of contrast enhancement, distinguishing tumor vs. abscess, degree of surrounding edema), the full extent of a stroke (also, strokes show up on the diffusion weighted sequence within minutes, whereas it can take up to 6 hours to clearly see them on CT), underlying causes of an ICH, degree of injury in traumatic and anoxic brain injury, degree of ligamentous injury in spinal cord trauma as well as lesions in the spinal cord. MR angiogram can also further characterize vessels. In patients with renal failure, vessel imaging can be obtained without giving IV contrast (time of flight sequence).

C. **Transcranial Doppler (TCDs):** dynamic study assessing the velocity of blood flow through the intracranial vasculature. It does not require contrast, is inexpensive and fast, and can be performed as a bedside study, but results can vary based on the operator. It is used to monitor patients with SAH to assess for vasospasm (manifesting as increased velocities), identify pathology within the circle of Willis (such as vascular stenoses, occlusions, turbulences, and retrograde flow) as well as an ancillary test for brain death evaluation (confirming absence of flow).

D. **Cerebral Angiography:** gold standard to evaluate the intracranial and neck vessels in detail. It is performed to better characterize aneurysms and other vascular malformations (such as AVMs and dural AVFs, whereas cavernomas are low-flow lesions that are not seen on angiography), to assess for suspected vasculitis and vasospasm. In some cases vascular malformations or vasospasm can be treated during the procedure (e.g. through coiling of the aneurysms or embolization of AVMs, or intra-arterial administration of calcium channel blockers, respectively).

E. **Nuclear Medicine Blood Flow Imaging:** useful for assessing cerebral perfusion in cases of suspected brain death, especially when factors that confound the clinical evaluation are present.

F. **Positron Emission Tomography (PET) and Single Photon Emission Computed Tomography (SPECT):** radioactive studies, used as adjunct tests to detect epileptic foci, assess the cerebral vasculature and perfusion and screen for dementia.

IV. BLOOD PRESSURE MANAGEMENT

A. **Ischemic Stroke:** In patients who suffer an acute ischemic stroke, in particular those with a proximal vessel occlusion (PVO), consider to allow blood pressures (BP) to autoregulate (stop antihypertensive agents on admission) at least for the first 24 to 48 hours. Assess carefully whether patients with a PVO or critical neck vessel stenosis have exam changes with varying blood pressures, and treat with vasopressors as needed to maintain perfusion of the penumbra.

After administration of IV tPA, systolic blood pressures (SBPs) should be maintained at <180 and diastolic blood pressures at <110 mmHg.

B. **Intracranial Hemorrhage:**
1. *Subdural and epidural hemorrhage, traumatic SAH:* SBP goal <140 mmHg
2. *Aneurysmal SAH:* Maintain SBP <140 mmHg until the aneurysm is secured (coiled or clipped) and then liberalize. If the patient develops vasospasm, vasopressors are used to further increase the BP in an effort to maintain perfusion.
3. *Intraparenchymal hemorrhage:* The optimal blood pressure goal is not clear with recent studies (INTERACT, INTERACT-2) suggesting that an SBP <140 mmHg is probably safe and may be effective in improving functional outcome. In some patients with chronically elevated BPs, SBPs should be controlled more cautiously to avoid end-organ damage due to decreased perfusion.

C. Hypertensive Encephalopathy and Posterior Reversible Encephalopathy Syndrome:
Maintain SBP <140 mmHg (with slower BP reduction in patients with chronically elevated BPs); start magnesium infusion in patients with eclampsia.

V. MANAGEMENT OF ELEVATED ICP

Treatment of increased ICPs should be initiated for sustained ICPs >25 mmHg or in patients with relevant clinical pathology at risk for herniation. In general, the head of bed should be elevated at 30° in patients at risk for high ICPs. Prior to central line placement, patients should be kept in that position until the last possible moment prior to puncture.

A. Osmotherapy: To date, mannitol is used more commonly than hypertonic saline (HTS); few studies have been performed to compare the two agents, with one recent article suggesting that HTS is more effective in lowering the ICP burden, leading to fewer days in the ICU. Avoid mannitol in patients with renal failure. HTS should be used with caution in patients with congestive heart failure as it can result in worsening volume overload: refer to Section VI.C. for formula to calculate plasma osmolality.

1. **Mannitol** (0.5–1.0 g/kg IV bolus every 4–6 hours) should be given to attain the minimum serum osmolality sufficient to produce the desired effects on the ICP, which often results in a stepwise increase in osmol gap (osmol gap = measured osm − calculated osm; normal <10). The goal of therapy can be continued until the osmol gap is equal to or greater than 15. Also, osmolality in excess of 320 mOsm/kg with mannitol does not produce incremental benefits and is often associated with an increased osmol gap and acute renal failure.

2. **Hypertonic saline (HTS)** may also be used to reach the desired osmolality by directly affecting plasma sodium levels. When administering HTS solutions, frequent serum Na assessments are required to avoid a rapid change in plasma Na concentration (which can result in central pontine myelinolysis). **NaCl at 3% concentration** can be given as either a bolus of 150 mL every 4 to 6 hours or as a continuous infusion of 0.5 to 1.0 mL/kg/h; **23.4% NaCl** is administered as a 30-to-60-mL IV bolus every 6 hours.

B. CSF Drainage: Draining even a small amount of CSF via the EVD catheter can significantly reduce ICP, especially with impaired intracranial compliance, although there is limited utility when the ventricles are collapsed.

C. Heavy Sedation and Paralysis: While sedation and paralysis are initially avoided in order to preserve the neurological examination, they can be used in patients with increased ICP refractory to hyperosmolar therapy. Agitation, posturing, and coughing are subsequently diminished. Barbiturate coma should only be considered as a last resort because of the serious potential side effects and because the neurological examination cannot be performed for several days or even longer.

D. Hypothermia: There is no clear data to suggest improvement of neurological outcomes when cooling patients with high ICP, but some studies demonstrate a reduction of ICP. Although not a first-line therapy (given the need for increased sedation and hemodynamic changes, and potential effects on the clotting cascade), it can be used as an adjunctive treatment for increased ICP refractory to other medical managements.

E. Hyperventilation: Hyperventilation decreases $PaCO_2$, which can induce constriction of cerebral arteries by alkalinizing the CSF. The resulting reduction in cerebral blood volume decreases ICP. However, with prolonged hyperventilation CBF returns toward normal as the pH in the CSF is restored. Therefore, hyperventilation should only be used as a bridge to more definitive therapies.

F. **Surgical Intervention:**
   1. If an underlying mass lesion (bleed, tumor, abscess, tension pneumocephalus) is contributing to the increase in ICP, urgent evacuation should be considered.
   2. Decompressive hemicraniectomy, allowing for herniation of the swollen brain through the bone window to relieve pressure, should be considered with rapidly increasing ICP despite aggressive medical therapy.

G. **Steroids:** While corticosteroids are useful in the management of vasogenic edema associated with brain tumors or other conditions that disrupt the blood–brain barrier, their utility in treating other causes of increased ICP is quite limited. Studies of steroids in stroke, intracerebral hemorrhage, and head injury have not demonstrated benefit.

H. **Medications That Influence ICP:**
   1. **Vasodilators** such as **hydralazine, sodium nitroprusside (SNP), nitroglycerin,** and, to a lesser degree, **nicardipine** can induce cerebral vasodilation. In patients with poor intracranial compliance, this can increase ICP.
   2. **Barbiturates** such as **thiopental** and **pentobarbital,** although typically administered to lower ICP, are also potent antihypertensive agents, decreasing venous tone and cardiac contractility. This usually undesirable side effect may require the use of adrenergic agonists such as **phenylephrine** and **norepinephrine** to maintain adequate cerebral perfusion pressure (CPP).
   3. **Hypo-osmolar and iso-osmolar solutions** such as lactated Ringer's solution and half normal saline in 5% dextrose (D_5 ½ NS) may exacerbate brain edema in the setting of osmotic diuretic therapy. **Glucose-containing solutions** may produce hyperglycemia and may lead to neurologic worsening after brain ischemia.

VI. SODIUM AND WATER HOMEOSTASIS

A. **Hyponatremia:** In patients with elevated ICP, hyponatremia can significantly contribute to additional swelling and potentially increase the risk of herniation. It is therefore important to maintain an appropriate Na goal, determined by the patient's baseline Na level, degree of intracranial injury, and evolution in exam. Check urine electrolytes (*before* initiating hyperosmolar therapy), volume status, fluid intake, and urine output to determine the underlying cause (volume depletion vs. syndrome of inappropriate antidiuretic hormone [SIADH] vs. salt wasting vs. other etiologies).
   1. **Intravascular volume depletion** remains a common cause of hyponatremia in the neurocritical care unit. Bladder catheterization and monitoring of CVP and plasma sodium are essential.
   2. Cerebral injury may cause release of **natriuretic factors,** leading to profound **salt wasting** that may require up to 200 mL/h of normal saline replacement or use of 3% solution in continuous infusion in addition to fludrocortisone (0.1–0.3 mg by mouth once or twice a day). This is seen most often in vasospasm after subarachnoid hemorrhage.
   3. **SIADH** should be treated aggressively with normal or hypertonic saline (3%) solution and loop diuretics when intravascular volume repletion is essential and fluid restriction is contraindicated.

B. **Hypernatremia due to Diabetes Insipidus (DI)** may be seen after pituitary tumor resection, traumatic brain injury, central herniation syndromes, and, occasionally, vasospasm following subarachnoid hemorrhage. **Hypotonic fluids** and **vasopressin** therapy may be indicated, and hourly monitoring of urine output and specific gravity is required.

C. **Osmotic Balance**

$$\text{Plasma osmolality} = (2 \times [\text{Na}^+]) + [\text{BUN}]/2.8 + [\text{Glucose}]/18$$

where BUN is blood urea nitrogen and is normally 280 to 290 mOsm/kg.

VII. TEMPERATURE REGULATION

A. The occurrence of **hyperthermia** after brain injury is very common and has been shown to increase the release of excitatory neurotransmitters, further the breakdown of the blood–brain barrier, and worsen clinical outcomes. The source of fever should be properly investigated and appropriate therapy initiated. Antipyretic measures such as the administration of acetaminophen 650 mg every 4 to 6 hours, surface cooling (cooling blankets, ice packs), and/or intravascular cooling catheters, should be instituted. **Normothermia** (temperature 37°C) should be maintained in all patients in the neuro ICU.

B. **Induced hypothermia** has been shown to be neuroprotective in global ischemic brain injury after cardiac arrest but not in focal brain injury, such as traumatic brain injury, ischemic stroke, and intracerebral hemorrhage. A large recent multicenter trial demonstrated that aggressive targeted temperature management at 36°C showed equivalent results in cardiac arrest patients compared with hypothermia at 33°C. Relative contraindications to cooling include intracranial hemorrhage, coagulopathies, active bleeding systemically, and hemodynamic instability.

VIII. GLUCOSE MANAGEMENT

Elevated blood glucose levels after acute brain and spinal cord injuries can increase tissue acidosis and edema in and around injured tissue and impair endogenous anti-inflammatory mechanisms of repair. **Hyperglycemia** has been shown to be a predictor of poor outcome in the intensive care unit (ICU) population and in many forms of acute brain injury. Hypoglycemia (<60 mg/dL) can also lead to focal neurologic deficits as well as anoxic brain injury, and glucose levels should be acutely restored with a bolus of **50% dextrose solution (D_{50})** along with 100 mg IV **thiamine** to the severely malnourished patient to avoid the complication of Wernicke's encephalopathy. Overall, the goal for care is to achieve normoglycemia (80–140 mg/dL) with the administration of insulin.

IX. MECHANICAL VENTILATION IN THE NEURO ICU

A. **Indications for Endotracheal Intubation:** Impairment of airway reflexes occurs frequently in the patients with neurological compromise and predisposes the patient to aspiration as well as poor clearance of secretions. Also, **neuromuscular respiratory failure** may be seen in amyotrophic lateral sclerosis, myasthenia gravis, AIDP, and critical care myopathy or polyneuropathy. **Transient apnea** in the setting of a self-limited generalized convulsion is not an indication for intubation or assisted ventilation.

B. **Complications of Endotracheal Intubation** include hypotension from anesthetic induction agents, reduced CBF, and increased ICP due to agitation or discomfort, or as a result of an increased transthoracic pressure. To avoid worsening cerebral ischemia, particularly in the setting of acute stroke and a proximal vessel occlusion, the BP goals for the patient should be clarified and ideally maintained even during induction.

    C. Considerations in Extubation: The ability to prevent aspiration and protect the airway is of utmost concern when extubating a neurologically ill patient. After confirming adequate cuff-leak oxygenation and spontaneous ventilation to support independent respiratory function, the clinician should evaluate the capacity for adequate airway protection. Ideally cough and gag reflexes should be present, and pharyngeal suctioning to keep the airway clear should not be needed more frequent than hourly and should not be increasing. In addition, careful evaluation of the swallowing and oral function should occur, especially in patients with facial weakness. Ask the patient to protrude the tongue, lick the lips, pucker the lips, and cough volitionally. While the patient does not need to be neurologically intact for a successful extubation, poor oral control may lead to rapid failure of extubation. Factors associated with successful extubation of neurological patients in a prior study include intact gag, normal eye movements, ability to close eyes, and cough to command. In addition, since hypercapnia may be poorly tolerated in patients with significant brain edema or disturbed autoregulation, the patient should be able to maintain normocapnia without ventilatory assistance, and the period of peak anticipated brain swelling should have passed.

    D. Permissive Hypercapnia is generally contraindicated in patients with intracranial hypertension or blood–brain barrier injuries because hypercapnia may result in unacceptable elevations of the ICP.

    E. Spontaneous or Induced Hyperventilation causes acute cerebral vasoconstriction if the CO_2 reactivity is preserved, decreasing **cerebral blood volume (CBV)** and thereby ICP. If autoregulation is preserved, an increased CPP may restore the CBF. **The brain quickly equilibrates** to changes in P_{CO_2}. A new steady state is established within hours in most patients. **With excessive hypocapnia,** excessive vasoconstriction may produce regional or generalized cerebral ischemia. Lack of response to hyperventilation is a poor prognostic sign.

    F. Neurogenic Pulmonary Edema: Within minutes to hours of CNS injury, there can be increased pulmonary interstitial and alveolar fluid (frequently seen in patient with SAH). This entity can be clinically difficult to distinguish from aspiration; however, fever and focal infiltrates are often absent. Although its precise pathophysiology is not completely understood, it is suggested that a massive sympathetic surge at the time of acute CNS injury may cause dramatically elevated pulmonary artery pressures and lead to capillary fracture with subsequent pulmonary edema, even though the pressures at the later time of measurement are no longer elevated. Supportive care and careful fluid management are required.

X. BRAIN DEATH DETERMINATION: Driven by advances in critical care medicine such as mechanical ventilation as well as the evolution of organ donation, the concept of brain death was first established in the 1950–1960 and further defined over the following decades. In 1995, the AAN published evidence-based practice parameters, updated in 2010, providing an algorithmic, unified, step-by-step approach to brain death determination. The key portions of brain death determination include the neurological exam, confirming coma and absent brainstem reflexes, as well as the apnea test, demonstrating absence of spontaneous respirations despite an elevated P_{CO_2} after inducing apnea (Figure 10.3). In some cases, when the exam and/or apnea test are equivocal or cannot be performed properly, ancillary tests are used, including electroencephalogram, nuclear medicine scan, CT angiogram, MRI, or transcranial Doppler. When performing the examination, the effect of sedatives and metabolic derangements should be taken into account as confounding factors.

Checklist for determination of brain death

Date and time_____

Prerequisites (all must be checked)

o   Coma, irreversible and cause known
o   Neuroimaging explains coma
o   CNS depressant drug effect absent (toxicology screen/serum levels if indicated)
o   No evidence of residual paralytics (electrical stimulation if paralytics used)
o   Absence of severe acid-base, electrolyte, or endocrine abnormality
o   Normothermia or mild hypothermia (core temperature $\geq$ 36° C/96.8° F)
o   Systolic blood pressure > 100 mmHg
o   No spontaneous respirations

Examination (all must be checked)

o   Pupils nonreactive to bright light
o   Corneal reflex absent
o   Oculocephalic reflex absent (tested only if C-spine integrity ensured)
o   Oculovestibular reflex absent (30-50 mL ice water each ear, observe 1 min, 5 min between ears)
o   No facial movement to noxious stimuli at supraorbital nerve, temporo-mandibular joint
o   Gag reflex absent
o   Cough reflex absent to tracheal suctioning
o   Absence of motor response to noxious stimuli in all 4 limbs (spinally-mediated reflexes are permissible, posturing is not)

Apnea testing (all must be checked)

o   Patient is hemo-dynamically stable and euvolemic
o   Ventilator adjusted to provide normocarbia ($PaCO_2$ 35–45 mmHg)
o   Patient preoxygenated with 100% FiO_2 for > 10 min to PaO_2 > 200 mm Hg
o   Patient well-oxygenated with a PEEP of 5 cm H_2O
o   Provide oxygen via a suction catheter to the level of the carina at 10 L/min or attach T-piece with CPAP at 10 cm H_2O
o   Disconnect ventilator
o   Spontaneous respirations absent
o   ABG drawn at 5 minutes
o   ABG drawn at 10 minutes (reconnect ventilator)
o $PaCO_2 \geq$ 60 mmHg **or** $\geq$ 20 mmHg rise from baseline

Pre-test ABG: pH___ pCO_2____pO_2____**Post-test ABG:** pH___ pCO_2____ pO_2____@____min

OR:

¤   Apnea test aborted (cardiac ectopy, O_2 sat < 90%, SBP < 100 mmHg)

Ancillary testing (only 1 needs to be performed; to be ordered only if clinical examination cannot be fully performed due to patient factors, or if apnea testing inconclusive or aborted)

¤   Cerebral angiogram   ¤   EEG
¤   SPECT   ¤   TCD

Time of death (MM/DD/YY & 00:00) _____**due to**_____

                                                                     (etiology of coma)

Name of physician and signature

                                        ¤   attending neurologist/neurosurgeon
_____   ¤   neurocritical care fellow

FIGURE 10.3 Checklist for brain death determination criteria, excerpt from the MGH Brain Death Protocol, most recently revised 03/2011.

Selected Readings

Adams RD, Victor M. *Principles of neurology.* New York: McGraw-Hill, 1993.

Anderson CD, Bartscher JF, Scripko PD, et al. Neurologic examination and extubation outcome in the neurocritical care unit. *Neurocrit Care* 2011;15(3):490–497.

Fisher CM. The neurological examination of the comatose patient. *Acta Neurol Scand* 1969;45(suppl 36):1–56.

Guarantors of Brain. *Aids to the examination of the peripheral nervous system.* London: Bailliere Tindall, 1986.

Mangat HS, Chiu YL, Gerber LM, et al. Hypertonic saline reduces cumulative and daily intracranial pressure burdens after severe traumatic brain injury. *J Neurosurg* 2015;122(1):202–210.

Nielsen N, Wetterslev J, Cronberg T, et al; TTM Trial Investigators. Targeted temperature management at 33ºC versus 36ºC after cardiac arrest. *N Engl J Med* 2013;369(23):2197–2206.

Plum F, Posner JB. *Diagnosis of stupor and coma*. 3rd ed. Philadelphia: FA Davis, 1982.

Ropper AH. *Neurological and neurosurgical intensive care*. 4th ed. New York: Raven, 2003.

Schwamm LH, Koroshetz WJ, Sorensen AG, et al. Time course of lesion development in patients with acute stroke: serial diffusion- and hemodynamic-weighted magnetic resonance imaging. *Stroke* 1998;29:2268–2276.

Suarez JI, ed. *Critical care neurology and neurosurgery*. New York: Humana Press, 2004.

Wijdicks EF. *The clinical practice of critical care neurology*. New York: Lippincott-Raven, 1997.

Wijdicks EF. Determining brain death in adults. *Neurology* 1995;45:1003–1011.

Wijdicks EF, Varelas PN, Gronseth GS, et al; American Academy of Neurology. Evidence-based guideline update: determining brain death in adults: report of the Quality Standards Subcommittee of the American Academy of Neurology. *Neurology* 2010;74:1911–1918.

11

Nutrition in Critical Illness

Rebecca I. Kalman and D. Dante Yeh

I. **INTRODUCTION.** The delivery of calories and protein to a critically ill patient should be considered a high priority that is integral to care, rather than a supportive afterthought. The goals of nutrition therapy include prevention of infectious morbidity, preservation of muscle mass, and prevention of metabolic complications. Choosing the appropriate route, timing, and dose of nutrition are crucial to achieving these goals.

II. **PATHOPHYSIOLOGY OF NUTRITION IN CRITICAL ILLNESS.** Postsurgical and critically ill patients are at risk for calorie–protein malnutrition. The response to illness includes increased energy expenditure, increased secretion of certain hormones (glucagon, glucocorticoids, catecholamines, vasopressin), and increases in inflammatory mediators (cytokines, acute-phase proteins).
   A. Fluid shifts occur due to water retention and increased vascular permeability.
   B. Increased glycogenolysis, gluconeogenesis, and insulin resistance result in hyperglycemia.
   C. Skeletal muscle protein is catabolized for gluconeogenesis, resulting in protein depletion.
   D. Resting energy expenditure remains elevated, and catabolism can continue for up to 3 weeks, even after resolution of the initial insult and despite adequate nutrition support.

III. **ASSESSMENT OF NUTRITIONAL STATUS.** The patients' medical history, nutritional intake history, physical exam, and laboratory data must be taken into account.
   A. **Clinical History.** Preexisting conditions such as unintentional weight loss, chronic disease, and alcohol abuse increase a patient's risk for protein–calorie malnutrition. The severity of the current illness, including the presence of fevers, burns, sepsis, or trauma, is associated with varying degrees of hypermetabolism and increased nutritional requirements.
   B. **Body Weight Measurements**
      1. Body mass index (BMI) = weight (kg)/height (m^2)
      2. Ideal body weight (IBW)
         a. Men (kg) = 50 + 2.3 (height [inches] − 60)
         b. Women (kg) = 45.5 + 2.3 (height [inches] − 60)
      3. Adjusted body weight (ABW) = IBW + 0.4 (actual weight − IBW)
         a. Calculate ABW if actual body weight is >30% of IBW
   C. **Nutritional Laboratory Indices**
      1. Baseline electrolytes, glucose, and liver function tests should be obtained prior to initiation of nutrition therapy.
      2. Albumin is a long-term marker of nutritional status with a half-life of approximately 21 days.
      3. Prealbumin and transferrin are serum proteins with short half-lives (2–3 days and 8 days, respectively).

4. It is increasingly recognized that low albumin and prealbumin are more reflective of acute inflammation in the critically ill patient. For this reason, initially low levels should be interpreted with caution and should always be measured concomitantly with C-reactive protein.

5. Trends over time are much more informative than single data points.

D. **Resting Energy Expenditure.** Energy requirements are difficult to estimate in the critically ill population. Predictive equations are commonly used but may over- or underestimate caloric requirements. Difficulties inherent in the surgical critically ill population include inaccurate weight assessments secondary to fluid resuscitation-related weight gain, inability to obtain an accurate nutrition history, and fluctuating metabolic needs throughout the course of illness.

1. Indirect calorimetry, also referred to as metabolic cart, measures the ratio of carbon dioxide eliminated ($\dot{V}CO_2$) to the oxygen consumed ($\dot{V}O_2$) by the body. This is measured over a 10-to-30-minute period to calculate a respiratory quotient (RQ). Patients must be intubated, breathing low FIO_2 (<50%), and without chest tube leaks for this to be accurate. They also should be hemodynamically stable and on a stable nutrient regimen.

2. Indirect calorimetry is recognized as more accurate than predictive equations and is recommended by the Society of Critical Care Medicine (SCCM) and the American Society of Parenteral and Enteral Nutrition (ASPEN) to determine caloric need.

3. A recent study (TICACOS) demonstrated superior outcomes when caloric prescription was guided by indirect calorimetry measurements, and a recent review concluded that "appropriately performed indirect calorimetry is really the only true means to set accurate goals for nutrition therapy."

4. With the use of noninvasive cardiac output monitors, indirect calorimetry may be obtained at minimal incremental time, effort, and expense. Best practice should include CO_2 production measurement for all mechanically ventilated patients *at the initiation* of enteral nutrition, *weekly thereafter*, and *as clinically indicated* to more accurately match caloric delivery to caloric needs.

5. The Harris–Benedict equation estimates basal metabolic rate (BMR) using a calculation based on gender, weight (kg), height (cm), and age (years).

E. **Protein Requirements.** Nitrogen balance can be calculated by measuring 24-hour urine urea nitrogen (UUN) to assess adequacy of protein intake.

1. Nitrogen loss (g/d) = 1.2 [UUN (g/dL) × urine output (mL/d) × (1 g/1,000 mg) × (1 dL/100 mL)] + 2 g/d.

2. Nitrogen balance (g/d) = [total protein intake (g/d)/6.25 (g protein/nitrogen)] − [Nitrogen loss (g/d)]

3. The goal is a positive nitrogen balance (anabolic state). Negative nitrogen balance indicates muscle breakdown (catabolic state), and protein intake should be increased.

4. An estimate calorie-to-nitrogen ratio is 150:1 and is provided in most isotonic enteral formulas.

IV. **COMPONENTS OF NUTRITION.** Caloric requirements should be fulfilled with protein, carbohydrates, and fat.

A. Protein provides 4 kcal/g. Protein intake is critical for muscle anabolism and maintenance of a positive nitrogen balance. It should consist of both essential and nonessential amino acids. The following are some general guidelines when calculating protein requirements.

1. Nonstressed patient = 0.8 to 1.0 g/kg/d
2. Postsurgical, mild *trauma* = 1.0 to 1.5 g/kg/d
3. Severe *trauma, sepsis*, organ failure = 1.5 to 2.0 g/kg/d
4. *Burn* (>20% TBSA) or severe *head injury* ≥2.0 g/kg/d

B. Carbohydrates should fulfill between 40% and 60% of total caloric needs. They provide 3.4 kcal/g.

C. Fat should provide 20% to 30% of total calories. Fat provides 9 kcal/g. Polyunsaturated fats are essential fatty acids and must be obtained from a dietary source.

V. INDICATIONS AND TIMING OF NUTRITIONAL SUPPORT

A. In previously healthy, well-nourished patients, nutritional therapy should be initiated if the expected illness duration without nutrition is expected to exceed 7 days or if the patient has gone without nutrition for 7 days.

B. In critically ill patients, nutrition should be initiated earlier due to the hypermetabolism and the catabolic consequences of the disease process. In the absence of contraindications, enteral feeding should be initiated within 24 to 48 hours of ICU admission.

1. Early enteral nutrition has been shown to be beneficial in patient populations in whom it was previously thought to be harmful: severe acute pancreatitis, hemodynamically unstable requiring vasopressor support, and open abdomen.

2. Current evidence suggests that enteral nutrition is safe and beneficial in these settings as luminal nutrients have been demonstrated to enhance splanchnic perfusion.

3. Feeding in patients with cardiogenic shock or rapidly escalating vasopressor requirements is more controversial, as increased splanchnic blood flow may compromise systemic perfusion. There patients should be monitored closely for hemodynamic and gastrointestinal tolerance. Caution is advised.

4. Patients with preexisting malnourishment or severe weight loss will also benefit from early nutritional support utilizing supplemental parenteral nutrition (PN) if unable to deliver >80% of nutrient requirements by ICU day 3.

VI. ENTERAL NUTRITION VERSUS PARENTERAL NUTRITION

A. Enteral nutrition (EN) is preferred over parenteral nutrition (PN) in patients with a functional GI tract. EN reduces infectious complications, improves wound healing, decreases GI mucosal permeability (and bacterial translocation), and is more cost effective than PN.

B. Even in patients unable to tolerate enteral nutrition at sufficient rates to fulfill their caloric needs, "trophic" tube feeds (10–20 cc/h) can provide non-nutritional benefits such as maintaining muscosal integrity, immune function, and preventing ileus.

C. For patients who cannot tolerate enteric feeds (i.e., prolonged ileus, intestinal obstruction or perforation, high-output enterocutaneous fistula) parenteral nutrition may be required. For previously well-nourished patients with these conditions, late initiation of PN (day 8 vs. day 3) has been shown to be associated with fewer infections, enhanced recovery, and decreased cost compared to early initiation.

VII. DELIVERY ROUTE OF ENTERAL NUTRITION. Nasogastric or nasoenteric tubes may be used for short-term enteral nutritional support (<1 month).

Postpyloric tubes may be helpful if gastroparesis prevents tolerance of gastric feeds, but have not been associated with lower rates of aspiration or delayed gastric emptying when compared with gastric feeding.

A. Placement of postpyloric tubes may be done blindly, endoscopically, or with fluoroscopic guidance.

  1. Blind **placement of stiletted postpyloric tubes** must be done cautiously and by experienced clinicians. When inserted in sedated, mechanically ventilated patients, these soft and sharp-tipped tubes may enter the airway instead of the GI tract. Complications include pneumothorax and lung infection/abscess secondary to infusion of tube feeds into the airway.

  2. Confirmatory radiographs must *always* be performed prior to initiation of enteral nutrition through a newly inserted feeding tube, as other methods confirmation, such as aspiration of gastric contents and auscultation are insufficiently accurate.

  3. Surgical placement of a gastric or jejunal feeding tube (i.e., nonoral access) is indicated for long-term nutritional support (>1 month) and may be achieved endoscopically, fluoroscopically, or surgically.

VIII. **IMMUNONUTRITION** is the modulation of the immune system through the supplementation of select nutrients. Several nutrients have been studied; however, data have been conflicting regarding the use of immune-enhancing formulas in critically ill patients.

A. **Glutamine:** the most abundant nonessential amino acid. It is synthesized predominantly in skeletal muscle and is involved in numerous essential functions such as nitrogen transport, neutrophil function, acid–base balance and is the preferred fuel source for rapidly dividing cells in the intestinal tract and the immune system. In a randomized trial (REDOX study), early provision of glutamine was associated with an increase in mortality in patients with multiorgan failure. Data on glutamine supplementation in specific patient subsets have been conflicting. For these reasons, supplementation with glutamine in critically ill patients is not recommended.

B. **Arginine:** a conditionally essential amino acid in periods of stress and has important roles in nitrogen metabolism and formation of nitric acid. Arginine may exacerbate the systemic inflammatory response syndrome (SIRS) and is not recommended in septic patients.

C. **Fatty Acids:** although some fatty acids have been hypothesized to have anti-inflammatory or proinflammatory effects, there is no high-quality evidence supporting the routine use of specific lipids in critically ill patients.

D. **Micronutrients:** administration of trace elements (selenium, copper, manganese, zinc, iron, vitamins E and C) has been proposed to reduce oxidative cellular damage. Standard enteral formulas and parental preparations are usually sufficient, and additional supplementation is rarely required.

IX. **PARENTERAL NUTRITION (PN)** is indicated in patients who require aggressive nutritional support but cannot tolerate enteral nutrition.

A. Peripheral parenteral nutrition (PPN) provides partial nutritional support and can be administered through a peripheral vein due to lower osmotic solutions (<900 mOsm/L). Dextrose, lipids, and proteins can all be given peripherally, but require a large volume of infusion and will not meet total metabolic demands. PPN is rarely utilized in the SICU.

B. Total parenteral nutrition (TPN) contains higher concentrations of dextrose and amino acids to meet total metabolic demands and is therefore hypertonic (requires central venous access).

C. The risk–benefit ratio of PPN has been questioned because it is associated with the same risk of immunosuppression and increased risk of infections as TPN, but without the benefit of total nutritional support.

D. Components of TPN include the following:

1. D-glucose (dextrose) the major source of non-protein calories (3.4 kcal/g). Maximum daily administration is 5 to 7 g/kg/d. Exceeding this maximum rate of glucose oxidation may result in lipid synthesis with CO_2 accumulation and hepatic steatosis.

2. Lipid emulsion is another source of nonprotein calories (9 kcal/g) and also provides essential fatty acids (ω-6 and ω-3 polyunsaturated fats). Maximum administration of lipid emulsion is 2.5 g/kg and should comprise <30% of total calories. Lipid emulsions provide 1.1 kcal/mL (for 10% IV emulsion), 2.0 kcal/mL (for 20% IV emulsion), and 3.0 kcal/mL (for 30% IV emulsion). Avoid infusion >110 mg/kg/h because of neutrophils and monocytes impairment and worsening gas exchange.

3. Amino acids (essential and nonessential) are needed to build muscle and maintain a positive nitrogen balance, but also are a source of calories (4 kcal/g). As in EN, protein requirements should be calculated on the basis of stress level and monitored with weekly UUN and nitrogen balance.

E. Calculation of TPN Formulation (Table 11.1)

1. Calculate total calorie requirements.

2. Estimate protein requirements.

3. Calculate maximum carbohydrate and lipid amounts and provide these "nonprotein calories" in a ratio of 70:30 (ideal).

4. Fluid/volume requirements average 30 mL/kg/d, but daily weight and strict measurement of fluid losses (urine, stool, insensible losses) help monitor fluid status.

5. Electrolytes, minerals, vitamins, and trace elements should be added according to usual or recommended doses (Table 11.2). Adjustments may be needed in critical illness, or with certain disease states

TABLE 11.1   Calculation of Total TPN

Component	Calorie Conversion	RQ	Maximum Daily Administration	% Total Calories
Amino acids	4 kcal/g	0.8	0.8–1.0 g/kg (normal) 1.25–1.5 g/kg (postsurgery, mild trauma) 1.5–2.0 g/kg (severe trauma, sepsis, organ failure) >2.0 g/kg (>20% TBSA burn, severe head injury)	15%–25%
Dextrose	3.4 kcal/g	1.0	5–7 g/kg (350–500 g or 1,190–1,700 kcal in 70 kg)	40%–60%
Lipids	9 kcal/g	0.7	2.5 g/kg[a] (175 g or 1,575 kcal in 70 kg)	20%–30%[b]
Total calories			25 kcal/kg plus stress factor (1,750 + kcal in 70 kg)	
Fluid/volume			25 kcal/kg plus stress factor	

[a] Critically ill patients may not be able to oxidize more than 1–1.5 g/kg/d.
[b] 70:30 ratio of nonprotein calories (carbohydrate:lipid).
RQ, respiratory quotient; TBSA, total body surface area.

TABLE 11.2	Additives to TPN

Additive	Recommended or Usual Daily Dose
Electrolytes	
Sodium	100–150 mEq/d
Potassium	60–120 mEq/d
Calcium gluconate	10–20 mEq/d
Phosphate	15–30 mM/d
Magnesium	8–24 mEq/d
Chloride or acetate[a]	Anion for sodium and potassium
Vitamins	
Vitamin C (ascorbic acid)	75–70 mg/d
Vitamin A	3,300 IU/d
Vitamin D	400 IU/d
Thiamine (B_1)	1.1–1.2 mg/d
Pyridoxine (B_6)	1.3–1.7 mg/d
Riboflavin (B_2)	1.1–1.3 mg/d
Niacin	14–16 mg/d
Pantothenic acid	5 mg/d
Vitamin E	15 mg/d
Biotin	30 µg/d
Folic acid	400 µg/d
Vitamin B_{12}	2.4 µg/d
Vitamin K	90–120 µg/d
Trace Elements	
Zinc	8–11 mg/d
Copper	900 µg/d
Manganese	1.8–2.3 mg/d
Chromium	20–35 µg/d
Selenium	55 µg/d

[a] Chloride can produce a metabolic acidosis; use acetate for patients with metabolic acidosis (converted to bicarbonate in the liver).

(i.e., renal failure or high-output fistula), and serum levels should be monitored routine.
6. Insulin can be added directly to TPN solution (up to half of daily sliding scale insulin requirement)

X. **ENTERAL FORMULAS.** Common enteral formulas used at the Massachusetts General Hospital are shown in Table 11.3. They vary by proportion of carbohydrate, protein, and fat, as well as caloric concentration, osmolality, elemental components, and various additives. Several formulas are particularly designed for certain patient populations (i.e., pulmonary or renal disease).

XI. **NUTRITIONAL MODIFICATIONS IN DISEASE.** Routine use of disease-specific formulas has not been shown to improve outcomes. However, there are nutrition-specific considerations in certain disease states.
A. **Diabetes:** low simple sugar, high fiber, and high fat to minimize hyperglycemia

B. Renal Failure: high concentration, low volume (to prevent volume overload), low electrolytes (phosphorus, potassium)

C. Acute Kidney Injury (AKI): a metabolic stressor that increases protein requirements. Deliberate underprovision of protein to a patient with AKI in order to avoid renal replacement therapy (RRT) is inappropriate. Up to 20% of serum amino acids are lost across the dialysate membrane and thus must be compensated for. For this reason, patients on continuous RRT should be given standard enteral formulas and not renal failure-specific formulas.

D. Liver Failure. Low-protein, high-branched chain amino acids have been developed to prevent encephalopathy, though their efficacy is questionable in critically ill patients. In general, protein delivery should not be restricted in the ICU for fear of precipitating hepatic encephalopathy.

E. Respiratory Failure. Overfeeding can lead to increased CO_2 and difficulty with ventilator weaning. Low-carbohydrate formulas have been developed, though they should not be used routinely. Concentrated formulas may be considered in patients at risk for pulmonary edema.

F. Pancreatitis. Enteral feeding is currently considered superior to TPN in severe acute pancreatitis. Though the majority of patients will tolerate gastric feeding, some will require postpyloric feeding or even more distal feeding beyond the ligament of Treitz. In the setting of exocrine insufficiency, some patients may better tolerate iso-osmolar or elemental tube feeds. Pancreatic enzyme replacement (e.g., Creon, Pancrease) may be required to assist in digestion.

G. Trauma. An "open abdomen"/temporary abdominal closure should not preclude enteral nutrition as long as the GI tract remains in continuity. Evidence suggests that early enteral nutrition with an open abdomen is associated with higher rates of facial closure and decreased infectious complications.

H. Burns. There is markedly elevated protein loss and may require up to 2.5 g/kg/day. Trace elements should be provided in higher-than-standard doses.

I. Obesity. Obesity and malnutrition can and often coexist. Calculations should be based on adjusted body weight (ABW) as ideal body weight (IBW), and actual body weight may under- or overestimate nutrient needs. Adequate protein delivery (>2.0 g/kg/d) is required even if a "hypocaloric" feeding strategy is undertaken.

XII. MONITORING OF NUTRITION. After initiation of nutritional support, basic laboratory values should be monitored to assess adequacy of nutrition and detect potential complications.

A. Baseline laboratory data should include the following:
   1. Glucose, electrolytes, liver function tests, albumin, prealbumin, transferrin, CRP
   2. UUN: to ensure adequacy of protein intake and prevent catabolic state (muscle breakdown)
   3. Triglyceride levels in patients receiving fat in emulsions. Levels greater than 500 mg/dL should prompt a decrease rate of infusion due to risk of pancreatitis.
   4. Low phosphate is usually indicative of benign refeeding hypophosphatemia but may indicate refeeding syndrome. In malnourished patients, initiation of nutrition can lead to increased utilization and depletion of phosphate, potassium, and magnesium, which in extreme cases can lead to arrhythmias, heart failure, and neurologic disturbances.

TABLE 11.3

Enteral Formulas

Massachusetts General Hospital Enteral Formulas

	Osmolite	Osmolite HN	Jevity Plus	Ensure Plus HN	Twocal HN	Glucerna	Promote with Fiber
Calories/mL	1.06	1.06	1.2	1.5	2.0	1.0	1.0
Protein (g/L) (% cal)	37.1 (14.0%)	44.3 (16.7%)	55.5 (18.5%)	62.6 (16.7%)	83.7 (16.7%)	41.8 (16.7%)	62.5 (25%)
Fat (g/L) (% cal)	34.7 (29%)	34.7 (29%)	39.3 (29.0%)	50 (30%)	89.1 (40.1%)	54.4 (49%)	28.2 (25%)
Carbohydrate (g/L) (% cal)	151.1 (57%)	143.9 (54.3%)	172.7 (52.5%)	199.9 (53.3%)	216.1 (43.2%)	95.6 (34.3%)	138.3 (50%)
Osmolality (mOsm)	300	300	450	650	690	355	380
Comments	Isotonic	Isotonic	Moderate protein, 12 g/L fiber	High calorie, high protein	Hypermetabolic fluid restricted patients	Low carbohydrates, 14.4 g/L fiber	High protein, low fat, 14.4 g/L fiber

	Pulmocare	Suplena	Nepro	Peptamen	Alitraq	Tolerex	Vital HN	Vivonex Plus
Calories/mL	1.5	2.0	2.0	1.0	1.0	1.0	1.0	1.0
Protein (g/L) (% cal)	62.6 (16.7%)	30.0 (6%)	69.9 (14%)	40.0 (16%)	52.5 (21%)	21 (8.0%)	41.7 (16.7%)	45 (18%)
Fat (g/L) (% cal)	93.3 (55.1%)	95.6 (43%)	95.6 (43%)	39 (33%)	15.5 (13%)	1.5 (1.0%)	10.8 (9.5%)	6.7 (6%)
Carbohydrate (g/L) (% cal)	105.7 (28.2%)	255.2 (51%)	222.3 (43%)	127 (51%)	165 (66%)	230 (91%)	185.0 (73.8%)	190 (76%)
Osmolality (mOsm)	475	600	665	380	575	550	500	650
Comments	High protein, high fat, low carbohydrate (to minimize CO_2 production)	Renal failure–predialysis (low protein, low electrolyte), high calorie.	Renal failure–on dialysis (moderate protein, low electrolyte)	Peptide based, gluten free, glutamine (3 g/L)	Elemental, glutamine (14.2 g/L)	Elemental, low protein	Elemental, higher protein	Elemental, glutamine (10 g/L)

In the absence of clinical signs of refeeding syndrome, nutrition therapy should continue with frequent monitoring and replacement of electrolytes.

XIII. **GASTRIC RESIDUAL VOLUME (GRV).** Though routinely used as a marker of enteral tube feeding tolerance, GRV measurements are technique dependent and may not reliably measure gastric contents. Data on the association between high residuals and increased risk of aspiration pneumonia is conflicting. Allowing high GRV, or even eliminating GRV measurements altogether, has not been associated with worse outcome in mechanically ventilated medical patients. See Figure 11.1 (gastric residual figure) for protocol used at MGH.

Starting Tube Feeds:
- Use of tube feeds and ability to advance tube feeds should be evaluated for every patient.
- Consult dietician for every patient regarding type and goal of tube feeds.
- Assess patient every shift for recent bowel movements, abdominal pain or distention, nausea, and vomiting.
- Start a bowel regimen in all patients unless contraindicated.

Advancing Tube Feeds:
- Begin tube feeds at 10 cc/h and advance by 10 cc/h every 2 hours to goal

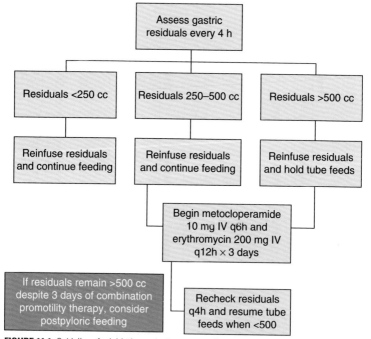

FIGURE 11.1 Guidelines for initiation and advancement of tube feeds.

XIV. COMPLICATIONS OF PARENTERAL NUTRITION
A. Catheter-Placement Complications (Pneumothorax, Hemothorax, or Arrhythmia)
B. Catheter Infection
C. Other Infections (Immune Suppression from TPN)
D. Metabolic Derangements (Hyperglycemia, Hypoglycemia, Electrolyte Imbalances, Fluid Overload)

Selected Readings

Bertolini G, Iapichino G, Radrizzani D, et al. Early enteral immunonutrition in patients with severe sepsis: results of an interim analysis of a randomized multicentre clinical trial. *Intensive Care Med* 2003;29(5):834–840.

Casaer MP, Mesotten D, Hermans G, et al. Early versus late parenteral nutrition in critically ill adults. *N Engl J Med* 2011;365(6):506–517.

Casaer MP, Van den Berghe G. Nutrition in the acute phase of critical illness. *N Engl J Med* 2014;370(13):1227–1236.

de Aguilar-Nascimento JE, Dock-Nascimento DB, Bragagnolo R. Role of enteral nutrition and pharmaconutrients in conditions of splanchnic hypoperfusion. *Nutrition* 2010;26(4):354–358.

Dissanaike S, Pham T, Shalhub S, et al. Effect of immediate enteral feeding on trauma patients with an open abdomen: protection from nosocomial infections. *J Am Coll Surg* 2008;207(5):690–697.

Heyland D, Muscedere J, Wischmeyer PE, et al. A randomized trial of glutamine and antioxidants in critically ill patients. *N Engl J Med* 2013;368(16):1489–1497.

Hurt RT, McClave SA. Gastric residual volumes in critical illness: what do they really mean? *Crit Care Clin* 2010;26(3):481–490, viii–ix.

McClave SA, Martindale RG, Kiraly L. The use of indirect calorimetry in the intensive care unit. *Curr Opin Clin Nutr Metab Care* 2013;16(2):202–208.

McClave SA, Martindale RG, Vanek VW, et al. Guidelines for the provision and assessment of nutrition support therapy in the adult critically ill patient: Society of Critical Care Medicine (SCCM) and American Society for Parenteral and Enteral Nutrition (A.S.P.E.N.). *JPEN J Parenter Enteral Nutr* 2009;33(3):277–316.

McClave SA, Snider HL. Clinical use of gastric residual volumes as a monitor for patients on enteral feeding. *JPEN J Parenter Enteral Nutr* 2002;26(6 suppl):S43–S48; discussion S49–S50.

Plank LD, Hill GL. Sequential metabolic changes following induction of systemic inflammatory response in patients with severe sepsis or major blunt trauma. *World J Surg* 2000;24(6):630–638.

Reignier J, Lascarrou JB. Residual gastric volume and risk of ventilator-associated pneumonia—reply. *JAMA* 2013;309(20):2090–2091.

Singer P, Anbar R, Cohen J, et al. The tight calorie control study (TICACOS): a prospective, randomized, controlled pilot study of nutritional support in critically ill patients. *Intensive Care Med* 2011;37(4):601–609.

White H, Sosnowski K, Tran K, et al. A randomised controlled comparison of early post-pyloric versus early gastric feeding to meet nutritional targets in ventilated intensive care patients. *Crit Care* 2009;13(6):R187.

Infectious Disease

Craig S. Jabaley

 Obtaining Blood Cultures

I. INTRODUCTION

A. The management of **infectious disease** is a crucial skill for the intensivist. Epidemiological studies suggest that more than 70% of adult patients in an ICU receive antibiotics, and about 50% demonstrate overt signs of infection during their stay. Infection is a major contributor to mortality among the most critically ill patients, especially following trauma, burns, and extensive surgical insults.

B. Critically ill patients have numerous potential **sources** of infection as outlined in Table 12.1. Table 12.2 summarizes the common bacterial pathogens referred to herein.

C. Chapter 27 reviews empiric and disease-specific **treatment**.

D. Please see the video regarding how to obtain blood cultures.

II. HOSPITAL-ACQUIRED INFECTION (HAI) increases health care costs, extends hospital stays, and contributes to excess mortality. A sizeable percentage of these infections are preventable through multifaceted measures; accordingly, HAI has become the focus of worldwide surveillance and practice-improvement measures.

A. The estimated **prevalence** varies, but approximately 4% to 5% of hospital patients are affected by HAI. Patients in an ICU are about three times more likely to contract HAI than are patients on a general care ward.

TABLE 12.1 Potential Sites of Infection in Intensive Care Unit Patients

Central nervous system	Epidural or brain abscess, encephalitis, meningitis
Head and neck	Sinusitis, pharyngitis, parotitis
Chest	Pneumonia, tracheobronchitis, endocarditis, empyema, mediastinitis, pericarditis
Abdomen	Peritonitis, cholecystitis, cholangitis, appendicitis, diverticulitis, *C. difficile* colitis
Genitourinary	Pyelonephritis, cystitis, prostatitis
Musculoskeletal and vascular	Cellulitis, abscess, pressure ulcers, osteomyelitis, deep venous thrombosis
Surgical	Wound, implanted hardware, anastomotic failure, abscess
Device-associated infections	Intravascular catheter, urinary catheter, epidural or spinal catheter, intracranial pressure monitor, any drain site or tract

TABLE 12.2	Classification of Common Pathogenic Bacterial Genera and Species
Gram-positive aerobic cocci	*Staphylococcus*
Gram-positive aerobic bacilli	*Bacillus, Corynebacterium, Listeria*
Gram-negative nonenteric bacilli	*Acinetobacter, Pseudomonas, Burkholderia, Neisseria, H. influenzae, Legionella*
Gram-negative enteric bacilli	(Enterobacteriaceae family) *E. coli, Klebsiella, Enterobacter, Proteus, Citrobacter, Serratia, Salmonella*
Gram-positive anaerobic cocci	*Peptostreptococcus*
Gram-positive anaerobic bacilli	*Bacteroides*
Gram-negative anaerobic bacilli	*Clostridium* (sporulating), *Actinomyces, Lactobacillus*

1. **Device-associated infections**, including central line–associated blood stream infection, catheter-associated urinary tract infection, and ventilator-associated pneumonia, have come under intense scrutiny despite contributing to only about 25% of all HAI. Efforts led by the CDC and other worldwide regulatory bodies are targeted at both surveillance and development of preventative strategies.
2. All critical care practitioners must be familiar with **guidelines** aimed at reducing the incidence of HAI (see Selected Readings).
3. Efforts at incentivizing improved hospital performance are continuing to develop and largely based around **pay for performance** models linked to HAI, including **surgical site** infections.
4. **Prevention** strategies have been bolstered by the JCAHO mandate that hospitals have an active program for the surveillance, prevention, and control of HAI. Strategies include the following:
   a. **Infection control measures** including universal precautions, isolation, and **hand hygiene** are fundamental (see Chapter 40).
   b. **Surveillance** should be implemented to gauge trends, identify problematic organisms, and alert clinicians to new trends in resistance or areas for improvement.
   c. Limiting the **duration** of care in an ICU helps to reduce patient exposure to the highest risk environment for HAI.
   d. The physical **design** of an ICU can help to reduce foot traffic, maximize availability of hand hygiene stations, facilitate easy cleaning, and provide adequate space for the routine care of isolated patients.
   e. **Invasive procedures** and **devices** should be **minimized** to the extent possible.
   f. **Device-specific procedures** should be implemented and monitored for the placement and maintenance of intravenous lines, urinary catheters, etc. Clinicians must be familiar with established protocols for their placement, use, and maintenance (see Selected Readings).
   g. Routine **cleaning** of the ICU environment, including multiuse diagnostic equipment, helps to reduce colonization.
   h. **Decolonization** of patients via daily chlorhexidine baths is somewhat controversial but has been proven beneficial in several studies.
5. Educating clinicians about **responsible antibiotic prescribing** is of the utmost importance.
B. Patterns of nosocomial pathogens are shifting as **gram-negative organisms** are beginning to overtake gram-positives as the most common pathogens worldwide (Table 12.3). However, broad epidemiological data are not substitutes for local trends in infection and resistance, which should be tracked to improve empiric treatment.

TABLE 12.3	Most Common Organsisms Isolated in Hospital-Acquired Infections (2009–2010)		
All Hospital-Associated Infection		**Device-Associated**	
Pathogen	% total	Pathogen	% total
C. difficile	12.1	S. aureus	15.6
S. aureus	10.7	Enterococcus spp	13.9
Klebsiella spp	9.9	E. coli	11.5
Enterococcus spp	8.7	CoNS	11.4
P. aeruginosa	7.1	Klebsiella	8
Candida spp	6.3	Pseudomonas	7.5
Streptococcus spp	5.0	Candida spp	9.5
CoNS	4.8	Enterobacter spp	4.7

HAI, hospital-associated infection; spp, species; CoNS, coagulase-negative staphylococci.
Data from: Magill SS, Edwards JR, Bamberg W, et al. Multistate point-prevalence survey of health care–associated infections. *N Engl J Med* 2014;370:1198–1208 and Sievert DM, Ricks P, Edwards JR, et al. Antimicrobial-resistant pathogens associated with healthcare-associated infections: summary of data reported to the National Healthcare Safety Network at the Centers for Disease Control and Prevention, 2009–2010. *Infect Control Hosp Epidemiol* 2013;34:1–14.

C. Although not the focus of similar regulatory attention at present, **gastrointestinal infection** is the third most common HAI (17%) behind pneumonia (22%) and surgical site infection (22%). **Clostridium difficile** is the main contributor to these underappreciated GI infections and warrants heightened clinical suspicion.

III. ANTIBIOTIC RESISTANCE AND INFECTION PREVENTION

A. Resistance represents a growing global challenge. Critically ill patients are highly susceptible to HAI owing to environmental colonization, immunosuppression, malnutrition, and the use of invasive devices. Coupled with higher rates of resistant organisms in critical care settings (Fig. 12.1), it is unsurprising that intensivists and their patients must frequently combat this problem.

1. The **etiologies** of bacterial resistance are diverse and differ widely depending on organism; however, they are the result of selective pressures that favor survival of robust organisms. Widespread antibiotic use, ineffective or inappropriate treatment, environmental contamination, incomplete patient isolation, and inadvertent transmission all contribute to the development and spread of resistant organisms.

2. Epidemiological studies suggest that **more than 50%** of nosocomial pathogens demonstrate some degree of resistance. The CDC estimates that the worldwide impact of antibiotic resistance in the United States alone exceeds $20 billion in addition to excess mortality and the societal impact of prolonged treatment among affected patients.

IV. Attention to **basic principles of antimicrobial therapy** is a key component of reducing antibiotic resistance and improving clinical outcomes.

A. The **diagnosis** of infection in the ICU is a nontrivial task. Fever, leukocytosis, respiratory disturbances, hemodynamic perturbations, and other markers of inflammation are nonspecific. Patients demonstrating these symptoms should also be evaluated for noninfectious sources of inflammation. In short, not all patients with fever are infected.

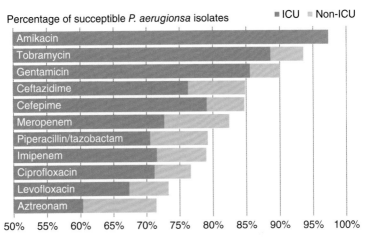

Percentage of succeptible *P. aerugionsa* isolates   ■ ICU   ■ Non-ICU

Amikacin
Tobramycin
Gentamicin
Ceftazidime
Cefepime
Meropenem
Piperacillin/tazobactam
Imipenem
Ciprofloxacin
Levofloxacin
Aztreonam

50% 55% 60% 65% 70% 75% 80% 85% 90% 95% 100%

FIGURE 12.1 Percentage of susceptible *Pseudomonas aeruginosa* isolates in US ICU versus non-ICU health care settings (2009–2011). (Data from: Sader HS, Farrell DJ, Flamm RK, et al. Antimicrobial susceptibility of gram-negative organisms isolated from patients hospitalized in intensive care units in United States and European hospitals (2009–2011). *Diagn Microbiol Infect Dis* 2014;78:443–448.)

B. **Testing** in the setting of a suspected infection should be directed toward identification of the **source** and obtaining specimens for **culture** and **susceptibility**. Ideally, specimens should be collected before the initiation of antibiotic therapy to improve their yield. Colonizing organisms often complicate culture results. Quantitative analysis and consultation with the microbiology lab can be useful adjuncts. Quite frequently the source of infection and associated pathogens are never identified.

C. **Empiric** antibiotics must be selected on the basis of suspected site of infection, likely pathogens at that site, local resistance patterns, prior antibiotic therapy (if any), and any comorbidities that may heighten risks of toxicity.

1. The initiation of empiric therapy should **not be delayed** unreasonably for diagnostic testing in the setting of a high clinical suspicion for sepsis, meningitis, or pneumonia. Increased latency from diagnosis to treatment leads to heightened mortality with these clinical entities.

2. Do not overlook the potential contribution of anaerobic and fungal organisms to clinically significant infections, especially in the setting of prior or ongoing antibiotic therapy.

D. **Documentation** of suspected infection, rationale for drug selection, and duration of proposed treatment is critical and reduces confusion during the course of treatment and turnover among the care team.

E. **Continuous Reassessment** of antibiotic therapy is complicated by the fact that many critically ill patients will be slow to improve despite selection of appropriate therapy.

a. **Deescalation** can be accomplished in one of three ways:

1. Transitioning from a broad-spectrum to a narrower-spectrum agent following the return of culture and sensitivity data

2. Shortening the duration of therapy on the basis of clinical response when the location of infection can be identified

3. In the familiar scenario of unhelpful culture data but obvious infection, antimicrobials can be discontinued in a stepwise fashion on the basis of the likely pathogen involved as judged by local patterns, clinical experience, and patient response.
    b. Consider **oral therapy** in patients with a functioning GI tract that are responding to treatment. Fluoroquinolones, linezolid, and fluconazole have excellent oral bioavailability.
    c. **Adverse effects** may not emerge until well into a course of therapy.
    d. **Superinfection** is a well-recognized consequence of broad-spectrum antimicrobial therapy, namely, with *C. difficile* and *Candida*.
    e. **Persistent fever** despite other signs of resolving infection should prompt reevaluation of other causes rather than escalation or unnecessary continuation of therapy.
  F. **Limit the Duration** of treatment whenever possible on the basis of type of infection and patient response. The ideal duration of treatment for many infections has not been concretely determined. Empiric therapy often must be stopped empirically.

V. **ANTIBACTERIALS** comprise a wide range of pharmaceuticals with variable microbial targets. A review of the most clinically relevant agents is presented herein.
  A. **Aminoglycosides** (gentamicin, tobramycin, amikacin) provide unique bactericidal activity among the inhibitors of protein synthesis. Owing to **toxicity**, their role is largely confined to a few specific indications often in combination with other agents.
    1. **Spectrum:** Aminoglycosides are most effective against aerobic gram-negative bacilli, including ***Pseudomonas*** (see Fig. 12.1), *Acinetobacter*, and members of the Enterobacteriaceae.
    2. **Resistance** to aminoglycosides is multifactorial but due largely to modifying enzymes. Amikacin is the least affected by these enzymes and often reserved for the treatment of resistant organisms.
    3. **Considerations**
       a. Aminoglycosides **penetrate poorly** into the CNS, secretions, pleural fluid, infected tissue, and anaerobic environments owing to their cationic structure and need for active transport.
       b. **Nephrotoxicity** almost invariably develops within the first week of treatment and can progress to nonoliguric renal failure that reverses upon discontinuation of therapy. Superimposed hypovolemia and chronic kidney disease, both common in the ICU, contribute to increased susceptibility.
       c. The incidence of **ototoxicity**, especially with concomitant loop diuretic administration, has been estimated at 3% to 15% and may manifest insidiously as ataxia, disequilibrium, or nystagmus.
       d. Rare but potentially life-threatening **neuromuscular blockade** has been reported in the setting of myasthenia gravis, hypocalcemia, or hypomagnesaemia. Aminoglycosides also potentiate nondepolarizing neuromuscular blockers.
       e. **Aerosolized** tobramycin and gentamicin have been studied for treatment of *Pseudomonas* in patients with cystic fibrosis and bronchiectasis. Although the role for inhalational administration in the ICU is less clear, it may be useful to help minimize toxicity or treat resistant isolates.
    4. **Dosage** must be adjusted on the basis of renal function and age, and **monitoring** of serum levels is recommended.

B. Anaerobic Agents

1. **Metronidazole** works via radical-mediated DNA disruption to exert bactericidal effects against anaerobic bacteria and is used in the treatment of *Clostridium difficile* and *Bacteroides*. It lacks efficacy against aerobes, facultative organisms, and nonsporulating gram-positive anaerobic bacilli. *Listeria* and *Lactobacillus* are resistant. Metronidazole has excellent oral bioavailability and is largely well-tolerated, with nausea and dyspepsia being the most common side-effects. Despite over five decades of clinical use, the estimated rate of anaerobic resistance is less than 5%.

2. **Clindamycin** interferes with bacterial protein synthesis and is bacteriostatic. Owing to its activity against both aerobic gram-positive cocci and most anaerobes, clindamycin can be used for treatment of skin or soft tissue infections. However, its strong association with the development of *C. difficile* and rising rate of resistance among *Bacteroides* spp. limit clindamycin's utility in a critical care setting.

3. **Tigecycline** is the sole member of the novel glycylcylines and demonstrates activity against not only anaerobes but also most multidrug-resistant (MDR) organisms. Initial enthusiasm was tempered by an association between tigecycline and increased mortality in patients treated for VAP. Subsequent analyses suggested that the underlying cause was likely worsening infection secondary to treatment failure, which is puzzling given its spectrum of activity. Tigecycline is largely reserved for salvage therapy when faced with resistant organisms, especially when anaerobes are involved.

C. β-Lactams comprise a diverse and frequently utilized group of antibiotics that inhibit bacterial cell wall synthesis.

1. The numerous **penicillins** currently used in clinical practice are reviewed in Table 12.4. They are often used in combination with β-lactamase inhibitors to overcome microbial resistance.

   a. **Spectrum:** While the penicillins possess a relatively broad spectrum of microbial coverage, patterns of resistance mandate sensitivity-directed treatment when considering their use for nosocomial infections. Nafcillin or oxacillin are used to treat methicillin-sensitive *S. aureus* (MSSA). The combination of ampicillin/sulbactam (**Unasyn**) offers broad coverage of gram-positives, Enterobacteriaceae, and anaerobes in the setting of maxillofacial pathology. Piperacillin in combination with tazobactam (**Zosyn**) offers the broadest spectrum of parenteral penicillin/β-lactamase combinations and is the most widely used penicillin in the ICU. As a part of empiric treatment regimens, it offers broad gram-positive and gram-negative coverage with efficacy against *B. fragilis* and (to a diminishing extent as outlined in Fig. 12.1) *Pseudomonas*.

   b. **Resistance** is a major hurtle that limits the clinical utility of many penicillins. Methicillin-resistant *S. aureus* (**MRSA**), and other gram-positive organisms, expresses **modified penicillin binding proteins** (PBPs) with low affinity for β-lactams. Many gram-negative organisms produce inducible β-**lactamases** that are able to render many β-lactam compounds ineffective. While the development of β-lactamase inhibitors has extended the utility of the penicillins, resistance continues to develop. For example, piperacillin-tazobactam is vulnerable to **extended-spectrum β-lactamases** (ESBLs), which are not inhibited by tazobactam.

   c. **Considerations**

      1. **Hypersensitivity** is the most common adverse reaction following penicillin administration and can range in severity from a rash

TABLE 12.4   Review of Selected β-Lactam Antibiotics

β-Lactam Class	β-lactam (& β-lactamase inhibitor)	Gram Pos[a]	Gram Neg	*Pseudomonas*	Covered Organisms
Natural	Penicillin G	+/−	−	−	*T. pallidum*, meningococcal meningitis
Penicillinase-resistant	(Methicillin) Nafcillin Oxacillin	++	−	−	MSSA, streptococci
Amino-penicillins	Ampicillin, Amoxicillin	+	+/−	−	Streptococci, enterococci
	With Sulbactam or Clavulanate	++	+	−	Above & MSSA, anaerobes, some Enterobacteriaceae
Ureido-penicillins	Piperacillin	+	+	+	Streptococci, enterococci
	With Tazobactam	++	++	+	Above & MSSA, anaerobes, some Enterobacteriaceae

[a]Therapy with Beta-lactams in the setting of gram-positive nosocomial infections should be guided by culture data owing to variable rates and patterns of resistance.

Pos, positive; Neg, negative; ++, highly active; +, active; +/−, limited activity; −, not active; MSSA, methicillin-sensitive *Staphylococcus aureus*.

to angioedema and anaphylaxis. Patients who are candidates for penicillin therapy but report a history of allergy should be questioned to elucidate the details of the adverse reaction. **Skin testing** for penicillin allergy is unreliable. Accordingly, **desensitization** via escalating doses may be considered when the benefits to treatment outweigh the possible risks in patients with a true history of severe hypersensitivity. These protocols should be conducted by specialists in an ICU setting with the assumption that fulminant anaphylaxis could develop.

2. Intravenous administration of all penicillins has been associated with **phlebitis**.

d. **Dosage** varies widely by drug and indication. Of note, piperacillin-tazobactam dosing must be adjusted for renal function, and extended infusion regimens have been associated with improved clinical outcomes. No specific **monitoring** is required.

2. **Cephalosporins** are a diverse class of antibiotics organized by generation that are structurally related to the penicillins. Table 12.5 outlines the cephalosporins currently used in clinical practice.

a. **Spectrum: Cefazolin**, a first-generation cephalosporin, remains popular for surgical site prophylaxis owing to its gram-positive coverage. Subsequent generations have improved activity against gram-negative aerobes and the Enterobacteriaceae. Accordingly, the third-generation **Ceftriaxone** is used for the treatment of community-acquired pneumonia. **Cefepime**, a fourth-generation agent, is often employed as first-line

TABLE 12.5 Review of Slected Cephalosporin Antibiotics

Gen	Agent	Gram Pos	Gram Neg	Anaerobes	ESBL	MRSA	CNS	Covered Organisms
1	Cefazolin	++	+/−	−	−	−	−	MSSA, streptococci
2	Cefuroxime	+	+	−	−	−	−	MSSA, streptococci, *H. influenzae*
	Cefoxitin, Cefotetan	+/−	+	+	−	−	−	Some Enterobacteriaceae & *B. fragilis*
3	Ceftriaxone, Cefotaxime	+	++	−	−	−	+	+/− MSSA, streptococci, Enterobacteriaceae
	Ceftazidime	+/−	++	−	−	−	+	Enterobacteriaceae, *Pseudomonas*
4[a]	Cefepime	++	++	−	+/−	−	+/−	MSSA, Streptococci, Enterobacteriaceae, *Pseudomonas*
5	Ceftobiprole[b], Ceftaroline	++	++	+/−	+/−	+	?	MRSA

[a]First through fourth generation cephalosporins demonstrate no activity against methicillin-resistant staphylococci or enterococci.
[b]Ceftobiprole is under review by the FDA at the time of publication.
Pos, positive; Neg, negative; ++, highly active; +, active; +/−, limited activity; −, not active; ?, unknown; ESBL, extended-spectrum β-lactamase organisms; MRSA, methicillin-resistant *Staphylococcus aureus*; MSSA, methicillin-sensitive *Staphylococcus aureus*.

empiric treatment of nosocomial infections. First- through fourth-generation cephalosporins are **not active** against **methicillin-resistant** staphylococci or enterococci. So-called **fifth-generation** cephalosporins have been introduced with activity against MRSA; however, their role in critical care settings is not yet well defined.

   b. Bacterial **resistance** is achieved through both expression of altered PBPs and β-lactamases. Despite initial hopes, third-generation cephalosporins perform poorly against ESBL-producing organisms, which commonly include *Klebsiella* and *Enterobacter*. Cefepime is both relatively resistant to common β-lactamases and typically does not induce their production. However, certain strains of *Acinetobacter, Pseudomonas,* and Enterobacteriaceae have become resistant.

   c. Considerations

   1. Classic teaching has been that patients with a history of true hypersensitivity reactions to penicillins demonstrate up to a 10% incidence of **cross-reactivity**. However, third- and fourth-generation agents pose less of a risk.

   2. Cefotetan has been linked with **hypoprothrombinemia** owing to competitive inhibition of vitamin K–dependent factor synthesis.

   3. Case reports suggest that failure to adjust **cefepime** dosage in the setting of renal insufficiency can lead to **neurotoxicity**, including myoclonus, seizures, encephalopathy, and coma.

   d. With the exception of ceftriaxone, all cephalosporins require **dosing modification** on the basis of **renal function**. Although dosage regimens vary by drug and indication, most require frequent dosing owing to short half-lives. **Monitoring** is not required.

3. Carbapenems (imipenem/cilastain, meropenem, ertapenem)

   a. Spectrum: Carbapenems offer the **broadest spectrum** of antimicrobial activity among not only the β-lactams but all antibiotics. **Imipenem** and **meropenem** are effective against all common gram-positive, gram-negative, and anaerobic pathogens, including *Pseudomonas* and *Acinetobacter*. (**Ertapenem** does not offer coverage of these latter two organisms.) Their spectrum of coverage does not extend to MRSA (like all β-lactams). *Legionella, Chlamydia, Mycoplasma, Burkholderia cepacia,* and *Stenotrophomonas maltophilia* are also not reliably covered. Carbapenems are currently used in the **empiric** treatment of nosocomial infections **with suspected resistance** and in the setting of polymicrobial infections.

   b. Resistance to carbapenems is usually the result of multiple mechanisms. While fortunately rare, carbapenem-resistant Enterobacteriaceae (CRE) sepsis is fatal in up to 50% of cases.

   1. Carbapenems are robust against most ESBLs; however, plasmid-encoded *K. pneumoniac* carbapenemase (KPC) causes weak hydrolysis and can contribute to resistance, especially among CRE species.

   2. Multidrug efflux pumps and porin channel mutations have both been implicated in resistant *Pseudomonas* strains.

   c. Considerations

   1. Seizures during treatment with imipenem have a reported incidence of 1% to 3%. Underlying renal dysfunction, failure to adjust dosage, and underlying structural neurological disease increase the risk of seizures. Meropenem appears less likely to cause seizures but can reduce levels of valproic acid.

    2. There is only a small risk of **cross-reactivity** in patients with penicillin allergies, and reactions are usually mild.

    3. Meropenem readily crosses the blood–brain barrier.

  d. **Dosage** of imipenem and meropenem must be adjusted on the basis of renal function. No **monitoring** is required. Ertapenem does not require adjustment for renal function and can be dosed once daily. These features make it attractive in cases of documented microbial sensitivity.

4. **Aztreonam**, the only commercially available **monobactam**, is active only against aerobic gram-negative bacteria. Its primary use is in the treatment of sensitive gram-negative organisms in patients with a history of allergy to other β-lactams owing to exceedingly rare cross-reactivity.

D. Gram-Positive Agents

1. **Vancomycin**, a glycopeptide antibiotic, inhibits bacterial cell wall synthesis.

  a. **Spectrum:** Vancomycin is active against nearly all aerobic and anaerobic gram-positive bacteria, including *Staphylococcus*, streptococci, and *C. difficile*. It has bactericidal effects against most susceptible organisms except for the enterococci. Given the high prevalence of staphylococcal infections in the ICU, vancomycin is a popular antibiotic; however, this enthusiasm must be tempered with an appreciation for its drawbacks.

  b. **Resistance**

    1. The emergence of vancomycin-resistant enterococci (**VRE**), which utilize an altered cell wall precursor without glycopeptide binding sites, has posed a growing treatment challenge. Among the enterococci, *E. faecium* is typically the most resistant strain.

    2. While true resistance among staphylococci is rare, isolates that require a minimum inhibitory concentration of greater than 2 μg/mL can be difficult to treat due to the aggressive dosing required to achieve the necessary trough levels of 15 to 20 μg/mL and are currently deemed "**intermediately susceptible**." Treatment with an alternative agent should be considered in this circumstance.

  c. **Considerations**

    1. Treatment of MSSA with vancomycin has been associated with longer courses of therapy, higher rates of failure, and increased mortality when compared with nafcillin or oxacillin.

    2. Rapid infusion causes clinically significant **histamine release**, which can include the "red man syndrome" marked by cutaneous flushing, erythema, and hypotension. Histaminergic symptoms do not represent a true allergy and can be mitigated by slow infusion, dose reduction, dilution, or premedication.

    3. The true incidence of **nephrotoxicity** is unclear; however, the risk is increased with concomitant administration of other nephrotoxins and when trough levels exceed 10 μg/mL (as is often desired). This risk must be balanced against the benefit of antimicrobial treatment.

    4. Vancomycin is an underappreciated cause of **DRESS syndrome** (drug reaction with eosinophilia and systemic symptoms). Diagnosis is complicated by the similarity of DRESS symptoms to those associated with infection or histamine release. Latency of 2 to 3 weeks between onset of treatment and symptomatology should prompt further investigation.

    5. Rare toxicities include ototoxicity, neutropenia, and thrombocytopenia.

    d. Dosage of vancomycin must be adjusted on the basis of renal function, age, and weight. Many hospitals have adopted nomograms to assist clinicians with dosing. The **monitoring** of trough concentrations (30 minutes prior to administration of the fourth dose), while contentious, is generally recommended.

    e. Dalbavancin, a novel second-generation glycopeptide was approved by the FDA in May 2014 for the treatment of complicated skin infections. Its role, if any, in the critical care environment has yet to be defined.

  2. Linezolid interrupts bacterial protein synthesis via a novel mechanism of action and has a similar spectrum of activity to that of vancomycin with the addition of **VRE.** In addition to excellent oral bioavailability, linezolid also benefits from high concentrations in the pulmonary epithelium. While it may offer a hypothetical benefit in the treatment of pneumonia, clinical data supporting this claim are sparse. Resistance remains rare at present. Numerous adverse reactions have been noted, including reversible myelosuppression and GI disturbances. Transient optic neuropathy and sometimes permanent peripheral neuropathy are rare but important considerations.

  3. Daptomycin is a naturally occurring cyclic lipopeptide that destabilizes bacterial membranes. Its spectrum is similar to that of vancomycin. It is comparatively less active, but still effective against, staphylococci with resistance to vancomycin. Interestingly, pulmonary surfactant deactivates daptomycin, rendering it ineffective for the treatment of pneumonia. Myopathy with elevated CPK is the primary toxicity, which warrants monitoring during treatment. Dosage must be adjusted in the setting of renal insufficiency.

  4. Quinupristin/dalfopristin demonstrates broad activity against gram-positives, including MRSA, vancomycin-resistant staphylococci, and vancomycin-resistant *E. faecium* (but not *E. faecalis*). Its use is often accompanied by the development of arthralgias and myalgias. Quinupristin/dalfopristin inhibits CYP3A4, which complicates its use in the setting of critical care polypharmacy. These considerations limit its utility to the treatment of otherwise resistant organisms.

E. Fluoroquinolones (ciprofloxacin, levofloxacin, moxifloxacin) exert rapid bactericidal activity through interference with DNA synthesis.

  1. Spectrum: Ciprofloxacin, the oldest fluoroquinolone still in active use, is active against a broad spectrum of both gram-positive and gram-negative organisms, especially enteric gram-negative aerobes. Newer agents such as **moxifloxacin** and, to a lesser extent, **levofloxacin** are more active against MSSA, streptococci, *Legionella,* and *Mycoplasma.*

  2. Resistance occurs largely through alterations in the genetic coding of enzymes responsible for DNA synthesis and the development of efflux mechanisms. These adaptations increasingly limit the clinical utility of fluoroquinolones following their initial widespread adoption. Their efficacy against *Pseudomonas* (ciprofloxacin, levofloxacin—see Fig. 12.1) and anaerobes (moxifloxacin) has been compromised, and plasmid-mediated resistance among mixed gram-negative species is on the rise.

  3. Considerations

    a. Preferential distribution into the lungs, urine, and bile leads to markedly increased efficacy at these sites.

    b. The enteral absorption of fluoroquinolones can be attenuated by numerous substances frequently administered in a critical care setting, including enteral nutrition formulas and minerals.

    c. Although generally **well tolerated**, common side effects include GI disturbance, CNS effects, and transient alterations in liver function tests.

    d. While rare, alterations in glucose metabolism, prolongation of the QT interval, and tendonitis leading to rupture have all been reported.

  4. Dosage of ciprofloxacin and levofloxacin (but not moxifloxacin) must be adjusted for renal function. Fluoroquinolones variably impair the metabolism of **warfarin** and **theophylline**; accordingly, careful monitoring thereof is warranted.

F. Macrolides (erythromycin, clarithromycin, azithromycin) inhibit bacterial protein synthesis.

  1. Spectrum: Macrolides demonstrate activity mainly against streptococci, including *S. pneumoniae*, in addition to *H. influenzae*. They are ineffective against many nosocomial pathogens, including the Enterobacteriaceae. Their role in the ICU is largely confined to the treatment of so-called atypical organisms, such as *Legionella, Lysteria, Chlamydia,* and *Mycoplasma.*

  2. Resistance to macrolides occurs via mutation of their ribosomal target, drug efflux, production of hydrolysis esterases, and protective methylase enzymes.

  3. Considerations

    a. Macrolides have long-recognized anti-inflammatory properties; however, concrete clinical applications for this effect have not been clearly elucidated.

    b. Erythromycin and its analogues are useful intestinal prokinetics.

    c. GI disturbance is the most common adverse effect associated with macrolides, and QT prolongation is the most serious.

    d. CYP3A4 is variably inhibited: erythromycin is the most potent followed by clarithromycin and azithromycin.

  4. Dosage is not affected by renal function, and no drug-specific **monitoring** is required.

G. Polymyxins are cationic detergents whose use to treat gram-negative infections was gradually abandoned starting in the 1970s as the less toxic aminoglycosides and antipseudomonal penicillins were introduced. However, the emergence of MDR gram-negatives has led to a resurgence of interest in these long-neglected agents thus necessitating refamiliarization for a new generation of practitioners.

  1. Colistin, more so than its other polymyxin counterparts, has seen renewed clinical utilization. It is active against most clinically relevant gram-negative aerobic bacilli, including the multidrug-resistant isolates of the Enterobacteriaceae, *Pseudomonas,* and *Acinetobacter.*

  2. Resistance to colistin is rare but has been reported among numerous organisms. Several mechanisms have been described, including cell wall adaptations, encapsulation, and efflux pumps.

  3. Considerations

    a. Although colistin is a known **nephrotoxin**, progression to overt renal failure with need for renal replacement therapy appears to be rare. Furthermore, renal insufficiency most always improves slowly after conclusion of treatment. As colistin is reserved for treatment in the absence of alternatives, its benefits typically outweigh this risk.

    b. In addition to a parenteral formulation, colistin can also be delivered via inhalation, which may help to avoid systemic toxicity. Bronchoconstriction has been described following nebulized administration.

    c. Polymyxins are **neurotoxic**, which may manifest as paresthesias or, more threateningly, neuromuscular blockade. The latter may progress to frank apnea in the setting of inadvertent overdose with superimposed renal insufficiency or in patients with disorders of neuromuscular junction.

4. **Dosage** must be adjusted in the setting of renal insufficiency. No drug-specific **monitoring** is indicated.

VI. **ANTIFUNGALS** are a mainstay of antibiotic therapy in immunocompromised patients.

A. **Amphotericin B** binds to sterol compounds in the membranes of sensitive fungi thus compromising their structural integrity.

1. **Spectrum:** Amphotericin B is active against multiple relevant organisms, including nearly all *Candida* species and *Aspergillus*. Owing to toxicity, amphotericin is reserved for treatment of resistant isolates or clinically serious infections.

2. **Resistant** isolates of both *Candida* and *Aspergillus* have been identified; however, resistance during treatment is rare.

3. **Considerations**

a. **Lipid formulations** have largely replaced the traditional Amphotericin B deoxycholate but are more expensive.

b. Although the **nephrotoxicity** of lipid compounds is reduced compared with the classic formulation, progression to overt **renal failure** is not uncommon and care should be taken to avoid further renal insults.

c. Fever and chills during administration are common but can be attenuated by pretreatment.

4. **Dosage** must be adjusted on the basis of renal function. No drug-specific **monitoring** is required; however, close monitoring of renal function is prudent.

B. **Azoles** (fluconazole, itraconazole, voriconazole) variably inhibit fungal cell wall synthesis via deprivation of essential sterols.

1. **Spectrum:** Azoles are active against most relevant *Candida* species (except for *C. krusei*), *Cryptococcus neoformans*, and *Histoplasma capsulatum*. Voriconazole and itraconazole demonstrate acceptable activity against *Aspergillus*. The primary clinical role for the azoles is for both prophylaxis and treatment of mild to moderate infections.

2. **Progressive resistance** during treatment is a common occurrence owing to fungal modification of drug targets. *C. glabrata* and *C. albicans* are often resistant.

a. Notably, patterns of fungal resistance are unpredictable in practice, and isolates with documented sensitivity are candidates for treatment despite the typical spectrum.

3. **Considerations**

a. Most azoles inhibit CYP3A4 at a minimum, and many interact with multiple **hepatic CYPs**. Care must be taken in patients receiving warfarin, digoxin, benzodiazepines, phenytoin, and cyclosporine. Consultation with a pharmacist can be helpful to avoid dangerous drug interactions.

b. Rashes, GI disturbances, and transient transaminitis are relatively common.

c. Voriconazole produces transient visual alterations in about one-third of patients.

4. **Dosage** of some azoles is adjusted on the basis of renal function. **Monitoring** of serum levels is inconsistently recommended but often performed during treatment with voriconazole. Otherwise, secondary monitoring is governed by possible drug interactions as noted previously.

C. Echinocandins (caspofungin, micafungin) inhibit the synthesis of glucan in fungal cell walls.
  1. **Spectrum:** Both caspofungin and micafungin are active against *Candida* (including fluconazole-resistant isolates) and are used in the treatment of clinically serious or refractory candidiasis, especially *C. glabrata*. They are also an alternative to amphotericin B in patients with renal failure. Although evidence is building that micafungin is active against *Aspergillus*, caspofungin is better established in that role.
  2. **Resistance** remains relatively rare; however, isolates of *C. glabrata* resistant to both the azoles and echinocandins have been identified.
  3. **Considerations**
     a. Capsofungin is well tolerated overall. Histaminergic reactions following rapid infusion have been described.
     b. Micafungin mildly inhibits CYP3A4 and is also well tolerated.
D. 5-Flucytosine is the sole member of the pyrimidine class and is typically used in **combination** with amphotericin B for the treatment of *Cryptococcus* or candidiasis. Resistance during therapy limits its utility as monotherapy. Flucytosine leads to bone marrow depression with concomitant leukopenia and thrombocytopenia, especially in patients with underlying susceptibility or with high serum levels.

Selected Readings

Blumenthal KG, Patil SU, Long AA. The importance of vancomycin in drug rash with eosinophilia and systemic symptoms (DRESS) syndrome. *Allergy Asthma Proc* 2012;33:165–171.

Cannon JP, Lee TA, Clark NM, et al. The risk of seizures among the carbapenems: a meta-analysis. *J Antimicrob Chemother* 2014;69:2043–2055.

Dellit TH, Owens RC, McGowan JE Jr, et al. Infectious Diseases Society of America and the Society for Healthcare Epidemiology of America guidelines for developing an institutional program to enhance antimicrobial stewardship. *Clin Infect Dis* 2007;44:159–177.

Dudeck MA, Weiner LM, Allen-Bridson K, et al. National Healthcare Safety Network (NHSN) report, data summary for 2012, device-associated module. *Am J Infect Control* 2013;41:1148–1166.

Falagas ME, Rafailidis PI, Ioannidou E, et al. Colistin therapy for microbiologically documented multidrug-resistant gram-negative bacterial infections: a retrospective cohort study of 258 patients. *Int J Antimicrob Agents* 2010;35:194–199.

Gilbert DN, Chambers HF, Eliopoulos GM, et al. *The Sanford guide to antimicrobial therapy.* 44 ed. Sperryville: Antimicrobial Therapy, 2014.

Legendre DP, Muzny CA, Marshall GD, et al. Antibiotic hypersensitivity reactions and approaches to desensitization. *Clin Infect Dis* 2014;58:1140–1148.

Magill SS, Edwards JR, Bamberg W, et al. Multistate point-prevalence survey of health care-associated infections. *N Engl J Med* 2014;370:1198–1208.

Sader HS, Farrell DJ, Flamm RK, et al. Antimicrobial susceptibility of gram-negative organisms isolated from patients hospitalized in intensive care units in United States and European hospitals (2009–2011). *Diagn Microbiol Infect Dis* 2014;78:443–448.

Sievert DM, Ricks P, Edwards JR, et al. Antimicrobial-resistant pathogens associated with healthcare-associated infections: summary of data reported to the National Healthcare Safety Network at the Centers for Disease Control and Prevention, 2009–2010. *Infect Control Hosp Epidemiol* 2013;34:1–14.

van Hal SJ, Lodise TP, Paterson DL. The clinical significance of vancomycin minimum inhibitory concentration in Staphylococcus aureus infections: a systematic review and meta-analysis. *Clin Infect Dis* 2012;54:755–771.

Vincent JL, Rello J, Marshall J, et al. International study of the prevalence and outcomes of infection in intensive care units. *JAMA* 2009;302:2323–2329.

Yokoe DS, Anderson DJ, Berenholtz SM, et al. A compendium of strategies to prevent healthcare-associated infections in acute care hospitals: 2014 updates. *Am J Infect Control* 2014;42:820–828.

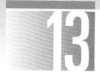

Critical Care Management of Ebola Virus Disease

Daniel W. Johnson

This chapter provides recommendations on the ICU care of Ebola virus disease in resource-rich environments. Prior to the 2014–2015 West African Ebola outbreak, the disease was thought to be nearly universally fatal. Recent clinical experience in West African nations, the United States, and Europe have shown that with aggressive supportive care, many patients infected with Ebola are able to make a complete recovery. In 2014, a small number of hospitals in the United States gained experience in the care of patients with Ebola primarily as a result of repatriation of U.S. citizens who contracted the disease in West Africa. The primary source of information in this chapter is the clinical experience of the Biocontainment Unit (BCU) at the University of Nebraska Medical Center (UNMC), where three patients received comprehensive care for confirmed Ebola virus disease.

I. **BACKGROUND ON EBOLA VIRUS / 2014 OUTBREAK**
   A. Ebola virus disease (EVD) is an infectious disease caused by the Ebola virus of the Filoviridae family. The Ebola virus is most likely animal-borne, with bats as the likely reservoir. Humans contract Ebola through direct contact with the body fluids of a person or animal that is sick with or has died from Ebola or from contact with an object contaminated with infected fluid.
   B. Ebola was discovered in 1976 in what is now the Democratic Republic of the Congo. A few small outbreaks of EVD have occurred in Africa since 1976, and in 2014 a large epidemic began in Liberia, Guinea, and Sierra Leone.
   C. The 2014 West African Ebola epidemic was the largest of all time and resulted in more than 27,000 cases and more than 11,000 deaths.

II. **COLLABORATIVE CARE**: Optimal care of the patient with EVD requires intense collaboration by multiple teams.
   A. **Strategic Planning** by the leadership of the following teams is essential: infectious disease, critical care, emergency medicine, hospital administration, nursing, clinical laboratory, respiratory care, infection control, pharmacy, radiology, clinical research, media relations, security, and public health departments.
   B. An **Infectious Disease specialist** and a **Critical Care physician** should be clearly identified as the attending physicians responsible for the overall care of a patient with EVD.

III. **DIAGNOSIS OF EVD** requires a high index of suspicion on the part of the clinician.
   A. **Identification of Patients at Risk** for EVD involves analysis of the following:
      1. **Recent travel** to areas with active EVD (e.g., West Africa in 2014–2015) or **known contact with EVD**.

2. History and physical findings may include fever, headache, myalgias, fatigue, diarrhea, emesis, abdominal pain, unexplained bleeding, or bruising. It is notable that in the 2014 outbreak, EVD was rarely associated with bleeding despite its former name "Ebola hemorrhagic fever."

B. The **diagnostic workup** for detection of Ebola should be directed by an infectious disease specialist and the public health authorities at the local, state, and federal levels.

   1. **Assays for Ebola** include ELISA, PCR, IgG, and IgM analyses. Optimal testing depends on timing and clinical situation.

C. **A Differential Diagnosis** must be constructed, as the vast majority of patients with these signs and symptoms have a disease other than EVD. Routine diagnostic testing for other possible diseases (e.g., malaria) should not be delayed for persons under investigation for EVD.

IV. **FACILITIES:** The care of a patient with EVD requires a significant amount of dedicated physical space capable of enabling full critical care services. While most hospitals lack a prededicated BCU, space can be created within an existing ICU provided that other patients can be located elsewhere and traffic within that ICU can be strictly controlled (Fig. 13.1).

A. **At Least Four Rooms** are needed to provide care for an individual with EVD:

   1. A **private isolation room** for the patient

   2. A room for the **storage of clean supplies** and **personal protective equipment (PPE)**. The following equipment should be dedicated to the unit (most equipment can be safely decontaminated by special cleaning procedures): portable X-ray, ultrasound machine, code blue cart, and an airway cart with a video laryngoscope.

   3. A room for **point-of-care laboratory** testing

   4. A room for the processing of **contaminated supplies and equipment**

B. **Video and Audio Monitoring** between the patient room and the nurses station is very useful as it allows clinicians and family members to observe the patient without coming into direct contact.

   1. To minimize exposure, one physician can examine the patient and call out physical findings while a colleague remains at the video monitor to act as a scribe.

   2. Frequent video and audio contact between the patient and family members are helpful for both as they endure the stress of battling a high-mortality illness.

V. The **initial workup** of a patient with confirmed EVD should include a comprehensive metabolic panel, calcium, magnesium, phosphorus, complete blood count with differential, PT-INR, PTT, fibrinogen, blood culture (aerobic and anaerobic), venous blood gas, portable chest X-ray, 12-lead EKG, and blood type. A complete antibody screen creates a high risk for splash exposure and thus should be omitted.

A. Laboratory testing should be performed with **point-of-care** equipment whenever possible. Any laboratory samples removed from the immediate patient care area must be handled with extreme caution so as to minimize the risk of transmission to a health care worker or to another patient. Extensive coordination with directors of clinical laboratories is necessary for optimal and timely utilization of laboratory tests.

B. Point-of-care **ultrasonography** can be especially helpful in the care of patients with EVD, as advanced imaging modalities such as CT and MRI are unavailable. Bedside ultrasonography can be used to assess for cardiac function, volume status, extravascular lung water, pleural effusion,

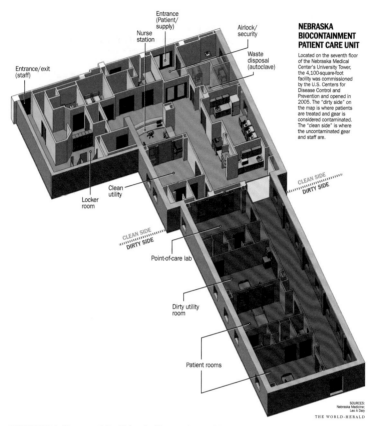

FIGURE 13.1 Diagram of the Nebraska Biocontainment Unit.

atelectasis, pneumonia, abdominal fluid, and deep venous thrombosis, in addition to guidance for invasive procedures such as central venous and arterial line placement. A standard ICU ultrasound system can be successfully decontaminated after use on a patient with EVD.

VI. **ENTRY TO THE PATIENT CARE UNIT** should be tightly restricted to essential personnel and should only take place after *all* personal items are stowed outside of the care area and the health care worker has changed into scrubs, closed-toed washable footwear, a gown, gloves, and standard mask.

VII. **PERSONAL PROTECTIVE EQUIPMENT (PPE)** is of critical importance and should be donned and doffed with a partner who is experienced in the use of PPE. The following PPE is recommended for all persons entering the room of a patient with EVD: fluid-impervious surgical gown, surgical cap (hair cover), N95 respirator mask, full-face shield, surgical hood (to cover the neck up to the chin), long surgical boot covers, standard gloves, long-cuff nitrile gloves with cuff edge duct taped to the surgical gown, covered by an additional pair of long-cuff nitrile gloves (three pairs of gloves in total).

A. The outer nitrile gloves should be considered to be the clinician's "gloves" while the inner pair of nitrile gloves should be considered to be the clinician's "skin."

   1. All members of the team must be vigilant for possible fluid exposures by colleagues and must speak up in the event they suspect exposure.

   2. In the event of significant glove contact with body fluids, the health care worker must wipe the outer gloves liberally with bleach wipes and then change the outer pair of gloves to reduce the likelihood of transmission of disease.

B. **Doffing** of PPE represents the highest risk time for contact with Ebola-infected fluids. Close observation by a doffing partner and strict adherence to published doffing protocols reduce this risk.

   1. Meticulous **hand/arm hygiene** with alcohol-based cleansers followed by thorough washing with soap and water is required after doffing PPE.

   2. A full-body shower with soap and water after departing the patient's room may be helpful in further reducing the likelihood of transmission.

VIII. **CLINICAL COURSE AND SUPPORTIVE CARE FOR EVD.** With the timely provision of full supportive care, the mortality rate of EVD appears to be well below 50% in resource-rich environments.

A. **Infectious Disease**: Symptoms begin about 8 to 10 days after exposure, and patients are considered noninfectious prior to the onset of symptoms. The high mortality rate of EVD is likely related to direct and indirect effects of the virus on cells and tissues vital to the immune system response.

B. **Neurologic/Musculoskeletal**: Patients generally develop severe fatigue, myalgias, and encephalopathy (likely related to dehydration and metabolic abnormalities). Standard delirium prevention measures should be performed. As soon as the patient can participate in physical therapy, this should be provided.

C. **Respiratory**: In the setting of likely capillary leak due to inflammatory response, rapid fluid administration has been observed to result in acute pulmonary edema and hypoxemia. While fluid resuscitation is necessary for all patients with EVD, patients must be closely monitored for changes in their respiratory status. Supplemental oxygen is often (but not always) necessary, and invasive mechanical ventilation has been necessary in several cases.

   1. If **tracheal intubation** is necessary, a rapid-sequence induction with neuromuscular blockade and video-laryngoscopy likely reduces the risks to patient and physician. PPE for intubation should consist of *enhanced* precaution PPE as recommended by the American Society of Anesthesiologists.

   2. Noninvasive positive pressure ventilation and flexible bronchoscopy are not recommended due to the high likelihood of aerosolization of secretions.

D. **Cardiovascular**: Patients vary widely with regard to hemodynamics, some demonstrating well-compensated hypovolemia and normal vital signs with others suffering from profound multifactorial shock. All patients have fluid deficits due to GI losses. Some exhibit systemic inflammatory response syndrome (SIRS) with loss of vascular tone while others do not. Orthostatic hypotension has been observed in multiple patients. In its severest form, EVD results in complete cardiovascular collapse secondary to low vascular tone, hypovolemia, and cardiac pump dysfunction with or without dysrhythmia. It is currently unknown whether this degree of hemodynamic derangement is seen with isolated EVD or is the result of bacterial superinfection exacerbating sepsis. Massive doses of vasopressors, inotropes, and fluids are, at times, indicated in the care of patients with EVD.

E. **Gastrointestinal, Hepatic, and Nutrition:** Patients generally suffer from severe diarrhea (sometimes with liters of liquid stool output per day), emesis, and inadequate oral intake. Early attempts at oral intake can be unsuccessful as they induce nausea and emesis. Total parenteral nutrition (TPN) is indicated in cases of ongoing inadequate intake. When patients improve enough to tolerate a moderate- to high-calorie diet, TPN should be replaced with oral intake. Elevated transaminases and bilirubin are common. This resolves among survivors, but in fatal cases liver laboratory values progressively worsen throughout the course, indicative of persistent hepatic necrosis.

F. **Renal, Fluids, and Electrolytes**

   1. **Dehydration, multiple electrolyte derangements (including hypokalemia, hyponatremia, hypocalcemia, and hypomagnesemia), and metabolic acidosis** are common. Fluid and electrolyte therapy should be started immediately, and the patient's volume status and electrolyte levels must be monitored closely. With initiation of nutrition, hypophosphatemia can become problematic and phosphorus must be repleted.

   2. **Acute kidney injury** may be absent, mild, or severe with complete anuria, depending on the severity of EVD and the timing of diagnosis.

      a. The underlying insult is likely prerenal due to dehydration, though a direct viral effect on kidney tissue is also possible.

      b. In cases of severe AKI, **renal replacement therapy** can be safely provided with continuous venovenous hemodialysis. Care should be taken to disinfect effluent from the dialysis machine prior to disposal.

G. **Hematologic Course:** Anemia, thrombocytopenia, and mild coagulopathy are common. Most patients do not require transfusion of blood products.

   1. Blood transfusion should follow accepted evidence-based practice guidelines.

   2. An ample supply of packed red blood cells that are type-specific for the patient and **negative for the Kell antigens** allows the intensivist to transfuse when necessary while minimizing the risk of a hemolytic transfusion reaction. This approach obviates the need for a full antibody screen on the patient's blood.

   3. Chemical prophylaxis against deep venous thrombosis may be precluded by thrombocytopenia and concern for possible hemorrhage.

IX. **VASCULAR ACCESS** must be established immediately after admission to allow for serial laboratory testing and for the administration of fluids and medications.

   A. If the patient is not severely critically ill, a **peripherally inserted central venous catheter (PICC)** is probably sufficient.

   B. Severely ill patients with organ system dysfunction should have **a multilumen internal jugular venous line and arterial line** placed.

      1. Obtaining advanced vascular access while wearing full PPE can be challenging. Ultrasound guidance is especially helpful because landmarks are difficult to palpate while wearing three pairs of gloves. Full sterile barrier precautions should be used as with any ICU patient—the outer layer of PPE should be a sterile surgical gown and sterile surgical gloves (in lieu of the outermost pair of nitrile gloves).

X. **EBOLA-SPECIFIC TREATMENTS** are all considered experimental at present, as no traditional clinical trials have been completed to assess efficacy and risks. Clinical trials are underway to evaluate these questions. Treatments administered during the 2014 outbreak include **ZMapp, TKM-Ebola, brincidofovir, and convalescent plasma.** Timely acquisition of plasma from EVD survivors requires rapid communication with the CDC, UNMC, and Emory University Hospital.

XI. **A STRICT ISOLATION POLICY,** prohibiting any movement of the patient outside of the isolation room for any reason, reduces the likelihood of disease transmission and should be strongly considered for all patients with confirmed EVD.

XII. **CODE STATUS** must be addressed immediately after admission to the patient care area. Clinicians and medical ethicists continue to engage in difficult debate on the issue of full cardiopulmonary resuscitation for patients with confirmed EVD. Each element of advanced cardiovascular life support (ACLS) must be considered in the context of the individual patient and then weighed against the very real risk of transmission of Ebola to a health care worker. Considering the low likelihood of survival when EVD has progressed to cardiac arrest and the risks of body fluid exposure to health care workers during chest compressions, a policy of "no chest compressions" is very reasonable while a patient is known to be currently infected with Ebola. Code status issues must be discussed with the patient and the family to ensure that all parties understand and agree to the current status at any given time. The intensivist can be especially helpful in these discussions, as end-of-life communication is a daily reality in the ICU environment.

XIII. **WASTE MANAGEMENT** during the care of a patient with EVD is challenging and must be thoroughly planned prior to patient admission. A single hospital stay for a patient with EVD can generate over 450 kg of solid waste, mostly due to the large amount of PPE utilized.
   A. Waste produced in the care of a patient with EVD cannot be managed in the same manner as standard medical waste, as the US Department of Transportation (DOT) classifies Ebola waste as Category A, which requires far more stringent methods for its removal.
   B. Two main options exist for the handling of Ebola solid medical waste:
      1. Dedicated biocontainment units benefit from **on-site autoclaves,** which can sterilize solid waste, allowing the waste to then be handled as standard medical waste.
      2. In the absence of on-site autoclave capabilities, a hospital must apply to the US DOT for a **special permit to handle Category A** waste.
   C. Liquid waste can be placed in the toilet with hospital-grade disinfectant, held for greater than the recommended contact time, and then flushed.

XIV. **THE PATIENT DISCHARGE PROCESS** must be conducted in conjunction with local, state, and federal public health authorities.
   A. Discharge requires consecutive blood samples drawn 24 hours apart to be **negative for Ebola virus RNA by qPCR** testing at the CDC.
   B. Prior to discharge the patient should **shower with chlorhexidine gluconate** (CHG) within a clean patient room, then shower again with CHG in the unit's shower. This process ensures that any contact between the Ebola-free patient and the contaminated environment does not result in the transmission of disease to people outside of the unit.

XV. ENVIRONMENTAL DECONTAMINATION OF THE ISOLATION ROOM AND ENTIRE UNIT should be conducted in full PPE according to the guidelines created by the UNMC College of Public Health.

XVI. MONITORING OF HEALTH CARE WORKERS WHO ENTER THE PATIENT ROOM should be conducted for 21 days following last patient contact. Different states and counties require different levels of monitoring, and the CDC provides guidelines on optimal monitoring practices and the appropriateness of travel restrictions.
   A. All health care workers exposed to patients with EVD should immediately contact an infectious disease specialist at the onset of classic symptoms: fever, headache, myalgias, fatigue, diarrhea, emesis, abdominal pain, unexplained bleeding, or bruising within the 21-day monitoring period.
   B. A predetermined plan must exist for the care of health care workers with suspected or confirmed EVD.

XVII. FREQUENT COMMUNICATION/COLLABORATION WITH OTHER CENTERS AND AGENCIES is necessary throughout the care of a patient with EVD. Resources to utilize include the CDC, NIH, local public health officials, the University of Nebraska Medical Center, and Emory University Hospital.

Acknowledgments

The author would like to acknowledge the entire Biocontainment Unit team at the University of Nebraska Medical Center, BCU patients and families, and every person worldwide who has worked to end the 2014–2015 Ebola crisis.

This chapter is dedicated to Dr. Martin Salia, a physician hero who bravely went to Sierra Leone to heal his fellow human beings while others fled. His courage and compassion will never be forgotten.

Selected Readings

Iwen PC, Smith PW, Hewlett AL, et al. Safety considerations in the laboratory testing of specimens suspected or known to contain Ebola virus. *Am J Clin Pathol* 2015;143(1):4–5.
Johnson DW, Sullivan JN, Piquette CA, et al. Lessons learned: critical care management of patients with Ebola in the United States. *Crit Care Med* 2015;43(6):1157–1164.
Kraft CS, Hewlett AL, Koepsell S, et al. The use of TKM-100802 and convalescent plasma in two patients with Ebola virus disease in the United States [published online ahead of print April 22, 2015]. *Clin Infect Dis.* doi:10.1093/cid/civ334
Lowe JJ, Gibbs SG, Schwedhelm SS, et al. Nebraska Biocontainment Unit perspective on disposal of Ebola medical waste. *Am J Infect Control* 2014;42(11):1152–1156.
Lowe JJ, Olinger PL, Gibbs SG, et al. Environmental infection control considerations for Ebola [published online ahead of print April 29, 2015]. *Am J Infect Control.* doi:10.1016/j.ajic.2015.03.006.
Nebraska Ebola Method App, available on iTunes U. Accessed May 22, 2015.
Smith PW, Boulter KC, Hewlett AL, et al. Planning and response to Ebola virus disease: an integrated approach. *Am J Infect Control* 2015;43(5):441–446.
Sueblinvong V, Johnson DW, Weinstein GL, et al. Critical care for multi-organ failure secondary to Ebola virus disease in the United States [published online ahead of print 2015]. *Crit Care Med.* doi:10.1097/CCM.0000000000001197
The Centers for Disease Control and Prevention. Ebola resource site. http://www.cdc.gov/vhf/ebola/. Accessed May 22, 2015.
The University of Nebraska Medical Center Biocontainment Unit. Ebola resource site. http://www.nebraskamed.com/biocontainment-unit/ebola. Accessed May 22, 2015.
The American Society of Anesthesiologists. Ebola resource site. http://www.asahq.org/resources/clinical-information/ebola-information#3. Accessed May 22, 2015.

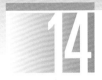

Transporting the Critically Ill Patient

Matthew J. G. Sigakis and Jeremi R. Mountjoy

I. **INTRODUCTION.** Critically ill patients often require transfer between or within hospitals when advanced levels of care, diagnostics, and/or procedures are required. The anticipated benefits of relocating a critically ill patient must be weighed against the potential risks involved during a transfer.

   A. **Interhospital Transport** refers to the relocation of a patient from one health care institution to another in order to provide more timely or additional specialized care. Issues associated with air transport and specialized teams are covered later in this chapter. Many of the principles learned from interhospital transfer may be applied to intrahospital transport.

   B. **Intrahospital Transport** is the movement of a patient to various sites *within* a health care facility for diagnostic or therapeutic procedures that cannot be performed at the primary location. For example, patients may be transported between locations of specialized resources such as the interventional radiology suite, operating room, or the intensive care unit.

II. **RISKS ASSOCIATED WITH TRANSPORT.** Whether the destination is near or far, the perceived benefit of transporting a patient must be balanced with the associated risks. These risks range from minor complications to major mishaps resulting in severe hypoxia, hypercarbia, or death. Hemodynamic and respiratory problems are most common. Patients who require transport out of the intensive care unit (ICU) have an increased rate of mortality, likely related to their severity of illness as opposed to transport alone.

   A. Risks of patient transport can be categorized as either *systems* or *patient* based (Tables 14.1 and 14.2). System errors may arise from equipment problems or human factors, such as poor provider communication or lack of sufficient training. These errors and circumstances may result in delay of problem recognition and amelioration. Any deterioration of a patient's condition may increase the risk of adverse events during transport. Sicker patients have low physiologic reserve and are exposed to more frequent intrahospital transfers. Compared with elective transport, emergent transport is associated with an increase in adverse events.

   B. Schwebel et al. reviewed 3,000 intrahospital transports in 1,700 ventilated ICU patients (18 years or older from April 2000 to November 2010). They matched transported patients with controls who had similar likelihoods of being transported but were not. Intrahospital transport was associated with an increased risk of several complications (Table 14.3).

III. **MINIMIZING RISKS OF TRANSPORT.** Various critical care and emergency medicine societies throughout the world have established criteria for managing patients during intrahospital transport (Table 14.4). Institutions should have written protocols for transporting patients within and between health care facilities.

   Each organ system must be assessed and specific plans made for transport and potential complications that may be encountered. A checklist is recommended (Appendices 1 and 2, supplemental material).

Systems-Based Complications

Equipment

Battery failure of portable equipment
Monitor malfunction
Depletion of portable oxygen supplies
Ventilator failure/disconnect
Disruption in portable medication infusions/pumps
Disconnection or loss of intravenous access
Chest tube failure/disconnect
Inaccurate calibration of hemodynamic monitors

Human

Inadequate training or experience
Poor planning and anticipation
Failure in hand-off and communication
Lack of vigilance and monitoring
Unintended/unrecognized extubation or loss of airway
Under-/Overventilation
Under-/Overresuscitation
Failure to secure or protect patient extremities

 Patient-Based Complications

Neurological—change in need for sedation or pain management, increased ICP, seizure
Respiratory—secretions, aspiration, de-recruitment, increased oxygen consumption
Cardiac—hypertension, hypotension, arrhythmia, ischemia
Increased bleeding
Hypothermia leading to shivering, hypercarbia, and inadequate ventilation

 Schwebel et al. 2013 *Crit Care Med*

Deep venous thrombosis
Pneumothorax
Ventilator-associated pneumonia
Atelectasis
Hypoglycemia
Hyperglycemia
Hypernatremia
Increased hospital length of stay

Essential Components of Safe Patient Transport

Stabilization of patient prior to transport
Risk assessment prior to patient transfer
Coordination and detailed communication between clinicians
Training and experience for managing patient condition and support mechanisms
Equipment adapted for transport and monitoring
Documentation—indication for transport and status pre-, during, and posttransport
Continuous patient and equipment checks
Establishing protocols and regular evaluation of transport processes
Minimize transport time
Close proximity of diagnostic and therapeutic units to ICU and emergency room
Adequate number of personnel

A. **Airway**. The stability of the patient's airway must be assessed prior to any movement. The position, function, and stability of an endotracheal tube (ETT) must be confirmed and, if necessary, resecured. Studies show that intubation can be safely accomplished during transport, yet certain patients may benefit from elective intubation prior to transport (Table 14.5). For both intubated and nonintubated patients, backup airway materials such as a bag valve mask, oral airway, intubation kit, and full oxygen tank are essential.

B. **Breathing and Ventilation**. Adequate oxygenation and ventilation must be substantiated prior to transport. An arterial blood gas should reflect a reasonable partial pressure of arterial oxygen (PaO_2), alveolar-to-arterial gradient (A-a) and partial pressure of arterial carbon dioxide ($PaCO_2$). Patients with a low PaO_2 or high A-a gradient may benefit from increased positive end-expiratory pressure (PEEP), increased fraction of inspired oxygen (FIO_2), suctioning, diuresis, or bronchoscopic evaluation. Elevated $PaCO_2$ can be addressed by optimizing minute ventilation, inspiratory-to-expiratory time or other ventilator mechanics. Paralysis may improve ventilator synchrony and prevent auto-PEEPing. Compared with manual ventilation, mechanical ventilation may be more appropriate in patients

 Indications for Pretransport Tracheal Intubation

Glasgow Coma Score less than 9
Respiratory acidosis and impending failure
Status asthmaticus
Shock (septic, hemorrhagic, cardiogenic, neurogenic)
Multitrauma
Recurrent seizures or status epilepticus
Facial or extensive burns
Acute epiglottitis
Angioedema
Anaphylaxis
Laryngeal-tracheal trauma
Combative patients

with complex medical issues, long transport distances, or specialized modes of ventilation. A chest tube for pneumothorax may be warranted, especially for air transport in which a small pneumothorax could expand into a tension pneumothorax.

C. **Circulation and Cardiovascular Support.** Adequate and functioning intravenous access must be established. Actively infusing medications for hemodynamic support must be noted and include a discussion of prior and anticipated trends in hemodynamics. Additional medications should accompany transport to ensure continual supportive care in anticipation of patient deterioration. All infusion pumps and monitors should be accurately calibrated, reliably functioning, and have sufficient battery life.

D. **Neurologic Status, Sedation, and Pain Management.** Neurologic status and preexisting deficits should be evaluated and documented before and after transport. Providers must anticipate the potential for decline in mental status and loss of airway. Adequate sedation and pain management should be provided to ensure patient comfort and to prevent patient from self-extubation or self-injury; restraints may be warranted. Often critically ill patients lack the muscle strength to generate sufficient respiratory effort due to myopathy of critical illness, steroid myopathy, or injury. If neuromuscular blocking drugs have been administered, sedation is usually required to prevent awareness.

E. **Temperature Regulation.** Patient transport from a temperature-controlled operating room (OR) or ICU through cooler hospital corridors or diagnostic suites may lead to hypothermia and significant patient consequences such as coagulopathy or increased $Paco_2$ due to shivering. Warm blankets can be used during transport to minimize heat loss.

F. **Patient Position.** Repositioning patients, such as from the OR table to transport bed, may lead to hemodynamic instability (particularly in hypovolemic patients). Ensure all patient extremities are within the confines of the transport vehicle to avoid incidental injury when moving through narrow walkways. Advance the patient bed in a "feet-first direction." The anesthesia provider should be positioned at head of bed, directing the movement and speed of transport, and maintain a clear and constant vision of monitors. There must be sufficient personnel to assist transport to allow for division of duties (pushing versus airway management or medication administration). The ability to call for help must be immediately available, such as with a mobile telephone.

G. **Consent and Legal Issues.** Disclosure of risks and consent to transport is usually implied, but should be delineated as separate from the risks associated with a planned procedure. Current guidelines require the patient or authorized health care proxy provide consent to interfacility transport.

1. Under the Emergency Medical Treatment and Active Labor Law (EM-TALA, 1986), transfer of patients to other care facilities must not be prejudiced by race or gender and must not be financially motivated. According to a landmark case in Maryland, *Sterling v. Johns Hopkins Hospital* in 2002, and consistent with the American College of Emergency Physicians regarding interfacility transfers, the treating physician at the sending hospital is responsible for assessing the patient condition, ascertaining need for transfer and determining a safe mode of relocation to the receiving care center. The receiving physician is mainly responsible for ensuring his or her institution's ability to provide the level of care requested. It is important to emphasize that the legal framework governing physician and hospital liability during interfacility transfer

TABLE 14.6	Verbal Hand-off between Sending and Receiving Care Providers

Patient demographics
Reason for transport
History of present illness
Active medical issues
Current vital signs
Airway management
Hemodynamic support
Critical medications
Access and monitoring
Critical laboratory and diagnostic studies
Pending information
Code status
Emergency family contact/health care proxy
Referring physician name
Accepting physician name
Exchange of contact information between care providers

varies between states and the particular circumstances related to the transfer. This emphasizes the importance of formal interfacility transfer agreements that delineate assignment of duty between the sending and receiving facilities.

H. Hand-offs. Almost two-thirds of adverse events in hospitals are a direct result of communication and hand-off failures. Implementation of a standardized hand-off bundle reduces medical errors and preventable adverse events among hospitalized patients. A standardized written and verbal hand-off between sending and receiving teams within or between institutions must be performed prior to transport. In addition, a posttransfer hand-off should occur between the transport and receiving care teams. Communication must occur physician-to-physician and nurse-to-nurse (Table 14.6). A provider familiar with the patient's medical course, along with the patient's medical record/chart, should accompany the patient during transport. Appropriately trained personnel and adequate care resources at the receiving site should be confirmed prior to patient transport (e.g., high-frequency oscillatory ventilation, extracorporeal membrane oxygenation, cardio-pulmonary bypass).

IV. USE OF CHECKLISTS: Implementation of checklists that emphasize safety guidelines before, during, and after transport is widely recommended. Various protocols developed for intrahospital transfer are *hospital specific*, but generally strive to achieve a balance between being too vague or too detailed. Our institution uses a practical and focused list of checks from the onset to conclusion of patient transport (see supplemental material, for example). Simulation improves the efficacy of transport protocols.

V. SPECIAL PATIENT POPULATIONS: In any patient, the airway, ventilation, and circulation should be assessed and stabilized. The progression of disease or complicating comorbidities may dictate preemptive endotracheal intubation and invasive monitoring prior to transfer.

A. **Pediatric Patient:** Adverse events during interhospital transport of critically ill pediatric patients are reduced with the use of specialized pediatric transport teams. Orr et al. illustrated that transport with a nonspecialized team was associated with increased unplanned events during transport and 28-day mortality. In this study, airway-related events were most common, followed by cardiopulmonary arrest, sustained hypotension, and loss of crucial intravenous access. Previously, the notion of the "golden hour" supported early transfer of critically ill pediatric patients to centers of specialized care. However, several more recent studies support physiologic stabilization with specialized pediatric critical care teams prior to transfer. Although retrospective in nature, these studies indicate adverse events during transport were reduced compared with early transfer. Delay of definitive treatment provided by the receiving specialized pediatric care center should always be considered. Intrafacility transport of complex patients such as those with congenital heart disease or receiving therapies such as extracorporeal membrane oxygenation or high-frequency oscillatory ventilation can be performed safely with the use of specialized teams and checklists.

B. **Obstetric Patient:** Maternal morbidity and mortality may be related to complications of the pregnancy itself, preexisting illness, or fetal delivery—operative or nonoperative. The most common causes of obstetric maternal morbidity, mortality, and ICU admission are obstetric hemorrhage and hypertensive (eclampsia) disorders. Trauma is the most common nonobstetric cause. Transport may occur if the primary location of delivery does not have the resources to care for the maternal or neonatal condition. Neonatal outcomes are improved when the mother is transported to a tertiary care center prior to delivery, as opposed to transporting a distressed neonate. Air transport is generally regarded as safe for the obstetric patient and fetus.

   1. The parturient airway is impacted by the physiology of pregnancy such as venous engorgement and increased soft tissue edema, leading to increased pharyngeal volume and potentially difficult mask ventilation, laryngoscopy, or intubation. When resuscitating and transporting an obstetric patient after approximately 20-week gestation, left uterine displacement must be maintained to prevent aortocaval compression leading to hypotension and uteroplacental insufficiency. Fetal heart rate monitoring may also be appropriate when the gestational age supports extrauterine viability.

C. **Burn Patient:** Burns to the face, soot in the airway, singed facial hair, and dark sputum suggest inhalation injury. Immediate application of high-flow oxygen and consideration of intubation is warranted. Carbon monoxide poisoning can lead to hypoxia that is unidentified by standard pulse oximetry. The inflammatory response to injury leads to rapid airway edema and histamine release causing bronchospasm, threatening airway patency. Prophylactic intubation or cricothyrotomy should be considered prior to transporting a burn patient.

   1. The inflammatory response after burn injury can lead to a significant distributive, hypovolemic, and cardiogenic shock, requiring aggressive fluid resuscitation. High urine output must be maintained if myoglobinuria is present secondary to rhabdomyolysis. Furthermore, lack of intact skin leads to significant heat and fluid loss. Warming blankets, clean sheets, fluid warmers, and elevated ambient temperature are employed throughout the transport process.

2. Chemical burns require copious irrigation of affected area. Contaminated clothing must be removed from patient, and health care personnel may require protective equipment to safely care for the patient during transport.

3. Positioning of the patient for transport after burn injury can have an important impact on outcome. To minimize contractures, patients with burns to the neck should be positioned with slight neck extension, provided there is no neck injury. Patients with burns to the axilla should be positioned with arms abducted in an "airplane position." Distal extremity burns should be splinted and wrapped in clean dressings.

D. **Neurologically Compromised Patient:** Neurologic injuries requiring transport for specialized care include trauma, ischemic stroke, hemorrhage, status epilepticus, and spinal cord injuries.

1. In acute ischemic stroke, extensive collateral sources of blood flow allow brain tissue to last substantially longer relative to a global ischemic state (such as cardiac arrest). When deemed appropriate, thrombolytic therapy may be used up to 3 hours (and in some patient populations 4.5 hours) after stroke symptom onset to restore blood flow to the ischemic penumbra. It is essential to minimize delays in inter- and intrahospital transport of the patient eligible for thrombolytic therapy. Avoiding hyperthermia and maintaining euglycemia are also important goals in minimizing brain ischemia.

2. In patients with elevated intracranial pressure (ICP), several methods may be employed to address acute elevations in ICP prior to or during transfer. Hyperventilation to drive $Paco_2$ less than 35 mmHg (maintenance typically <40 mmHg), elevating the head of bed, avoiding excessive PEEP, administering hyperosmolar therapy in the form of hypertonic saline or mannitol, or increasing drainage from an intraventricular catheter may be employed. Intracranial pressure may be monitored via an intracranial-pressure-monitoring bolt or intraventricular catheter, also known as an external ventricular drain (EVD). A pressure-monitoring bolt is a sensor placed directly into the brain parenchyma to transduce ICP. An EVD is placed directly into the ventricle and is attached to a pressure transducer. The EVD can monitor ICP and offer therapeutic cerebrospinal fluid (CSF) drainage. Care must be taken to ensure appropriate calibration and management of these devices during transport. Improper height of the EVD may prevent therapeutic (or lead to excess) CSF drainage, causing catastrophic injury.

3. During prehospital transport, spinal stabilization is achieved with a cervical collar and long backboard to prevent movement of a potentially unstable spinal column injury, leading to further injury of the spinal cord and nerve roots. The 2013 Congress of Neurological Surgeons (CNS) and the American Association of Neurological Surgeons (AANS) consensus statements recommend optimizing spinal cord perfusion pressure by avoidance of hypotension and maintenance of MAP between 85 and 90 mmHg for the first 7 days after injury. Avoidance of hypoxia is also important to minimize secondary neurologic injury. The updated guidelines specifically emphasize intravenous steroids (methylprednisolone) are NOT recommended for the treatment of acute spinal cord injury.

VI. MODES OF TRANSPORT

A. **Air-Based Interfacility Transport:** Transportation by air may be accomplished via fixed wing or rotor wing (helicopter). Rotor-wing transport is generally more efficient than ground transport for distances more than 45 miles and operates at an altitude below 5,000 ft. Fixed-wing transport is best utilized for distances more than 250 miles and cabins are pressurized between 5,000 and 7,000 ft despite true altitude often greater than 20,000 ft. Mobilizing an appropriately trained team for transport is needed to address patient-specific issues in-flight. Air-based in-transit critical events are as high as 5.0% in some studies, with hemodynamic deterioration the most common critical event.

1. **Air pressure:** Boyle's law indicates that at a constant temperature, the volume of air will increase as pressure decreases. Thus, it is important to consider patient injuries that could expand with aircraft altitude (Table 14.7). Decompression tubes should be placed prior to takeoff. It is also important to consider endotracheal tube cuff pressure and IV fluid bag volume that could also expand with increased altitude. Cabin pressures can be maintained at sea level, but this requires lower flying altitude and, thus, longer flight time. Some patients may require low-level altitude transfer <500 ft above sea level. For example, divers who ascend too quickly or fly shortly after a dive (particularly deep dives) may be at risk for nitrogen decompression sickness (bends). Until arrival at a specialized center with hyperbaric therapy, minimizing inflight altitude to avoid precipitation or exacerbation of symptoms is recommended.

2. **Oxygen:** The arterial partial pressure of oxygen, PaO_2, decreases with altitude secondary to decreased barometric pressure (Dalton's law) and can lead to hypoxia. Therefore, supplemental oxygen is required for patients in-flight. For patients with a high oxygen requirement, increases in PEEP may be more effective than further increases in inspired oxygen.

3. **Noise and Motion:** In-flight communication between transport personnel may be difficult without microphone-headset. Auscultation of heart and breath sounds may also be challenging. There is increased reliance on visual alarms rather than audible alarms. Supine patients with a fixed visual horizon may develop nausea and emesis, threatening an unprotected airway. Vibration may prevent effective palpation of pulses, noninvasive blood pressure cuff monitoring, and performance of procedures (e.g., intubation, IV access). Acceleration and deceleration forces can lead to changes in intracranial pressure and intravascular volume

| TABLE 14.7 | Medical Conditions Potentially Worsened by Altitude |

Pneumothorax
Pneumopericardium
Subcutaneous emphysema
Gas gangrene
Decompression sickness
Systemic air emboli
Gastric distention or pneumoperitoneum
Pneumocephalus
Eye or tympanic injury

and must be anticipated to ensure proper patient immobilization. Patient pain and anxiety may also be exacerbated.

   4. **Temperature and humidity**: Altitude may lead to patient hypothermia and dehydration requiring warming blankets and close assessment of the patient's temperature and intravascular volume status.

B. **Land-Based Interfacility Transport**: The advantages of ground transport include lower cost, better monitoring, and rapid mobilization. The transferring physician should be aware of the scope of practice of the transporting personnel. Land-based in-transit critical events are as high as 6.5% in some studies, with new hypotension being the most common critical event. Patients with mechanical ventilation, baseline hemodynamic instability, and longer transport duration are associated with the highest rate of critical events. Ground transport is usually faster than air transport for distances less than 10 miles.

APPENDIX 1. ICU PATIENT HOSPITAL TRANSPORT CHECKLIST

1. Patient
   a. Identify Patient (name, medical record number)
   b. Stable/appropriate for transport?
2. Care Team
   a. Identify team members planning to travel
   b. At least one team member familiar with patient history
   c. Identify receiving care team members and hospital
3. Medications/Transfusions
   a. Current infusions (e.g., vasopressors, blood product transfusions, epidural)
   b. Anticipated or scheduled medications
   c. Backup emergency medications
4. Airway
   a. Airway status appropriate for travel and planned procedure
   b. Planned mode of ventilation during travel and at receiving site
   c. Is there paralysis or insufficient respiratory effort?
   d. Backup airway equipment (e.g., ambu bag, backup tracheostomy kit)
5. Monitoring
   a. Standard monitor check (e.g., SpO_2, $ETCO_2$, blood pressure, telemetry, temperature)
   b. Other monitor check (e.g., intracranial pressure, arterial line, CVP/PA line)
6. Tubes/Line/Drains
   a. Chest tube check (e.g., leak/no leak, remain on suction)
   b. Spinal drain and/or endoventricular drain check (e.g., open/close, height)
   c. Other drain check (e.g., urinary, surgical drains, NG tube)
7. Additional Safety Checks
   a. Sufficient oxygen and electrical reserves (e.g., full oxygen tank, pump battery)
   b. If mechanically ventilated, pressure alarm active
   c. Sufficient intravenous access
   d. Patient extremities in safe position to avoid trauma or pressure point injury

APPENDIX 2. ICU PATIENT HOSPITAL TRANSPORT STATUS CHECKLIST

1. Airway—secure ventilation system
2. Breathing—bilateral chest rise and auscultation, insufflation pressure, SpO_2, end-tidal CO_2

3. Circulation—vital signs on monitor, palpable pulse
4. Disconnect—airway, oxygen supply, IV lines, infusions, drains, electrical supply
5. Ergonomics—patient position and support

Selected Readings

American College of Emergency Physicians. Interfacility transportation of the critical care patient and its medical direction, revised and approved by the ACEP April 2012. http://www.acep.org/Clinical---Practice-Management/Interfacility-Transportation-of-the-Critical-Care-Patient-and-Its-Medical-Direction/. Accessed June 20, 2014.

Australasian College for Emergency Medicine, Australian and New Zealand College of Anaesthetists, Joint Faculty of Intensive Care Medicine. Minimum standards for intrahospital transport of critically ill patients. *Emerg Med (Fremantle)* 2003;15(2):202–204.

Borrows EL, Lutman DH, Montgomery MA, et al. Effect of patient- and team-related factors on stabilization time during pediatric intensive care transport. *Pediatr Crit Care Med* 2010;11:451–456.

Cancio LC. Airway management and smoke inhalation injury in the burn patient. *Clin Plast Surg* 2009;36:555–567.

Day D. Keeping patients safe during intrahospital transport. *Crit Care Nurse* 2010;30:18–32.

Edge WE, Kanter RK, Weigle CG, et al. Reduction of morbidity in interhospital transport by specialized pediatric staff. *Crit Care Med* 1994;22:1186–1191.

The Emergency Medical Treatment and Active Labor Act, as established under the Consolidated Omnibus Budget Reconciliation Act (COBRA) of 1985 (42 USC 1395 dd) and 42 CFR 489.24; 42 CFR 489.20 (EMTALA regulations).

Fanara B, Manzon C, Barbot O, et al. Recommendations for the intra-hospital transport of critically ill patients. *Crit Care* 2010;14:R87.

Goss C, Ugarte J, Vadukul K, et al. Cool the burn: burn injuries require quick identification, treatment & transport. *JEMS* 2012;37:34–40.

Hurlbert RJ, Hadley MN, Walters BC, et al. Pharmacological therapy for acute spinal cord injury. *Neurosurgery* 2013;72(suppl 2):93–105.

Intensive Care Society. *Guidelines for the transport of the critically ill adult.* 3rd ed. London: Intensive Care Society, 2011.

Jauch EC, Saver JL, Adams HP Jr, et al. Guidelines for the early management of patients with acute ischemic stroke: a guideline for healthcare professionals from the American Heart Association/American Stroke Association. *Stroke* 2013;44:870–947.

Johnson D, Luscombe M. Aeromedical transfer of the critically ill patient. *JICS* 2011;12:307–312.

Joint Commission. Sentinel event statistics data: root causes by event type. http://www.jointcommission.org/assets/1/18/Root_Causes_by_Event_Type_2004-2Q2013.pdf. Accessed June 20, 2014.

Kodali BS, Chandrasekhar S, Bulich LN, Topulos GP, Datta S. Airway changes during labor and delivery. *Anesthesiology* 2008;108:357–362.

Lahner D, Nikolic A, Marhofer P, et al. Incidence of complications in intrahospital transport of critically ill patients: experience in an Austrian university hospital. *Wein Klin Wochenschr* 2007;119:412–416.

Lawless N, Tobias S, Mayorga MA. FiO$_2$ and positive end-expiratory pressure as compensation for altitude-induced hypoxemia in an acute respiratory distress syndrome model: implications for air transportation of critically ill patients. *Crit Care Med* 2001;29:2149–2155.

Low RB, Martin D, Brown C. Emergency air transport of pregnant patients: the national experience. *J Emerg Med* 1988;6:41–48.

Orr RA, Felmet KA, Han Y, et al. Pediatric specialized transport teams are associated with improved outcomes. *Pediatrics* 2009;124:40–48.

Prodhan P, Fiser RT, Cenac S, et al. Intrahospital transport of children on extracorporeal membrane oxygenation: indications, process, interventions, and effectiveness. *Pediatr Crit Care Med* 2010;11:227–233.

Quenot JP, Milési C, Cravoisy A, et al. Intrahospital transport of critically ill patients (excluding newborns) recommendations of the Société de Réanimation de Langue Française (SRLF), the Société Française d'Anesthésie et de Réanimation (SFAR), and the Société Française de Médecine d'Urgence (SFMU). *Ann Intensive Care* 2012;2:1.

Ryken TC, Hurlbert RJ, Hadley MN, et al. The acute cardiopulmonary management of patients with cervical spinal cord injuries. *Neurosurgery* 2013;72(suppl 2):84–92.

Schwebel C, Clec'h C, Magne S, et al. Safety of intrahospital transport in ventilated critically ill patients: a multicenter cohort study. *Crit Care Med* 2013;41:1919–1928.

SIAARTI Study Group for Safety in Anesthesia and Intensive Care. Recommendations on the transport of critically ill patient. *Minerva Anestesiol* 2006;72(10):XXXVII–LVII.

Singh JM, MacDonald RD, Bronskill SE, et al. Incidence and predictors of critical events during urgent air-medical transport. *CMAJ* 2009;181:579–584.

Singh JM, MacDonald RD, Ahghari M. Critical events during land-based interfacility transport. *Ann Emerg Med* 2014;64:9–15.e2. doi:10.1016/j.annemergmed.2013.12.009.

Sterling v. Johns Hopkins Hosp., 802 A. 2d 440 (Md. Ct. Spec. App. 2002).

Warren J, Fromm RE, Orr RA, et al. Guidelines for the inter- and intra-hospital transport of critically ill patients. *Crit Care Med* 2004;32:256–262.

Zeeman GG. Obstetric critical care: a blueprint for improved outcomes. *Crit Care Med* 2006;34(9 suppl):S208–S214.

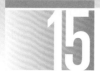

Coronary Artery Disease

Stephen D. Wilkins, Corry "Jeb" Kucik and
Michael G. Fitzsimons

I. **INTRODUCTION**: Coronary artery disease (CAD) is the most common type of heart disease and is the leading cause of adult morbidity and mortality in the United States, accounting for ~17% of deaths. The accumulation of atheromatous plaques within coronary arteries over time results in ischemia and/or infarction of the myocardium. Medical treatment focuses on identifying at-risk patients and preventing sequelae through risk modification. The major **risk factors** of CAD are hypertension (HTN), diabetes mellitus (DM), smoking, dyslipidemia (high LDL or low HDL), age above 45 (for men), age above 55 (for women), obesity or metabolic syndrome, physical inactivity, elevated homocysteine levels, and a family history of CAD. African American, Mexican American, and Native American patients also tend to have higher incidences of CAD. Aggressive risk factor modification and coronary interventions with stenting have resulted in marked improvements in the outcomes of these patients.

A. **Definitions**

1. **Angina pectoris** is substernal pressure or pain that occurs at rest or with physical or emotional stress, lasting up to 10 minutes. It can radiate to the back, jaw, arm, or shoulder, usually on the left. Angina usually reflects compromise of at least one epicardial coronary artery and implies ischemia, but not necessarily myocardial infarction (MI). Angina is the initial manifestation in 50% of patients with ischemic heart disease. Symptoms also include nausea, vomiting, diaphoresis, and shortness of breath. Angina may present in valvular heart disease, hypertrophic cardiomyopathy, or uncontrolled HTN. The Canadian Cardiovascular Society Classification System grades angina from Class I (ordinary physical exertion does not cause angina) to Class IV (angina with minimal exertion or at rest).

   a. **Stable angina** demonstrates a pattern that has not changed in frequency, duration, or ease of relief for several months. Predictable symptoms present with exertion and abate with rest. A fixed coronary atheroma with a fibrous cap is generally the culprit lesion.

   b. **Variant (Prinzmetal's) angina** occurs at rest, is often worse in the morning, lasts several minutes, and is accompanied by transient ST-segment elevation and/or ventricular dysrhythmias. It can be induced by exercise and stems from vasospasm in a coronary artery that may not have significant atheromatous disease. Smoking is a major risk factor. Hyperventilation, hypocalcemia, cocaine, pseudoephedrine, and ephedrine have also been implicated.

2. **Acute coronary syndromes (ACS)** are three conditions associated with acute myocardial ischemia secondary to poor myocardial perfusion: unstable angina **(UA)**, non–ST-segment elevation myocardial infarction **(NSTEMI)**, and ST-segment elevation myocardial infarction **(STEMI)**.

   a. **Unstable angina** indicates ischemia, has a recent onset (1–2 months), has increasing frequency and intensity, and recurs at progressively lower levels of stress, even at rest. The prognosis is poor, as 10% of patients have significant disease of the left main coronary artery and approximately 20% of patients will suffer an acute MI within 3 months. Plaque rupture, platelet aggregation, thrombosis, and vasospasm are the underlying causes.

  b. **NSTEMI** indicates more severe myocardial ischemia in the setting of suggestive angina, resulting in a release of cardiac biomarkers. NSTEMI presents with ST-segment depressions or prominent T-wave inversions. The management of NSTEMI focuses on improving oxygen (O_2) supply and reducing demand in at-risk myocardium, thus preventing progression of damage. It must always be borne in mind that **a nondiagnostic electrocardiogram (ECG) does not rule out MI**.

  c. STEMI is defined by characteristic symptoms of myocardial ischemia with associated ST-segment elevation and subsequent release of cardiac biomarkers. There is severe, possibly irreversible damage to the myocardium, with the appearance of a new ST-segment elevation at the J-point in at least two contiguous leads ≥ 2 mm (0.2 mV) in men or ≥ 1.5 mm (0.15 mV) in women in leads V_2–V_3 and/or ≥ 1 mm (0.1 mV) in other contiguous leads. New or presumably new LBBB has traditionally been considered a STEMI equivalent; however, recent evidence finds that most patients with chest pain and a "new" LBBB do not have a STEMI, calling into question the validity of this practice. Left ventricular hypertrophy, hyperkalemia, pericarditis, early repolarization, or paced rhythms can complicate the diagnosis. Treatment focuses on timely reperfusion.

3. **Noncardiac chest pain** is not related to coronary ischemia, but may be life threatening. Aortic dissection, pulmonary embolism, and pneumothorax must be ruled out immediately. Diagnosing chest pain as cardiac or noncardiac can be challenging, and cardiac risk factors, past medical history, physical exam, and radiologic and laboratory results must be considered. Gastrointestinal and esophageal pathology, pleuritic or costochondritic causes, and recent physical or emotional stress are frequent causes of noncardiac chest pain.

4. **Perioperative MI** is one of the most significant threats in major noncardiac surgery. Patients who suffer MI after surgery have a 15% to 25% risk of in-hospital death and a significant increase in 6-month morbidity and mortality. While there is controversy over accepted definitions of perioperative MI, the incidence may be up to 6% in patients with CAD. While an MI is normally diagnosed on the basis of three criteria (chest pain, biomarker levels, ECG changes), a perioperative MI may be obscured by pain or pain-control techniques to the point of being "silent." A high index of suspicion is critical, and increased consideration should be given to the ECG and cardiac enzymes.

B. **Pathophysiology**

1. **Myocardial O_2 supply–demand balance.** The myocardium has the highest O_2 consumption per tissue mass of all human organs. At rest, the myocardial O_2 extraction ratio is near maximum at 70% to 80% leaving minimal O_2 extraction reserve for increased demand. During exertion, increased O_2 demand must be met with an increase in O_2 delivery. Myocardial ischemia and infarction occur when O_2 demand exceeds O_2 delivery.

   a. **Myocardial O_2 supply** is determined by the following:

      1. **Coronary blood flow** is determined by the aortic root pressure at the beginning of diastole minus the resistance of transmural

pressure. As transmural resistance is low in diastole, myocardial blood flow is higher during this period. Tachycardia, which minimizes diastolic time, can thus induce ischemia. Normal coronary arteries compensate by sympathetically or metabolically mediated dilation, which can increase blood flow four- to fivefold during exercise or stress. However, stenosis can reduce ability of the coronary artery to dilate and thus limit O_2 supply downstream. Polycythemia, hyperviscosity, and sickle cell disease may further compromise coronary blood flow.

2. **O_2 content** is dependent on hemoglobin (Hgb) concentration and saturation with O_2 (Sao_2), and to a lesser extent on dissolved O_2 concentration (see **Chapter 2**). An ideal Hgb level is not known, but compensation through increased cardiac output (CO) occurs with anemia. Hyperbaric oxygen therapy may be useful to augment O_2 supply in patients with severe anemia or ACS.

b. **Myocardial O_2 demand** is influenced by the following:
1. **Ventricular wall tension (T),** which according to Laplace's law is $T = PR/2h$, where P is transmural pressure, R is ventricular radius, and h is wall thickness. Ventricular dilation and increased afterload both increase wall tension and myocardial O_2 demand. Concentric hypertrophy can decrease wall tension, but also increases the amount of myocardium to be perfused.
2. **Heart rate (HR)** increases O_2 demand by increasing O_2 consumption. Tachycardia shortens diastole and limits coronary perfusion in atherosclerotic vessels thereby limiting O_2 supply. Hyperthyroidism, sympathomimetics (e.g., cocaine), or anxiety can increase HR and O_2 demand.
3. An increase in **contractility,** which is the intrinsic property of the myocyte to contract against a load, increases O_2 demand. Positive inotropes (e.g., epinephrine, digoxin) increase the O_2 demand of myocardium that may already be at risk.

2. **Etiologies of myocardial O_2 demand imbalance.** More than 90% of myocardial ischemia and infarction result from atherosclerosis. Accordingly, most perioperative MIs stem from abrupt, unpredictable occlusion (partial or complete) secondary to acute atherosclerotic plaque rupture. Other causes include coronary vasospasm or thromboembolism, stent thrombosis, vasculitis, trauma, valvular heart disease (e.g., aortic stenosis), hypertrophic or dilated cardiomyopathies, and thyrotoxicosis.

II. ANGINA

A. **History** should ascertain whether risk factors (DM, smoking, HTN, family history of early coronary disease) exist. Pain is characterized by character, location, duration, radiation, and exacerbating (emotional stress, eating, cold weather) or alleviating (rest, medications) factors. Pain is often a "pressure" described as "heavy" or "grip-like" and may radiate to the arm or jaw. Women, elderly, and diabetic patients may present with atypical symptoms including nausea, vomiting, mid-epigastric pain, or sharp chest pain. An unstable, escalating constellation of symptoms must be differentiated from a stable anginal pattern. Severe angina of recent onset, angina at rest, or angina of increasing duration, frequency, or intensity is classified as unstable and considered a part of the spectrum of ACS.

B. **Physical Examination** is often nonspecific. Findings of distress, anxiety, tachycardia, HTN, an S4 gallop, pulmonary rales, xanthomas, or peripheral atherosclerosis may be evident. Pulmonary edema, a new or worsening murmur of mitral regurgitation, and angina with hypotension are associated with a high risk of progression to nonfatal MI or death.

C. Noninvasive Studies

1. The sensitivity of **resting ECG** abnormalities for coronary heart disease events is low. The prevalence of the most common ECG abnormalities (Q waves, left ventricular hypertrophy, bundle-branch blocks, and ST-segment depression) ranges from 1% to 10%. ECG changes indicative of myocardial ischemia that may progress to MI include new ST-segment elevations at the J-point in two or more contiguous leads that are $\geq$0.2 mV in leads V_2–V_3 and $\geq$0.1 mV in all other leads. Ischemia from coronary vasospasm may present with ST-segment elevation. ST-segment depression or T-wave inversions may also signal risk for MI. Isolated J-point elevation or early repolarization may occur as a normal variant in young, healthy adults. Significant Q waves are suggestive of a prior MI. A bundle branch block (BBB) or artificial pacer may complicate detection of ST-segment or T-wave abnormalities. Serial ECGs in 15-to-20-minute intervals can determine whether ischemia is evolving. In general, reversibility of ECG changes after therapeutic interventions is highly suggestive of ischemia. Table 15.1 outlines the ECG changes associated with specific regions of ischemic myocardium.

2. **Exercise ECG.** Exercise stress testing involves monitoring HR, blood pressure (BP), and ECG while the patient performs a standardized exercise protocol on a treadmill or bicycle. Indications for exercise testing include presumptive obstructive CAD, risk assessment and prognosis in suspected or known CAD, the presence of multiple risk factors in asymptomatic patients, and certain postrevascularization situations. Each level of exercise reflects increased O_2 uptake or metabolic equivalents (METs). A single MET is 3.5 cm^3 O_2/kg/min. Most protocols initiate exercise at 3 to 5 METs and increase by several METs every 2 to 3 minutes. The test is discontinued for moderate to severe angina, significant arrhythmias, exhaustion, CNS symptoms, decrease in BP > 10 mmHg from baseline, severe hypertensive response (SBP > 250 mmHg or DBP >115 mmHg), significant ECG changes, or evidence of poor peripheral perfusion. In general, achievement of a predicted maximal HR of 85% or a double product (HR $\times$ SBP) of 20,000 is necessary for

TABLE 15.1	Location of Ischemia or Infarct by Electrocardiographic Criteria	
Region	**Leads**	**Coronary Artery**
Anteroseptal	V_1–V_2	Left anterior descending
Anterior	V_2–V_5	Left anterior descending
Apical	V_5–V_6	Left anterior descending
Lateral	I, aVL	Circumflex
Inferior	II, III, aVF	Right coronary artery
Posterior (Inferolateral)[a]	Large R wave in V_1, V_2, or V_3 with ST depression	Right coronary artery
Right ventricular	V_3R, V_4R	Right coronary artery

[a]The posterior and inferolateral designate the same segment of the left ventricle. A posterior myocardial infarction may be the result of compromise of the right coronary artery or an obtuse marginal branch of the circumflex artery.

a diagnostic negative test. A **positive test** (i.e., one which demonstrates ST-segment elevation or depression, a fall in BP with exercise, development of serious arrhythmias, or the development of anginal chest pain with exercise) indicates a high likelihood of significant CAD. Sensitivity for obstructive CAD increases with the severity of stenotic disease. ECG changes occurring at lower workloads are generally more significant than those at higher workloads. Positive tests should prompt consideration of cardiac catheterization and revascularization. Absolute contraindications to exercise stress testing include a recent MI (within 2 days), high-risk unstable angina, symptomatic severe aortic stenosis, symptomatic heart failure, arrhythmia causing hemodynamic compromise, acute pulmonary embolus, aortic dissection, inability to exercise, and an uninterpretable ECG. Relative contraindications include uncontrolled HTN (SBP >200 mmHg or DBP >110 mmHg), moderate stenotic valvular disease, tachy- or bradyarrhythmias, hypertrophic cardiomyopathy, left main coronary stenosis, high-grade atrioventricular block, and a physical or mental limitation to exercise.

3. **Myocardial injury enzymes.** Biomarker analysis is undertaken immediately to help determine whether angina is stable or unstable. Negative results within 6 hours of symptom onset necessitate further testing at 6-hour intervals if ACS is suspected. When damaged (e.g., by trauma or infarction), cardiac myocytes release various proteins such as **creatine kinase-MB fraction** (CK-MB), **troponin,** and myoglobin into the blood. Myocardial troponin is the most accurate marker. Troponin is substantially more sensitive than CK-MB related to the fact that more troponin is found in the heart per gram of myocardium and a greater percentage released from tissue arrives in the blood stream. Troponin is highly specific for cardiac injury, and rare false positives are inherent to any immunoassay testing. In the setting of renal failure, troponin levels may be chronically elevated, and the trend from baseline is key to diagnosing acute injury. Other causes of troponin elevation include advanced heart failure, subarachnoid hemorrhage, acute pulmonary embolism, acute critical illness, acute pericarditis, direct trauma, and myocarditis. Troponin levels may be especially valuable in the perioperative period where CK-MB may be elevated for other reasons and may not reflect myocardial necrosis.

4. **Radionuclide perfusion imaging** assesses both myocardial perfusion and function in a patient with stable angina.
   a. **Exercise myocardial perfusion imaging.** Thallium-201 is a radioactive potassium analog that is avidly extracted by viable myocardium in proportion to regional myocardial blood flow during exercise. Regions of decreased uptake correlate with the severity of coronary stenosis supplying the regions. Imaging after rest may show a "fixed defect" that takes up no tracer at all, which represents an area of prior infarct, while a "reversible defect," a region that regains uptake, is considered to be myocardium at risk of ischemia.
   b. **Exercise radionuclide ventriculography.** Intravenous technetium-99m sestamibi accumulates in myocardium in proportion to myocardial blood flow, and multiple ventricular images that are synchronized to the cardiac cycle are acquired at rest and during stress. Ischemia is suggested by regional wall motion abnormalities and the inability to increase left ventricular ejection fraction (LVEF) during exercise.
   c. **Pharmacologic stress perfusion imaging.** Patients not able to undergo exercise testing due to inability to perform moderate physical

activity or disabling comorbidity can undergo pharmacological stress imaging. **Adenosine** and **dipyridamole** are coronary vasodilators commonly used in stress imaging. Adenosine increases blood flow in disease-free coronary vessels. Dipyridamole inhibits cellular uptake and degradation of adenosine, indirectly increasing coronary flow in disease-free vessels. Since stenotic areas are already maximally dilated, the dilation of disease-free vessels creates differential flow patterns upon coronary imaging. Both drugs may cause angina, headache, or bronchospasm, and must be used with caution in patients with obstructive pulmonary disease. The inotrope **dobutamine** increases HR, SBP, and contractility, causing increased blood flow secondarily. Imaging after dobutamine administration may show heterogeneous flow due to nondilating stenotic areas.

D. Invasive Studies. Coronary angiography remains the gold standard for quantifying the extent of CAD and guiding percutaneous coronary intervention (PCI; e.g., angioplasty, stenting, atherectomy) or coronary artery bypass grafting (CABG). Coronary angiography will reveal cardiac and coronary anatomy, wall motion abnormalities, and hemodynamic parameters (e.g., ejection fraction). A coronary obstruction is clinically significant when more than 70% of the luminal diameter is narrowed or when more than 50% of the luminal diameter of the left main coronary artery is narrowed. Coronary angiography is not without risk; the mortality rate is approximately 0.5% to 1%. Complications associated with PCI include coronary dissection or perforation, coronary intramural hematoma, distal embolization, myocardial ischemia and infarction, access site bleeding or hematoma, retroperitoneal hematoma, acute kidney injury, stroke, thrombocytopenia, arrhythmias, infection, and effects of radiation exposure.

E. Medical Management. Once it has been determined that angina is stable, appropriate management should be initiated.
1. Smoking cessation
2. **BP control** to a goal of $<140/90$ mmHg
3. Dietary modification
4. Medically supervised physical activity and weight reduction
5. **Aspirin (ASA)** acts by irreversibly inhibiting cyclooxygenase-1 (COX-1) in platelets thereby preventing formation of thromboxane A2 and decreasing platelet aggregation. ASA should be started at 81 to 325 mg daily if no contraindications exist (e.g., allergic reaction, bleeding disorder, coagulopathy).
6. **Angiotensin-converting enzyme (ACE) inhibitors** reduce sympathetic tone, control HTN, and have a survival benefit in heart failure (HF). In the absence of contraindications (e.g., angioedema, renal artery stenosis), ACE-inhibitors should be started in all patients with an ejection fraction less than 40%, especially if HTN, DM, or renal disease coexists. The benefit of ACE-inhibitors in patients with stable CAD without HF is uncertain in the literature.
7. **β-Blockers** should be initiated in all patients with a history of MI or ACS unless contraindicated (Table 15.2).
8. **HMG-CoA reductase inhibitors ("statins")** improve lipid profiles, limiting progression of atherosclerotic disease and coronary calcium deposition while stabilizing existing plaques. Statin therapy lowers the risk of coronary heart disease death, recurrent MI, stroke, and the need for revascularization. Contraindications include allergic reaction and active liver disease.

TABLE 15.2 Contraindications to β-blockers in ACS

- Marked first-degree AV block
- Any form of second- or third-degree AV block
- Active asthma or history of reactive airway disease
- Evidence of left ventricular dysfunction, heart failure, or low output state
- High risk for shock (e.g., time delay to presentation, lower blood pressure)

F. Invasive Management for stable angina consists of PCI or CABG and depends upon the patient's response to medical management as well as the underlying coronary artery disease found on coronary angiography (see **Section II.B.**)

III. **ACUTE CORONARY SYNDROMES.** Regardless of whether ACS is due to unstable angina (UA), NSTEMI, or STEMI, the goal is to minimize ischemic time and, when appropriate, initiate reperfusion therapy with thrombolysis, PCI, or CABG.

  A. The **history** should attempt to differentiate UA from an acute MI. Symptoms are often indistinguishable (see **Section II.A**).

  B. The **physical examination** is unlikely to distinguish UA from an acute MI (see **Section II.B**).

  C. As for angina, noninvasive studies include the ECG and cardiac enzymes.

   1. A **12-lead ECG** should be obtained as soon as possible to determine whether a STEMI is occurring and immediate revascularization is needed. Transient ST-segment elevations (>0.05 mV) that resolve with rest likely indicates true ischemia and severe underlying CAD. ST-segment elevation <0.05 mV, ST-segment depression, or T-wave inversion is more often associated with NSTEMI or UA. A normal ECG does **not** rule out MI, as up to 6% of patients later confirmed to have had MIs may present as such. Serial ECGs are more accurate than an isolated study.

   2. The best **biomarker** confirmation is a rise in cardiac troponin I or T ($>$99th percentile). If clinical suspicion for MI is high, cardiac troponin should be drawn at 0, 6 to 9, and 12 to 24 hours. Cardiac troponin I and T are highly specific for myocardial damage but do not indicate the mechanism of damage. CK-MB is less sensitive, but may be substituted if troponin measurement is not available (see **Section II.C.3**).

   3. The **chest x-ray (CXR)** can detect MI complications such as pulmonary venous congestion and can help to rule out aortic dissection, pneumonia, pleural effusion, and pneumothorax. Pulmonary venous congestion and increased cardiothoracic ratio ($>50\%$) found on initial CXR is a marker for increased mortality in acute MI.

   4. **Transthoracic echocardiography (TTE)** can help establish the diagnosis, prognosis, location, extent, and complications related to acute MI. Findings may include regional wall motion abnormalities, ventricular septal defect (VSD), papillary muscle rupture, free wall rupture, valvular pathology, thrombus formation, and changes in global ventricular function. If TTE is available and the echocardiographer is experienced, this modality offers a convenient method by which a more complete clinical picture can be obtained.

D. Management of Acute MI

1. The general approach to acute MI focuses on minimizing total ischemic time (onset of symptoms to start of reperfusion). In a PCI-capable hospital, **primary PCI should be accomplished within 90 minutes of STEMI.** Initiation of thrombolysis within 30 minutes is the system goal for STEMI when PCI is not available. Early invasive strategy (diagnostic angiography, PCI) is indicated in UA/NSTEMI in the setting of refractory angina or hemodynamic and/or electrical instability. Patients initially stabilized on medical therapy with UA/NSTEMI for whom an initial invasive (PCI) strategy is chosen, early angiography and intervention within 24 hours reduces ischemic complications.

2. **Supportive measures.** Supplemental O_2, IV access, routine vitals, and continuous ECG should be initiated. Few data exist to support or refute the value of routine O_2 in ACS. Supplemental O_2 is indicated for patients with HF or hypoxemia (Spo_2 <90%). Patients with severe HF or cardiogenic shock may need either noninvasive positive pressure ventilation or intubation and mechanical ventilation. Laboratory studies include electrolytes with magnesium, lipid profile, and complete blood count to detect anemia. Continuous pulse oximetry is critical to evaluate oxygenation, especially in patients with HF or cardiogenic shock.

3. **Treatments.** Unless contraindicated, a β-blocker, ASA, anticoagulation, ACE-inhibitor, statin, and possibly a thienopyridine (e.g., clopidogrel) should be administered.

   a. **β-BLOCKADE** appears to reduce myocardial O_2 consumption by slowing the HR and reducing cardiac contractility. However, there is evidence that β-blockers may be detrimental in patients with acute HF (**Table 15.2**). If no contraindications exist, β-blockers should be initiated in the first 24 hours. Initially, **metoprolol** 5 mg IV every 5 minutes up to a total of 15 mg may be given, titrating to HR and BP. If tolerated, metoprolol 25 to 50 mg orally every 6 hours can be administered for 2 days and then increased up to 100 mg orally twice daily as tolerated. **Carvedilol** 6.25 mg administered orally twice a day, titrated up to a maximum of 25 mg twice a day, may reduce mortality in patients with an acute MI and LV dysfunction.

   b. The benefit of **calcium-channel blockers (CCBs)** in ACS is related to symptom reduction in patients already receiving β-blockers and nitrates or who cannot tolerate these agents. There is no beneficial effect on infarct size or the rate of reinfarction when CCBs are initiated during the acute phase of STEMI. **Nifedipine** 30 to 90 mg orally can be administered. If tolerated, a longer-acting agent such as **Diltiazem** (slow release) 120 to 360 mg once daily or **Verapamil** (slow release) 120 to 480 mg by mouth once a day may be initiated.

   c. **Nitrates** increase venous capacitance, thus decreasing preload and cardiac work. Nitrates dilate epicardial coronary arteries and collateral circulation, and also inhibit platelet function. Evidence does not support routine long-term nitrate therapy in MI unless pain persists. IV **nitroglycerin (NTG)** is started at 10 μg/min and titrated to symptom relief or BP response. Patients with acute MI or HF, large anterior infarcts, persistent ischemia, or HTN may benefit from IV NTG for the first 24 to 48 hours. Those with continuing pulmonary edema, recurrent ischemia, or recurrent angina may benefit from even more prolonged use of NTG. Ideally, IV NTG should be changed to an oral route within 24 hours; for instance, **isosorbide dinitrate** 5 to 80 mg orally 2 to 3 times per day. NTG is generally contraindicated in patients with hypotension, marked bradycardia or tachycardia, RV infarction, or 5'phosphodiesterase inhibitor use within 24 to 48 hours.

d. ACE-inhibitors should be initiated within 24 hours to all patients with anterior MI, HF, or ejection fraction $\leq 40\%$ unless contraindicated. An **angiotensin II receptor blocker (ARB)** can be substituted in patients intolerant of ACE-inhibitors. ACE-inhibitors reduce fatal and nonfatal major cardiovascular events in patients with STEMI independent of the use of other pharmacotherapies (e.g., ASA, β-blocker). Lisinopril 2.5 to 5 mg per day can be administered initially with higher titration as tolerated. Caution should be taken in patients with renal failure, hyperkalemia, or hypotension.

e. HMG-CoA reductase inhibitors ("statins") should be initiated in all patients with ACS without contraindications. Statin therapy lowers the risk of coronary heart disease death, recurrent MI, stroke, and the need for revascularization. **Atorvastatin** 80 mg daily has been shown to reduce death and ischemic events in patients with ACS.

f. Analgesia. Morphine sulfate (1–5 mg IV) for analgesia and anxiolysis is reasonable unless contraindicated by hypotension or history of morphine intolerance. Associated modest reductions in HR and BP decrease O_2 consumption. Side effects include hypotension, respiratory depression, bradycardia, and nausea. Except for ASA, **nonsteroidal anti-inflammatory drugs (NSAIDs)** and selective **cyclooxygenase II enzyme (COX-2) inhibitors** may be associated with an increased risk of death, reinfarction, cardiac rupture, HTN, renal insufficiency, and HF. NSAIDs and COX-2 inhibitors are contraindicated in patients with STEMI and should be discontinued in patients taking them prior to hospitalization.

g. Antiplatelet therapy should be considered in all patients presenting with ACS. Agents are chosen on the basis of whether the proposed management will be conservative or invasive (e.g., CABG or PCI, which yield an increased risk of hemorrhage). A combination of **ASA** and **clopidogrel** has been shown to reduce recurrent coronary events in the posthospitalized ACS population. For UA/NSTEMI patients treated medically without stenting, ASA should be prescribed indefinitely and clopidogrel should be prescribed for up to 12 months in the absence of contraindications. For ACS patients treated with a bare metal stent (BMS) or drug-eluting stent (DES), **ASA should be prescribed indefinitely** and **clopidogrel should be prescribed for at least 12 months** (continuation may be considered past 12 months). For patients receiving **DES** for a non-ACS indication, **clopidogrel should be given for at least 12 months** and continuation may be considered past 12 months. For patients receiving **BMS** for a non-ACS indication, **clopidogrel should be given at least 1 month** and ideally up to 12 months. If bleeding risks outweigh the benefits of platelet inhibitors, earlier discontinuation should be considered.

1. **ASA** 325 mg by mouth should be given to all patients, unless contraindicated by hypersensitivity or a history of major GI bleeding. ASA acts by irreversibly inhibiting cyclooxygenase-1 (COX-1) in platelets thereby preventing formation of thromboxane A2 and decreasing platelet aggregation.

2. If a contraindication to using ASA exists, a 300-mg oral loading dose of **clopidogrel** followed by 75 mg once a day can be started.

Clopidogrel and ASA are given together if PCI management is planned.

3. **Glycoprotein IIb/IIIa inhibitors** may be added as a third agent as part of a triple antiplatelet therapy in select high-risk patients. The risk of using these agents as a part of triple antiplatelet therapy may outweigh their potential benefit when there is concern for increased bleeding risk or in non–high-risk patients.

h. Further **anticoagulation** depends upon whether conservative or invasive management is pursued. Unfractionated heparin (UFH), low-molecular-weight heparin (LMWH), a direct thrombin inhibitor (e.g., bivalirudin), or a factor Xa inhibitor (e.g., fondaparinux) may be chosen.

1. **UFH** has the advantage of common use but the disadvantage of a risk of heparin-induced thrombocytopenia (HIT). Initial dosing should be titrated to target an aPTT of 1.5 to 2 × normal. A normal dose is a 60-unit-per-kilogram bolus followed by a 12-unit-per-kilogram-per-hour infusion.

2. **LMWH** has a lower risk of HIT and, being given subcutaneously, it is generally thought to be easier to administer. Concerns about the ability to monitor the effectiveness of LMWH compared with UFH, as well as a concern that reversal with protamine may be difficult in the setting of planned PCI, have limited its use.

3. **Direct thrombin inhibitors** have no risk of HIT but are associated with more bleeding complications and an inability to reverse effects with either protamine or FFP. **Bivalirudin** is a direct-acting synthetic antithrombin that acts against clot-bound thrombin with a very short half-life (25 minutes). Bivalirudin can be useful in patients with HIT.

4. **Fondaparinux**, a **factor Xa inhibitor**, is efficacious in anticoagulation management after ACS and confers a lower risk of bleeding when compared with UFH and GP IIb/IIIa inhibitors. The lack of antidote and catheter thrombosis during PCI limit its use.

i. **Magnesium** dilates coronary arteries, inhibits platelet activity, suppresses automaticity, and may protect against reperfusion injury. Prophylactic administration in acute MI does not improve mortality but may reduce arrhythmias at the cost of an increased incidence of hypotension, bradycardia, and flushing. Current evidence does not support magnesium as an effective treatment in ACS. However, supplemental magnesium is indicated for hypomagnesemia and torsades de pointes. Hypomagnesemia is corrected with magnesium sulfate 2 g IV over 30 to 60 minutes, while torsades de pointes is treated with 1 to 2 g IV over 5 minutes. Since most magnesium in the body is intracellular, hypomagnesemic patients may require multiple replacement doses to achieve normal levels.

j. **Insulin** should be administered to patients presenting with ACS and hyperglycemia to maintain blood glucose levels <180 mg/dL while avoiding hypoglycemia.

k. Pharmacologic or mechanical **reperfusion therapy** reduces infarct size and mortality and improves function, even after a prolonged period. Transient myocardial impairment ("stunned myocardium") may exist after the injury is reversed. In general, PCI is preferred for STEMI with a goal to be performed within 90 minutes of initial presentation to a PCI-capable hospital. Immediate transfer to a PCI-capable hospital is recommended if initial presentation is at a non-PCI-capable hospital with the goal of first medical contact to reperfusion time of <120 minutes. If the anticipated time to PCI is >120 minutes, thrombolysis is preferred in the absence of contraindications.

1. **Thrombolysis** is only indicated in the presence of ST-segment elevation >0.1 mV in at least two contiguous leads when PCI cannot be performed within 120 minutes of first medical contact and no contraindications exist. Thrombolysis yields the greatest benefit when initiated within 6 hours of symptom onset, although definite benefit exists even at 12 hours. Patients presenting within 12 to 24 hours but with continuing symptoms may also benefit. Response to therapy results in improvement in ST-segment elevation and resolution of chest discomfort. Persistent symptoms and ST-segment elevation 60 to 90 minutes after thrombolysis are indications for urgent angiography and possible PCI. Thrombolysis offers no benefit in patients without ST-segment elevation or in those with MI complicated by HF or cardiogenic shock. Table 15.3 shows a comparison of the commonly used thrombolytic agents. Side effects are bleeding, hypotension, and allergic-type reactions. **Absolute contraindications** are any prior intracranial hemorrhage, cerebral vascular malformation or malignant intracranial neoplasm, suspected aortic dissection, active bleeding, intracranial or intraspinal surgery within the past 2 months, significant head trauma or ischemic stroke within the past 3 months (does not include an acute CVA within 4.5 hours), or severe uncontrolled HTN unresponsive to medical therapy.

TABLE 15.3 Fibrinolytic Agents (adapted from 2013 ACC/AHA STEMI Guidelines)

Fibrinolytic Agent	Administration	Fibrin Specificity[a]	Patency Rate (90-min TIMI 2 or 3 flow)
Fibrin-specific			
Alteplase (tPA)	90 min. weight-based infusion[b]	+ +	73%–84%
Reteplase (rPA)	10 units + 10 unit IV boluses given 30 min apart	+ +	84%
Tenecteplase (TNK-tPA)	Single IV weight-based bolus[c]	+ + + +	85%
Non-fibrin-specific			
Streptokinase[d]	1.5 million units IV given over 30–60 min	None	60%–68%

[a]Strength of fibrin specificity, "+ + + +" is more specific, "+ +" is less specific.
[b]Bolus 15 mg, infusion 0.75 mg/kg for 30 min (max. 50 mg), then 0.5 mg/kg (max. 35 mg) over the next 60 min; total dose not to exceed 100 mg.
[c]Bolus 30 mg for weight <60 kg; 35 mg for 60–69 kg; 40 mg for 70–79 kg; 45 mg for 80–89 kg; 50 mg for ≥90 kg.
[d]Streptokinase is no longer marketed in the United States, but is available in other countries.

Relative contraindications include chronic, severe, poorly controlled HTN, significant HTN on presentation (SBP >180 mmHg or DBP >110 mmHg), history of prior ischemic stroke more than 3 months ago, dementia, known intracranial pathology not covered in absolute contraindications, traumatic or prolonged cardiopulmonary resuscitation (>10 minutes), major surgery within the past 3 weeks, internal bleeding within the past 2 to 4 weeks, concurrent anticoagulation, noncompressible vascular puncture sites, pregnancy, or active peptic ulcer disease.

   a. **Alteplase (tPA)** is a recombinant tissue plasminogen activator with a serum half-life of 5 minutes. By increasing plasmin binding to fibrin, it provides relative clot-selective fibrinolysis without inducing a systemic lytic state. When given with heparin, its early reperfusion rate is slightly better than other agents.

   b. **Reteplase (rPA)** is a recombinant nonglycosylated form of human tissue plasminogen activator that has a modified amino acid structure. These modifications give rPA a longer half-life of 13 to 16 minutes, improved ability to penetrate into clots, and a more convenient administration which may lead to faster thrombolysis.

   c. **Tenecteplase (TNK)** is a recombinant tissue plasminogen activator derived from tPA by modifications at three amino acid sites. These modifications produce a longer half-life of 18 to 20 minutes, a greater resistance to inactivation by plasminogen activator inhibitor, and more fibrin specificity than tPA or rPA. TNK has the advantage of convenient single-bolus administration.

   d. **Streptokinase** is a bacterial protein produced by β-hemolytic streptococci. It induces activation of free and clot-associated plasminogen, eliciting a nonspecific systemic fibrinolytic state. Streptokinase has largely been supplanted by the recombinant tissue plasminogen activators listed above.

2. **PCI** has replaced percutaneous transluminal coronary angioplasty as atherectomy and stenting have improved patency rates above that of angioplasty alone. In addition to the absence of a sternotomy and associated complications, there are fewer neurological sequelae with PCI compared with CABG. The primary constraint of PCI is the availability of personnel and support facilities that are only available in PCI-capable hospitals. Adjuncts to PCI that reduce coronary reocclusion include **IV heparin, ASA, clopidogrel,** and **GP IIb/IIIa inhibitors**. The benefit of LMWH compared with UFH in PCI is unclear at this time. A glycoprotein IIb/IIIa inhibitor (e.g., abciximab) may decrease mortality, MI recurrence, and the need for urgent revascularization.

   a. **PCI** reduces the incidence of angina, but has not been demonstrated to improve survival in stable, non-ACS patients. PCI may increase the short-term risk of MI and does not lower the long-term risk of MI. Despite improvements in PCI technology and pharmacology over the past several decades, PCI has not been demonstrated to reduce the risk of death or MI in patients without recent ACS.

   b. When **comparing CABG and PCI**, rates of survival and MI have been found to be similar while procedural stroke is more common with CABG. However, relief of angina is superior with CABG and requirement for repeat revascularization is significantly higher with PCI. Outcomes of patients undergoing PCI or CABG with relatively uncomplicated and lesser degrees of CAD are comparable. In patients with more complex and diffuse CAD, CABG appears to be preferable, especially in patients with diabetes. Revascularization is complete in most patients undergoing CABG, while <70% of PCI patients receive complete revascularization. The need for subsequent CABG is usually higher in those with incomplete revascularization after PCI.

c. In-hospital mortality among patients undergoing PCI is ~1.2% (ranging from 0.65% in elective PCI to 4.8% in STEMI PCI). Causes of periprocedural MI include acute arterial closure, embolization, side branch occlusion, and acute stent thrombosis. The rate of emergency CABG after PCI is ~0.4%. The common indications for emergency CABG are coronary dissection, acute artery closure, perforation, and failure to cross the lesion. The rate of PCI-related stroke is ~0.22%, and in-hospital mortality among these patients is 25% to 30%. The rate of vascular complications ranges from 2% to 6%. Vascular complications are primarily related to vascular access and include access site hematoma, retroperitoneal hematoma, pseudoaneurysm, arteriovenous fistula, and arterial dissection or occlusion.

3. **Acute surgical reperfusion** may be emergently indicated for patients with operable coronary anatomy who have failed medical management but (1) are not candidates for PCI; (2) have failed PCI; (3) have persistent ischemia, hemodynamic instability, or cardiogenic shock; (4) have surgically correctable complications of MI (e.g., severe mitral regurgitation or VSD); or (5) have life-threatening arrhythmias in the presence of severe left main or three-vessel CAD. Mortality from emergent CABG is high.

I. **Intra-aortic balloon counterpulsation** with an intra-aortic balloon pump (**IABP**) may be indicated in patients awaiting PCI or CABG who have low CO unresponsive to inotropic support or who demonstrate refractory pulmonary congestion. The effects of IAB counterpulsation include diastolic BP augmentation (which increases coronary perfusion) and systolic BP reduction (which decreases impedance to ejection). Recent evidence questions the utility of IABP for patients with acute MI complicated by cardiogenic shock. As a result, the European Society of Cardiology downgraded the IABP recommendation from 1C to 2B in their 2012 STEMI guidelines while the most recent 2013 ACC/AHA STEMI guidelines did not incorporate these data and were not changed. The use of IABP in acute MI complicated by cardiogenic shock remains controversial.

IV. COMPLICATIONS OF MI

A. **Recurrent Ischemia and Infarction.** Common causes of chest pain after MI are pericarditis, ischemia, and reinfarction. Up to 58% of patients show early recurrent angina after reperfusion. Reinfarction occurs in approximately 4% of patients within 10 days of thrombolysis and ASA. Patients with reinfarction are at risk of cardiogenic shock and fatal dysrhythmias. The initial approach optimizes medical therapies and may include repeat thrombolysis or PCI. Emergency CABG may benefit those who have failed or are not candidates for medical treatment or PCI. Patients with active ischemia unresponsive to medical therapy may receive an IABP while awaiting angiography.

B. Mechanical Complications

1. **Mitral regurgitation (MR)** can occur from papillary muscle rupture, often presenting 3 to 5 days postinfarct, and is commonly associated with an inferior MI. Findings may include pulmonary edema, hypotension, cardiogenic shock, and a new apical systolic murmur. A pulmonary artery occlusion pressure waveform may exhibit large V-waves. A ruptured papillary muscle and MR may be evident on echocardiography. Treatment includes afterload reduction, inotropes, IABP, and emergent surgical repair. An IABP improves multiple cardiac parameters including a decrease in pulmonary capillary wedge pressure, a decrease in V-wave amplitude, and a decrease in the severity of acute MR largely via afterload reduction and augmentation of forward systemic flow. Medical management alone yields a mortality of roughly 75% in the first 24 hours.

2. **Ventricular septal defect (VSD)** most commonly occurs 3 to 5 days after an anterior MI. Clinical signs include a new holosystolic murmur with systolic thrill and cardiogenic shock. A septal defect will be seen on echocardiography. An increased SaO_2 between blood sampled from the right atrium and right ventricle can confirm an interventricular shunt. Treatment includes afterload reduction, inotropic support, and IABP. An IABP improves the clinical scenario for the same reasons it improves acute papillary muscle rupture MR as discussed above, but it has also been shown decrease the Qp/Qs ratio via afterload reduction and augmentation of forward systemic flow. Hemodynamically stable patients may not require immediate surgical repair, but mortality in patients with cardiogenic shock is up to 90% without surgical intervention.

3. **Ventricular free wall rupture** accounts for approximately 10% of peri-infarct death. Risk factors include sustained HTN after MI, a large transmural MI, late thrombolysis, female sex, advanced age, and exposure to steroids or NSAIDs. It is most common in the first 2 weeks after MI, with peak incidence 3 to 6 days postinfarct. Recurrent chest pain, acute HF, and cardiovascular collapse suggest free wall rupture. Death can occur rapidly and overall mortality is high. Diagnosis is by echocardiography. Volume expansion, tamponade decompression, and IABP temporize prior to emergent surgical repair.

4. **Ventricular aneurysm** is usually due to thinning of the infarcted ventricular wall. It is characterized by a protrusion of scar tissue in association with HF, malignant dysrhythmias, and systemic embolism. Persistent ST-segment elevation may be evident, while echocardiography confirms the diagnosis. Anticoagulation is required, especially in patients with documented mural thrombus. Surgical correction of ventricular geometry may be necessary.

5. **Pericarditis,** due to extension of myocardial necrosis to the epicardium, occurs in approximately 25% of patients within weeks of MI. Pleuritic chest pain or positional discomfort, radiation to the left shoulder, a pericardial rub, diffuse J-point elevation, concave ST-segment elevation, reciprocal PR depression, and pericardial effusion on echocardiography may be evident. Treatment includes **ASA** 162 to 325 mg daily, increased to 650 mg every 4 to 6 hours if necessary. Indomethacin,

ibuprofen, and corticosteroids are avoided, as wall thinning in the zone
of myocardial necrosis may predispose to ventricular wall rupture.

C. **Dysrhythmias,** including premature ventricular contractions, bradycardia,
atrial fibrillation, atrioventricular blocks, ventricular fibrillation,
ventricular tachycardia, and idioventricular rhythms, are common
in the setting of MI. Multiple etiologies may include HF, ischemia,
reentrant rhythms, reperfusion, acidosis, electrolyte derangements (e.g.,
hypokalemia, hypomagnesemia, intracellular hypercalcemia), hypoxemia,
hypotension, drug effects, and heightened reflex sympathetic and vagal
activity. Treatment of any precipitating cause should be undertaken
immediately. **Chapter 17** discusses these dysrhythmias and their treatments
in detail.

D. **Heart Failure and Cardiogenic Shock.** The incidence of cardiogenic shock
after MI is approximately 7.5%. Mortality is extremely high. Contractility
of approximately 40% of the ventricular myocardium must be lost for
cardiogenic shock to develop. Causes include VSD, acute MR, tamponade,
and right ventricular failure. Management includes hemodynamic support
with inotropes and immediate revascularization. An IABP has traditionally
been advocated; however, recent evidence questions the benefit of its use.
The pulmonary artery catheter can assist with management and trend the
response to other therapies. ECMO and ventricular assist devices have
emerged as therapies in the management of cardiogenic shock and are
discussed further in **Chapter 18**.

E. **Hypertension** increases myocardial O_2 demand and may worsen ischemia.
Causes of HTN after MI include premorbid HTN, HF, and elevated
catecholamines due to pain and anxiety. Treatment includes adequate
antianginal therapy, analgesia, anxiolysis, IV NTG, β-blockade, and
ACE-inhibitors. Calcium-channel blockers (verapamil or diltiazem) may
be indicated in patients who have contraindications to other agents.
Nitroprusside may be required if HTN is severe.

V. PERIOPERATIVE MYOCARDIAL ISCHEMIA AND INFARCTION

A. **Definition, Incidence, and Implications.** As medical and surgical therapies
for cardiovascular disease continue to improve, more patients with these
conditions are living longer, healthier lives. However, as a result, more
patients with CAD or related risk factors (advanced age, HTN, DM, HF,
decreased exercise tolerance, and renal disease) are presenting for cardiac
and noncardiac surgery than ever before, and this number continues to
rise. Normal risks of surgery and anesthesia (pain, tachycardia, HTN,
increased sympathetic tone, coronary vasoconstriction, hypoxemia,
anemia, shivering, hypercoagulability) place this population at increased
risk for ischemia and perioperative MI. Of more than 27 million patients
undergoing noncardiac surgery each year, approximately 1 million suffer
some form of perioperative cardiac complication, contributing to added
health care costs. In patients with preexisting CAD, roughly 6% will
experience a perioperative MI. Patients who suffer MI after surgery have a
15% to 25% risk of in-hospital death and a significant increase in 6-month
morbidity and mortality. The benefit of revascularization prior to vascular
surgery has been evaluated in the Coronary Artery Revascularization before
Elective Major Vascular Surgery (CARP Trial). Coronary revascularization
before elective vascular surgery among patients with stable cardiac
symptoms did not significantly alter long-term outcomes and cannot be
recommended. In general, coronary revascularization prior to noncardiac
surgery is recommended for patients in which revascularization would be

indicated according to existing clinical practice guidelines independent of surgery. However, the cumulative risks and benefits of both the coronary revascularization procedure and the noncardiac surgery should be weighed. Coronary revascularization prior to noncardiac surgery is not recommended for the exclusive goal of reducing perioperative cardiac events.

B. **Perioperative Monitoring and Diagnosis.** Under normal conditions, MI is diagnosed on the basis of history (see **Sections I.A.1, II.A**), increased biomarkers (see **Section III.C.2**), and characteristic ECG changes (see **Section III.C.1**). However, postoperative pain and pain-control techniques may render a perioperative MI "silent." As perioperative MI occurs most often on the day of surgery or postoperative day 1, increased diagnostic weight must be given to ECG changes and cardiac enzymes early in the postoperative course. A high index of suspicion, especially in a population likely to have preexisting ECG abnormalities (e.g., arrhythmias, bundle branch blocks, left ventricular hypertrophy, pacemakers), should be maintained. Comparison of a daily ECG to baseline is a cost-effective monitoring plan. Biomarkers should be obtained for confirmation rather than for surveillance, bearing in mind that these enzymes may be elevated as a direct result of surgery (e.g., in CABG). Transthoracic and transesophageal echocardiography (see **Chapter 3**) are excellent investigative modalities when an adverse cardiac event is suspected, as regional wall motion abnormalities will precede both ECG changes and biomarker increases.

C. **Perioperative Preventive Strategies.** Surgical stress and anesthesia provoke myriad physiologic and biochemical changes that can be influenced to the betterment of postoperative care.

1. **β-Blockade.** Current evidence suggests the use of perioperative β-blockade reduces perioperative cardiac events, but this benefit is offset by higher relative risk of perioperative stroke and an uncertain mortality benefit or risk. Perioperative β-blockade started within 1 day or less before noncardiac surgery can prevent nonfatal MI but increases the risk of stroke, death, hypotension, and bradycardia. There are insufficient data on β-blockade started 2 or more days prior to noncardiac surgery. For patients undergoing surgery who have been on β-blockade chronically, the 2014 ACC/AHA Guideline on Perioperative Cardiovascular Evaluation and Management of Patients Undergoing Noncardiac Surgery (hereafter 2014 ACC/AHA Perioperative Guidelines) recommend continuation of perioperative β-blockade. The guidelines state that the risks and benefits of perioperative β-blockade appear to favor use in patients with intermediate or high-risk ischemia found on preoperative stress testing. Additionally, patients with ≥3 Revised Cardiac Risk Index (RCRI) risk factors appear to benefit from perioperative β-blockade. In the absence of multiple RCRI risk factors, the safety and benefit of perioperative β-blockade is unclear. Decisions regarding initiation of perioperative β-blockade should include consideration of risk factors for stroke or other contraindications (e.g., decompensated HF). If perioperative β-blockade is initiated, it may be reasonable to initiate therapy long enough in advance to assess safety and tolerability. Initiation of therapy ≤1 day prior to or on the day of surgery in β-blocker-naïve patients is at a minimum ineffective and may be harmful. Initiation of therapy 2 to 7 days prior to surgery may be preferred, and few data support the need to initiate therapy >30 days prior. Postoperatively, the management of perioperative β-blockade should

be guided by clinical circumstances. Hypotension, bradycardia, bleeding, or other contraindications to β-blockade may necessitate down-titration or temporary discontinuation.

2. **Clonidine.** As an α-2 agonist, clonidine inhibits presynaptic norepinephrine release and produces beneficial effects on HR, BP, and thrombosis. While clonidine had previously been thought to be beneficial in preventing perioperative ischemia, the recent POISE-2 trial revealed that perioperative clonidine did not reduce the risk of death or nonfatal MI for noncardiac surgery. Instead, clonidine was found to increase the risk of nonfatal cardiac arrest and clinically significant hypotension. Therefore, the 2014 ACC/AHA Perioperative Guidelines state α-2 agonists are **not recommended** for prevention of cardiac events in the perioperative period of noncardiac surgery.

3. **Statins** should be continued perioperatively in patients currently taking them who are scheduled for noncardiac surgery (2014 ACC/AHA Perioperative Guidelines). In addition, perioperative statin initiation is reasonable in patients undergoing vascular surgery. Perioperative statin initiation may be considered in patients with clinical indications according to goal-directed medical therapy who are undergoing elevated-risk procedures. Current evidence suggests a protective effect of perioperative statins against cardiac complications during noncardiac surgery.

4. **CCBs** have been investigated for prevention of cardiac events during noncardiac surgery, although additional data are needed. The available data suggest CCBs reduce both ischemia and supraventricular tachycardia and produce a trend toward reduced death and MI. The majority of these benefits are attributable to diltiazem. Dihydropyridines and verapamil did not decrease the incidence of myocardial ischemia. CCBs with significant negative inotropic effects, such as diltiazem and verapamil, can precipitate or worsen HF in susceptible patients.

5. **ACE-inhibitors** have been found to increase the incidence of perioperative hypotension but have no effect on important cardiovascular outcomes (death, MI, stroke, kidney failure) when taken on the day of surgery. There are limited data on the impact of discontinuing ACE-inhibitors before noncardiac surgery. The 2014 ACC/AHA Perioperative Guidelines state continuation of ACE-inhibitors is reasonable. In addition, if ACE-inhibitors are held before surgery, it is reasonable to restart as soon as clinically feasible postoperatively. Evidence is also sparse regarding ARBs, but it is reasonable to treat such drugs as equivalent to ACE-inhibitors.

6. **ASA** inhibits production of thromboxane and has analgesic, anti-inflammatory, antipyretic, and antiplatelet effects. The value of ASA in preventing perioperative ischemic events in nonstented patients for noncardiac and noncarotid surgery remains uncertain. Observational data suggest withdrawal of ASA preoperatively leads to an increase in perioperative thrombotic complications. However, the recent POISE-2 trial revealed that neither continuation nor initiation of low-dose ASA reduced the risk of death or nonfatal MI for noncardiac surgery but instead increased the risk of major bleeding. For these reasons, the 2014 ACC/AHA Perioperative Guidelines state that for nonstented patients, continuation of ASA may be reasonable when the risk of potential cardiac events outweighs the increased risk of bleeding such as in patients with high-risk CAD or cerebrovascular disease. Additionally, initiation or continuation of ASA in nonstented patients presenting for elective

noncardiac surgery is not beneficial unless the risk of ischemic events outweighs the risk of surgical bleeding. For patients with stents, the protective effect of ASA is discussed in **Section V.D.**

7. Anticoagulation. Surgery can induce a protective hemostatic state that may be detrimental to the patient with CAD. Decreased fibrinolysis, increased platelet count and function, and increased fibrinogen and coagulation factor levels may cause intracoronary thrombosis. The risks of bleeding perioperatively must be weighed against the benefit of remaining on anticoagulation. There have been no studies on the benefit of anticoagulants on the prevention of perioperative myocardial ischemia or MI.

8. **NTG.** The 2014 ACC/AHA Perioperative Guidelines assert intravenous NTG administered prophylactically is not effective in reducing myocardial ischemia in patients undergoing noncardiac surgery.

9. **Anesthetic technique.** Currently, there is no evidence to suggest that the use or addition of neuraxial anesthesia reduces perioperative cardiac events. The surgical procedure, patient comorbidities, and patient preferences must be considered on a case-by-case basis. Evidence relating to neuraxial analgesia for postoperative pain control is discussed in **Section V.C.9.**

10. **Postoperative pain control** should be carefully planned and continually assessed. Patients may not be able to accurately report postoperative or ischemic pain due to sedation, intubation, or pain control modalities. Surgical pain may cause tachycardia, HTN, sympathetic discharge, and coronary vasoconstriction, all of which can raise myocardial O_2 consumption while compromising supply. Adequate sedation and analgesia (using opioids, benzodiazepines, propofol, or regional anesthesia) are mainstays of postoperative care that may contribute to improved cardiac outcomes. There are limited data comparing perioperative epidural and intravenous analgesia with many studies showing no difference in perioperative cardiac events. However, epidural analgesia has been shown to reduce the incidence of perioperative MI in patients undergoing abdominal aortic procedures. Additionally, *preoperative* epidural analgesia has been shown to reduce the incidence of *preoperative* MI, HF, and atrial fibrillation in elderly patients with hip fracture.

11. **Anemia** can limit O_2 delivery to at-risk myocardium contributing to perioperative cardiac events. While transfusion practices vary widely, the 2012 American Association of Blood Banks Clinical Practice Guidelines advocate a restrictive transfusion strategy in hospitalized patients with cardiovascular disease, as well as consideration of transfusion for symptomatic patients (e.g., chest pain, orthostasis, CHF) or those with a hemoglobin (Hgb) <8 g/dL. The TRICC trial revealed that a restrictive transfusion strategy (transfusion threshold of 8 g/dL vs. 10 g/dL) was not associated with worse outcomes. The FOCUS trial also favored a restrictive transfusion strategy (threshold of 7 g/dL vs. 10 g/dL) as evidenced by lower mortality. Therefore, consideration for transfusion in asymptomatic patients with stable CAD seems reasonable at Hgb levels <8 g/dL.

12. **Temperature regulation.** Perioperative hypothermia has been associated with major adverse cardiac events, death, coagulopathy, increased blood loss, transfusion requirement, and wound infection. Maintenance of normothermia may reduce perioperative cardiac events in patients undergoing noncardiac surgery. Hypothermia can be prevented by means of forced air warmers, warmed IV fluids and blood products, and limiting unnecessary exposure.

13. Glucose homeostasis. Surgical stress can exacerbate preexisting DM or impaired glucose tolerance. High glucose levels can worsen to endothelial dysfunction. An insulin infusion or sliding scale should maintain a goal of <180 mg/dL.

D. Perioperative Management of Patients with Coronary Stents. Patients undergoing noncardiac surgery who have coronary stents are at increased risk of major adverse cardiac events. Perioperative care should be co-managed by the perioperative team including the cardiologist, the surgeon, and the anesthesiologist.

1. **Timing.** Elective noncardiac surgery should be delayed for 14 days after balloon angioplasty, 30 days after BMS implantation, and 1 year after DES implantation. Elective noncardiac surgery should not be performed within 30 days of BMS or 1 year of DES if dual antiplatelet therapy (DAPT) will need to be discontinued perioperatively. Similarly, elective noncardiac surgery should not be performed within 14 days of balloon angioplasty if ASA will need to be discontinued perioperatively. If noncardiac surgery is likely to be required within 1 to 12 months of PCI, a strategy of BMS and 4 to 6 weeks of DAPT consisting of ASA and clopidogrel with continuation of ASA perioperatively may be appropriate. If noncardiac surgery is likely to be required within 2 to 6 weeks of PCI, consideration of balloon angioplasty with provisional BMS implantation is reasonable.

2. For **urgent noncardiac surgery**, within 4 to 6 weeks of BMS or DES implantation, DAPT should be continued unless the risk of bleeding outweighs the benefit of prevention of stent thrombosis. In situations that require discontinuation of clopidogrel within this time frame, continuation of ASA is strongly recommended if possible. Clopidogrel should be restarted as soon as possible postoperatively.

3. The risk of **perioperative stent thrombosis** for BMS and DES is highest in the first 4 to 6 weeks after implantation. Discontinuation of DAPT, especially within this early time frame, is the most important risk factor for stent thrombosis and adverse cardiac events. The incidence of perioperative stent thrombosis and adverse cardiac events is inversely related to the time interval between PCI and surgery. If urgent or emergent noncardiac surgery is required, the risks and benefits of continuing ASA or DAPT should be considered. The risk of bleeding is higher with DAPT than with ASA alone or with no antiplatelet therapy, but the magnitude of the increase is uncertain. There is no convincing evidence that "bridging therapy" with warfarin, antithrombotic agents, or glycoprotein IIb/IIIa inhibitors reduce the risk of stent thrombosis after discontinuation of oral antiplatelet agents. Perioperative management includes vigilant monitoring for ischemia or MI. If perioperative stent thrombosis is suspected, rapid PCI is critical for restoration of coronary blood flow.

E. Perioperative Ischemia Management

1. **Consultation** with a cardiologist, the primary surgical team, and when indicated, a cardiac surgeon should begin the moment a perioperative MI is suspected, as emergent reperfusion by PCI or CABG may be warranted (see **Section III.D.3.j**). Because of the patient's recent surgery, thrombolysis will likely be contraindicated.

2. **Supportive measures** include continued ECG, biomarker, and invasive monitoring as appropriate, as well as intervention in all parameters listed under "Perioperative Preventive Strategies" (see **Section V.C**).

3. Current **medications** (as discussed in **Sections II.E, III.D.3, and V.C**) should be reviewed in light of the change in clinical status. If not begun already,

ASA, β-blockade, ACE-inhibitors, and statins should be started if no contraindications exist. Again, thrombolysis will likely not be an option.
4. **Invasive management** strategies such as PCI or CABG may be warranted, and an IABP may be considered for improving coronary blood flow, though device placement may be complicated in vasculopathic patients.

Selected Readings

Alpert JS, Thygesen K, Jaffe A, et al. The universal definition of myocardial infarction: a consensus document. *Heart* 2008;94(10):1335–1341.

Barash P, Akhtar S. Coronary stents: factors contributing to perioperative major adverse cardiovascular events. *Br J Anaesth* 2010;105(suppl 1):i3–i15.

Battler A, Karliner JS, Higgins CB, et al. The initial chest x-ray in acute myocardial infarction. Prediction of early and late mortality and survival. *Circulation* 1980;61(5):1004–1009.

Bennett MH, Lehm JP, Jepson N. Hyperbaric oxygen therapy for acute coronary syndrome. *Cochrane Database Syst Rev* 2011;8:CD004818.

Butterworth J, Furberg CD. Improving cardiac outcomes after noncardiac surgery. *Anesth Analg* 2003;97(3):613–615.

Devereaux PJ, Mrkobrada M, Sessler DI, et al. Aspirin in patients undergoing noncardiac surgery. *N Engl J Med* 2014;370(16):1494–1503.

Devereaux PJ, Sessler DI, Leslie K, et al. Clonidine in patients undergoing noncardiac surgery. *N Engl J Med* 2014;370(16):1504–1513.

Devereaux PJ, Goldman L, Yusuf S, et al. Surveillance and prevention of major perioperative ischemic cardiac events in patients undergoing noncardiac surgery: a review. *Can Med Assoc J* 2005;173(7):779–788.

Fleisher LA, Fleischmann KE, Auerbach AD, et al. 2014 ACC/AHA guideline on perioperative cardiovascular evaluation and management of patients undergoing noncardiac surgery: executive summary: a report of the American College of Cardiology/American Heart Association Task Force on Practice Guidelines. *Circulation* 2014;130(24):2215–2245.

Gold HK, Leinbach RC, Sanders CA, et al. Intra-aortic balloon pumping for ventricular septal defect or mitral regurgitation complicating acute myocardial infarction. *Circulation* 1973;47(6):1191–1196.

Greaves SC. Role of echocardiography in acute coronary syndromes. *Heart* 2002;88(4):419–425.

Hillis LD, Smith PK, Anderson JL, et al. 2011 ACCF/AHA guideline for coronary artery bypass graft surgery. A report of the American College of Cardiology Foundation/American Heart Association Task Force on Practice Guidelines. Developed in collaboration with the American Association for Thoracic Surgery, Society of Cardiovascular Anesthesiologists, and Society of Thoracic Surgeons. *J Am Coll Cardiol* 2011;58(24):e123–e210.

Jneid H, Anderson JL, Wright RS, et al. ACCF/AHA focused update of the guideline for the management of patients with unstable angina/non-ST-elevation myocardial infarction (updating the 2007 guideline and replacing the 2011 focused update): a report of the American College of Cardiology Foundation/American Heart Association Task Force on Practice Guidelines. *Circulation* 2012;126:875–910.

Landesberg G, Beattie WS, Mosseri M, et al. Perioperative myocardial infarction. *Circulation* 2009;119(22):2936–2944.

Levine GN, Bates ER, Blankenship JC, et al. 2011 ACCF/AHA/SCAI guideline for percutaneous coronary intervention: a report of the American College of Cardiology Foundation/American Heart Association Task Force on Practice Guidelines and the Society for Cardiovascular Angiography and Interventions. *Circulation* 2011;124(23):e574.

Li J, Zhang Q, Zhang M, et al. Intravenous magnesium for acute myocardial infarction. *Cochrane Database Syst Rev* 2007;2:CD002755.

Ludbrook G, Webb R, Currie M, et al. Crisis management during anaesthesia: myocardial ischaemia and infarction. *Qual Saf Health Care* 2005;14(3):e13.

O'Gara PT, Kushner FG, Ascheim DD, et al. 2013 ACCF/AHA guideline for the management of ST-elevation myocardial infarction: a report of the American College of Cardiology Foundation/American Heart Association Task Force on Practice Guidelines. *J Am Coll Cardiol* 2013;61(4):e78–e140.

Podgoreanu MV, White WD, Morris RW, et al. Inflammatory gene polymorphisms and risk of postoperative myocardial infarction after cardiac surgery. *Circulation* 2006;114(1 suppl):I275–I281.

Priebe H-J. Perioperative myocardial infarction––aetiology and prevention. *Br J Anaesth* 2005;95(1):3–19.

Saenger AK, Jaffe AS. Requiem for a heavyweight: The demise of creatine kinase-MB. *Circulation* 2008;118(21):2200–2206.

Schiele F. Fondaparinux and acute coronary syndromes: update on the OASIS 5–6 studies. *Vasc Health Risk Manage* 2010;6:179.

Sorbets E, Labreuche J, Simon T, et al. Renin–angiotensin system antagonists and clinical outcomes in stable coronary artery disease without heart failure. *Eur Heart J* 2014;35(26):1760–1768.

Thiele H, Zeymer U, Neumann FJ, et al. Intra-aortic balloon support for myocardial infarction with cardiogenic shock. *N Engl J Med* 2012;367(14):1287–1296.

Thiele H, Zeymer U, Neumann FJ, et al. Intra-aortic balloon counterpulsation in acute myocardial infarction complicated by cardiogenic shock (IABP-SHOCK II): final 12 month results of a randomised, open-label trial. *Lancet* 2013;382(9905):1638–1645.

Wijeysundera DN, Duncan D, Nkonde-Price C, et al. Perioperative beta blockade in noncardiac surgery: a systematic review for the 2014 ACC/AHA guideline on perioperative cardiovascular evaluation and management of patients undergoing noncardiac surgery: a report of the American College of Cardiology/American Heart Association Task Force on Practice Guidelines. *J Am Coll Cardiol* 2014;64(22):2406–2425.

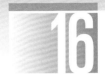

16

Valvular Heart Disease

Alexander S. Kuo and Justin M. Poltak

The prevalence of valvular heart disease is an increasingly burdensome problem and a common complicating comorbidity in the critically ill patient.

I. **AORTIC STENOSIS (AS)** refers to a narrowing of the valvular orifice, restricting flow from the left ventricle (LV) into the ascending aorta during systole. Etiologies of AS include senile degeneration (calcific), congenital bicuspid or unicuspid valves, and, rarely in North America, rheumatic disease.

A. **Pathophysiology**
   1. A narrowing of the aortic valve orifice leads to restriction of flow from the LV into the ascending aorta. This obligates increased LV chamber pressures, resulting in increased LV wall tension, myocardial oxygen demand, and compensatory LV concentric hypertrophy with increased **susceptibility to ischemia and arrhythmias**.
   2. Adequate coronary perfusion pressure becomes dependent on maintenance of diastolic pressure through preservation of systemic vascular resistance.
   3. Increasing LV wall thickness subsequently leads to impairment of active relaxation and passive ventricular filling during diastole.

B. **Diagnosis**
   1. **Physical exam:** Auscultation reveals a loud, late peaking systolic murmur best heard at the right upper sternal border, radiating to the carotids, with delayed carotid upstroke.
   2. **Symptoms:** Patients present with dyspnea on exertion, angina, or presyncope/syncope. The onset of symptoms strongly correlates to disease progression and dramatic increase in risk of sudden cardiac death.
   3. **Diagnosis:** Echocardiography is used to diagnose aortic stenosis but cardiac catheterization may also be used. Pressure gradients obtained via catheterization are typically lower than echo-derived gradients.

C. **Severe Aortic Stenosis:** Aortic valve area (AVA) **less than 1.0 cm^2**, or 0.6 cm/m^2 when normalized to BSA for extremes in body size. Mean gradients **greater than 40 mmHg**, or peak flow velocity greater than 4 m/s. Pressure gradients are flow dependent, and the severity may be underestimated in patients with decreased LV function.

D. **Hemodynamic Management**
   1. **Heart Rate: Reduction is essential** in patients with severe aortic stenosis. Tachycardia leads to significantly increased myocardial oxygen demand and decreased diastolic filling time. Extremes of bradycardia can be deleterious due to fixed stroke volume of the thickened ventricle or when it leads to decreased coronary perfusion.
   2. **Rhythm:** Sinus rhythm becomes imperative as the hypertrophied LV becomes dependent on atrial contraction to maintain LV filling. In the setting of impaired LV relaxation, up to 40% of LV end diastolic volume is contributed by atrial contraction.

3. **Afterload:** Hypotension is poorly tolerated and should be **treated immediately** due to the high susceptibility of the hypertrophied myocardium to ischemia. First-line treatment is a **pure vasoconstrictor such as phenylephrine** to avoid tachycardia while improving coronary perfusion. In patients with decompensated heart failure and severe aortic stenosis, afterload reduction can be very carefully titrated with intensive hemodynamic monitoring to improve forward flow. In moderate or asymptomatic aortic stenosis, hypertension can be treated following standard medical guidelines.

4. **Preload:** Diastolic dysfunction from concentric hypertrophy may require elevated filling pressure for adequate stroke volume. However, in decompensate AS, aggressive fluid administration may lead to pulmonary edema.

5. **Contractility:** Inotropic support may be need in decompensated severe AS. However, inodilators such as dobutamine and milrinone can lead to dangerous decreases in systemic blood pressure and tachyarrhythmias.

E. **Treatment**

1. For mild to moderate asymptomatic aortic stenosis, medical therapy aimed at blood pressure and heart rate control following established guidelines is generally sufficient.

2. The definitive treatment for severe aortic stenosis is aortic valve replacement (AVR). Indications for surgical AVR or transcatheter aortic valve replacement (TAVR) include symptomatic severe AS or severe AS with heart failure. Surgical AVR is recommended for patients who are at low to intermediate surgical risk. TAVR may be considered in patients who meet indications for AVR but are at prohibitive surgical risk and have an expected survival of greater than 12 months.

3. Percutaneous balloon dilation: results in a modest reduction in the severity of AS, but is often complicated by severe AR, restenosis, and clinical deterioration. Percutaneous aortic balloon dilation as a bridge to AVR is controversial. Palliative balloon dilation is not recommended due to the associated morbidity and lack of improved mortality.

F. **Postoperative AS Treatment Care:** Although LV outflow resistance and LV cavity pressures should improve following AVR, LV hypertrophic remodeling may not resolve for months. Persistent LV hypertrophy requires higher filling pressures to maintain cardiac output, and the thickened myocardium remains susceptible to ischemia at low coronary perfusion pressures.

G. **Hypertrophic Obstructive Cardiomyopathy** (HOCM) is subvalvular dynamic obstruction of the left ventricular outflow tract (LVOT) caused by regional hypertrophy of the myocardium. Patients with HOCM are prone to lethal ventricular arrhythmias. Dynamic LVOT obstruction can lead to refractory hypotension and is exacerbated by ventricular underfilling, increased inotropy, decreased afterload, and tachycardia. Acute management includes **increasing preload**, increasing afterload with pure α-agonists such as **phenylephrine**, and administration of β-**blockers, such as esmolol**, to decrease inotropy and chronotropy.

II. AORTIC REGURGITATION

Aortic regurgitation (AR) is caused by incompetence of the aortic valve, resulting in retrograde blood flow from the ascending aorta into the LV during diastole.

A. **Acute Aortic Regurgitation:** Acute severe or moderate AR can lead to LV volume overload, decreased effective systemic output, and terminal ventricular arrhythmias. It is considered a surgical emergency. Acute AR is often a result of aortic dissection, infective endocarditis, trauma, or as a consequence of surgical or percutaneous intervention.

B. Chronic Aortic Regurgitation: Chronic AR is generally progressive. It may be the result of degenerative calcification, a bicuspid aortic valve, rheumatic fever, or aortic root dilatation. Chronic LV volume overload leads to LV remodeling. Initial eccentric LV hypertrophy will often progress to LV dilation in end-stage disease. Symptoms of severe disease include angina, congestive heart failure, and dyspnea on exertion.

C. Diagnosis
   1. **Physical exam:** decrescendo diastolic murmur along left sternal border; widened pulse pressure; visible capillary pulsation with nail bed compression
   2. Diagnosis and grading is made by echocardiography or catherization. Echocardiographic evidence of holo-diastolic flow reversal in the descending thoracic aorta by spectral Doppler, an AR vena contracta width of >0.6 cm, and an AR jet width/LVOT diameter ratio of >65% by color m-mode are consistent with severe AR by echocardiography.

D. Hemodynamic Management
   1. **Afterload: Reduction is critical** and improves forward cardiac output when patient is acutely decompensated. In chronic AR, treatment of chronic hypertension is recommended; however, it does not alter the natural disease progression.
   2. **Heart rate: Elevation is beneficial** to the management of decompensated AR. An elevated heart rate decreases regurgitant time, promotes forward flow, and may reduce diastolic volume overload. However, judicious β-blocker use may be indicated in the setting of aortic dissection to minimize propagation of the dissection.
   3. **Contractility:** Inotropic support is often necessary to support heart failure in AR. Dobutamine and milrinone are often used for afterload reduction and for their positive chronotropic effect.
   4. **Preload:** Fluid administration should be carefully regulated to prevent volume overload.

E. Treatment
   1. Acute AR is often poorly tolerated and is considered a surgical emergency. Aortic valve replacement may be indicated for treatment of chronic severe AR when patients are symptomatic or have indications of LV systolic dysfunction or severe LV dilatation.

F. Anticoagulation after Aortic Valve Replacement
   1. Mechanical valves—Long-term anticoagulation with low-dose aspirin 75 to 100 mg daily, plus warfarin with a targeted INR goal of 2.0 to 3.0 is recommended. If anticoagulation needs to be interrupted, the time with subtherapeutic INR should be minimized. Bridging with heparin is not generally required.
   2. AVR with additional risk factors: hypercoagulable state, atrial fibrillation, prior thromboembolic event, or older-generation AVR—A higher INR goal of 2.5 to 3.5 is recommended. **Use of heparin to bridge** interruptions of anticoagulation is recommended.
   3. Bioprosthetic AVR—Long-term, low-dose aspirin 75 to 100 mg daily, with warfarin—INR goal of 2.5 for the first 6 months after AVR.
   4. Bioprosthetic TAVR—Clopidogrel 75 mg and low-dose aspirin 75 to 100 mg daily for the first 6 months.

III. MITRAL STENOSIS

Mitral stenosis (MS) results from obstruction of LV inflow through the mitral valve during diastole. Common etiologies of MS include rheumatic heart disease and senile calcific stenosis. MS commonly leads to elevated left atrial and pulmonary arterial pressures, which may lead to pulmonary edema and right ventricular (RV) dysfunction.

A. Diagnosis
1. **Physical Exam:** loud S1, opening snap after the S2, with a diastolic murmur best heard at the apex
2. MS may present with atrial fibrillation from left atrial distension, orthopnea, dyspnea on exertion, or heart failure. Hemoptysis is also a possible presentation from pulmonary hypertension. The appearance of symptoms is an indicator of significantly increased mortality in untreated disease.
3. Assessment with echocardiography or angiography is recommended. Exercise testing is also performed because transvalvular pressures are highly dependent on heart rate and hemodynamic loading. RV and LV performance and assessment for left atrial thrombus is also important. Severe MS is defined as a valve area < 1.5 cm^2 and very severe as < 1.0 cm^2.

B. Hemodynamic Management
1. **Heart Rate: Lowering the heart rate** facilitates diastolic filling of the LV. This improves forward flow and reduces pulmonary congestion. If pacing is needed, a longer PR time (0.2 seconds) may allow for better filling across the mitral valve.
2. **Preload:** Maintenance of adequate preload is critical for adequate filling through the stenotic mitral valve. Pulmonary artery occlusion pressures will be elevated but **will not accurately reflect LV end diastolic filling pressure**. However, the pulmonary vascular congestion resulting from the MS predisposes the patient to pulmonary edema so preload must be titrated carefully.
3. **Contractility:** If inotropic support for RV or LV failure is needed, use of drugs without increased chronotropy, such as digoxin or milrinone are advantageous.
4. **Arrhythmia:** Atrial fibrillation is common in MS and may be difficult to control. Unfortunately, ventricular filling may be highly dependent on atrial contraction in these patients. Rapid ventricular rates should be avoided and if rapid rates are associated with hemodynamic instability, the rates need to be treated aggressively.

C. Treatment
1. Percutaneous mitral balloon commissurotomy can be considered for symptomatic patients with severe MS and favorable anatomy. Mitral valve replacement or repair is considered for patients who have failed or are not candidates for percutaneous mitral balloon commissurotomy.

D. Anticoagulation with MS
1. Because of the high risk of embolic events, long-term anticoagulation is recommended in patient with MS and one of the following: atrial fibrillation, prior embolism, or left atrial thrombus. INR goal 2–3.

IV. MITRAL REGURGITATION
Mitral regurgitation (MR) is insufficiency of the mitral valve resulting in backflow during systolic ejection of the LV into the left atrium. This causes elevated pulmonary hypertension and ultimately right heart failure. The compensatory response of the LV results in dilation and eventually systolic dysfunction.

A. Acute Mitral Regurgitation is poorly tolerated and often presents with sudden hemodynamic decompensation. The sudden regurgitant flow of blood into the pulmonary circulation leads to pulmonary edema. The loss of forward flow leads to systemic shock. Acute MR can occur with papillary muscle or cordae tendinea rupture or dysfunction, often in the setting of an inferior myocardial infarction or valvular damage secondary to infective endocarditis. Early surgical repair is often indicated for severe acute MR.

B. **Chronic Mitral Regurgitation:** results in eccentric hypertrophy of the LV allowing it to accept the volume overload without major increases in LV end diastolic pressure. Chronic MR is characterized as primary if it is the result of dysfunction in the valvular apparatus, or secondary due to severe LV dilation and dysfunction. The etiology of disease has significance for definitive treatment. Because a fraction of the stroke volume is regurgitant, a normal ejection fraction (EF) is elevated in MR, 70%. When **EF declines to 60%** or end-systolic diameter is greater than 40 mm, **LV dysfunction is inferred**.

C. **Diagnosis**
1. **Physical exam:** Holo-systolic murmur is best heard at the apex with radiation to the left axilla. A hyperdynamic point of maximal impulse is often palpable. In severe acute MR, the murmur may be absent due to the rapid equilibration of pressure between the left atrium and LV.
2. Echocardiography is the primary method for diagnosis of acute MR, with transesophageal imaging indicated if transthoracic echocardiography is equivocal.

D. **Hemodynamic Management**
1. **Afterload: reduction is essential** for the management of MR. Reduced afterload promotes forward flow and reduces regurgitant fraction of the stroke volume. Nitroglycerin or calcium-channel blockers are often used in acute management. In severely unstable patients, intra-aortic balloon pumps (IABP) can be very effective by reducing effective afterload while preserving coronary perfusion.
2. **Heart rate: higher heart rates** decrease regurgitant time and reduce end diastolic volume preventing LV overdistension.
3. **Preload:** Volume status must be carefully balanced between adequate filling and overdistension of the LV that may dilate the MV annulus and worsen the MR.
4. **Contractility:** Inotropic agents that also have chronotropic and afterload-reducing effects, such as milirinone or dobutamine, can be effective in improving forward flow in patients with heart failure from LV dysfunction.
5. **Pulmonary hypertension:** often occurs in severe MR and may lead to right heart failure. Avoidance of factors that elevated pulmonary artery pressures is important, such as hypoxia, hypercarbia, and acidosis. Use of pulmonary artery dilators such as inhaled nitric oxide or prostaglandin E1 may be considered.

E. **Treatment**
1. Mitral valve replacement or repair is indicated for patients with primary severe MR who are symptomatic or has signs of LV dysfunction. The treatment for secondary MR is less defined. It involves treatment of the underlying heart failure and possible cardiac resynchronization therapy.

F. **Postoperative MVR Care**
1. After repair or replacement of MR, the entire LV stroke volume ejected against the high systemic pressures results in higher effective afterload. This **may unmask LV dysfunction** and result in heart failure. Inotropic or IABP support may be required. Atrial fibrillation is poorly tolerated and antiarrhythmic or atrial overdrive pacing may be needed.

Valvular Lesion	Heart Rate	Preload	Afterload	Contractility
		Qualitative Summary of Acute Hemodynamic Goals of Left-Sided Valvular Lesions		
Aortic stenosis	↓↓	↑	↑	↔
Mitral stenosis	↓	↔	↔	↔
HOCM	↓↓	↑↑	↑	↓
Aortic regurgitation	↑	↔	↓↓	↑
Mitral regurgitation	↑	↓	↓↓	↑

G. Anticoagulation after MVR
  1. **Mechanical mitral valve:** Long-term anticoagulation with low-dose aspirin 75 to 100 mg daily and warfarin to INR goal of 2.5 to 3.5 is recommended. If anticoagulation needs to be interrupted, bridging with heparin is recommended.
  2. **Bioprosthetic mitral valve:** Long-term low-dose aspirin with warfarin anticoagulation for the first 3 months to an INR goal of 2.0 to 3.0 (Table 16.1).

V. TRICUSPID STENOSIS
Tricuspid stenosis is the narrowing of the tricuspid valve impeding the inflow of blood into the right ventricle. It is rare compared with the previously discussed valvular lesions. It is most often secondary to rheumatic fever but can also be the result of carcinoid syndrome, systemic lupus erythematosus, or endomyocardial fibroestosis. As the disease progresses, right atrium (RA) becomes distended from elevated pressures and predisposes the patient to arrhythmias.
A. Diagnosis
  1. **Physical exam:** Diasystolic murmur may be difficult to detect on exam. Patient may present with venous congestion, jugular distention, hepatomegaly, peripheral edema, and/or ascites.
  2. First presenting sign may also be palpitations or decreased exercise tolerance.
  3. It is often diagnosed with echocardiography while evaluating coexisting valvular disease. Severe disease is considered when the valve area is less than 1.0 cm^2.
B. Hemodynamic Management
  1. **Preload:** Elevated central venous filling pressures may be needed to maintain adequate cardiac output. In hemodynamically stable patients, diuresis can help relieve symptoms of peripheral venous congestion.
  2. **Heart rate:** Lower heart rates allow adequate filling of the RV.
C. Treatment
  1. Severe symptomatic TR can be alleviated by repair or replacement. Outcomes are dependent on the underlying RV function. Often tricuspid repair or replacement is undertaken when the patient is indicated for surgery for a left-sided valvular lesion.
D. Postoperative Care after Tricuspid Valve Repair or Replacement for Stenosis
  1. Increase in RV filling may provoke right ventricular failure. Inotropic support for the RV and pulmonary artery pressure reduction may be required. It is **inadvisable to float a pulmonary artery catheter** blindly after tricuspid valve replacement or repair.

VI. TRICUSPID REGURGITATION

Tricuspid regurgitation (TR) is insufficiency of the tricuspid valve allowing backflow during systole from the RV to RA. It is usually associated with other valvular lesions. Isolated TR is often well tolerated. Primary TR can be caused by chest trauma, endocarditis, or carcinoid syndrome. TR can also be secondary to pulmonary hypertension or ventricular dysfunction. Volume overload of the RA predisposes to atrial fibrillation.

A. Diagnosis

1. **Physical Exam:** systolic murmur accentuated by inspiration; S3 gallop. There may be pulsatile jugular venous flow. Venous congestion, including congestive hepatopathy and peripheral edema, may be present in severe cases.
2. Doppler evidence of systolic flow reversal in the hepatic veins or annular diameter >4 cm indicates severe TR.

B. Hemodynamic Management

1. **Afterload:** Reduction in pulmonary vascular resistance decrease regurgitation and facilitate forward flow.
2. **Heart rate:** Higher heart rates decrease diastolic regurgitant time and reduce RV volume overload.
3. **Contractility:** With RV failure, inotropic agents like dobutamine and milrinone can be used without significant increases in pulmonary vascular resistance.
4. **Preload:** Adequate preload is important to maintaining cardiac output. Diuresis may be needed in patients with severe congestive heart failure.

C. Postoperative Care after Tricuspid Repair or Replacement for TR

1. After correction of TR, the entire stroke volume is ejected forward, effectively increasing RV afterload. This may precipitate RV failure requiring inotropic support and minimizing pulmonary vascular resistance.

VII. PULMONIC VALVE DISEASE

Congenital pulmonic stenosis presents as right heart failure. Acquired pulmonic stenosis is rare, and pulmonic regurgitation is usually well tolerated. Surgical intervention on the pulmonic valve often consists of excision of the valve without prosthetic replacement.

VIII. INFECTIVE ENDOCARDITIS

Infective endocarditis can be caused by bacteremia due to oral infections or other infections, including those associated with intravenous drug abuse. Patient's with endocarditis may present with acute valvular dysfunction caused by destructive lesions, large vegetations, or papillary muscle dysfunction. Infectious endocarditis is reviewed in more detail in Chapter 28.

IX. ANTIBIOTIC PROPHYLAXIS FOR ENDOCARDITIS/RHEUMATIC HEART DISEASE

A. **Antibiotic prophylaxis for endocarditis before dental procedures** is reasonable in high-risk patients, including those with prosthetic valves, a past history of endocarditis, cardiac transplants with structural valve abnormalities, unrepaired cyanotic congenital heart disease, repaired congenital heart disease with prosthetic material within 6 months, or with defects near prosthetic site.

B. Antibiotic prophylaxis is **not recommended in patients for nondental procedures** without active infection. Recurrent rheumatic fever can worsen rheumatic heart disease. Patients with prior history of rheumatic heart disease are often prescribed **long-term prophylaxis**, typically with penicillin.

X. PROSTHETIC VALVE THROMBOSIS

A. Prosthetic valve thrombosis can be a dangerous complication that should be emergently investigated. Evaluation is typically done using echocardiography with transesophageal echocardiography indicated for suspected left-sided thrombosis. Anticoagulation or fibrinolytic therapy for right-sided thrombosis is reasonable. For large or hemodynamically significant left-sided thrombosis, emergent surgery is often required.

Selected Reading

Nishimura RA, Otto CM, Bonow RO, et al. 2014 AHA/ACC guideline for the management of patients with valvular heart disease: a report of the American College of Cardiology/American Heart Association Task Force on Practice Guidelines. *J Am Coll Cardiol* 2014;63:2438–2488.

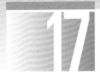

Cardiac Dysrhythmias

Yasuko Nagasaka and Kenneth Shelton

I. INTRODUCTION

Perioperative arrhythmias and conduction disturbances increase morbidity and mortality. New onset arrhythmias affect about 7% of patients following major noncardiothoracic surgery and up to 60% of post–cardiac-surgery patients. Atrial fibrillation (AF) is the most common postoperative arrhythmia.

In this chapter, we review the classification, etiology, and treatment of the arrhythmias most frequently encountered in critical care medicine.

II. CLASSIFICATION AND MANAGEMENT

A. The cardiac conduction system consists of three main parts: the sinus node, the atrioventricular (AV) node, and the His–Purkinje system.

B. There is not just one pacemaker system; instead, there are multiple mechanisms in cardiac pacing. Pathology of the sinus node and atrioventricular conduction system, as well as the right and left atrioventricular rings/right ventricular outflow tract, contribute to arrhythmias in the adult heart.

III. BRADYARRHYTHMIA

A. Pulseless Electrical Activity (PEA)

1. PEA is cardiac arrest with the presence of spontaneous organized cardiac electrical activity in the absence of adequate organ perfusion sufficient to maintain consciousness.

   a. *Management:* Cardiopulmonary resuscitation (CPR) with uninterrupted chest compressions and standard pharmacological interventions provide the basis of the treatment. Primary management involves treating the underlining cause (significant hypoxia, profound acidosis, severe hypovolemia, tension pneumothorax, electrolyte imbalance, drug overdose, sepsis, large myocardial infarction, massive pulmonary embolism, cardiac tamponade, hypoglycemia, hypothermia, etc.). Extracorporeal life support with prolonged failure of return to spontaneous circulation should also be considered.

B. Abnormal Sympathetic Tone and the Cardiovascular Reflexes

Arrhythmias secondary to cardiovascular reflexes are commonly seen (Table 17.1).

TABLE 17.1 Cardiovascular Reflexes

Reflex	Trigger	Receptor	Afferent limb	Nucleus	Efferent limb	Response
Arterial baroreceptor reflex	Increased BP	Baroceptors in aortic arch and carotid sinus	Glossopharyngeal (IX, carotid sinus) and vagus (X, aortic arch) nerves	Medulla (nucleaus solitarius)	The autonomic nervous system	Decreased HR, BP, and contractility
Bezold–Jarisch reflex	Hypotension	Mechanical and chemosensitive receptors in ventricular walls	Nonmyelinated vagal (X) C-fiber	Medulla	Inhibition of sympathetic outflow	Triad: decreased HR, decreased BP, and apnea
Bainbridge reflex	Changes in volume in the central thoracic compartment	Stretch receptors at junction of the vena cava and right atrium, junction of the pulmonary vein and left atrium, and vessel wall of carotid sinus and aortic arch	Vagus (X) nerve	Medulla	Inhibition of vagal outflow and enhancement of sympathetic outflow to sinoatrial node	Increased HR
Chemoreceptor reflex	Low O_2 and hydrogen ion, high CO_2	Chemoreceptors in carotid sinus and aortic body	Fibers in glossopharyngeal (IX, carotid sinus) and vagus (X, aortic arch) nerves	Medulla oblongata	Decrease parasympathetic nerve flow (vagal: X), increase sympathetic nerve flow (sympathetic nerve system)	Increased HR and stroke volume
Cushing reflex	Increased ICP	α-1 adrenergic receptors followed by vagus nerve stimulation	Arterioles of cerebrum	N/A	Sympathetic response activates α-1 adrenergic receptors, followed by vagus nerve parasympathetic response	Increased HR, BP, and contractility
Trigeminal reflex	Any stimulus to the trigeminal nerve	Mechanical and chemosensitive receptors in ventricular walls	Trigeminal nerve	Trigeminus nucleus—nucleus ambiguous in the brain stem	Premotor parasympathetic cardio-inhibitory neurons of the vagal nerve	Systemic hypotension, cardiac dysrhythmia (bradycardia), apnea, gastric hypermotility, and coronary vasospasm

C. Sinoatrial (SA) Node Abnormality

1. *Sick sinus syndrome (SSS):* SSS indicates bradyarrhythmias with or without tachyarrhythmias. More than 50 percent of patients with SSS develop tachy–brady syndrome with atrial fibrillation or flutter, leading to an increased risk of embolic stroke. The etiology includes intrinsic dysfunction of the SA node including degenerative fibrosis, an infiltrative process, or inherited dysfunction of ion channels within the SA node. Extrinsic conditions, that is, metabolic, infectious, autonomic, or pharmacologic conditions may also cause SSS (for a review, see Selected Readings).

   a. *Management:* Chronic bradycardia may lead to ventricular electrical remodeling, and symptomatic SSS is a class I indication for a permanent pacemaker.

D. Conduction Delay and Bundle Branch Block (Congenital, Acquired)

1. **Conduction delay:** First degree A-V block is not an entirely benign condition. Instead, it may indicate worse clinical prognosis, especially among the elderly population. Second- and third-degree A-V block warrants pacemaker implantation.

   a. *Management:* Cardiac pacing/resynchronization therapy for the patients with/without coexisting SSS, but the optimal pacing (as measured using the aortic flow time velocity integral measured on cardiac ultrasound) depends on intrinsic AV interval and desired pacing frequency.

2. **Bundle branch block:** Bundle branch block occurs secondary to a wide range of cardiac pathology. Compared with right bundle branch block (RBBB), left bundle branch block is considered to have high-diffuse disease, underlying ischemia, and dyssynchrony.

   a. *Management:* Both RBBB and LBBB may benefit from biventricular pacing to restore synchrony of right/left ventricular contraction.

IV. TACHYRRHYTHMIAS

A. Sinus Tachycardia

1. The etiology may include sepsis, hypovolemia, cardiac ischemia/CHF, pain, and endocrine pathology (hyperthyroidism).

B. Atrial Fibrillation

1. Atrial fibrillation (AF) is characterized by a lack of organized P-wave activity and an irregularly irregular ventricular response on the ECG. AF is the most common arrhythmia requiring treatment, affecting around 5 million Americans, with the prevalence expected to double by 2050.

2. Atrial fibrillation is a complex molecular process. Atrial fibrillation may induce rapid atrial rates and promote increased sympathetic nerve activity, which augments β-adrenergic tone. This leads to an increase in protein kinase A–mediated hyperphosphorylation of atrial ryanodine receptors (RyR2). Increased RyR2 phosphorylation promotes sarcoplasmic reticulum calcium release that induces calcium-mediated inhibition of voltage-dependent L-type calcium currents. This leads to shortening of atrial myocyte action potential duration (ADP) and effective refractory periods (ERP). The electric remodeling promotes further AF and increased sympathetic nerve output, myocyte apoptosis, and fibrosis and promotes atrial dilatation and structural remodeling (reviewed by Wickramasinghe and Patel).

3. **Management**

   a. **Treatment of stable AF** consists of pharmacologic intervention or overdrive pacing. Pharmacological treatment for hemodynamically stable AF includes class I and III medications (Table 17.2).

TABLE 17.2 Current Antiarrhythmic Drug Therapy for Atrial Fibrillation

Class	Examples	Proarrhythmia	Other Significant Side Effects	Contraindications
IC	Flecainide and propafenone	VT/VF; rapid atrial flutter	Rapidly conducting AF	CAD, hypertrophy
III	Sotalol and dofetilide	Torsade des pointes		Prolonged QT (at baseline or QTc>500 on treatment); heart failure (sotalol)
III	Dronederone	Torsade des pointes (rare), VT/VF	Heart failure exacerbation and death (in those with CHF); hepatic injury (rare)	NYHA class IV CHF or class II/III with recent exacerbation; prolonged AT (QTc>500); and permanent AF
III	Amiodarone	Torsade des pointes (rare)	Lung toxicity, hepatic toxicity, thyroid toxicity, and optic neuritis (rare)	Liver failure and existing lung disease

AF indicates atrial fibrillation; CAD, coronary artery disease; CHF, congestive heart failure; NYHA, New York Heart Association; VF, ventricular fibrillation; and VT, ventricular tachycardia.
Adapted from 2014 Circulation Research: Woods and Olgin "Atrial Fibrillation Therapy Now and in the Future" (permission pending)

b. Unstable AF (altered mental status, hypotension of systolic <90 mmHg, chest pain, shortness of breath) warrants synchronized cardioversion. For maintaining sinus rhythm after cardioversion, several class IA, IC, and III drugs, as well as class II (β-blockers), are moderately effective in maintaining sinus rhythm after conversion of atrial fibrillation.

c. Pharmacological interventions

1. **Amiodarone:** Amiodarone prophylaxis significantly reduces the incidence of atrial fibrillation after lung resection, transthoracic esophagectomy, and cardiac surgery. Amiodarone may reduce the incidence of AF to 23% (range: 12%–31%), with a number needed to treat of 4.4 (range: 3.1–7.8) (PASCART trial).

2. **Diltiazem:** In a randomized, double-blinded, placebo-controlled study of 330 patients, diltiazem almost halved the incidence of clinically significant postoperative atrial arrhythmias (P = 0.023) following pneumonectomy.

d. Ablations

1. **Radiofrequency ablation for paroxysmal AF** (vs. pharmacological therapy): The pulmonary vein–left atrial junction and an enlarged atrium harboring fibrosis and inflammation serve as the substrate for sustaining wavelets of atrial fibrillation. In radiofrequency ablation, low-voltage, high-frequency electricity is used to target focal areas thought to be responsible for AF. In a multicenter randomized trial at 24 months posttreatment, atrial fibrillation was significantly lower in the ablation group compared with the drug-therapy group (9% vs. 18%).

C. **Ventricular Tachyrrhythmias (VT)**
The key findings that suggest VT are atrioventricular dissociation, fusion or capture beats, QRS width (LBBB >160 ms, RBBB >140 ms), northwest axis, concordance, and LBBB morphology with right-axis deviation.

D. **Perioperative Torsades de Pointes**
   1. Risk factors for perioperative torsades de pointes are hypokalemia, hypomagnesemia, hypocalcemia, bradycardia, medications, and congenital long QT syndrome.
   2. Risk factors for drug-induced torsades de pointes include female sex, hypokalemia, bradycardia, recent conversion from atrial fibrillation (particularly with a QT-prolonging drug), congestive heart failure, digitalis therapy, high drug concentrations (with the exception of quinidine), baseline QT prolongation, subclinical long-QT syndrome, ion-channel polymorphisms, and severe hypomagnesemia.

V. **ETIOLOGY**
   A. **Cardiac Etiologies**
      1. **Abnormal QT syndromes and channelopathies:** Prolonged QTc affects short-term and long-term outcomes in patients with normal left ventricular function undergoing cardiac surgery. Mutations (inherited or acquired) in ion channels or associated proteins are the cause of a variety of cardiac arrhythmias. The genetics of sudden cardiac death caused by arrhythmias has been widely studied.
         a. Cardiac dysrhythmias may also be due to several genetic mutations:
            1. Alteration of slow delayed-rectifier potassium current (Iks) leads to life-threatening cardiac arrythmias, long QT syndrome, short QT syndrome, sinus bradycardia, and atrial fibrillation.
            2. Congenital sodium channelopathies leads to Brugada syndrome.
            3. Increased RyR2 activity has been shown to cause arrhythmias and increased CaMKII activity and phosphorylation of RyR2 at Ser2814. This may play a role in the pathogenesis of atrial fibrillation and ventricular arrhythmias.
      2. **Cardiomyopathy**
         a. **Inherited arrhythmogenic diseases**
            1. Cardiomyopathy (hypertrophic cardiomyopathy, arrhythmogenic right ventricular cardiomyopathy, dilated cardiomyopathy)
            2. *Channelopathy* (long QT syndrome, short QT syndrome, Brugada syndrome, and catecholaminergic polymorphic ventricular tachycardia)
         b. **Ischemic cardiomyopathy**
         c. **Frequent premature ventricular contractions**
            1. PVCs are being recognized as a cause of cardiomyopathy and suboptimal response to cardiac resynchronization therapy.
         d. **Extrinsic cardiomyopathy**
            1. Alcoholic, cirrhotic, metabolic, chemotherapy induced, radiation
         e. **Infiltrative cardiomyopathy**
            1. Amyloidosis, sarcoidosis, iron (thalassemia, hemochromatosis, hemosiderosis), autoimmune (rheumatic arthritis, systemic lupus erythematosus, systemic sclerosis, polymyocitis, dermatomyocitis, ankylosing spondylitis, celiac disease), Fabry's disease, G6PD deficiency, idiopathic fibrosis
   B. **Drug-Induced QT Prolongation (Table 17.3)**
   Drug-induced QT prolongation due to cardiovascular therapies (especially medications that delay QT interval) or noncardiovascular therapies

(i.e., anesthetics, psychotropic medications, etc.) have been shown to prolong the QT interval and may lead to cause torsades de pointes. Inhibition of the cardiac K^+ channels may selectively block the rapidly activating delayed rectifier channel Ikr (i.e., repolarizing potassium current) and is a common mechanism across drug classes.

C. Metabolic

1. Perioperative torsades de pointes can be fatal, and a major risk factor is QT prolongation secondary to metabolic disarray.
   a. *Management:* Treat hypokalemia, hypomagnesemia, hypoxemia, hypothermia, hypoglycemia, and hypothyroidism.

D. Spinal Cord Injury

1. Bradycardia is the most commonly seen arrhythmia in the acute phase of SCI (1–14 days after injury).

E. Infection

1. Bacterial, viral, and parasitic infections are known to cause cardiac arrhythmias. Viral (coxackie B, HIV), community acquired pneumonia (up to 5% may develop arrhythmias), Lyme disease, and Chagas disease are known to induce dysrhythmias. After the initial acute phase (<1% of patients will develop acute myocarditis), chronic disease can lead to upward of 33% of patients developing progressive cardiomyopathy-associated arrhythmias.

VI. ANESTHESIA-RELATED TOPICS

A. Inhalational anesthetics predispose the heart to arrhythmias. Classically, this has included halothane and methoxyflurane. However, even more modern anesthetics (sevoflurane, isoflurane) have been reported to prolong the QT interval.

B. The risk of arrhythmias associated with tracheal intubation was significantly reduced with preinduction administration of local anesthetics, calcium-channel blockers, β-blockers, and narcotics compared with placebo.

C. Thoracic epidural analgesia: The use of thoracic epidural analgesia in patients undergoing coronary artery bypass graft surgery may reduce the risk of postoperative supraventricular arrhythmias and respiratory complications. There were no beneficial effects of TEA with general anesthesia on the risk of mortality, myocardial infarction, or neurological complications compared with general anesthesia alone (*The Cochrane Database of Systematic Reviews*).

VII. EPILEPSY

Sudden, unexpected death has been reported in patients with epilepsy. Primary etiologies include channelopathies that involve both the brain and the heart (long-QT syndrome type 2). Syncope, seizure-induced bradycardia, and asystole may be secondary to an activated sympathetic system, increased compensatory responses (elevated adenosine levels), hypoxemia, hypercarbia, and pulmonary edema.

VIII. CONCLUSION

Arrhythmias predispose patients to increased morbidity and mortality. A thorough preoperative assessment, appropriate monitoring, and perioperative vigilance may reduce the inherent risks associated with these arrhythmias. As perioperative practitioners, we are often the first clinicians to intervene when lethal dysrhythmias occur.

Drug Classification	Drugs
Cardiovascular	Amiodarone, arsenic trioxide, bepridil, cisapride, calcium-channel blockers, disopyramide, dofetilide, flecainide, ibutilide, procainamide, quinidine, sotalol
Anesthetics	Volatile anesthetics (halothane, isoflurane, sevoflurane, desflurane)
	Intravenous anesthetics (etomidate, ketamine, propofol, thiopental)
	Local anesthetics
	Opioid receptor agonists or antagonists (alfentanyl, buprenorphine, fentanyl, meperidine, methadone, morphine, oxycodone, remifentanyl, sufentanyl, tramadol)
Neuromuscular blocker	Depolarizing (succinylcholine)
	Nondepolarizing (atracurium, cisatracurium, rocuronium, vecuronium)
Neuromuscular reversal agents	Anticholinesterases plus anticholinergics (neostigmine + atropine/glycopyrrohate, edrophonium + atropine), sugammadex
Perioperative adjuvants	Benzodiazepine (midazolam, etc.), dexmedetomidine, domperidon, droperidol, metoclopramide, promethazine, 5HT-3 antagonists (ondansetron, dolasetron, tropisetron)
Psychotropic medications	Antipsychotic drugs (amisulpride, aripiprazole, chlorprothixen, clozapine, flupenthixol, haloperidol, levomepromazine, olanzapine, palperidone, perphenazine, pimozide, quetiapine, risperidone, sertindole, sulpiride, ziprasidone, zuclopenthixole)
	TCA and MAO inhibitors (amitriptyline, clomipramine, doxepin, imipramine, isocarboxazid, moclobemide, nortriptyline)
	Neurotransmitter uptake inhibitors (agomelatine, bupropion, citalopram, duloxetine, escitalopram, fluoxetine, mianserin, mirtazapine, paroxetine, reboxetine, sertraline, venlafaxine)
	Mood stabilizers (lithium)
	Antiseizure (carbamazepine, lamotrigine, valproate)
	Anxiolytic drugs (benzodiazepines, gabapentin, pregabaline)
	Anticholinergic drugs (biperiden, orphenadrine)
Drugs can cause low K	Diuretics (loop diuretics)
Drugs can cause low Mg	PPI (lansoprazole)
Antibiotics and antivirals	Fluoroquinolones
	Macrolides (azithromycin, erythromycin, clarithromycin)
	Chloroquines
	Protease inhibitors
Chemotherapy agents	Anthracycline, capecitabine (5-FU), cisplatin, histone deacetylase inhibitor (vorinostat)
Toxins	Mad honey intoxication (diterpene grayanotoxins), hydrocarbon, alcohol
Energy drinks	Caffeine
Other medications	Albuterol, cholchicine, tosylchloramide

Selected Readings

Fleisher LA, Beckman JA, Brown KA, et al. ACC/AHA 2007 guidelines on perioperative cardiovascular evaluation and care for noncardiac surgery: executive summary: a report of the American College of Cardiology/American Heart Association Task Force on Practice Guidelines (Writing committee to revise the 2002 guidelines on perioperative cardiovascular evaluation for noncardiac surgery) developed in collaboration with the American Society of Echocardiography, American Society of Nuclear Cardiology, Heart Rhythm Society, Society of Cardiovascular Anesthesiologists, Society for Cardiovascular Angiography and Interventions, Society for Vascular Medicine and Biology, and Society for Vascular Surgery. *J Am Coll Cardiol* 2007;50(17):1707–1732.

Frendl G, Sodickson AC, Chung MK, et al. 2014 AATS guidelines for the prevention and management of perioperative atrial fibrillation and flutter for thoracic surgical procedures. *J Thorac Cardiovasc Surg* 2014;148(3):e153–e193. doi:10.1016/j.jtcvs.2014.06.036

January CT, Wann LS, Alpert JS, et al. 2014 AHA/ACC/HRS guideline for the management of patients with atrial fibrillation: a report of the American College of Cardiology/American Heart Association Task Force on Practice Guidelines and the Heart Rhythm Society. *J Am Coll Cardiol* 2014;64(21):e1–e76. doi:10.1016/j.jacc.2014.03.022

Link MS. Clinical practice. Evaluation and initial treatment of supraventricular tachycardia. *N Engl J Med* 2012;367(15):1438–1448.

Peretto G, Durante A, Limite LR, et al. Postoperative arrhythmias after cardiac surgery: incidence, risk factors, and therapeutic management. *Cardiol Res Pract* 2014;2014:615987.

Roden DM. Drug-induced prolongation of the QT interval. *N Engl J Med* 2004;350(10):1013–1022.

Szelkowski LA, Puri NK, Singh R, et al. Current trends in preoperative, intraoperative, and postoperative care of the adult cardiac surgery patient. *Curr Probl Surg* 2015;52(1):531–569. doi:10.1067/j.cpsurg.2014.10.001

Vardas PE, Simantirakis EN, Kanoupakis EM. New developments in cardiac pacemakers. *Circulation* 2013;127(23):2343–2350.

Woods CE, Olgin J. Atrial fibrillation therapy now and in the future: drugs, biologicals, and ablation. *Circ Res* 2014;114(9):1532–1546.

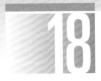

ECMO and Ventricular Assist Devices

Gaston Cudemus and Jose P. Garcia

I. EXTRACORPOREAL LIFE SUPPORT (ECLS/ECMO)

A. The development of ECLS/ECMO as a temporary assist device is a direct extension of the principles of cardiopulmonary bypass, which usually involves intrathoracic venoarterial (VA) cannulation. The use of ECMO allows time for treatment and recovery from severe heart and lung failure.

B. ECMO is most commonly used in patients with inadequate oxygen delivery resulting from ineffective oxygenation due to severe lung disease or low cardiac output due to severe circulatory failure, or both.

C. There are a number of key differences between cardiopulmonary bypass and ECMO. The most obvious difference is the duration of required support. Whereas cardiopulmonary bypass typically is employed for several hours during cardiac surgery, ECMO is designed for a longer duration of support. Also, ECMO involves a closed system without a reservoir for blood collection. These differences are thought to reduce the inflammatory response and the more pronounced coagulopathy that can be seen with cardiopulmonary bypass, although there is generally a rapid rise of inflammatory cytokines with the initiation of ECMO support.

II. BACKGROUND.
In May 1953, Gibbon used artificial oxygenation and perfusion support for the first successful open heart operation. Then, in 1975 Bartlett et al., were the first to successfully use ECMO in neonates with severe respiratory distress.

A. There have been two randomized trials in adults with acute respiratory distress syndrome (ARDS) and neither has shown a survival benefit. Both used ECMO techniques that are now outdated and had complication rates considerably higher than those reported recently by high-volume ECMO centers. ECMO can fully support and save the lives of some patients with severe respiratory or cardiac failure, and the best results are obtained in centers with established programs and well-trained, experienced staff.

B. Indications and Contraindications to the initiation of ECLS in adults were carefully reviewed by the ECMO committee at Massachusetts General Hospital. These include the following:

1. *Indications for VA ECMO*:

    a. Cardiogenic shock with end-organ hypoperfusion including the following:

        1. Poor LV or RV function on echocardiogram

        2. Cardiac Index <2.2 L/min/m^2 or SVO$_2$ $<60\%$ on two inotropes

        3. High biventricular filling pressures (PCW >20, CVP 15)

        4. Rising lactate

        5. Worsening metabolic acidosis

    b. Hypotension (systolic BP <100 mmHg) with significant vasopressor requirement (two or more of the following): norepinephrine ≥50 mcg/min, vasopressin ≥0.04 units/min, and/or phenylephrine ≥100 mcg/min, and epinephrin ≥5 mcg/min

    c. On maximal medical therapy: IABP or percutaneous VAD (e.g., TandemHeart or Impella) plus inotropic support (milrinone ≥0.3 mcg/kg/min, dopamine ≥5 mcg/kg/min, dobutamine ≥10 mcg/kg/min, and/or epinephrine ≥2 mcg/min) with adequate heart rate (>80 but <120)

    d. Contraindication to inotropic support (e.g., VT)

    e. Unstable arrhythmias requiring multiple cardioversion (e.g., AF, VT)

  2. *Indication for VV ECMO (Lung Support)*:

    a. Acute respiratory failure (hypoxemic or hypercarbic)

    b. Failure of maximal medical therapy despite optimization of the ventilator settings:

      1. FIO_2 100%

      2. PEEP ≥15 cmH_2O for plateau <30 cmH_2O

      3. Recruitment maneuvers attempted

      4. Inhaled nitric oxide or epoprostenol (optional)

    c. Persistent hypoxemia/hypercarbia (oxygen saturation <90% or $PaCO_2$ >100 mmHg for 1 hour with respiratory acidosis pH <7.20)

    d. Normal biventricular function

    e. Significant vasopressor or inotrope requirement

    f. Murray Score ≥3.

  3. Absolute contraindications. To be screened by ECMO Team

    a. Acute intracranial hemorrhage or massive stroke.

    b. Mechanical ventilation >7 days.

    c. Paralytics and steroids >48 hours (if patient is intubated).

    d. CPR more than 60 minutes in-hospital, otherwise more than 30 minutes outside of the hospital.

    e. Severe aortic insufficiency.

    f. Acute aortic dissection.

    g. End-stage liver disease.

    h. BMI >40 kg/m^2.

    i. Contraindication to anticoagulation, or refusal to receive blood products.

  4. Relative contraindications

    a. Age >70 years.

    b. Active cancer.

    c. Suicide.

    d. Chronic kidney disease.

    e. Multi-organ system failure(≥3 organs).

    f. Lack of social support or inability to identify healthcare proxy.

III. ECMO CIRCUIT

  An **ECMO circuit** contains several key components including a drainage (venous) cannula, a return (arterial) cannula, a driving force (pump), a gas exchange unit (oxygenator), a heat exchanger, and connection tubing. There are also devices to maintain the safety of, and measure the functioning of, the circuit. The cannulas are sized between 21 and 28 French for adults and smaller for newborns and children. Circuit components should be chosen to enable a blood flow of at least 50 to 60 mL/kg/min. The $PaCO_2$ is determined by the oxygenator gas flow (or sweep speed). In practice, CO_2 is efficiently cleared by ECMO and usually $PaCO_2$ is easily controlled. The determinants of PaO_2 are more complex, but the most important determinant is the circuit blood flow.

  A. ECLS can support patient's gas exchange and hemodynamic function, with two basic strategies of **circulatory access: venovenous (VV) and venoarterial**

(VA) ECMO. Technological advances have led to improved cannula flows and mechanics, and VV ECMO has begun to replace the VA approach, unless concomitant severe cardiac failure exists. (Fig. 18.1)

B. In general, VV ECMO is used for respiratory failure and VA ECMO for both lung and cardiac failure. Low-frequency positive–pressure ventilation extracorporeal CO_2 removal (LFPPV-ECCO2R) uses VV extracorporeal circulation. CO_2 can be removed with a low extracorporeal blood flow (around 20% of the patient's cardiac output).

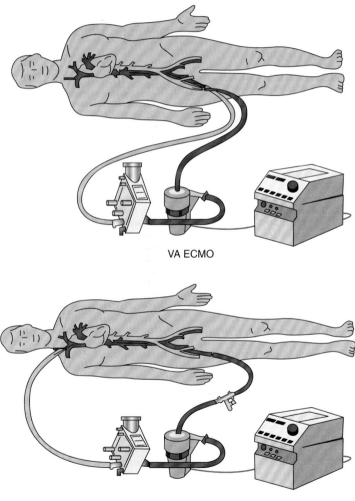

VA ECMO

VV ECMO

FIGURE 18.1 VA ECMO and VV ECMO.

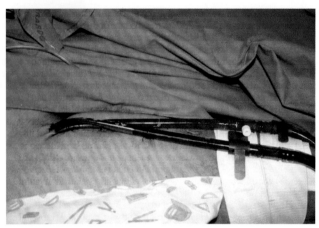

FIGURE 18.2 Peripheral VA ECMO. If ECMO is started at the end of cardiac surgery, the right atrium and ascending aorta may be used as cannulation sites. With VA ECMO, the patient's heart and lungs are bypassed, normal arterial blood gases and hemodynamics can be obtained, and full cardiac and respiratory support can be provided.

1. **Venoarterial ECMO.** Systemic venous blood is drained via a cannula placed in one of the vena cava, most commonly the right internal jugular vein or the femoral vein, and is returned to the arterial system via a cannula placed in the femoral, axillary, or carotid artery (Fig. 18.2).

2. **Venovenous ECMO** involves venous blood from the patient being accessed from a large central vein and returned to the venous system near the right atrium after passing through an oxygenator. It provides support for severe respiratory failure when no major cardiac dysfunction exists. When flow through a single access cannula is insufficient to support the high ECMO flow rate that may be required in severe respiratory failure, a second venous access cannula may be required (Fig. 18.3).

C. **Selecting the Form of ECMO; VV or VA.** VV ECMO is a low-pressure circuit compared with VA, resulting in less stress on the circuit tubing and oxygenator, and may therefore improve their longevity. The major advantage of VA over VV ECMO is the management of cardio-respiratory failure or cardiac failure where use of a ventricular assist device (VAD) is inappropriate. It may be indicated for cardiac decompensation following cardiac surgery either as a bridge to recovery or to another destination therapy.

D. **Components of the Circuit (Fig. 18.4)**

1. The size of the venous cannula will determine blood flow, and therefore the largest possible cannula should be placed. Sizes 23 F through 29 F have been used successfully. For the return cannula, a 19 F through a 21 F is used for arterial cannulation and a 21 F through a 23 F for venous cannulation. In the majority of cases, venous cannulas can be placed percutaneously. To minimize limb complications from ischemia, one strategy is to place a 5 to 7 F perfusion cannula in the superficial femoral artery distal to the primary arterial inflow cannula to perfuse the leg. This cannula is connected to a tubing circuit that is spliced into the arterial circuit with a Y-connector. The distal cannula directs continuous flow into the leg and significantly reduces the incidence of leg

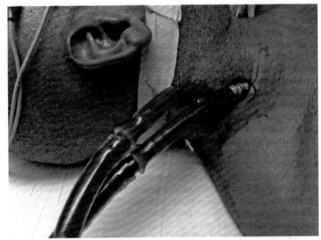

FIGURE 18.3 Avalon cannula VV ECMO. VV ECMO improves patients' oxygenation by reducing the amount of blood that passes through the lung without being oxygenated and in addition, removes CO_2 from patients' blood. This is the appropriate mode of support for virtually all patients with primary respiratory failure, even when there is significant hemodynamic instability. The requirement for high doses of vasoactive drugs is not a contraindication to VV ECMO because once oxygenation improves and mechanical ventilation is reduced, the circulation usually improves dramatically.

    ischemia. It should be noted, however, that limb ischemia associated with long-term peripheral cannulation relates not just to arterial perfusion, but also to the relative venous obstruction that can occur with large venous lines. In such circumstances, distal venous drainage can be established by placing another small venous cannula into the circuit.

2. Cannulas used for VV ECMO are either single or double lumen. The right IJ vein is used for cannulation with a double-lumen cannula. This double-lumen cannula is placed so that the distal end of the cannula is in the inferior vena cava, the proximal drainage port is in the superior vena cava, and the reinfusion port is in the low right atrium directed at the tricuspid valve. Another option is placement of the drainage cannula in the femoral vein and the return cannula in the jugular vein; this provides higher flow rates and less recirculation than the reverse situation. With this arrangement, the tip of the drainage cannula should sit below the level of the diaphragm and the tip of the return cannula in the proximal superior vena cava above the level of the right atrium. Preventing air embolism is essential. Heparin is used prior to cannulation, and the position of the cannula is confirmed by TEE and x-rays.

3. **Oxygenators** consist of a series of hollow fibers with an integrated heat-exchange system through which the blood passes. Control of oxygenation and ventilation is relatively easy; increasing the total gas flow rate increases CO_2 removal (increasing the "sweep") by reducing the gas-phase CO_2 partial pressure and promoting diffusion. Blood oxygenation is controlled simply by changing the fraction of O_2 in the gas supplied to the oxygenator.

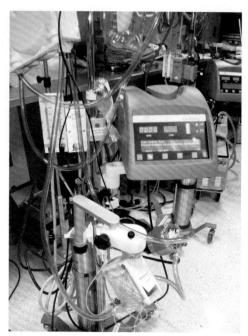

FIGURE 18.4 Circuit components.

4. **Blood pump** may be either a centrifugal pump (most common) or a roller pump. Both are acceptable, and the choice will be determined by institutional experience.

5. Roller pumps compress the plastic tubing and physically push blood forward. This requires a reservoir between the venous cannula, and the pump utilizes gravity for drainage into the reservoir. Venous drainage is passive and can be assisted by raising the height of the patient's bed above the ECMO base.

6. Centrifugal pumps have been popular in Europe and are becoming more popular in the United States; they utilize the spinning action of cones to create an effect similar to a tornado, pulling blood into the pump head and expelling it from the outer edge. These pumps do not require gravity, so they can be placed at any height in relation to the patient. Centrifugal pumps can generate very high negative pressures, which may cause hemolysis. This problem is reduced with newer generation pumps (e.g., Rotaflow [Maquet], Centrimag [Levotronix], and BioConsole550 [Medtronic perfusion]).

7. **Heat exchangers** allow for maintenance of normothermia given the potential heat loss that can occur through the long circuit.

IV. MANAGEMENT OF ECMO

A. Following cannulation, ECMO is started by gradually increasing blood flow until venous return is limited by venous drainage. For most adults, a flow of 4 to 5 L/min is ideal. Once the initial respiratory and hemodynamic goals have been achieved, the blood flow is maintained at that rate. If the circuit blood flow is significantly less than ideal and the patient's blood volume is adequate, there is likely to be a problem with the position of the drainage cannula. Once adequate flow has been achieved, ventilator settings are reduced during ECMO in order to avoid barotrauma and volutrauma (FIO_2 <0.5, peak inspiratory pressure <20 cmH_2O, PEEP <10 cmH_2O). It is important to remember that the goal of VV ECMO is not to accomplish normal oxygenation but to achieve similar levels found in a mechanically ventilated patient with severe ARDS (SaO_2 of 85%–92%) and to rest the lungs. Once the ventilator settings have been achieved, circuit blood flow should be adjusted to SaO_2 of 85% to 92%. The circuit venous saturation will usually be 80% to 85%. When the venous oxyhemoglobin saturation is below target, interventions that may be helpful include increasing blood flow, intravascular volume, or hemoglobin concentration. The oxygenator fresh gas flow should be altered to achieve a $PaCO_2$ of 40 to 50 mmHg, which is often easily obtained. If, despite good positioning of cannulas and adequate intravenous volume, flow remains inadequate and mechanical ventilation cannot be reduced, a second drainage cannula is required.

B. With VA ECMO, blood flow is adjusted according to blood pressure and signs of adequate systemic blood flow. This includes a falling lactate level and a circuit venous saturation of approximately 75%, which will usually produce SaO_2 greater than 90%.

C. Supportive therapy is continued, including appropriate antivirals and antibiotics, nutritional support, and volume management to the patient's approximate dry weight. Systemic anticoagulation with heparin to prevent circuit clotting is required and is titrated by bedside anticoagulation monitoring. The use of continuous renal replacement therapy for fluid overload or renal failure is common.

D. Adequate **sedation** (midazolam/fentanyl) to inhibit respiratory movement is required initially. Addition of ketamine or propofol may be necessary. Muscle relaxation is not routinely administered unless patient movement interferes with venous return. In some patients, VV ECMO sedation may be lightened but this should only be attempted at the discretion and in the presence of the treating ECMO physicians.

E. Based on our experiences the use of ambulatory single-venous VV ECMO is safe and effective in ARDS and CF patients. Our belief is that a key step in the treatment course is early application of VV ECMO after development of acute respiratory failure, requiring mechanical ventilation. VV ECMO avoids the use of mechanical ventilation while allowing patients to participate in physical therapy and to eat normally while receiving respiratory support. The majority of our patients are awake, liberated from the ventilator, ambulating on a treadmill or hallway, and up in a chair up to 6 hours a day.

F. Continuous **circuit monitoring** includes circuit blood flow, pump speed, pressures in the drainage cannula, pressures on both sides of the oxygenator, oxygen saturation on the arterial and venous side of the oxygenator, and blood temperature. With a centrifugal pump, inlet pressures are commonly –50 to –100 mmHg. The higher the pressure, the more likely the oxygenator and circuit leaks.

V. LABORATORY TESTING AND ANTICOAGULATION

A. Blood gases should be measured every 4 to 8 hours, and **anticoagulation** should be monitored hourly by examining activated clotting times (ACTs). This should be supplemented with standard coagulation tests and a complete blood count 2 to 4 times daily. Some centers also measure antithrombin III levels daily and perform regular thromboelastography. Anticoagulation is achieved with a continuous infusion of unfractionated heparin adjusted to maintain an ACT of 160 to 180 seconds. The ACT target is decreased if bleeding develops. Platelets are continuously consumed during ECMO because they are activated by exposure to the foreign surface area and therefore should be transfused to maintain the count above 100,000/mm^3. Hematocrit must be maintained above a minimum of 30% to 40%. Plasma-free hemoglobin should be measured daily to monitor for hemolysis related to either circuit thrombus or excessive negative pressure. Daily circuit blood cultures should be obtained.

VI. **CONTINUOUS RENAL REPLACEMENT THERAPY (CRRT OR CVVHD).** Ideally, the CVVHD circuit is connected to the ECMO circuit to prevent risk associated with dialysis catheter insertion. The most common way to connect the CVVHD circuit to the ECMO circuit is to attach the access and return lines for CVVHD to the two three-way taps between the outlet of the pump head and the oxygenator. The CVVHD-circuit return blood can be connected to an alternative venous access. In central ECMO (no backflow cannula), the return line could be attached to a peripheral line. If there is no alternative, separate dialysis catheter access may be required. CVVH off the ECMO circuit should be monitored for LDH increase.

   A. A range of **complications and problems** can occur during ECMO. Some of them are common to all forms of ECMO and some are specific to VV or VA ECMO or to certain types of circuit components. Some mechanical **circuit problems** are life threatening (e.g., massive blood loss from the circuit or air embolism) and may require immediate clamping of the cannulas and removal of the patient from ECMO support. Backup ventilator settings should always be prescribed for such emergencies.

   B. Because a large artery must be cannulated on VA ECMO, a surgical cutdown is sometimes required, which may cause **bleeding** at the insertion site. Percutaneous cannulation can be performed as long as a lower extremity cannula can also be placed percutaneously. Minor bleeding should be managed by making sure that the platelet count is over 100,000/mm^3 and that the coagulation panel is normal. When major bleeding occurs, coagulation should be managed by increasing the platelet count to more than 150,000/mm^3 and confirming that the fibrinogen concentration is more than 200 mg/L and that the prothrombin ratio is less than 1.5. If bleeding continues, the target ACT range must be lowered (e.g., to 140–160 seconds). The most serious bleeding complication is intracranial hemorrhage. A risk factor is a platelet count less than 50,000/mm^3. Minor procedures can cause significant bleeding, and the need for such procedures should be carefully reviewed.

   C. The formation of **clots in the circuit** is the most common mechanical complication. Small clots and fibrin strands adhering to the tubing are almost inevitable with prolonged ECMO and do not necessarily pose a risk for the patient. Larger clots can cause systemic embolization, hemolysis, oxygenator failure, and disseminated intravascular coagulation.

   D. If a small volume of **air** enters the circuit, it may be able to be moved to the venous reservoir or the oxygenator and then aspirated. If a large volume of air enters the circuit, an **air embolism** or venous airlock develops. In this situation, the drainage and return cannulas should be clamped immediately and primary attention directed to maintaining the patient's circulation and ventilation.

E. In a patient with minimal or no native cardiac function, sudden **hemodynamic deterioration** implies loss of circuit flow, usually due to hypovolemia or venous cannula displacement. Loss of circuit flow should be managed by giving IV fluids. Hemodynamic deterioration despite normal circuit function implies deteriorating cardiovascular function. Causes for sudden, severe hemodynamic deterioration include tension pneumothorax, hemothorax, pericardial tamponade, massive bleeding, myocardial ischemia, arrhythmias, and sepsis.

F. Acute **hypoxemia** in a previously stable patient should be assessed first by reviewing the ECMO circuit flow. If it has fallen, management is the same as for loss of pump flow. If it is unchanged, the oxygenator may be failing or the oxygenator fresh gas flow may have become disconnected.

G. Oxygenator failure may be recognized by deterioration in gas exchange, an increasing pressure gradient across the membrane, and signs of clot in the membrane.

H. ECMO will unload the right ventricle but not the **compromised left ventricle**, even though left ventricular preload is reduced. If the heart is dilated and poorly contracting, the marked increase in afterload provided by the ECMO system offsets any change in end-diastolic left ventricular volume produced by bypassing the heart, resulting in cardiac damage and pulmonary edema. The heart remains dilated because the left ventricle cannot eject sufficient volume against the increased afterload to reduce either end-diastolic or -systolic volume. ECMO may increase left ventricular wall stress and myocardial oxygen consumption unless an IABP, decreased ECMO flow, switch from femoral to central ECMO, atrial septostomy, or other means is used to unload the left ventricle and reduce left ventricular wall stress.

I. If VA ECMO is used inappropriately for respiratory failure in a patient with good cardiac function, the coronary arteries and cerebral vessels may be perfused by deoxygenated blood. This is why VA ECMO should be reserved for patients with profound cardiac failure. Other important complications associated with ECLS using heparin-coated circuits included renal failure (requiring dialysis), bacteremia or mediastinitis, and leg ischemia.

VII. WEANING FROM ECMO

A. Venovenous ECMO. Improvement of lung function is suggested when lower ECMO circuit flow is required to achieve a patient arterial oxygen saturation of 85% to 92%. An increase in arterial oxygen saturation above the mixed venous and circuit venous saturation will be seen. Circuit flow is then gradually reduced to maintain the patient's arterial oxygen saturation above 90%. When the flow is less than 1.5 to 2 L/min, the patient is ready for a trial period without ECMO, done by ventilating the patient and then stopping the circuit gas flow. Patients are observed for several hours, during which the ventilator settings that are necessary to maintain adequate oxygenation and ventilation off ECMO are determined. If the blood gases are marginal and there are no ECMO-related complications, it is better to return to full support for a further 24 to 48 hours. If blood gases and lung compliance are satisfactory, the patient can then be decannulated.

B. Venoarterial ECMO. Saturation provides a good measure of lung function while flows give you an indication of right ventricular function. VA ECMO trials require temporary clamping of both the drainage and infusion lines, while allowing the ECMO circuit to circulate through a bridge between the arterial and venous limbs. Patients are usually weaned from VA ECMO onto modest inotropic support. The planned inotropic regimen should be started 6 to 12 hours before attempting to wean. Blood flow is slowly reduced to around 1 L/min, and cardiac function is reviewed clinically and by TEE. In addition, the arterial and venous lines should be flushed continuously with heparinized saline or intermittently with heparinized blood from the circuit. Native heart ejection may be seen on the arterial waveform before flows are reduced, indicating some myocardial recovery. VA ECMO trials are generally shorter in duration than VV ECMO trials because of the higher risk of thrombus formation.

C. Other Indications. Nowadays, more reports evidence the successful use of ECMO in **lung transplantation**, either in graft failure after lung transplantation or in bridging to lung transplantation with good post–lung transplant outcomes. In cases of persistent, severe pulmonary graft dysfunction refractory to mechanical ventilatory maneuvers, ECMO have been used successfully to stabilize gas exchange. Urgent retransplantation can also be considered if other interventions fail. Cardiopulmonary bypass and/or ECLS are rarely needed, but in patients with severe pulmonary contusions, intrathoracic tracheal injuries with concomitant great vessel injury, cardiac injury, and complex cranial disruption, they can be lifesaving.

VIII. FUTURE. Applications for ECMO may expand in the future to include percutaneous temporary left ventricular assistance and low-flow ECMO for CO_2 removal (ECOOR). In addition, new technologies will improve the simplicity and safety of ECMO, including new oxygenators, pumps, and surface coatings.

A. Mechanical Circulatory Support (MCS)

1. Over the past few decades, much progress has been made in the development and refinement of ventricular assist devices (VADs), medical devices capable of maintaining circulatory output of the diseased ventricle.

2. VADs consist of a pump connected to the heart and aorta via an inflow cannula and an outflow cannula, respectively, an external driveline that powers the motor within the device, and a system controller. Power may be delivered through a power base unit or battery packs, allowing increased mobility. VADs support the failing heart by unloading the ventricle and generating flow to the systemic and/or pulmonary circulation.

3. MCS for patients with advanced heart failure has evolved considerably during the past 30 years and is now standard therapy at many medical centers worldwide.

B. Indications. Patients can have preexisting chronic heart failure or acute heart failure after viral illness, MI, or after unsuccessful surgery or intervention with cardiac index <2 L/min/m², SBP <90 mmHg, pulmonary capillary wedge pressure or CVP >18, SVR >2,100, decreased mental status, low urine output, and metabolic acidosis.

C. Contraindications are relative but include end stage renal disease, malignancy, severe PVD, sepsis, central nervous system injury, severe hepatic disease, and severe chronic pulmonary disease. These contraindications need to be evaluated individually.

1. Pulsatile or displacement pumps almost always work in asynchrony to the native heart and have been the most commonly used devices in the United States. Pulsatile devices approved by the FDA include the Abiomed BVS5000 and AB5000, Novacor (withdrawn from the market by the manufacturer), and the Thoratec PVAD and IVAD devices. These pumps consist of inflow and outflow conduits, unidirectional valves, a pumping chamber, a battery pack, and a system controller and may be

driven pneumatically or electrically. Recently published literature suggests that continuous compared with pulsatile VADs provide favorable hemodynamic circulatory assistance to support end-organ function and functional status.

2. The second-generation devices include implantable, continuous flow, rotary pumps with axial flow that offer several advantages over pulsatile flow pumps, like the smaller size that reduces the risk of infections and simpler implantation. Some of the limitations of this type of device are hemolysis, ventricular suction, and thrombus formation. Examples are the HeartMate™ II, the Jarvik 2000®, and the DeBakey® LVAD. Clinical experience shows that the HeartMate II LVAD provides excellent support in the outpatient setting, with significant improvement in functional capacity (Fig. 18.5).

3. The third-generation of devices includes centrifugal continuous-flow pumps with an impeller or rotor suspended in the blood flow path using a noncontact bearing design. The levitation systems suspend the moving impeller within the blood field without any mechanical contact, thus eliminating frictional wear and reducing heat generation. This feature promises longer durability and higher reliability with low incidence of device failure and need for replacement.

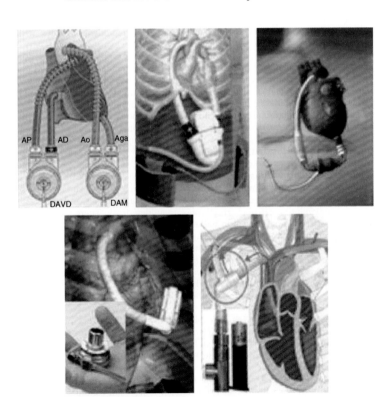

FIGURE 18.5 Different types of VADs.

D. Right Ventricular and Biventricular Assist Devices

1. The majority of patients with chronic heart failure require left ventricular assist device (LVAD) support. Isolated right ventricular dysfunction requiring insertion of a right ventricular assist device (RVAD) to support the failing ventricle is a rare event. Usually, a moderate amount of RV dysfunction can be managed perioperatively with milrinone and nitric oxide. Some LVAD patients need temporary mechanical RV support that can then be weaned.

2. The unique physiology created by a mechanical pump is further complicated if biventricular support is needed. Unlike a single VAD, biventricular mechanical devices create a complex system with two independent pumps, one right sided and the other left sided. Biventricular support is used for acute cardiogenic shock after an MI or post-open heart surgery. Chronic biventricular failure in some cases can be managed as a bridge to transplant with an implantable biventricular assist device (BiVAD) with either the Thoratec devices or the CardioWest Total Artificial Heart. The BiVAD device is approved for long-term use and is a bridge to transplant; patients with these can be discharged home.

3. The classification is typically broken down into three categories: bridge to recovery, bridge to transplantation, and destination therapy.

E. Bridge to Recovery was one of the first indications of VAD. The goal of this strategy is to unload the heart and improve the hemodynamic status with the hope of achieving sufficient myocardial recovery to permit device removal. The most common scenarios for this type of support is after an MI and after open heart surgery when ventricular performance is not adequate enough to allow weaning from CPB or to support the individual while the heart recovers. Patients who continue to be in shock despite opening an obstructed vessel are candidates for mechanical support. The IABP is the standard of care, along with inotropes and vasopressors. Those patients who are still in cardiogenic shock despite these measures are candidates for assist devices (Figs. 18.5 and 18.6).

F. Bridge to Transplant (BBT) is the most common in clinical practice. These patients are candidates for heart transplant, but are not predicted to survive the waiting-list period secondary to sequelae of cardiac failure, including worsening end-organ function, rising PA pressures, or those with refractory cardiogenic shock on escalating inotropes, and those with malignant ventricular arrhythmias or sudden death. There is equivalent posttransplant survival in patients coming to transplant on continuous inotropic support or on LVAD support. In BTT candidates, VADs typically improve organ function after implantation; therefore, patients are able to recover and be in a better situation at the time of transplant. However, the impact on posttransplant survival is controversial. Complications include infections of the drive line, pocket, and device itself; device malfunction; sepsis; multisystem organ failure; right heart failure; stroke; bleeding; and pulmonary complications.

G. Destination Therapy is applicable for advanced refractory heart failure patients who are not transplant candidates owing to the presence of contraindications, including older age, cancer, pulmonary hypertension, obesity, smoking, and advanced lung and kidney disease. This is a relatively new concept where the assist device is implanted as a permanent solution to end-stage heart disease. Initially, this has been reserved for patients with extremely limited life expectancy who were not candidates for heart transplant. The REMATCH trial showed a 48% reduction in mortality for

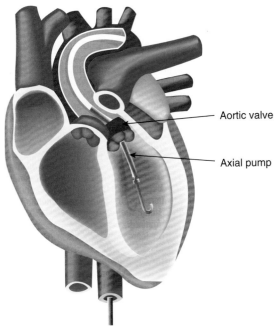

Aortic valve

Axial pump

FIGURE 18.6 Impella.

the LVAD group as compared with optimal medical management. Current indications include NYHA IV symptoms for >60 days, LVEF <25%, peak oxygen consumption <12 mL/kg per minute or inability to wean from inotropic support, and contraindications to heart transplant. With a fixed number of heart transplants being performed, interest in applications is quickly widening, and there are many devices in the development and testing phases.

H. Total Artificial Heart (TAH) will be the conceptual end solution for cardiac replacement of the failing heart. Assist devices work in parallel to the left ventricle, and are becoming simpler, smaller, and valveless, in contrast to the TAH, which displaces the heart and retains pulsatile flow. The original Jarvik TAH is still in use as is the CardioWest BiVAD and is used as a bridge to transplant, as well as the AbioCor. Current indications include patients <75 years of age with severe irreversible biventricular failure or end-stage heart disease who are not transplant or LVAD candidates and cannot be weaned from multiple inotropic support or mechanical biventricular support. Long-term risks include thromboembolic complications, the risk of infection, and trauma to components of blood.

I. Anticoagulation or antiplatelet therapy is a central component of outpatient management because thromboembolism is associated with all devices. International normalized ratios of 1.5 to 2.5 are currently targeted for pneumatically driven pulsatile devices. In patients with a continuous flow pump, some VAD centers are now recommending a lower international normalized ratio of 1.7 to 2.3. If an individual experiences a neurologic event, a higher international normalized ratio may be targeted.

Selected Readings

Avalon Laboratories. Avalon elite bi-caval dual lumen catheter. http://www.avalonlabs .com/html/pulmonary_support.html. Accessed November 25, 2011.

Cypel M, Keshavjee S. Extracorporeal life support as a bridge to lung transplantation. *Clin Chest Med* 2011;32(2):245–251.

Doll N, Kiaii B, Borger M, et al. Five-year results of 219 consecutive patients treated with extracorporeal membrane oxygenation for refractory postoperative cardiogenic shock. *Ann Thorac Surg* 2004;77:151–157.

Kirklin JK, Naftel DC, Kormos RL, et al. The fourth INTERMACS annual report: 4000 implants and counting. *J Heart Lung Transplant* 2012;31:117–126.

Koeckert MS, Jorde UP, Naka Y, et al. Impella LP 2.5 for left ventricular unloading during venoarterial extracorporeal membrane oxygenation support. *J Card Surg* 2011;26:666–668.

Park PK, Napolitano LM, Bartlett RH. Extracorporeal membrane oxygenation in adult acute respiratory distress syndrome. *Crit Care Clin* 2011;27:627–646.

Roy BJ, Rycus P, Conrad SA, et al. The changing demographics of neonatal extracorporeal membrane oxygenation patients reported to the Extracorporeal Life Support Organization (ELSO) Registry. *Pediatrics* 2000;106(6):1334–1338.

Thiagarajan RR, Brogan TV, Scheurer MA, et al. Extracorporeal membrane oxygenation to support cardiopulmonary resuscitation in adults. *Ann Thorac Surg* 2009;87:778–785.

Ziemba EA, John R. Mechanical circulatory support for bridge to decision: which device and when to decide. *J Card Surg* 2010;25:425–433.

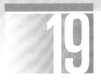

The Acute Respiratory Distress Syndrome

Lorenzo Berra and B. Taylor Thompson

I. **DEFINITION:** Acute respiratory distress syndrome (ARDS) is an inflammatory lung condition characterized by increased vascular permeability, pulmonary edema and consolidation, and hypoxemia. It can be triggered by direct and indirect injuries and is usually associated with signs of other organ dysfunction. Although histopathologically well defined (diffuse alveolar damage; DAD), the clinical diagnosis of ARDS has relatively poor specificity for the presence of DAD at postmortem. Recently, great effort has been put in redefining the diagnostic criteria of ARDS (**Berlin definition of ARDS,** Table 19.1); however, these new ARDS criteria still have relatively low specificity for DAD. It is unknown if patients meeting the clinical criteria for ARDS but without DAD behave differently than do patients with clinical ARDS with DAD.

II. **ETIOLOGY:** ARDS usually develops in patients that suffer from predisposing conditions that induce a systemic inflammatory response. ARDS can be caused by pulmonary conditions, such as pneumonia, aspiration pneumonitis, and contusions, or, less commonly, by extrapulmonary conditions, such as abdominal sepsis, acute pancreatitis, and multiple trauma. Trauma-associated ARDS is generally considered a less severe form of ARDS compared with pneumonia-associated ARDS (which is by far the most common cause

 The Berlin Definition of ARDS

	Acute Respiratory Distress Syndrome
Timing	Within 1 week of known clinical insult or new/worsening respiratory symptoms
Chest imaging[a]	Bilateral opacities—not fully explained by effusions, lobar/lung collapse, or nodules
Origin of edema	Respiratory failure not fully explained by cardiac failure or fluid overload; need objective assessment (e.g., echocardiography) to exclude hydrostatic edema if no risk factor present
	Oxygenation[b]
Mild	$200 < PaO_2/FiO_2 \leq 300$ with PEEP or CPAP ≥ 5 cmH$_2$O[c]
Moderate	$100 < PaO_2/FiO_2 \leq 200$ with PEEP ≥ 5 cmH$_2$O
Severe	$PaO_2/FiO_2 \leq 100$ with PEEP ≥ 5 cmH$_2$O

[a] Chest radiograph or computed tomography scan.
[b] If altitude is higher than 1,000 m, the correction factor should be calculated as follows: [PaO$_2$/FiO$_2$ × (barometric pressure/760)].
[c] This may be delivered noninvasively in the mild acute respiratory distress syndrome group.
ARDS, acute respiratory distress syndrome; FiO$_2$, fraction of inspired oxygen; PaO$_2$, partial pressure of arterial oxygen; PEEP, positive end-expiratory pressure; CPAP, continuous positive airway pressure.
Adapted from ARDS Definition Task Force; Ranieri VM, Rubenfeld GD, Thompson BT, et al. Acute respiratory distress syndrome: the Berlin definition. *JAMA* 2012;307(23):2526–2533.

of ARDS). Computed tomography may distinguish different patterns of ARDS. In Figure 19.1A, ARDS secondary to pneumonia (direct lung injury) shows most of the dense consolidations localized to the lower lung fields, and in **Figure 19.1B**, ARDS secondary to acute pancreatitis (indirect lung injury) shows a diffuse, almost homogeneous pattern of consolidation. However, there is substantial overlap in CT findings between ARDS caused by direct and indirect lung injury. Some pathogens causing direct lung injury (such as the H1N1 virus) may present with diffuse consolidation on CT.

III. **EPIDEMIOLOGY:** Nosocomial ARDS may be a "preventable" syndrome. Over the past 20 years, the incidence of nosocomial ARDS has declined remarkably. In a population-based cohort study (from 2001 to 2008) conducted in Olmsted

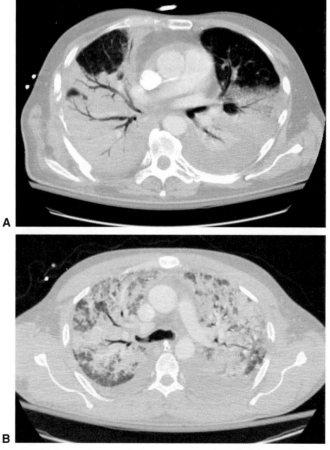

FIGURE 19.1 Computed tomography (CT) scans of two patients. **A:** Pulmonary ARDS due to pneumonia. **B:** Extrapulmonary ARDS due to acute pancreatitis.

County, Minnesota, Li et al. observed a steady decrease of nosocomial ARDS; however, the incidence of community-acquired ARDS was unchanged (as shown in Figure 19.2). These observations corroborate the hypothesis that ARDS can be prevented by improved care of critically ill patients. Important elements that might have contributed to a reduced incidence of nosocomial ARDS are lung-protective ventilation for patients at risk for ARDS, ventilator care bundles, goal-directed therapy in sepsis and septic shock, early antimicrobial administration, male donor plasma, and more cautious fluid administration and transfusions of blood products. Despite these encouraging findings, mortality among patients with ARDS remains high, up to 45% for severe disease. Recovery from severe ARDS and prolonged ventilation is slow and accompanied by muscle wasting and weakness. After 5 years from the ARDS episode, exercise limitation, impairment of memory, cognition, and ability to concentrate may persist.

IV. PATHOPHYSIOLOGY

A. Direct versus Indirect Lung Injury: The causes of ARDS are complex and variable but broadly fall within two clinical categories: direct and indirect injury to the lung. Direct injury to the lung includes trauma associated with mechanical ventilation (ventilation-induced lung injury), massive aspiration, infection (mainly pneumonia), near drowning, and pre-ICU chest and lung trauma. Indirect injuries include just about any type of systemic inflammatory process, such as sepsis and pancreatitis, that may lead to diffuse inflammatory lung injury. Identifying an underlying cause of ARDS is crucial, as ARDS may not recover if the underlying cause is not identified and treated.

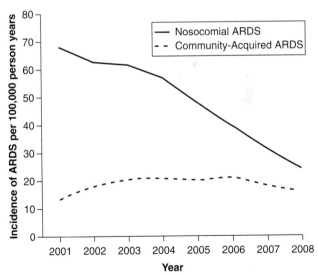

FIGURE 19.2 Note the decrease of incidence of "nosocomial ARDS" over time, while, the incidence of "community-acquired ARDS" did not change. From Li G, Malinchoc M, Cartin-Ceba R, et al. Eight-year trend of acute respiratory distress syndrome: a population-based study in Olmsted County, Minnesota. *Am J Respir Crit Care Med* 2011;183(1):59–66.

B. **Primary Immune Response**: Activation of resident macrophages, release of inflammatory mediators (cytokines and chemokines), recruitment of neutrophils into the lung with the release of additional inflammatory mediators and toxic products causes lung epithelial and endothelial injury. Activation of coagulation in the microcirculation contributes to additional endothelial injury. A number of inflammatory mediators have been associated with worse outcomes in patients with ARDS. Dysregulated apoptosis and autophagy as well as impaired function of T regulatory lymphocytes contribute to injury and/or delayed resolution. The disruption of the endothelial-epithelial barrier due to inflammation causes the accumulation of protein-rich edema fluid in the airspaces and interstitium as well as impaired lung edema clearance. Inactivation of the existing surfactant and production of abnormal surfactant may occur. Alveolar exudate, lung consolidation, and alveolar collapse produce low lung compliance and right-to-left intrapulmonary shunt, leading to arterial hypoxemia.

C. **Secondary Lung Injury**: Additional injury, such as from ventilator-induced lung injury (VILI) and/or ventilator-associated pneumonia (VAP), may lead to an increased severity of ARDS and prolonged time to recovery. VILI is caused by a mechanical stress and strain induced by positive-pressure ventilation. Overdistension of the lung when ventilating with an excessively high tidal volume or the recurrent recruitment and derecruitment of alveoli through insufficient application of PEEP can lead to lung damage. VAP may develop during mechanical ventilation due to micro-aspiration of bacterial-laden secretion into the lungs. Bacterial virulence (i.e., *Pseudomonas aeruginosa* and oxacillin-resistant *Staphylococcus aureus*) and inadequate initial antibiotic treatment have been shown to increase morbidity and mortality in ARDS patients.

D. **Physiologic Characteristics and Evolution of ARDS**: ARDS evolves in three different phases that do not represent discrete entities but are meant to describe a *continuum* of the same pathological process. During the **first phase,** alveolar damage is predominant, resulting in loss of surfactant production, atelectasis, and hypoxemia. The main feature of the second phase of ARDS, the **exudative phase**, is the disruption of the endothelial barrier with exudation of protein-rich fluid and blood cellular elements. The last phase of ARDS, the **fibroproliferative phase**, is characterized by an organizing inflammatory process fibroblast growth. All three phases may be completely reversible.

E. **Dead Space and Prognosis**: In a landmark study, Nuckton et al. showed that dead space is increased from early stage of ARDS and that it is independently associated with higher mortality. The increased dead space is probably due to pulmonary vascular injury though hyperinflation may also contribute. Pulmonary capillary microthrombi, inflammation, and obstruction of regional pulmonary blood probably result in areas of ventilated lung with no perfusion (increased dead-space ventilation), which results in hypercapnia for a given minute ventilation.

V. **TREATMENT**: Management of ARDS requires an intensive and systematic approach to diagnosing and treating the underlying cause of lung injury, preventing secondary injuries to the lungs and other organs, avoiding complications, and providing overall supportive care.

A. **Initial Diagnosis and Management**: In order to prevent progression and severity of ARDS, treatment of the underlying condition is a priority. Important early interventions include **early** and **appropriate** antibiotic administration and drainage and debridement of abscesses and necrotic tissue or burned tissue ("source control").

B. Hemodynamic Management: Conservative fluid management has been advocated in ARDS patients and has been shown to reduce the duration of mechanical ventilation as well as ICU stay. However, judicious fluid restriction should be balanced against inadequate organ perfusion (most commonly manifesting as prerenal kidney injury). There is no role for the routine use of pulmonary artery catheterization in the management of ARDS, although it may be useful in select populations, such as the presence of severe pulmonary hypertension and right ventricular dysfunction.

C. Treatment and Prevention of Infections: Early and appropriate antibiotic treatment for sepsis together with deescalation of antibiotics when no longer needed have been shown to decrease incidence of multidrug-resistant bacterial infection. Decrease of nosocomial ARDS incidence as observed by Li et al. can be attributed to the widespread adoption of clinical bundles designed to prevent health care–associated infections.

D. Early Nutrition is recommended. The enteral route is preferred either through nasogastric or jejunal access. Trophic enteral nutrition (providing 20%–40% of caloric needs) for the first 6 days appears to provide similar short- and long-term outcomes with less gastrointestinal intolerances than early full-calorie nutrition, at least in medical patients with ARDS. A combination of enteral and supplemental parenteral nutrition should be considered if meeting the nutritional target through enteral route is difficult later in the course. In patients with elevated dead space, special formulation should be administered to optimize Vco_2 and Vo_2 (i.e., low carbohydrates, high-lipid formulation). Immune-modulatory formulations (such as Omega-3 enriched) should be avoided.

E. Support of Other Organ System Functions is an integral part of the treatment of ARDS. Hemodynamic instability, acute renal failure gastrointestinal hemorrhage, coagulation abnormalities, and neuromuscular changes may complicate the course of these critically ill patients.

VI. MECHANICAL VENTILATION IN PATIENTS WITH ARDS: In ARDS, portions of the lungs are not available for normal gas exchange and ventilation occurs in a small fraction of the lung (the so-called baby lung). The ARDS-net trial showed that a ventilation strategy with a lower tidal volume (4–8 mL/kg of predicted body weight; PBW) was associated with lower mortality and shorter length of mechanical ventilation. This trial used a combination of volume and pressure limitation. For example, if the plateau airway pressures were higher than 30 cmH_2O, tidal volumes were reduced to 5 or 4 mL/kg PBW. This approach was designed to reduce the mechanical damage on lung tissue and the associated inflammatory response caused by overdistension of the alveolar wall. In order to obtain lung protective ventilation with low tidal volume and low plateau pressure, permissive hypercapnia is tolerated if pH is higher than 7.20. The optimal approach to patients with severe acidemia (pH <7.2) is not clear. One strategy for the management of severe, symptomatic acidemia is presented in Chapter 8. In case of lung resection, administration of volumetric ventilator support should be carefully adjusted according to the estimated lung volume. A recent multilevel mediation analysis on 3,562 ARDS patients found that the reduced driving pressure (plateau pressure minus positive end-expiratory pressure) was associated with increased survival and suggested that driving pressure could be used to titrate tidal volume to the size of the baby lung. Prospective validation of this approach is needed.

A. **PEEP Titration Techniques**: The optimal PEEP titration technique is controversial. In general, a higher PEEP strategy appears to be beneficial for patients with more severe ARDS and for those with evidence of improved mechanics or oxygenation on higher PEEP levels. One approach is to assess the oxygenation and respiratory system compliance response after a recruitment maneuver and during a decremental PEEP trial. PEEP is set 2 cmH_2O above the best PEEP identified and the respiratory system recruited again. Another approach to PEEP titration is based on the evaluation of end-expiratory transpulmonary pressure, defined as the difference between the pleural pressure and the pressure at the airways at end expiration. Pleural pressure can be estimated through the positioning of an esophageal balloon. PEEP should then be adjusted in order to achieve a positive end-expiratory transpulmonary pressure and then perform a recruitment maneuver. Another approach is to set PEEP using a PEEP/FIO_2 table. A prospective evaluation of four different PEEP titration techniques found similar levels of PEEP were applied, on average, with each technique, though important differences in the volume of recruitable lung were noted. However, hyperinflation by CT was seen at the level of "best PEEP" by all techniques, suggesting a fundamental limitation of low tidal volume ventilation and best PEEP for recruitment (e.g., trying to strike the balance between lung recruitment and hyperinflation) when patients are ventilated in the supine or semirecumbant position.

B. **Lung Recruitment**: Recruitment maneuvers can be performed by different methods. Recruitment maneuvers are used in order to open areas of atelectasis improving lung compliance and oxygenation. Due to heterogeneity of the disease, patients show different degrees of response to recruitment. It is important to note that increasing PEEP without lung recruitment may not provide much benefit since the pressures required to reopen atelectatic alveoli are greater than typical PEEP levels. In fact, increasing PEEP without recruitment may promote overdistention of the expanded portions of the lung.

   1. A sustained pressure of 30 to 40 cmH_2O is applied to the airways for 40 seconds to one minute. If improvement in respiratory system compliance and oxygenation occurs, a higher PEEP approach, such as the higher PEEP/FIO_2 tables used in the ALVEOLI or LOV studies would be applied.

   2. **Incremental recruitment**: Lung is incrementally recruited from lower to higher plateau pressure up to 40 to 50 cmH_2O. This would be followed by a decremental PEEP trial as noted above.

   3. A **sigh** is a cyclical large breath for about 3 seconds period to a plateau pressure of 30 to 40 cmH_2O.

C. **High-Frequency Oscillatory Ventilation (HFOV)**: HFOV has been used in ARDS treatment as a rescue therapy when lung-protective ventilation fails to maintain adequate oxygenation, or the pressure levels required for proper ventilation are too high. However, it requires specially designed mechanical ventilators and personnel expert on the use of HFOV. There is no current guideline for initiating HFOV—it has been suggested to consider HFOV after controlled mechanical ventilation, paralysis, and pronation have already been attempted in the setting of refractory hypoxemia (i.e., inability to adequately oxygenate or ventilate the patient while maintaining a plateau pressure <30 cmH_2O and an FIO_2 <0.6).

Suggested initial settings are 5 Hz of frequency, a power of 60 to 90 cmH$_2$O, an FiO$_2$ of 0.9, a target of 5 cmH$_2$O above the mPaw during conventional mechanical ventilation, 33% of inspiratory time, and a bias flow of 40 L/min. Recent trials have shown no superiority or increased mortality with the use of HFOV over the use of conventional lung-protective ventilation. At the present time, HFV cannot be recommended for routine use in patients with ARDS regardless of severity. Its role as a rescue therapy is unproven.

VII. ADDITIONAL STRATEGIES

A. Sedation and Paralysis: The compromise in gas exchange can induce a rise in respiratory rate, leading to patient–ventilator dyssynchrony. One of the possible interventions for reducing the respiratory drive is the administration of opioids. Opioids offer one of the best profiles, and continuous infusion can be titrated until ventilator–patient synchrony is restored and the optimal respiratory rate reached (up to 35 breaths/min). While recent studies have shown an immunosuppressing effect of carbon dioxide that could reduce the inflammatory response of ARDS and improve outcome, the overall risk-to-benefit profile of hypercapnia for patients with ARDS is unknown and could be deleterious in the setting of sepsis-related ARDS, as an acidotic pH has shown to promote bacterial growth. In addition, hypercapnia should be avoided in subjects with or at risk for increased intracranial pressure. In the setting of severe ARDS (P/F <100), paralysis and controlled mechanical ventilation has been reported to improve outcomes. Confirmatory studies are underway.

B. Prone Positioning: Ventilation in the prone position usually improves oxygenation in ARDS patients. Early studies of 12 hours/day of prone ventilation did not show a survival benefit. Subsequent trials of 17 hours per day suggested benefit in the subset of patients with P/F <100. Recently, an RCT of 17 hours of prone ventilation per day in patients with severe ARDS, continued until the supine P/F ratio exceeded 150 (mean 4 days), showed an impressive survival benefit. The maneuver requires team coordination and training, and, given recent data, major centers caring for patients with severe ARDS should acquire this expertise.

C. Pleural Effusion Drainage: ARDS patients frequently have pleural effusion as a result of fluid overload, septic heart failure, or altered pleural hydrostatic pressure due to pneumonia or atelectasis. The presence of a massive pleural effusion can alter the regional transmural pressure of the lung, causing passive atelectasis and possibly worsening gas exchange. However, no guidelines exist on pleural effusion management in ARDS. In the presence of a normally distensible abdomen, an adequately titrated PEEP level should compensate the increase in transmural pressure caused by the pleural effusion itself. Placement of a chest tube for drainage of the pleural effusion should be considered on a case-by-case basis and after other interventions (CMV, paralysis, pronation) have failed.

D. Extracorporeal Membrane Oxygenation (ECMO): With the epidemic of ARDS secondary to H1N1, venous–venous ECMO was shown to be a valuable therapeutic option in severe ARDS. The use of ECMO allows decreased minute ventilation, smaller tidal volumes, and low airway pressure allowing the lung to rest and recover. Nonetheless, despite the technological advances and the encouraging results, ECMO is a technique that should be confined to a few, highly specialized centers for limited indications.

E. Pharmacologic Adjuncts:

1. **Inhaled selective pulmonary vasodilators: Inhaled nitric oxide** (INO) does not reduce mortality in ARDS, and the beneficial effects on gas exchange (due to improved ventilation-perfusion matching) and pulmonary artery pressures may be transient. However, it might be a useful adjunct in limited cases of severe ARDS with pulmonary hypertension to reduce pulmonary vascular resistance and improve oxygenation as a bridge to another intervention such as prone ventilation or ECMO. INO is administered at a dose of 5 to 40 parts per million. **Inhaled epoprostenol** has similar effects on gas exchange and pulmonary artery pressures as INO and is substantially less expensive, although there is less data for its use in ARDS compared with INO. The dose ranges from 10 to 50 ng/kg/min.

2. **Corticosteroids:** Corticosteroids have been studied for both prevention and treatment of ARDS. However, systematic reviews and meta-analyses have produced ambiguous findings and demonstrate substantial heterogeneity. Current data do not support the use of corticosteroids as routine treatment for early- or late-phase ARDS.

3. **HMG CoA reductase inhibitors:** A recent multicenter double-blinded randomized clinical trial tested the efficacy of rosuvastatin administration in ARDS patients. No effect on mortality was observed; moreover, patients that received statin therapy had a higher incidence of hepatic and renal dysfunction compared with the placebo population. Thus, the use of statins in patients with ARDS is not recommended.

Selected Readings

Amato MB, Meade MO, Slutsky AS, et al. Driving pressure and survival in the acute respiratory distress syndrome. *N Engl J Med* 2015;372(8):747–755.
ARDS Definition Task Force; Ranieri VM, Rubenfeld GD, Thompson BT, et al. Acute respiratory distress syndrome: the Berlin Definition. *JAMA* 2012;307(23):2526–2533.
Chiumello D, Cressoni M, Carlesso E, et al. Bedside selection of positive end-expiratory pressure in mild, moderate, and severe acute respiratory distress syndrome. *Crit Care Med* 2014;42(2):252–264.
Ferguson ND, Cook DJ, Guyatt GH, et al. High-frequency oscillation in early acute respiratory distress syndrome. *N Engl J Med* 2013;368(9):795–805.
Gattinoni L, Caironi P, Cressoni M, et al. Lung recruitment in patients with the acute respiratory distress syndrome. *N Engl J Med* 2006;354(17):1775–1786.
Guérin C, Reignier J, Richard JC, et al. Prone positioning in severe acute respiratory distress syndrome. *N Engl J Med* 2013;368(23):2159–2168.
Herridge MS, Tansey CM, Matté A, et al. Functional disability 5 years after acute respiratory distress syndrome. *N Engl J Med* 2011;364(14):1293–1304.
Li G, Malinchoc M, Cartin-Ceba R, et al. Eight-year trend of acute respiratory distress syndrome: a population-based study in Olmsted County, Minnesota. *Am J Respir Crit Care Med* 2011;183(1):59–66.
Matthay MA, Ware LB, Zimmerman GA. The acute respiratory distress syndrome. *J Clin Invest* 2012;122(8):2731–2740.
National Heart, Lung, and Blood Institute Acute Respiratory Distress Syndrome (ARDS) Clinical Trials Network; Rice TW, Wheeler AP, Thompson BT, et al. Initial trophic vs full enteral feeding in patients with acute lung injury: the EDEN randomized trial. *JAMA* 2012;307(8):795–803.
National Heart, Lung, and Blood Institute ARDS Clinical Trials Network; Truwit JD, Bernard GR, Steingrub J, et al. Rosuvastatin for sepsis-associated acute respiratory distress syndrome. *N Engl J Med* 2014;370(23):2191–2200.
National Heart, Lung, and Blood Institute Acute Respiratory Distress Syndrome (ARDS) Clinical Trials Network; Wiedemann HP, Wheeler AP, Bernard GR, et al. Comparison of two fluid-management strategies in acute lung injury. *N Engl J Med* 2006;354(24):2564–2575.

Nuckton TJ, Alonso JA, Kallet RH, et al. Pulmonary dead-space fraction as a risk factor for death in the acute respiratory distress syndrome. *N Engl J Med* 2002;346(17):1281–1286.

Papazian L, Forel JM, Gacouin A, et al. Neuromuscular blockers in early acute respiratory distress syndrome. *N Engl J Med* 2010;363(12):1107–1116.

Talmor D, Sarge T, Malhotra A, et al. Mechanical ventilation guided by esophageal pressure in acute lung injury. *N Engl J Med* 2008;359(20):2095–2104.

The Acute Respiratory Distress Syndrome Network. Ventilation with lower tidal volumes as compared with traditional tidal volumes for acute lung injury and the acute respiratory distress syndrome. *N Engl J Med* 2000;342(18):1301–1308.

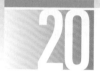

Asthma, Chronic Obstructive Pulmonary Disease

R. Scott Harris and Guido Musch

I. INTRODUCTION

Asthma and COPD are common clinical conditions that are characterized by airflow obstruction measured with spirometry. Obstruction is usually defined by a forced expiratory volume in 1 second (FEV_1) to forced vital capacity (FVC) ratio of <0.7 or the lower limit of normal based on a 95% confidence interval in population-based studies of healthy subjects of similar sex, height, age, and race. Asthma and COPD can lead to respiratory failure and ICU admission during acute exacerbations of these conditions, or they can complicate the ICU care of a patient who is admitted for other reasons or who is admitted from the operating room. Since the effect of each condition on lung physiology is very similar and they share many treatments, they are discussed together here.

A. Definitions

1. COPD—GOLD definition

The Global Initiative for Chronic Obstructive Lung Disease (GOLD) defines COPD as "a common preventable and treatable disease, characterized by persistent airflow limitation that is usually *progressive* and associated with an enhanced chronic inflammatory response in the airways and the lung to noxious particles or gases. Exacerbations and comorbidities contribute to the overall severity in individual patients."

2. Asthma—GINA definition

The Global Initiative for Asthma (GINA) defines asthma as "a chronic inflammatory disorder of the airways in which many cells and cellular elements play a role. The chronic inflammation is associated with airway hyperresponsiveness that leads to recurrent episodes of wheezing, breathlessness, chest tightness, and coughing, particularly at night or in the early morning. These episodes are usually associated with widespread, but variable, airflow obstruction within the lung that is often *reversible* either spontaneously or with treatment."

3. Status asthmaticus

Acute severe asthma, formerly known as status asthmaticus, is defined as severe asthma unresponsive to repeated courses of β-agonist therapy such as inhaled albuterol, levalbuterol, or subcutaneous epinephrine. We will use both terms interchangeably. Status asthmaticus is not a distinct condition, but rather the most severe manifestation of an asthma exacerbation along a continuous spectrum of severity, thus the preferred term *acute severe asthma*. These patients often require ventilatory assistance in addition to inhaled and intravenous medication. Treatments for acute severe asthma and all asthma exacerbations in general will be discussed together as they are essentially the same, except that more treatments are added as the patient's condition worsens.

B. Epidemiology
1. COPD
  a. Recent epidemiological studies report a prevalence of COPD in developed countries of 8% to 10% in adults older than 40 years, with 1.4% having severe COPD. While the prevalence of COPD has been stable in the United States in recent years, it is increasing in women and decreasing in men, as is mortality attributable to COPD. Acute exacerbation of COPD accounts for approximately 2.5 hospitalizations per 10,000 people per year and has an in-hospital mortality of approximately 5%. Currently, COPD is the third cause of death in the United States, where it affects more than 15 million people.
  b. A recent large study reported that approximately 9% of patients admitted to the ICU have a diagnosis of COPD and roughly one-third of them, corresponding to 2.5% of all admissions, are due to acute respiratory failure from COPD exacerbation.
  c. COPD is an independent risk factor for ICU mortality even when it is a comorbid condition rather than the primary cause for admission.
2. Asthma
  a. Asthma affects more than 25 million people in the United States and accounts for approximately 1.25 million hospitalizations per year, corresponding to an annual hospitalization rate of 13.5 per 10,000 individuals.
  b. About 10% of asthma hospitalizations result in admission to the ICU and approximately 2% require endotracheal intubation.
  c. Both ICU admission and intubation, as well as the presence of comorbidities, increase the odds of in-hospital death. In-hospital asthma mortality is approximately 0.5%.

C. Physiology
1. Airway inflammation
  Although both asthma and COPD are characterized by airway inflammation, there are important differences in the cause of the inflammation and the inflammatory cell composition in each condition. Asthma is most commonly caused by an allergic reaction to one or more airborne environmental allergens, whereas COPD is the result of chronic inhalation of smoke. The airway inflammation in asthma is dominated by eosinophils, whereas the inflammation in COPD is largely composed of neutrophils. In fact, in atopic asthma, uptake of $[^{18}F]$ fluorodeoxyglucose measured with positron emission tomography in inflamed lung regions, an index of inflammatory cell activation, correlates with eosinophil counts from those regions. In contrast, in COPD, pulmonary $[^{18}F]$ fluorodeoxyglucose uptake is related to neutrophil infiltration. Another major distinction between the two is that while both can have airway wall inflammation, edema, and constriction, COPD very often results in loss of lung tissue, termed emphysema. Thus, for COPD, there has historically been a distinction made between those patients who have primarily airway disease from those who have primarily emphysema, though there is great overlap between the two phenotypes. In fact, it is accepted that there are likely many different phenotypes, both in asthma and COPD, and recognition of these phenotypes may lead to important treatment decisions.
2. Phenotypes
  There is a growing appreciation that patients with asthma and COPD are very heterogeneous and likely have multiple causes for their intermittent airway obstruction. In asthma, at least five clinical phenotypes

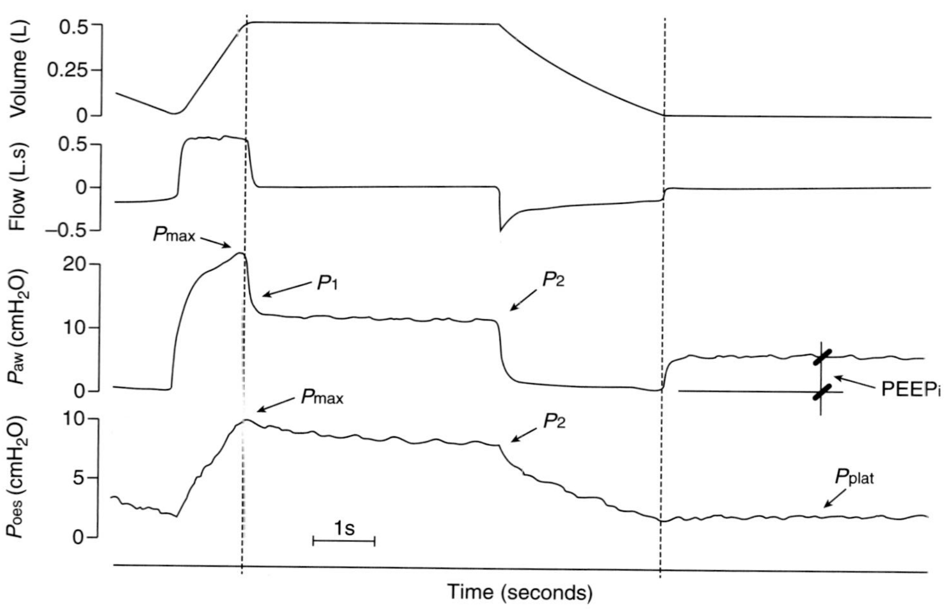

FIGURE 20.1 Tracings of volume (obtained by integration of the flow signal), flow, airway pressure (Paw) and esophageal pressure (Poes) in a representative patient with chronic obstructive pulmonary disease (COPD) during an end inspiratory occlusion followed by an end expiratory occlusion. Dashed lines indicate timing of occlusions. Pmax, maximum value; P_1, zero flow value; P_2, plateau value; PEEPi, intrinsic positive end-expiratory pressure is the static end-expiratory recoil pressure of the respiratory system; Pplat, plateau value of Poes after end-expiratory occlusion. Values of Paw, Pmax, used for calculations were corrected for the resistive pressure drop due to the artificial airway. (From Musch G, Foti G, Cereda M, et al. Lung and chest wall mechanics in normal anaesthetized subjects and in patients with COPD at different PEEP levels. *Eur Respir J* 1997;10:2545–2552, with permission.)

have been identified: (1) early-onset allergic, (2) late-onset eosinophilic, (3) exercise induced, (4) obesity related, and (5) neutrophilic. COPD also represents a heterogeneous syndrome with chronic bronchitis and emphysema being recognized early on as distinct phenotypes. Chronic bronchitis has classically been associated with cough, obesity, hypoxemia, and hypoventilation, whereas emphysema has been associated with muscle wasting and hyperinflation but preserved gas exchange. COPD can be further characterized by other factors, such as the degree, type, and distribution of emphysema, or nonspirometric physiologic parameters, such as diffusing capacity and hyperinflation. As with asthma, classification schemes of COPD phenotypes based on frequency of exacerbations, radiologic parameters, and inflammatory biomarkers are being developed. It is important to note that there is an "overlap" phenotype that is characterized by a positive bronchodilator response, sputum eosinophilia, a personal history of asthma before age 40, high total IgE level, and a history of atopy. These patients seem particularly prone to frequent exacerbations and lung function decline.

3. **Airflow obstruction**
   a. The pathophysiologic hallmark of both asthma and COPD is airway narrowing with ensuing increase in respiratory resistance and wheezing.
   b. In asthma, airway narrowing is due predominantly to contraction of smooth muscle cells in the airway wall, airway wall edema, and mucus plugging. Consequently, airway narrowing is present during *both* inspiration and expiration. The narrowed airways retard expiratory flow, resulting in dynamic hyperinflation, that is, an increase in end-expiratory lung volume above functional residual capacity due to lack of equilibration between alveolar pressure and pressure at the airway opening. In fact, bronchoconstriction can be so severe that airways completely occlude, trapping gas behind them. Interestingly, the size of these gas-trapping areas termed *ventilation defects* appears to be less in the prone than in the supine position, suggesting a rationale for the use of prone positioning in status asthmaticus.
   c. In COPD with emphysema, airway narrowing is due predominantly to intrapulmonary airway collapse during *expiration*. Because of the destruction of lung tissue, the tethering forces exerted by the parenchymal septae on the *intrapulmonary* airway wall are decreased. Consequently, during expiration, when the transmural pressure in these airways becomes negative (i.e., when the intraluminal airway pressure becomes lower than the surrounding extraluminal airway pressure), the airways collapse and interrupt flow. As flow is interrupted, upstream pressure rises and the airways reopen. As flow restarts, the transmural pressure becomes negative and flow again stops. This "flutter" pattern is responsible for the phenomenon of *expiratory airflow limitation*.
   d. Expiratory airflow limitation is defined as a state in which expiratory flow is independent of transpulmonary pressure and hence is maximal. In the presence of flow limitation, an increase in upstream pressure, for example, by activation of expiratory muscles, will *not* result in a higher expiratory flow. The point in the airway tree in which the transmural airway pressure turns negative is called *equal pressure point*. If this point localizes within the collapsible

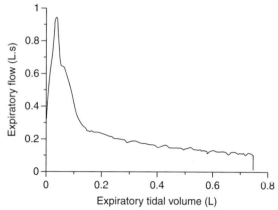

FIGURE 20.2 Expiratory flow volume curve during passive exhalation at zero end-expiratory pressure in a patient with chronic obstructive pulmonary disease. Notice the bowing toward the volume axis (i.e., upward concavity) especially during the first part of exhalation, which suggests the presence of flow limitation. (From Musch G, Foti G, Cereda M, et al. Lung and chest wall mechanics in normal anaesthetized subjects and in patients with COPD at different PEEP levels. *Eur Respir J* 1997;10:2545–2552, with permission.)

intrapulmonary airway, it will become a "choke point" that impedes further increases in expiratory flow. Equally ineffective in increasing flow will be a negative pressure applied at the opening of the airway during expiration.

e. Similarly, if pressure at the airway opening is raised, flow will not decrease until the applied pressure is sufficiently high to overcome flutter at the choke point, that is, to render transmural pressure positive along the entire collapsible airway. Levels of applied pressure higher than this critical threshold will decrease expiratory flow, causing further hyperinflation.

f. Consequently, in the presence of expiratory flow limitation, flow is maximal because neither an increase in upstream pressure nor a decrease in downstream pressure will result in higher flows, and an increase in downstream pressure will either not affect flow ("waterfall" effect) or decrease it if the increase is sufficiently high to overcome the critical threshold. In the presence of flow limitation, expiratory flow is thus independent of the pressure gradient along the airway and depends only on lung volume, being higher at higher volumes. However, while it is maximal, the absolute flow is quite minuscule, and prolonged expiratory times would be needed to reach functional residual capacity.

4. Risk factors for death in ICU

For patients admitted to the ICU with respiratory failure from an asthma or COPD exacerbation, the major risk factors for death are need for mechanical ventilation, hyperinflation and auto-PEEP causing hypotension (from decreased venous return), profound acidemia, and barotrauma.

II. ASSESSMENT
A. History
1. A history of poorly controlled asthma as evidenced by nocturnal awakening for asthma symptoms, increased dyspnea and wheezing, increased β-agonist use, increased peak flow variability (>20%), recent or frequent emergency room visits or hospitalizations and a previous history of intubation and mechanical ventilation, and glucocorticoid nonadherence are risk factors for fatal asthma. A history of current smoking also identifies high-risk patients with asthma. Patients with nonallergic asthma, asthma triggered by aspirin, or exercise-induced asthma or patients with asthma who use cocaine or heroin have a higher risk of mortality, and these factors should be assessed. A history of rapid improvement with intubation can often be a clue to an upper airway cause of respiratory failure, and in particular a condition termed *paroxysmal vocal cord motion*. Patients with this condition often have mild asthma and a history of frequent severe attacks, many times with intubation followed by rapid extubation.
2. For patients with COPD, risk factors for mortality include multiple admissions for exacerbations, intubation and mechanical ventilation, age (both younger and older age groups), lower BMI, history of lung cancer, and cardiovascular comorbidity. For COPD patients, it is important to establish the patient's baseline arterial $PaCO_2$ (or try to infer it from the patient's baseline bicarbonate level). This serves two purposes—a warning that the patient may be particularly susceptible to the hypercarbic effects of supplemental oxygen (discussed below) and as a target for setting minute ventilation should mechanical ventilation become necessary.

B. Physical Examination
1. **Appearance**
   Patients with severe exacerbations of asthma or COPD are often unable to lie down, so they are often sitting upright or leaning forward slightly. A patient who is unable to speak in full sentences may be nearing respiratory arrest. As with any patient in respiratory failure, it is important to note the patient's color to assess perfusion and oxygenation. A patient in respiratory failure without a previous diagnosis of COPD is likely to have a maximum laryngeal height (the distance from the sternal notch to the thyroid cartilage) of less than 4 cm at end exhalation. This is caused by hyperinflation of the lungs that pulls the trachea downward.

2. **Assess for intubation difficulty**
   a. While neither COPD nor asthma per se have been associated with increased incidence of difficult intubation, the association of obesity with asthma and early COPD can make the intubation of these patients more challenging than in the general population. In contrast, patients with moderate to severe COPD (GOLD stages 3 and 4) have a lower body mass index.
   b. Irrespective of body mass, a thorough assessment of the airway (e.g., Mallampati class, thyromental distance, receding mandible, protruding upper incisors) should be performed in all patients with obstructive pulmonary disease admitted to the ICU even if they do not yet require mechanical ventilation. In fact, these patients can deteriorate rapidly and require emergent intubation when gas exchange is already impaired.

3. **Auscultation**
   Wheezing may be audible even without a stethoscope and should be expiratory and polyphonic, indicating that it is coming from multiple

small airways. A monophonic wheeze might indicate a single large airway obstruction. Stridor indicates obstruction that is extrathoracic, usually at the vocal cords or above. In patients with COPD and asthma who appear to be in respiratory distress, lack of wheezing or vesicular (normal) breath sounds can be a sign of impending respiratory arrest as ventilation becomes so poor that very little sound is made with each breath. In COPD patients, it may be difficult to hear breath sounds normally, since they may have very little lung tissue left through which to transmit airway sounds.

4. **Accessory muscle use**

Patients with exacerbations of asthma and COPD are often anxious, sitting upright with arms extended, supporting the upper chest. This position allows the abdominal contents to pull downward on the diaphragm and expand the lungs. It also allows the rib cage to be expanded and the accessory muscles of the neck and shoulders to pull upward on the rib cage when inhaling. Accessory muscle use and retraction of the rib cage or of the intercostal muscles is an ominous sign and indicates increased mechanical work to ventilate. Even more ominous is "abdominal paradox" where the usual abdominal protrusion during inhalation is reversed, such that the abdomen pulls inward during inspiration. This indicates that the diaphragm is either not functioning (due to paralysis or paresis) or the lungs are so hyperinflated that the diaphragm is at a mechanical disadvantage and can no longer pull the lungs downward. Once this happens, only the accessory muscles are able to lower intrathoracic pressure and this draws the abdominal contents inward toward the thorax. Hyperinflation of the lungs with a flattened diaphragm can also result in "Hoover's Sign," where the lower costal margin is drawn inward during contraction of the diaphragm. Although often a sign of respiratory failure in COPD, it can be seen in stable outpatients, but indicates more severe disease.

C. **Laboratory**

1. **Arterial blood gas**

   a. Depending on the severity of disease, COPD patients may present a chronic respiratory acidosis (i.e., increased arterial $PaCO_2$) that is partially offset by renal tubular excretion of H^+ and reabsorption of HCO_3^-, resulting in a compensatory metabolic alkalosis. CO_2 retention is a result of *both* hypoventilation due to airflow obstruction and ventilation-perfusion mismatch due to heterogeneous parenchymal involvement in COPD. To preserve the equilibrium of the Henderson–Hasselbalch equation, these patients present a largely increased HCO_3^- concentration and base excess. A typical blood gas in this setting would be as follows: $PaCO_2 = 60$ mmHg, pH $= 7.36$, $HCO_3^- = 33$ mEq/L. PaO_2 and SaO_2 also depend on severity of disease and on whether the patient is on supplemental oxygen therapy, but are often moderately decreased ($PaO_2 = 60$–80 mmHg and $SaO_2 = 90\%$–95%).

   b. An acute on chronic exacerbation of COPD often results in further CO_2 retention and uncompensated respiratory acidosis, in addition to worsening hypoxemia. The presence of hypercapnia and acidosis despite markedly increased bicarbonate, and a base excess is indicative of acute decompensation in acid–base status of these patients.

   c. In asthmatics, blood gases are usually normal at baseline, except in very advanced stages of disease when chronic features of obstructive disease appear. During an acute attack, however, PaO_2 may decrease below 60 mmHg (SaO_2 <90%) and hypercapnia may also ensue. Importantly, because an asthma attack is accompanied by increased respiratory drive, a $PaCO_2$ only mildly elevated (e.g., >42 mmHg) could signify impending respiratory failure because for that level of drive the expected $PaCO_2$ in the absence of significant bronchoconstriction would be much lower.

2. **Complete blood count (CBC)**

    a. A CBC is not usually required during asthma exacerbations but may be warranted in patients with a fever or purulent sputum. Even in the absence of superimposed bacterial infection, these patients may show neutrophilia due to the stress response and concomitant therapy (corticosteroids and β_2-agonists). Furthermore, asthma can cause eosinophilia, which is usually mild to moderate, that is, 500 to 1,500 eosinophils/μL.

    b. During an acute exacerbation of COPD, the patient may present neutrophilia if the cause of the exacerbation is an acute bacterial infection. However, as for asthma, such leukocytosis could be simply the result of concurrent stress or therapy.

3. **Theophylline level**

    A serum theophylline level should be checked in patients with acute exacerbations who have been on this medication, especially if symptoms of toxicity, such as nausea and vomiting, are present.

4. **ECG**

    The electrocardiogram may show sinus tachycardia, right ventricular strain that may normalize with the relief of airflow obstruction, and right-axis deviation. Multifocal atrial tachycardia is associated with COPD, and its appearance may portend a poor outcome. Calcium-channel blockers and amiodarone can be used to treat supraventricular tachycardia. Nonselective β-blockers should be used with caution.

5. **Peak Expiratory Flow (PEF)**

    PEF monitoring can be useful in the acute care setting, where spirometry and FEV_1 measurement are hardly feasible. PEF is usually reduced to 40% to 70% of predicted in moderate obstruction and to 25% to 39% in severe obstruction. PEF can also be useful to monitor response to therapy.

D. **Imaging**

1. The value of routine chest radiography in both asthma and COPD is controversial. The prevalence of abnormalities on plain chest films in asthma was found to be 9% in one study of acute severe asthma patients who were admitted to the hospital. These were abnormalities that were felt to affect management and were not predicted on the basis of physical exam findings. In COPD, two studies found opposite results. One large study of 847 emergency room visits found abnormalities in 16% of patients and about 25% of those could not be predicted. A smaller study of 128 patients admitted for COPD exacerbations found that only in those with prespecified "complicated" presentations was management changed by the chest radiograph. In COPD and asthma, the main value of the chest radiograph may be to assess for changes that would alter the likelihood of pulmonary embolus (discussed below), a major confounding diagnosis for these patients, where shortness of breath and wheezing can be presentations of all three diagnoses (asthma, COPD, or pulmonary embolus).

2. If pulmonary embolus is suspected, a pulmonary embolus protocol CT scan can be performed and may even replace plain chest radiography.

Epidemiologic studies have shown that the presence of a diagnosis of asthma or COPD increases the risk of pulmonary embolus. In COPD, the risk of pulmonary embolus in those that present with a COPD exacerbation has been reported to be as high as 25%. In addition, those patients with inappropriately undiagnosed pulmonary embolus often had COPD or asthma. Given the high prevalence in COPD exacerbations, it is reasonable to obtain a pulmonary embolus protocol CT scan in these patients, even with a normal d-dimer. For asthma, the need for CT scanning is less clear as there have been no studies evaluating the risk of pulmonary embolus in patients presenting with an asthma exacerbation.

III. RESPIRATORY SUPPORT

A. Supplemental Oxygen

Supplemental oxygen should be administered to maintain Spo_2 >88% in both asthma and COPD. Asthma rarely leads to severe hypoxemia unless it is associated with another pulmonary condition such as lobar pneumonia or there is significant hypoventilation and hypercarbia. For patients with COPD, the administration of supplemental oxygen can lead to excessive hypercarbia, a condition termed *hyperoxic hypercarbia*. In addition to the well-known decrease in minute ventilation that can occur due to the relief of patient's hypoxic drive (or inducing sleep), it is thought that supplemental oxygen can cause hypercarbia by releasing CO_2 from hemoglobin (Haldane effect), increasing dead space fraction by releasing hypoxic pulmonary vasoconstriction in low $\dot{V}/\dot{Q}$ units (thus worsening high $\dot{V}/\dot{Q}$) and causing bronchodilation from a direct effect of CO_2 on the airway. When supplemental oxygen is given by face mask, these effects can be magnified as patients decrease their minute ventilation and entrain less air, thus effectively increasing their FIO_2.

B. Helium/Oxygen Gas Mixtures (Heliox)

Helium is less dense than nitrogen and has nearly the same viscosity, so, theoretically, a mixture of helium and oxygen should reduce turbulence in airways, thus moving more gas for the same pressure gradient. In both asthma and COPD, helium–oxygen mixtures have been used with varying success. Studies have been inconclusive when using helium–oxygen delivered by face mask or by ventilator, and no definite conclusions can be made regarding its efficacy in either condition. Overall, the evidence appears weaker in COPD than in asthma, either for improving ventilation, or when used to drive impact nebulizers. It should be noted that because of the differences in density of helium–oxygen mixtures versus nitrogen–oxygen mixtures, mechanical ventilator flow sensors need to be calibrated for helium–oxygen in order for proper functioning. A recent meta-analysis of 11 trials in adults and children of driving nebulizers with helium–oxygen mixtures appeared to show benefits in improvement of airflow limitation and hospital admission (number needed to treat to prevent one admission = 9) when given in the emergency room for acute asthma.

C. NPPV

1. Patients with COPD and asthma develop respiratory failure most often because of increased airway resistance and inefficient respiratory muscle mechanics from hyperinflation. Therefore, they cannot ventilate effectively. Noninvasive positive pressure ventilation (NPPV), delivered through a tight-fitting nasal or oronasal mask, has become an important tool for the prevention of intubation in many patients with respiratory failure. In obstructive lung disease, NPPV would be expected to

dilate airways (with the use of positive expiratory pressure) and assist the inspiratory muscles (with the use of positive inspiratory pressure).

2. For exacerbations of COPD, the data clearly show efficacy for NPPV on mortality, need for intubation, treatment failure, and hospital stay. Studies have consistently shown that improvements in pH, $Paco_2$, and respiratory rate are seen within the first hour of application. The number needed to treat to save one life with NPPV is 4, and the complications of the therapy are low. The indications for use in COPD exacerbations usually consist of patients with increased respiratory rate and hypercapneic respiratory failure. Contraindications are few, but consist of vomiting, unconsciousness, and inability to fit a mask to the patient's face.

3. NPPV has been used in asthma, but the studies are often small and potentially subject to publication bias. In a recent Cochrane Review, the authors conclude that given the paucity of data, the use of NPPV is controversial in this setting. Mortality from exacerbations of asthma is much lower than from exacerbations of COPD, so very large studies would be required to see any possible effect on mortality. To date, NPPV has not shown definitive efficacy on other important endpoints such as intubation, ICU length of stay, or hospital stay.

D. Intubation

1. **Timing**

   a. Compared with a few years ago, the availability of adjunct therapies such as helium–oxygen and NPPV has resulted in a postponement, on average, of the decision to intubate a patient with acute exacerbation of obstructive lung disease. While adjunct therapies have spared patients from avoidable intubations, their increased use has also resulted in patients often having exhausted their respiratory reserve by the time the decision to intubate is taken.

   b. Consequently, signs of impending respiratory failure such as intercostal retraction during inspiration and asynchronous movement of the abdomen and rib cage, use of accessory respiratory muscles (e.g., sternocleidomastoid and scalene muscles), inability to speak and altered mental status, hypercapnia, and hypoxemia should prompt the decision to intubate. Most studies of NPPV have determined that improvements in signs of respiratory failure should be seen within the first 2 hours and if these are not seen, intubation should be performed without delay.

   c. While the specific intubation technique (e.g., asleep direct or video laryngoscopy, awake or asleep fiberoptic intubation) is up to the individual provider, it is important to have an array of airway equipment readily available and a backup plan should the first intubation attempt fail, given the low respiratory reserve of these patients.

2. **Hypotension**

   a. After confirming intubation of the trachea with a CO_2 sensor, the provider should resist the instinct to aggressively ventilate these patients. The presence of dynamic hyperinflation and the consequent impediment to venous return, the abolition of inspiratory efforts, which favored venous return, and the increase in pulmonary vascular resistance due to positive pressure ventilation in patients that may already have pulmonary hypertension all contribute to systemic hypotension.

   b. Vasopressors (e.g., phenylephrine) and inotropic agents (e.g., norepinephrine or epinephrine) should be readily available at the time of intubation to treat hypotension, as should intravenous fluids and proper intravenous access.

E. Bronchoscopy

For asthma, where increased mucus production is part of the pathophysiology of the airway obstruction, it might seem that bronchoscopy would be a valuable treatment, especially in patients on mechanical ventilation. In fact, there was initial enthusiasm for the use of bronchoscopy in asthma, but this was tempered by a report of bronchoscopy inducing bronchospasm in asthma patients getting a bronchoscopy for reasons not related to their asthma. It was postulated that the severe bronchospasm was caused by mechanical stimulation of vagal afferents in the airway by the bronchoscope. A subsequent study found bronchospasm in only one of 10 mild asthmatics undergoing bronchoscopy and no change in FEV_1 after the procedure in any of the subjects. These subjects were pretreated with aminophylline prior to the procedure and all were mild asthmatics. Subsequent to this, there have been multiple case reports of successful bronchoscopic lavage, sometimes with acetlycysteine or DNAse, to improve lung function in intubated asthma patients. Overall, it appears from a limited number of cases that bronchoscopy with lavage in mechanically ventilated asthmatics was well tolerated and resulted in improvements in lung mechanics. However, data are too limited to make any definitive conclusions about the role of bronchoscopy in the routine care of patients in the ICU with an asthma exacerbation. For respiratory failure caused by COPD, there has not been any study showing benefit with the use of bronchoscopy as a therapeutic tool.

F. Mechanical Ventilation

Mechanical ventilation aims to decrease the patient's work of breathing and support gas exchange. Work of breathing is increased during acute exacerbation of asthma or COPD due to both increased resistive and elastic load. Airway narrowing increases resistive work. Furthermore, the resulting expiratory flow obstruction can lead to dynamic hyperinflation, placing the respiratory system on a less compliant part of its pressure–volume curve, with consequent increase also of the elastic component of the work of breathing. Ventilator management must balance the goal to achieve adequate oxygenation (SpO_2 = 88%–92%) and ventilation with avoidance of further hyperinflation and barotrauma.

1. Dynamic hyperinflation and auto-PEEP

Because of the increase in airway resistance and, in COPD, also compliance, the time constant of the respiratory system (equal to the product of resistance by compliance) is increased in patients with obstructive lung disease, especially during acute exacerbations. Consequently, the expiratory time may not be sufficient to allow complete lung emptying, resulting in an increase in end-expiratory lung volume above functional residual capacity (or equilibrium volume if PEEP is applied), that is, dynamic hyperinflation. Accordingly, alveolar pressure is higher than pressure at the airway opening at the end of expiration and this increase is termed "auto" (or "intrinsic") PEEP. Note that while dynamic hyperinflation is always accompanied by auto-PEEP, auto-PEEP can also occur without hyperinflation or even at an end-expiratory volume lower than functional residual capacity in a subject who is actively exhaling. For example, patients with very low respiratory compliance and impending respiratory failure (e.g., ARDS) may use the expiratory muscles to "push" the respiratory system below functional residual capacity at end exhalation, such that the first phase of the ensuing inspiration is passive because it is driven by the outer recoil of the respiratory system. This "work-sharing" is a protective mechanism to partly unload the fatigued inspiratory muscles at the expense of the expiratory muscles.

a. **Clinical assessment of auto-PEEP**

Signs of auto-PEEP include the following: (1) Inspiratory efforts by the patient that do not trigger the ventilator (patient–ventilator dyssynchrony), as auto-PEEP essentially acts as an additional pressure trigger; (2) Expiratory flow does not reach zero before the next inspiration. However, in the presence of flow-limitation end-expiratory flow can be minuscule despite significant auto-PEEP; or (3) A biphasic expiratory flow pattern (sharp spike followed by almost a plateau at a very low flow rate) caused by rapid emptying of a small volume of gas from the large airways followed by a very slow emptying of distal alveoli.

b. **Measurement of auto-PEEP**

1. **Controlled mechanical ventilation.** The easiest way to measure auto-PEEP in a muscle-relaxed patient is to perform an end-expiratory airway occlusion (Fig. 20.1). The occlusion interrupts flow and, consequently, pressure at the airway opening equilibrates with alveolar pressure, that is, auto-PEEP. Three to 5 seconds are usually sufficient to obtain a stable measurement of auto-PEEP. However, this method could underestimate the degree of auto-PEEP in patients with status asthmaticus because of complete closure of airways feeding to lung units with the highest alveolar pressure. The alveolar pressure in these units would then not be transmitted to the proximal airway. This interpretation is consistent with the observation that gas tracer delivered to alveoli through the bloodstream is retained in the alveolar airspace in acute asthma rather than being excreted by ventilation.

2. **Assisted breathing.** In a patient with spontaneous respiratory efforts, measurement of auto-PEEP requires esophageal manometry. Auto-PEEP corresponds to the deflection in esophageal pressure from the start of the patient's inspiratory effort to the start of inspiratory flow. In the absence of an esophageal balloon, a rough estimate of auto-PEEP can be obtained with an end-expiratory occlusion, provided the patient reaches a fairly relaxed state.

c. **Strategies to reduce dynamic hyperinflation**

Given that expiration is either passive or flow is not increased by activation of expiratory muscles in the presence of flow limitation, the only strategies to decrease dynamic hyperinflation at a given minute ventilation are (1) relief of bronchoconstriction (e.g., β_2-agonists); (2) reduction of the inspiratory-to-expiratory time ratio, with ensuing prolongation of expiratory time; and (3) possibly, helium–oxygen.

2. **Initial settings**

a. The fundamental concept in the initiation of mechanical ventilation in patients with acute exacerbation of asthma or COPD is to avoid aggressive ventilation, which can further worsen dynamic hyperinflation and hence cause barotrauma and cardiovascular collapse. Reasonable initial settings for most patients could be tidal volume of 6 to 8 mL/Kg predicted body weight and respiratory rate of 8 to 12 breaths/min with 25% inspiratory time (i.e., inspiratory-to-expiratory ratio of 1:3).

b. If pressure-controlled ventilation is chosen, tidal volume should be closely monitored because it can decrease over time if airway resistance worsens and auto-PEEP increases. With volume-controlled ventilation, peak and preferably plateau airway pressure should be closely monitored.

3. Setting PEEP

There is no general agreement as to whether PEEP should be used in airflow obstruction. Part of this lack of consensus stems from the fact that whether PEEP has a beneficial or detrimental effect on respiratory mechanics in this setting depends on the underlying mechanism of auto-PEEP:

a. Auto-PEEP with airflow limitation

When the underlying pathophysiologic mechanism for auto-PEEP is expiratory flow limitation, PEEP will not retard expiratory flow until the critical pressure at the "choke point" is reached. This pressure has been reported to range from 70% to 85% of auto-PEEP. Consequently, setting PEEP up to 70% of auto-PEEP measured at zero end-expiratory pressure will not cause substantial further hyperinflation and will instead decrease the work of breathing in a spontaneously breathing patient and the pressure that the inspiratory muscles must generate to trigger the ventilator. In a patient on controlled, rather than assisted, ventilation, applying PEEP up to 70% of auto-PEEP may still be beneficial because it favors a more uniform distribution of tidal volume. In fact, the value of auto-PEEP measured with an end-expiratory pause is the average of many different values of individual respiratory units. When inspiration starts from zero end-expiratory pressure, units with the lowest auto-PEEP receive proportionally more tidal volume than those with the highest auto-PEEP, which start to inflate only later during inhalation. In this setting, PEEP acts as an "equalizer" of individual units' auto-PEEP, promoting more uniform distribution of ventilation and improved ventilation-to-perfusion matching.

b. Auto-PEEP without airflow limitation

If instead auto-PEEP is due to airflow obstruction without flow limitation (i.e., there is no "flutter"/"waterfall" mechanism), then extrinsic PEEP will be transmitted all the way up to the alveoli and will result in further hyperinflation, increased (elastic) work of breathing, and hypotension.

c. Detecting the presence of airflow limitation

From the discussion above, it follows that the clinician must determine if the patient is flow-limited to decide if and how much PEEP to apply. The classical method of obtaining isovolume pressure–flow curves by changing pressure at the airway opening while measuring flow at a given absolute lung volume has been applied in mechanically ventilated COPD patients. Signs indicative of expiratory flow limitation include the following: (1) A biphasic expiratory flow-volume curve showing a sharp peak expiratory flow that falls abruptly to a much lower flow (Fig. 20.2), which then decreases linearly with exhaled volume at a very slow rate; (2) The value of end-expiratory flow does not decrease substantially when expiratory time is prolonged, that is, even with very long expiratory times it is hard to reach zero flow; (3) If PEEP is applied stepwise, inspiratory plateau pressure will not increase until the critical pressure threshold is achieved. This test can also be used to set PEEP at the highest value that will not cause significant increase in plateau pressure when an end-expiratory hold button is not available; (4) If an end-expiratory hold can be performed with the ventilator, stepwise application of PEEP will result in a decrease of auto-PEEP of similar magnitude to the increase in PEEP until flow limitation is reversed (usually 70%–85% of auto-PEEP at zero end-expiratory pressure).

4. **Permissive hypercapnia**

Permissive hypercapnia was originally conceived as a strategy for the ventilation of patients with status asthmaticus, in which the goal was no longer to restore adequate alveolar ventilation and $Paco_2$ but to limit airway pressures in order to avoid barotrauma (e.g., pneumothorax) and cardiocirculatory failure. It is implemented by reduction of tidal volume to 6 mL/kg and reduction of respiratory rate with prolongation of expiratory time. $Paco_2$ of 60 to 80 mmHg and pH as low as 7.15 are considered acceptable in the absence of contraindications such as intracranial hypertension. The main side effects of this strategy are:

a. Need for deep sedation and possibly neuromuscular blockade to prevent patient–ventilator dyssynchrony. Propofol is a sedative with bronchodilating properties. Atracurium is a neuromuscular blocker with predictable pharmacokinetics, a feature than can be helpful since neuromuscular blockers should be titrated carefully in these patients that are usually on high doses of corticosteroids and hence prone to myopathy. Sedatives and paralytics also reduce CO_2 production and hence dampen hypercapnia.

b. Increased intracranial pressure due to cerebral vasodilation. Consequently, permissive hypercapnia is contraindicated in patients with preexisting intracranial lesions. Subarachnoid hemorrhage has been reported after institution of permissive hypercapnia for status asthmaticus.

G. **ECMO and ECCO$_2$R**

For patients with status asthmaticus and hypoxemia or hypercapnia that is refractory to other therapies, extracorporeal membrane oxygenation (ECMO), or extracorporeal CO_2 removal (ECCO$_2$R) have been used successfully to maintain gas exchange. More recently, extracorporeal techniques have been used to allow early extubation, ambulation, and weaning and to prevent intubation in patients failing NPPV or awaiting lung transplantation.

IV. **PHARMACOLOGIC THERAPY**

Common (and less common) medications used in asthma and COPD are listed in Table 20.1.

A. **Bronchodilators**

1. **β_2-agonists**

a. Inhaled β_2-agonists are the primary treatment for acute asthma, and in nonintubated patients they can be given via metered-dose inhaler (MDI) or nebulizer. Studies have shown equivalence for the use of MDI with a valved holding chamber or nebulizer, provided that patients are able to use the MDI. One Cochrane Review of seven studies found that for nebulized albuterol or salbutamol, continuous nebulization provided greater improvement in PEF and FEV_1 and reduced hospitalization in the more severe acute asthma patients. For mechanically ventilated patients, either MDIs or aerosol provided by vibrating mesh nebulizer are efficacious. Levalbuterol, the R-enantiomer of albuterol that is responsible for bronchodilation, has been shown to be effective at half the dose of albuterol, but randomized trials comparing it with racemic albuterol have been mixed.

Medications used in Asthma or COPD

Drug	Dose	Interval
Albuterol MDI	108 µg, 2 inhalations	q4–6h
	4 inhalations	q10min for acute severe asthma
Albuterol nebulized	2.5 mg or 5 mg	q4–6h
		q20min or continuous for acute severe asthma
Levalbuterol MDI	45 µg, 2 inhalations	q4–6h
Levalbuterol nebulized	1.25 mg	q20min
Formoterol	12 µg, 2 inhalations	q12h
Arformoterol	15 µg in 2 mL	q12h
Salmeterol	50 µg, 1 inhalation	q12h
Olodaterol	2.5 µg, 2 inhalations	q24h
Indacaterol	75 µg, 1 inhalation	q24h
Ipratropium MDI	21 µg, 2 inhalations	q4–6h
Ipratropium nebulized	2.5 mL (500 µg)	q6–8h
Aclidinium	400 µg, 1 inhalation	q12h
Tiotropium	18 µg, 1 inhalation	q24h
Albuterol/ipratropium MDI	120 µg albuterol/21 µg ipratropium	q6h
Albuterol/ipratropium nebulized	3 mg albuterol/0.5 mg ipratropium in 3 mL	q4h
Umeclidinium/vilanterol	62.5/25 µg, 1 inhalation	q24h
Theophylline	300–600 mg	q12h
Aminophylline	380–760 mg	q6–8h
Terbutaline	0.25–0.5 mg sc	q15–30min
Epinephrine	0.1–0.5 mg sc	q3–4h
	0.25–2 µg/min IV	Continuous
Beclomethasone	40 or 80 µg, 1–4 inhalations	q12h
Fluticasone	44, 110, 220 µg, 2 inhalations	q12h
Mometasone	220 µg, 1–2 inhalations	q12h
Flunisolide	80 µg, 2–4 inhalations	q12h
Ciclesonide	80 or 160 µg, 1 inhalation	q12h
Budesonide	90 or 180 mcg, 1–4 inhalations	q12h
Budesonide nebulized	0.25–1 mg/2 mL	q12h
Salmeterol/fluticasone	100–500/50 µg, 1 inhalation	q12h
Fluticasone/vilanterol	100/25 µg, 1 inhalation	q24h
Mometasone/formoterol	100–200/5 µg, 2 inhalations	q12h
Prednisone	40–60 mg (1 mg/kg)	qD
Methylprednisolone	Up to 125 mg IV	X1, then lower doses q6h
Magnesium sulfate	Ped 25–75 mg/kg IV	
	Adult 2 mg IV over 20 min	
Ketamine	bolus dosing 0.5 mg/kg	q20min

  b. It has been noted that patients with acute asthma often have very elevated lactate levels. The origin of this lactate has been the source of debate, with respiratory muscles and altered metabolism from β_2-agonist therapy being some of the suggested sources. The elevated lactate can be so severe as to cause significant acidemia and prompt an investigation for sources of infection. In a recent study of 175 patients with acute asthma, plasma albuterol was significantly correlated with serum lactate concentration after adjusting for asthma severity. Elevated lactate was not associated with worse FEV_1, increased hospitalization, or relapse at 1 week. These data suggest that the elevated lactate is from treatment with β_2-agonists, but that it has no effect on outcome. Elevated lactate has been reported with other drugs with β_2-agonist activity, such as terbutaline and epinephrine.

  c. Inhaled β_2-agonist therapy is also used for acute management of COPD because of its rapid onset of action. As with asthma, MDIs or nebulized β_2-agonist therapy can be utilized, although nebulized therapy is often used in those patients that have difficulty with MDI technique. MDIs or nebulized β_2-agonist via vibrating mesh nebulizer can be used in patients on mechanical ventilation.

2. β_1-antagonists

  a. Many patients with asthma and COPD are either taking, or may require, β_1-antagonist therapy for heart conditions or for other conditions such as variceal bleeding prevention. In asthma, it has been known for a long time that nonselective β-blockers such as propranolol can precipitate asthma exacerbations, particularly at high doses and some, such as pindolol can increase airway resistance in small airways. For selective β_1-antagonists, two meta-analyses have demonstrated that most patients have only a modest reduction in FEV_1 (mean drop of 7.5% predicted), but that approximately 1 in 8 could have an acute drop of >20% in the absolute FEV_1. Interestingly, however, chronic, regular use of even nonselective β-blockers such as propranolol or nadolol may actually not change FEV_1 appreciably or even improve bronchodilator response to albuterol. Therefore, for acute asthma exacerbations, and certainly for acute severe asthma, the introduction of selective or nonselective β_1-antagonists should be avoided, if possible, but if asthma patients are on β_1-antagonists chronically, it is not necessary to stop them. Obviously, in some situations (acute MI), the benefits of selective β_1-antagonist therapy may outweigh the risks.

  b. For COPD, the beneficial effects of cardioselective β_1-antagonists greatly outweigh the risks of worsening lung function. The acute effects of cardioselective β_1-antagonists such as esmolol seem less or nonexistent in COPD compared with those in asthma, but noncardioselective β_1-antagonists such as propranolol have been shown to adversely affect lung function.

3. Ipratropium bromide

Inhaled ipratropium has a slower onset of action compared with albuterol and therefore is not as effective for acute asthma. However, it can be added to albuterol for a greater bronchodilator action. In patients with severe airflow obstruction, ipratropium and albuterol are superior to albuterol alone in terms of bronchodilation and rates of hospitalization. The results of combined albuterol and ipratropium therapy for acute exacerbations of COPD have been mixed, with some studies showing modest improvement and others showing no difference.

B. **Methylxanthines**

Intravenous aminophylline has been used for years for exacerbations of asthma and COPD. It is a weak bronchodilator that has been largely replaced by more effective β_2-agonists or ipratropium. Its major drawback is the narrow therapeutic window and risk of side effects such as nausea and vomiting, tachyarrhythmias, and seizures. A Cochrane Review from 2012 demonstrated no additional benefit in peak flow rate or hospital admission. For every 100 patients treated with aminophylline, 20 patients experienced vomiting and 15 experienced arrhythmias. For COPD, there is even less evidence for efficacy in acute exacerbations. Although oral theophylline may have benefits for reduction in exacerbations of COPD through anti-inflammatory effects, there is no evidence that either oral theophylline or IV aminophylline are useful for short-term treatment of exacerbations and, given the high frequency of side effects, their use cannot be recommended.

C. **Corticosteroids**

1. Treatment of exacerbations of COPD with systemic corticosteroids by the oral or parenteral route has been shown in multiple studies to reduce the likelihood of treatment failure and relapse at 1 month and shorten length of stay in hospital inpatients. There is no evidence for benefit of parenteral treatment over oral treatment when looking at treatment failure, relapse, or mortality. There is an increase in adverse drug effects with corticosteroid treatment, which is greater with parenteral administration compared with oral treatment. Although traditional treatment has been high-dose methylprednisolone (125 mg IV) followed by 60 mg every 6 hours for 3 days and then tapering over 2 weeks, recent data suggest that a short course starting with 40 mg of intravenous methylprednisolone followed by 5 days of oral prednisone has equivalent efficacy to 2 weeks of steroid therapy.

2. The data are very similar for asthma, with corticosteroids demonstrating improvements in meaningful outcomes and no difference in lower ($\leq$80 mg methylprednisolone) versus higher doses of intravenous steroids or in oral versus intravenous route when given in equipotent doses.

D. **Neuromuscular Blockade**

With the use of permissive hypercapnia in mechanically ventilated patients with asthma, neuromuscular blockade would seem particularly attractive in addition to deep sedation in the early treatment of status asthmaticus. However, asthma patients have been shown to be particularly prone to prolonged neuromuscular weakness when neuromuscular blockade has been used, even for periods as short as 12 hours. It is not entirely clear if this weakness is the direct effect of neuromuscular blockade or another effect, such as the deep sedation that is often required to achieve the low ventilatory goals. The effects of neuromuscular blockade and deep sedation in acute exacerbations of COPD are even less clear, although they might be expected to have even greater effects on prolonged weakness since COPD is often associated with lower body mass index and skeletal muscle weakness as part of its systemic effects.

E. **Antibiotics**

1. The use of antibiotics in acute exacerbations of asthma or COPD in the ICU should be guided by the acuity of the illness and the symptoms and signs of infection. Acute exacerbations of COPD are thought to

arise from direct bacterial or viral infection, or the immune response to changes in respiratory flora. When antibiotics are chosen, consideration should be given to covering *Haemophilus influenzae* since this organism is often recovered from bronchial secretions of COPD patients with acute exacerbations who do not have risk factors for hospital-acquired organisms. One small study of 93 intubated patients with acute exacerbation of COPD and clear chest radiographs randomized to a fluoroquinolone versus placebo showed a remarkable clinical benefit to giving the fluoroquinolone, with a number needed to treat six patients for each life saved. The procalcitonin level at admission is a promising biomarker for deciding who can have antibiotics safely stopped and does not result in increased rates of hospital readmission over the 6 month follow-up period. Predictors of COPD patients who may have infections with multidrug-resistant organisms are those with antibiotic exposure in the previous 2 weeks or intubation in the past 6 months.

2. For acute exacerbations of asthma, a randomized trial of telithromycin in hospitalized patients showed an improvement in symptoms but not in peak flow, and the symptom improvement was not related to the presence of *Chlamydophila pneumoniae* or *Mycoplasma pneumoniae*, two organisms that would be expected to be treated by a macrolide antibiotic. Similar to exacerbations of COPD, the use of procalcitonin for antibiotic management in hospitalized asthma patients reduced the use of antibiotics significantly without any change in length of hospital stay or readmission over the 12-month follow-up period. Asthma patients admitted to the ICU with respiratory failure should be tested and treated for influenza, as they are a high-risk group for respiratory failure, ARDS, and death from H1N1 infection.

F. Mucolytics

Mucolytic therapy may be beneficial for COPD or asthma patients with copious or retained secretions during acute exacerbations, but there are no data supporting their routine use.

G. Leukotriene-Receptor Antagonists

Leukotriene-receptor antagonists montelukast and zafirlukast are important controller medications for asthma, but have not been shown to improve outcomes in the treatment of hospitalized patients with asthma. Although some case series have reported benefit with intravenous leukotriene antagonists, currently these medications are only available in oral form in the United States. The 5-lipoxygenase inhibitor zileuton has been tried in a randomized trial for treatment of COPD exacerbations. This trial did not find a difference in length of hospital stay in patients treated with zileuton.

H. Magnesium Sulfate (MgSO$_4$)

Intravenous magnesium sulfate (2 g over 20 minutes), when given early in acute asthma, has been shown to prevent the need for mechanical ventilation in children and to improve spirometry and reduce hospitalizations in adults. In adults, the effect of magnesium seemed to be greatest in those with more severe airflow obstruction. Nebulized magnesium sulfate has also been used in combination with inhaled albuterol, but results have been mixed. Neither intravenous nor nebulized magnesium have been shown to be effective in acute exacerbations of COPD.

I. Ketamine

Ketamine has both adrenergic activity and anticholinergic activity through inhibition of vagal pathways. These effects lead to bronchodilation.

Despite numerous case reports and case series of improvement when used in status asthmaticus, in two randomized trials, one in nonintubated children and another in intubated adults, ketamine did not prove superior to conventional therapy. Ketamine has not been studied in acute exacerbations of COPD.

J. Inhaled Anesthetics

1. Halogenated inhaled anesthetics have both direct bronchodilator properties, by modulating Ca_2^+-dependent contractile mechanisms in airway smooth muscle, and indirect bronchodilatory effects, by reversing muscarinic receptor-mediated bronchoconstriction.
2. Clinical and experimental evidence suggests that isoflurane and sevoflurane improve respiratory mechanics in asthma.
3. Several case series have reported on the potential usefulness of halogenated anesthetics in the treatment of status asthmaticus both in adults and children, occasionally used in conjunction with ketamine.
4. Despite these anecdotal reports, a retrospective study has failed to associate improved outcome with use of inhaled anesthetics in severe asthma. Consequently, in the absence of definitive data from clinical trials, the use of these agents should be reserved for the treatment of severe asthma attacks refractory to maximal conventional treatment.

Selected Readings

Bateman ED, Hurd SS, Barnes PJ, et al. Global strategy for asthma management and prevention: GINA executive summary. *Eur Respir J* 2008;31:143–178.

Camargo CA, Spooner CH, Rowe BH. Continuous versus intermittent beta-agonists in the treatment of acute asthma. *Cochrane Database Syst Rev* 2003;(4):CD001115.

Funk G-C, Bauer P, Burghuber OC, et al. Prevalence and prognosis of COPD in critically ill patients between 1998 and 2008. *Eur Respir J* 2013;41:792–799.

Howton JC, Rose J, Duffy S, et al. Randomized, double-blind, placebo-controlled trial of intravenous ketamine in acute asthma. *Ann Emerg Med* 1996;27:170–175.

Jat KR, Chawla D. Ketamine for management of acute exacerbations of asthma in children. *Cochrane Database Syst Rev* 2012;11:CD009293.

Kimball WR, Leith DE, Robins AG. Dynamic hyperinflation and ventilator dependence in chronic obstructive pulmonary disease. *Am Rev Respir Dis* 1982;126:991–995.

Leatherman JW, Ravenscraft SA. Low measured auto-positive end-expiratory pressure during mechanical ventilation of patients with severe asthma: hidden auto-positive end-expiratory pressure. *Crit Care Med* 1996;24:541–546.

Leuppi JD, Schuetz P, Bingisser R, et al. Short-term vs conventional glucocorticoid therapy in acute exacerbations of chronic obstructive pulmonary disease: the REDUCE randomized clinical trial. *JAMA* 2013;309:2223–2231.

Lewis L, Ferguson I, House SL, et al. Albuterol administration is commonly associated with increases in serum lactate in patients with asthma treated for acute exacerbation of asthma. *Chest* 2014;145:53–59.

Lim WJ, Mohammed Akram R, Carson KV, et al. Non-invasive positive pressure ventilation for treatment of respiratory failure due to severe acute exacerbations of asthma. *Cochrane Database Syst Rev* 2012;12:CD004360.

Lindenauer PK, Pekow PS, Lahti MC, et al. Association of corticosteroid dose and route of administration with risk of treatment failure in acute exacerbation of chronic obstructive pulmonary disease. *JAMA* 2010;303:2359–2367.

Malhotra A, Schwartz DR, Ayas N, et al. Treatment of oxygen-induced hypercapnia. *Lancet* 2001;357:884–885.

Manser R, Reid D, Abramson M. Corticosteroids for acute severe asthma in hospitalised patients. *Cochrane Database Syst Rev* 2001;(1):CD001740.

Morales DR, Jackson C, Lipworth BJ, et al. Adverse respiratory effect of acute β-blocker exposure in asthma: a systematic review and meta-analysis of randomized controlled trials. *Chest* 2014;145:779–786.

Musch G, Foti G, Cereda M, et al. Lung and chest wall mechanics in normal anaesthetized subjects and in patients with COPD at different PEEP levels. *Eur Respir J* 1997;10:2545–2552.

Pendergraft TB, Stanford RH, Beasley R, et al. Rates and characteristics of intensive care unit admissions and intubations among asthma-related hospitalizations. *Ann Allergy Asthma Immunol Off Publ Am Coll Allergy Asthma Immunol* 2004;93:29–35.

Ram FS, Picot J, Lightowler J, et al. Non-invasive positive pressure ventilation for treatment of respiratory failure due to exacerbations of chronic obstructive pulmonary disease. *Cochrane Database Syst Rev* 2004;(1):CD004104.

Salpeter SR, Ormiston TM, Salpeter EE. Cardioselective beta-blockers in patients with reactive airway disease: a meta-analysis. *Ann Intern Med* 2002;137:715–725.

Vaschetto R, Bellotti E, Turucz E, et al. Inhalational anesthetics in acute severe asthma. *Curr Drug Targets* 2009;10:826–832.

Vestbo J, Hurd SS, Agustí AG, et al. Global strategy for the diagnosis, management, and prevention of chronic obstructive pulmonary disease: GOLD executive summary. *Am J Respir Crit Care Med* 2013;187:347–365.

Wenzel SE. Asthma phenotypes: the evolution from clinical to molecular approaches. *Nat Med* 2012;18:716–725.

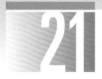

Deep Venous Thrombosis and Pulmonary Embolism in the Intensive Care Unit

Alison S. Witkin and Richard N. Channick

 RV clot

 McConnell's sign

I. **OVERVIEW**: Venous thromboembolic event (VTE) refers to both deep venous thrombosis and pulmonary embolism. Episodic thrombosis and/or embolism may appear to be discrete events, but increasingly they are considered to be manifestations of the same process.

A. **Deep Venous Thrombosis (DVT)** refers to clot in the deep vessels of the venous circulation. While local discomfort with limb swelling and postthrombotic syndrome can occur, the majority of morbidity and mortality results from embolization to the pulmonary circulation. While the proximal veins of the lower extremity are the most common site of involvement and have a higher risk of embolization, upper extremity DVT can also lead to pulmonary embolism. Without DVT prophylaxis, the incidence of DVT in the intensive care unit (ICU) is quite high with ranges of 10% to 30% in medical patients and up to 60% in trauma patients. This risk can be significantly reduced, but not eliminated, with prophylaxis.

B. **Pulmonary Embolism (PE)** occurs when the pulmonary artery or one of its branches becomes obstructed by material. While thrombus is the most common, air, fat, or tumor can also cause embolism. The clinical significance of PE is broad and ranges from an incidental finding with no signs or symptoms to catastrophic circulatory collapse leading to death. The incidence of PE is approximately 112 per 100,000 person-years. The mortality from PE approaches 20% with higher mortality rates in those who are unstable at the time of presentation.

C. **Risk Factors**. DVT and PE have similar risk factors. Some of the most common risk factors in ICU patients include the following:

1. **Recent surgical procedures**: The risk of VTE is highest in patients who have had major orthopedic or general surgery procedures. Specific procedures associated with a high risk of VTE include hip or knee replacement and coronary artery bypass. Major trauma also has a high risk of VTE.

2. **Spinal cord injury**: Risk is highest immediately following injury and decreases with time.

3. **Malignancy**: Risk is highest in patients with advanced solid organ malignancies. Certain chemotherapy regimens may also increase risk.

4. **Central venous lines**: can lead to line-associated DVT with potential for embolization to pulmonary vasculature

5. **Oral contraceptive pills**: also increased with hormone replacement therapy

6. **Pregnancy**: Greatest risk occurs in postpartum period.

7. **Immobility**: due to injury, travel, or hospitalization

8. **Thrombophilias:** including antiphospholipid antibody syndrome, heparin-induced thrombocytopenia, as well as hereditary causes, including antithrombin deficiency, Protein C and S deficiencies, Factor V Leiden mutations, and prothrombin gene mutation
9. **Previous VTE**

D. **VTE in the ICU.** The incidence of VTE in the ICU is difficult to determine as the diagnosis requires a high degree of suspicion in patients with other ongoing pulmonary processes, and obtaining confirmatory testing is not always feasible in a critically ill patient. Regardless of the reason for ICU admission, critically ill patients are at increased risk for VTE as most patients are immobile and many receive central venous catheters. The incidence in postmortem studies of ICU patients is 7% to 27%.

E. **Prophylaxis in ICU patients.** The use of pharmacologic prophylaxis with either low-dose heparin or low-molecular-weight heparin (LMWH) decreases but does not eliminate the risk of DVT in patients admitted to the ICU and thus should be used in patients without contraindications, such as active bleeding. Patients who cannot receive pharmacologic prophylaxis should receive mechanical prophylaxis. Intermittent pneumatic compression of the lower limbs is the mechanical intervention with the highest quality data. Regardless of the strategy used for prophylaxis, it is important to remember that no strategy provides complete protection against VTE.

II. DIAGNOSIS

A. **DVT**
1. **Exam:** Limb pain, edema, and palpable cord are suggestive of DVT. Sudden severe pain associated with cyanosis or evidence of compartment syndrome or impaired arterial circulation is suggestive of massive proximal thrombosis (phlegmasia cerluea dolens). Exam alone is not sufficient to rule in or rule out DVT.
2. **Ultrasound** utilizes vein compressibility and/or color flow imaging. It has high sensitivity and specificity for DVT although may miss clots in pelvic veins. Ultrasound is ideal in ICU patients as it can be done at the bedside without radiation exposure.
3. **Computed tomography (CT) venogram** can be done at the same time as a CT for evaluation of PE, eliminating the need for an additional imaging study; however, this test leads to increased radiation exposure and many protocols have higher doses of contrast material. CT-venogram, unlike ultrasound, can evaluate for pelvic thrombosis.
4. **Magnetic resonance (MR) venogram** can image the lower extremity veins, including pelvic veins, without use of contrast material or radiation. Disadvantages include availability and time required to obtain study.
5. **D-dimer:** The main utility of the D-dimer assay is in ruling out DVT in the emergency department setting. Due to a high degree of false positives in the setting of critical illness, this test has minimal utility in the ICU.

B. **Pulmonary Embolism**
1. **Clinical exam:** Although findings such as tachycardia, hypoxia, tachypnea, fever, and hypotension may raise clinical suspicion for PE, exam alone is not enough to rule in or rule out PE.
2. **Lab tests:** While brain natriuretic peptide (BNP) and troponin may be elevated, these tests lack the necessary specificity to be useful in diagnosis. Additionally, as in DVT, the D-dimer is often elevated even in ICU patients without PE, limiting its utility in diagnosis.

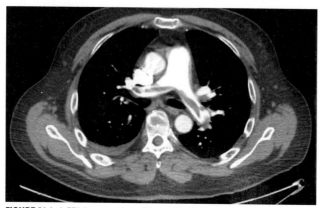

FIGURE 21.1 A CTA from a patient with a saddle PE. Clot can be seen extending into both the left and right main pulmonary arteries.

3. **EKG:** While EKG abnormalities, such as sinus tachycardia and evidence of right ventricular strain, are common, they lack both the specificity and sensitivity to make a diagnosis of PE.

4. **Chest x-ray (CXR):** The majority of patients have nonspecific abnormalities on CXR. If infarction has occurred, this may appear as a wedge-shaped opacity at the periphery.

5. **CT angiography (CTA)** (Fig. 21.1) has become the diagnostic imaging study of choice, as it can be performed in minutes and additionally allows for simultaneous evaluation of other pulmonary processes. Addition of venous imaging improves sensitivity. Disadvantages include the requirement that the patient be able to comply with a breath hold, radiation exposure, and need for iodinated contrast. Poor-quality imaging due to either motion artifact or poor timing of contrast bolus may decrease sensitivity.

6. **Ventilation/perfusion (V̇/Q̇) scan** is useful in patients who cannot tolerate CTA as it does not require iodinated contrast. However, its interpretation requires clinical correlation as a low-probability scan does not entirely rule out PE and a high-probability scan does not guarantee presence of PE. In addition, in patients with significant underlying pulmonary disease, perfusion scans are difficult to interpret and have a high false-positive rate.

7. **Pulmonary angiography:** As the quality of CTA has improved, the use of pulmonary angiography has decreased; however, it remains the gold standard for diagnosis of PE. Angiography is generally well tolerated with a low complication rate and has the additional benefit of allowing for direct assessment of pulmonary hemodynamics.

8. **Echocardiogram** is useful in assessing right ventricular function. Findings suggestive of PE include increased right ventricular (RV) chamber size with decreased function, although this finding can be seen in a variety of cardiac and pulmonary diseases. More specific findings include presence of RV clot (Online Video 1) and McConnell's sign (Online Video 2), in which there is akinesis of the mid-free RV wall with normal apical function. Although none of these findings are diagnostic of PE, as echocardiogram can be performed at the bedside, it can be used to

help confirm a clinical diagnosis in a patient too unstable to travel for more definitive testing.

III. INITIAL EVALUATION OF THE PATIENT WITH CONFIRMED OR SUSPECTED PE.

A. Assess Severity: The initial bedside assessment of a patient with PE is focused on assessing severity. Patients with hypotension and shock without other cause are considered to have massive PE (defined as systolic blood pressure of less than 90 mmHg or a drop of at least 40 mmHg from baseline for at least 15 minutes) and require immediate intervention.

1. The pathophysiology of massive PE is complex. When obstruction occurs by embolism, the RV experiences an acute rise in pressure and volume, causing shift of the interventricular septum toward the left ventricle. In addition, as RV output decreases, the left ventricular preload also falls. This combination of septal shift and decreased RV output can ultimately lead to decreased cardiac output, shock, and hemodynamic collapse (Fig. 21.2).

2. In patients without massive PE, it is important to distinguish between those at higher risk for hemodynamic collapse versus those with lower-risk PE. This is primarily accomplished through either direct or indirect assessment of RV compromise or strain. Those patients with hemodynamic stability but evidence of RV strain are considered to have intermediate-risk PE.

B. Physical Exam should focus on signs of shock, including hypotension and signs of end organ hypoperfusion, indicating massive PE. In the hemodynamically stable patient, hypoxia and tachycardia, particularly if worsened with activity, may suggest a patient is at risk for decompensation.

C. Lab Testing: Troponin elevation is seen in roughly one-third of patients with PE and is likely due to increased stretch on the right ventricle due to pressure overload in massive or intermediate-risk PE. Troponin elevation is associated with both presence of RV strain on transthoracic

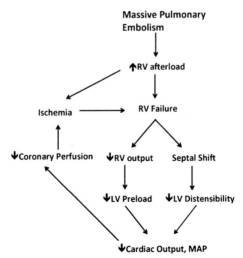

FIGURE 21.2 A schematic demonstrating the cycle by which massive PE leads to hemodynamic instability.

echocardiogram (TTE) and increased mortality. BNP or NT-pro-BNP elevation is seen in approximately one-half of patients with PE, reflecting RV myocyte stretch. Like troponin, an elevation is associated with RV strain on TTE and increased mortality when compared with patients with normal BNP and NT-pro-BNP levels.

D. CT Findings: In addition to the finding of the PE itself, the CTA chest can demonstrate findings of RV dysfunction and allow for assessment of clot burden. RV enlargement on CT (defined as the ratio of right ventricular to left ventricular diameter >0.9) is associated with increased thirty-day mortality. Additionally, the location of clot can be used to identify patients at higher risk of decompensation, as central emboli (saddle or at least one main pulmonary artery) are associated with increased risk of death or clinical deterioration when compared with more peripheral emboli.

E. TTE should be performed in most patients with concern for intermediate-risk pulmonary embolism as it provides visual assessment of RV function. At least one-third of hemodynamically stable patients with PE have evidence of RV dysfunction on TTE. High-quality data on mortality is sparse; however, there is a suggestion of increased in-hospital mortality in these patients. Additionally, TTE allows for evaluation of other cardiac abnormalities including patent foramen ovale, which increases concern for paradoxical embolus to the systemic circulation, and presence of RV thrombus, which is associated with worse prognosis and increased risk of hemodynamic instability.

F. ICU Considerations: Diagnosing DVT and PE in ICU patients may be challenging. As many of these patients are intubated and sedated and have other concurrent severe illnesses (ARDS, sepsis, etc.), it may be difficult to determine the cause of clinical decompensation. Relatively subtle changes, such as a swollen upper extremity (especially associated with an indwelling catheter), increasing dead space ventilation (rising $Paco_2$ or minute ventilation requirements), increased vasopressor needs, or worsening hypoxemia with no apparent cause, should raise suspicion for VTE. As mentioned, acute RV dysfunction in ICU patients may be due to several processes besides VTE, including sepsis, acute lung injury, or intrinsic PEEP.

IV. TREATMENT

A. Resuscitation. The first priority in treating a patient with pulmonary embolism is ensuring hemodynamic stability. Most patients with PE will have an increased A-a gradient due to both $\dot{V}/\dot{Q}$ mismatch combined with surfactant dysfunction due to release of inflammatory mediators, atelectasis, and shunt (particularly intracardiac in patients with a patent foramen ovale). Supplemental oxygen can be used to correct hypoxia, and inhaled nitric oxide may decrease shunting and improve pulmonary hemodynamics through pulmonary vasodilation. Caution should be used if a patient requires intubation, as severe hypotension may result in the presence of significant RV dysfunction.

1. For hypotensive patients, fluid should be given cautiously to correct any volume deficit, with typically no more than 1,000 mL of crystalloid given. Aggressive fluid resuscitation may worsen hypotension both by increasing RV stretch as well as worsening the interventricular shift, further impairing left ventricular function. If a vasopressor is required, there are no randomized controlled trials to guide management; however, norepinephrine, dopamine, or epinephrine, plus the consideration of dobutamine, are reasonable selections. If a patient is in refractory shock, the use of extracorporeal membrane oxygenation (ECMO) should

be considered. ECMO can provide both ventilatory and hemodynamic support while a patient is treated with more definitive therapy.

B. **Systemic Anticoagulation** should be promptly initiated when PE or DVT is diagnosed or strongly suspected. Unfractionated heparin (UFH), LMWH, and fondaparinux are all considered first line for the acute treatment of PE and DVT. As patients with VTE typically require anticoagulation for a minimum of 3 months, most patients without malignancy will be transitioned to an oral agent. Contraindications to anticoagulation include active bleeding and intracranial tumor. Patients with recent bleeding events, invasive procedures, or who are otherwise at increased risk of complications should be evaluated on an individual basis.

1. **UFH** has several advantages over other parenteral agents. Compared with LMWH and fondaparinux, UFH has the shortest half-life and can be reversed with protamine if needed, making it a good choice in patients with increased risks of bleeding. Due to the short half-life, it should be used in patients who are being considered for thrombolysis. Additionally, UFH does not rely on renal clearance, so it is ideal for use in renal failure. The main drawback to UFH use is that it requires frequent laboratory monitoring and can take time to reach therapeutic levels. Such delays have been associated with increased mortality from PE and higher rates of VTE recurrence.

2. **Low-molecular-weight heparins**: Multiple formulations of LMWH exist, with variations in dosing. Compared with UFH, LMWH is associated with decreased complications, lower incidence of bleeding, as well as decreased mortality. However, as LMWH is cleared renally and can be challenging to reverse, its use should be avoided in patients with decreased creatinine clearance or who are considered to be at increased bleeding risk.

3. **Factor Xa inhibitors**: Fondaparinux is an injectable factor Xa inhibitor that has similar efficacy to UFH and does not require drug level monitoring. Rivaroxaban and apixaban are oral factor Xa inhibitors that are approved for treatment of VTE. Although they have been studied in the acute setting, they are not considered a first-line treatment. There is no reversal agent for Factor Xa inhibitors and use should be avoided in patients with renal failure. This class of medication can be safely used in patients with a history of heparin-induced thrombocytopenia (HIT).

4. **Direct thrombin inhibitors**: Argatroban is an intravenous direct thrombin inhibitor approved for treatment of thrombosis when associated with HIT. Some centers may use Bivalirudin, a direct thrombin inhibitor approved for anticoagulation for percutaneous coronary intervention, in an off-label fashion for treatment of thrombosis with HIT. Dabigatran is an oral direct thrombin inhibitor approved for treatment of VTE. Its use has not been studied in the acute setting and thus is not recommended as initial therapy. Dabigatran should be avoided in patients with impaired renal function and cannot be reversed in the event of bleeding.

5. **Warfarin**: Due to the initial prothrombotic effects of warfarin, it should not be used alone in the acute setting; however, its efficacy in preventing recurrent VTE has been well established. Warfarin requires close monitoring of INR to avoid inadequate treatment while minimizing the risk of bleeding. In event of overdose or bleeding, fresh frozen plasma and Vitamin K can be used to reverse its effects.

C. **Systemic Thrombolysis**
1. **Overview.** Thrombolytic agents activate plasminogen to form plasmin, leading to increased lysis of thrombus. Due to increased bleeding

risk, including fatal intracranial bleeding, patients must be carefully screened for contraindications. Major and absolute contraindications include intracranial lesions, previous intracranial hemorrhage, ischemic stroke within 3 months, recent head trauma, recent brain or spine surgery, active bleeding and bleeding diathesis. Notable relative contraindications include systolic or diastolic hypertension, recent invasive procedures, recent bleeding, and history of ischemic stroke more than 3 months prior. Studied thrombolytic agents include tissue plasminogen activator (tPA), streptokinase, and urokinase.

2. **Indications.** Systemic thrombolysis is recommended for patients with massive pulmonary embolism without contraindications. Systemic thrombolysis is not recommended for the majority of patients with DVT, although it can be considered in patients with acute, extensive proximal clot. Systemic thrombolysis is also generally not recommended for patients with intermediate-risk PE. Several studies that examined the use of full dose thrombolytic therapy in patients with nonmassive PE and evidence of RV dysfunction found decreased rates of hemodynamic decompensation and need for escalation in treatment; however, there was no improvement in mortality and most studies reported increase in major bleeding. The MOPETT study gave patients with "moderate" PE, as defined by degree of involvement on angiography or $\dot{V}/\dot{Q}$ scan, no more than half-dose tPA and found that this regimen improved pulmonary artery pressures without an increase in bleeding. However, more studies are needed before lower dose therapy becomes a routine recommendation for intermediate-risk PE.

D. **Surgical Embolectomy** should be considered in patients with massive PE who either fail or are not candidates for systemic lysis. One advantage of surgical embolectomy is that it allows for simultaneous intervention on associated abnormalities, such as patent foramen ovale closure or removal of intracardiac clot. This intervention is limited to hospitals with appropriate staff resources and experience.

E. **Catheter-Directed Therapies** are emerging tools in the treatment of both massive and submassive PE, particularly when patients have contraindications to systemic lysis or have failed initial interventions. These techniques allow for clot fragmentation and removal as well as targeted delivery of reduced doses of lytic medications. The concurrent use of ultrasound-enabled devices enhances fibrinolysis by increasing drug penetration. Like surgical embolectomy, these interventions are limited to hospitals with appropriate staff and resources.

F. **Vena Cava Filters** should be used in patients who have DVT with contraindications to anticoagulation or who fail anticoagulation. Use of a filter is also considered in patients with residual lower extremity clot for whom another PE would likely be fatal. Filters appear to primarily decrease PE in the acute setting and their long-term use is associated with recurrent DVT, often at the filter site. Removable filters should be considered in those with only temporary indications for placement.

G. **Multidisciplinary Approach.** Treatment of patients with intermediate-risk and massive PEs often requires a multidisciplinary approach with collaboration between the emergency department, cardiology, surgery, radiology, and intensive care unit teams. Additionally, the ideal treatment for a particular patient will depend on available resources and patient-specific information. The use of a multidisciplinary pulmonary embolism response team to help coordinate these efforts has recently been described and may streamline the care for these patients.

V. FOLLOW-UP

A. Duration of Anticoagulation varies depending on the presence of reversible risk factors as well as if the patient has a history of VTE. Most patients require a minimum of 3 months of systemic anticoagulation, with prolonged or even life-long therapy in those with irreversible risk factors or recurrent VTE. The choice of the long-term anticoagulant agent should be tailored to the individual patient's risk factors and comorbidities.

B. Chronic Thromboembolic Pulmonary Hypertension occurs in approximately 3.8% of patients following acute PE. During outpatient follow-up, patients should be assessed for residual symptoms of dyspnea, particularly on exertion. Those who have persistent symptoms, had evidence of RV dysfunction on presentation, or had significant clot burdens should be considered for additional screening, including $\dot{V}/\dot{Q}$ scan and repeat TTE.

Selected Readings

Aklog L, Wiliams CS, Byrne JG, et al. Acute pulmonary embolectomy: a contemporary approach. *Circulation* 2002;105:1416–1419.

Anderson FA, Spencer FA. Risk factors for venous thromboembolism. *Circulation* 2003;107:I-9–I-16.

Attia J, Ray JG, Cook DJ, et al. Deep vein thrombosis and its prevention in critically ill adults. *Arch Intern Med* 2001;161:1268–1279.

Capellier G, Jacques T, Balvay P, et al. Inhaled nitric oxide in patients with pulmonary embolism. *Intensive Care Med* 1997;23:1089–1092.

Chan CM, Shorr AF. Venous thromboembolic disease in the intensive care unit. *Semin Respir Crit Care Med* 2010;31:39–46.

Decousus H, Leizorovicz A, Parent F, et al. A clinical trial of vena caval filters in the prevention of pulmonary embolism in patients with proximal deep-vein thrombosis. *NEJM* 1998;338:409–415.

Eid-Lidt G, Gaspar J, Sandoval J, et al. Combined clot fragmentation and aspiration in patients with acute pulmonary embolism. *Chest* 2008;134:54–60.

EINSTEIN-PE Investigators. Oral rivaroxaban for the treatment of symptomatic pulmonary embolism. *NEJM* 2012;366:1287–1297.

Engelberger RP, Kucher N. Catheter-based reperfusion treatment of pulmonary embolism. *Circulation* 2011;124:2139–2144.

Erkens PM, Prins MH. Fixed dose subcutaneous low-molecular-weight heparins versus adjusted dose unfractionated heparin for venous thromboembolism. *Cochrance Database Syst Rev* 2010;9:CD001100.

Geerts W, Selby R. Prevention of venous thromboembolism in the ICU. *Chest* 2003;124:357S–363S.

Goldhaber SZ, Visani L, De Rosa M. Acute pulmonary embolism: clinical outcomes in the international cooperative pulmonary embolism registry (ICOPER). *Lancet* 1999;353:1386–1389.

Ho KM, Tan JA. Stratified meta-analysis of intermittent pneumatic compression of the lower limbs to prevent venous thromboembolism in hospitalized patients. *Circulation* 2013;2013:1003–1020.

Horlander KT, Leeper KV. Troponin levels as a guide to treatment of pulmonary embolism. *Curr Opin Pulm Med* 2003;9:374–377.

Kanne JP, Lalani TA. Role of computed tomography and magnetic resonance imaging for deep venous thrombosis and pulmonary embolism. *Circulation* 2004;109:I-15–I-21.

Kearon C, Akl EA, Comerota AJ, et al. Antithrombotic therapy and prevention of thrombosis, 9th ed: American College of Chest Physicians evidence-based clinical practice guidelines. *Chest* 2012;141:e419S–e494S.

Kline JA, Nordenholz KE, Courtney DM, et al. Treatment of submassive pulmonary embolism with tenecteplase or placebo: cardiopulmonary outcomes at 3 months: multicenter double-blind, placebo-controlled randomized trial. *J Thromb Haemost* 2014;12:459–468.

Klock FA, Mos ICM, Huisman MV. Brain-type natriuretic peptide levels in the prediction of adverse outcome in patients with pulmonary embolism. *Am J Respir Crit Care Med* 2008;178:425–430.

Konstantinides S, Geibel A, Heusel G, et al. Heparin plus alteplase compared with heparin alone in patients with submassive pulmonary embolism. *NEJM* 2002;347:1143–1150.

Kucher N. Deep-vein thrombosis of the upper extremities. *NEJM* 2011;364:861–869.

Kucher N, Goldhaber SZ. Management of massive pulmonary embolism. *Circulation* 2005;112:e28–e32.

Lensing AW, Prandoni P, Brandjes D, et al. Detection of deep-vein thrombosis by real-time B-mode ultrasonography. *NEJM* 1989;320:342–345.

Matisse Investigators. Subcutaneous fondaparinux versus intravenous unfractionated heparin in the initial treatment of pulmonary embolism. *NEJM* 2003;349:1695–1702.

McConnell MV, Solomon SD, Rayan ME, et al. Regional right ventricular dysfunction detected by echocardiography in acute pulmonary embolism. *Am J Cardiol* 1996;78:469–473.

Meyer G, Vicaut E, Danays T, et al. Fibronolysis for patients with intermediate-risk pulmonary embolism. *NEJM* 2014;370:1402–1411.

Mismetti P, Rivron-Guillot K, Quenet S, et al. A prospective long-term study of 220 patients with a retrievable vena cava filter for secondary prevention of venous thromboembolism. *Chest* 2007;131:223 229.

Ogren M, Bergqvist D, Eriksson H, et al. Prevalence and risk of pulmonary embolism in patients with intracardiac thrombosis: a population-based study of 23796 consecutive autopsies. *Eur Heart J* 2005;26:1108–1114.

Pengo V, Lensing AWA, Prins MH, et al. Incidence of chronic thromboembolic pulmonary hypertension after pulmonary embolism. *NEJM* 2004;350:2257–2264.

PIOPED Investigators. Value of the ventilation/perfusion scan in acute pulmonary embolism. *JAMA* 1990;263:2753–2759.

Provias T, Dudzinski DM, Jaff MR, et al. The Massachusetts General Hospital Pulmonary Embolism Response Team (MGH PERT): creation of a multidisciplinary program to improve care of patients with massive and submassive pulmonary embolism. *Hosp Pract (1995)* 2014;42:31–37.

Rodger M, Makropoulos D, Turek M, et al. Diagnostic value of the electrocardiogram in suspected pulmonary embolism. *Am J Cardiol* 2000;86:807–809.

Schoepf UJ, Kucher N, Kipfmueller F, et al. Right ventricular enlargement on chest computed tomography: a predictor of early death in acute pulmonary embolism. *Circulation* 2004;110:3276–3280.

Schulman S, Kearon C, Kakkar AK, et al. Dabigatran versus warfarin in the treatment of acute venous thromboembolism. *NEJM* 2009;361:2342–2352.

Sharifi M, Bay C, Skrocki L, et al. Moderate pulmonary embolism treated with thrombolysis (from the "MOPETT" trial). *Am J Cardiol* 2013;111:273–277.

Smith SB, Geske JB, Maguire JM, et al. Early anticoagulation is associated with reduced mortality for acute pulmonary embolism. *Chest* 2010;137:1382–1390.

Stein PD, Athanasoulis C, Alavi A, et al. Complications and validity of pulmonary angiography in acute pulmonary embolism. *Circulation* 1992;85:462–468.

Stein PD, Fowler SE, Goodman LR, et al. Multidetector computed tomography for acute pulmonary embolism. *NEJM* 2006;354:2317–2327.

Stein PD, Hull RD, Patel KC, et al. D-dimer for the exclusion of acute venous thrombosis and pulmonary embolism: a systematic review. *Ann Intern Med* 2004;140:589–602.

ten Wolde M, Sohne M, Quak E, et al. Prognostic value of echocardiographically assessed right ventricular dysfunction in patients with pulmonary embolism. *Arch Intern Med* 2004;164:1685–1689.

Torbicki A, Galie N, Covezzoli A, et al. Right heart thrombi in pulmonary embolism results from the International Cooperative Pulmonary Embolism Registry. *J Am Coll Card* 2003;41:2245–2251.

Vedovati MC, Becattini C, Agnelli G, et al. Multidector CT scan for acute pulmonary embolism: embolic burden and clinical outcome. *Chest* 2012;142:1417–1424.

Wiener RS, Schwartz LM, Woloshin S. Time trends in pulmonary embolism in the United States: evidence of overdiagnosis. *Arch Intern Med* 2011;171:831–837.

Wood KE. Major pulmonary embolism: review of a pathophysiologic approach to the golden hour of hemodynamically significant pulmonary embolism. *Chest* 2002;121:877–905.

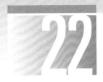

Discontinuation of Mechanical Ventilation

Crystal M. North and Ednan K. Bajwa

I. **INTRODUCTION:** The safe discontinuation of mechanical ventilation is the primary goal for physicians caring for patients with respiratory failure. Advancements in the understanding of sedation, delirium, and volume status management over the past 15 years, as well as modifications to ventilator strategies, have led to shorter time on mechanical ventilation and better hospital outcomes. A detailed understanding of the factors leading to respiratory failure and ways in which successful ventilator discontinuation can be achieved are paramount to the care of the intubated patient.

II. **DEFINITIONS**
   A. **SAT:** Spontaneous awakening trial. The cessation of all sedatives, or decreasing doses of sedative infusions in order to allow a patient to reliably interact and follow commands
   B. **SBT:** Spontaneous breathing trial. A decrease in the amount of support provided by a mechanical ventilator to test the patient's ability to breathe without support
   C. **Weaning:** Decreasing ventilator settings in a stepwise approach in order to determine the patient's minimal ventilator needs
   D. **Ventilator Dependence:** The inability to wean a patient from mechanical ventilation despite repeated attempts
   E. **Extubation:** Removal of the endotracheal tube
   F. **Decannulation:** Removal of the tracheostomy tube

III. **VENTILATOR DEPENDENCE**—can be due to a variety of reasons related to any component of the respiratory system. A thorough investigation into each of the etiologies described below is central to the care of ventilated patients.
   A. **Nervous System**
      1. **Primary brain injury**—can lead to damage to centers in the brain involved in the control and initiation of respiration. Examples include stroke, hemorrhage, mass effect, cerebral edema, seizures, and central apnea.
      2. **Sedating medications**—can decrease the respiratory drive
      3. **Spinal cord and peripheral nerves**—Damage to these structures can impair the function of the diaphragm and intercostal muscles.
      4. **Critical illness myopathy/polyneuropathy (CIM/CIP)**—Each is multifactorial, related to length of immobility, degree of critical illness, use of systemic steroids, and paralytic agents. The presence of CIM or CIP can lead to impaired function of the diaphragm and accessory muscles of inhalation, resulting in respiratory failure.
      5. **Psychological:** Untreated/undertreated anxiety or other psychiatric diseases may lead to unnecessary anxiety surrounding the removal of ventilator support. Reassurance or low-dose anxiolytics may be necessary, depending on the clinical scenario.

B. Respiratory Muscles
1. **Electrolyte imbalances**—Phosphate and magnesium are each central to muscular function. Severe depletions in each are associated with muscle weakness and may lead to difficulty with ventilator weaning.
2. **Nutritional factors**—Inadequate nutrition can lead to muscle catabolism, which may result in respiratory muscle weakness and prolonged reliance on mechanical ventilation. Conversely, overfeeding can result in excess CO_2 production and resultant increases in minute ventilation.
3. **Endocrine imbalances**—Cortisol, insulin, and glucagon have been implicated in normal respiratory muscle function, and deficiencies in each have been hypothesized to lead to compromised function. Hypothyroidism may result in diaphragmatic weakness.

C. Pulmonary Mechanics—Increased resistance and decreased compliance each increase the amount of work required during respiration. The degree to which resistance and compliance are abnormal determines the degree to which a patient will be reliant on the ventilator.
1. **Resistance**—the opposition to airflow in the respiratory system
   a. Increased airways resistance can be due to bronchospasm, increased respiratory secretions, airway inflammation, endotracheal or tracheostomy tube obstruction, or small diameter of endotracheal tube.
2. **Compliance**—the ability of the thorax and lungs to expand their volume as transmural pressure increases. Measured at end-inhalation during a breath hold; the reciprocal of elastic recoil.
   a. The compliance of the **chest wall** may be impaired due to morbid obesity, chest wall bony abnormalities, or intra-abdominal processes that interfere with diaphragm function.
   b. **Lung** compliance can be decreased as a result of consolidation, fibrosis, or pulmonary edema.
3. **Auto-PEEP**—increased end-expiratory intra-alveolar pressure caused by incomplete exhalation. Can be caused by increased resistance, rapid respirations, or by ventilator dyssynchrony. Of specific concern in patients with severe obstructive lung disease, which may make the patient dyssynchronous and complicate ventilator weaning
4. **Minute ventilation**—required to maintain normal acid–base status. Increased minute ventilation requirement may indicate increased CO_2 production or increased dead space. High minute ventilation requirements (particularly >10 L/min) may not be tolerated by the newly extubated patient and should suggest to the clinician that a search for undiagnosed underlying causes be undertaken.

D. Inadequate Gas Exchange—High levels of FIO_2 and PEEP may be required due to the compromise of the alveolar-arterial interface (i.e., significant pneumonia, ARDS, pulmonary edema, fibrosis).

E. Cardiovascular Disease—Patients for whom cardiac dysfunction is present may not tolerate the additional stress to the cardiovascular system that the removal of mechanical ventilation can cause. Underlying coronary artery disease may manifest as chest pressure or pain during an SBT or following extubation that is related to stress-induced cardiac ischemia. Patients with congestive heart failure may develop acute pulmonary edema due to the removal of all positive pressure and the subsequent increase in venous return.

IV. STANDARDIZED CARE OF THE INTUBATED PATIENT

A. The **"ABCDE"** bundle. Applied to all intubated patients on a daily basis

  1. **"AB"**: Daily SAT (**"A"**) and SBT (**"B"**) to assess for extubation readiness

  2. **"C"**: Choice of sedative

  3. **"D"**: Delirium monitoring and management

  4. **"E"**: Early mobilization of intubated patients

  5. www.icudelirium.org—useful reference for clinicians

B. Addition of the SAT to the usual care of intubated patients (as opposed to sedation management at the discretion of the clinician) lead to fewer days on mechanical ventilation and in the ICU, with no difference in complications such as self-extubation.

C. Early Mobilization—Physical therapy that begins while intubated, during periods of lightened sedation, has been shown to be safe and leads to decreased mortality, more functional independence after hospital discharge, less delirium, and more ventilator-free days.

V. SEDATION MANAGEMENT: This will be addressed in more detail in Chapter 7. Below is a brief overview of an approach to sedation in the intubated patient.

A. Consider an **"analgesia-first" strategy** to treat pain symptoms, adding a sedative only if the patient remains uncomfortable after pain control is achieved.

B. Short-acting agents are preferred to long-acting agents, due to both quicker onset of action and shorter duration of effect once discontinued. Frequent renal and liver dysfunction in medical ICU patients affect timely clearance of medications.

C. Use **lowest necessary continuous infusion rates**. When possible, use intermittent IV bolus dosing rather than continuous infusion.

D. Use a validated scale to set sedation targets, such as the **RASS** (Richmond Agitation Sedation Scale).

  1. Scale by which sedation is titrated, assessed by nursing frequently

  2. –5 (unarousable) to +4 (combative)

  3. Target: 0 (alert and calm) to –1 (drowsy)

E. Sedative Choices

  1. Propofol: GABA potentiation

   a. Side effects: Hypotension, propofol infusion syndrome (rare), hypertriglyceridemia

  2. Midazolam (Versed): GABA potentiation

   a. Hepatic metabolites are also active GABA potentiators.

   b. Side effects: Prolonged sedation once discontinued, delirium

  3. Dexmedetomidine (Precedex): Alpha-2 agonist

   a. Side effects: Hypotension, bradycardia

   b. Due to cost, generally restricted to patients within 24 hours of extubation

F. Analgesia—Intermittent boluses or continuous infusions of opiates are utilized for pain control in intubated patients. Common opiates in the ICU include the following:

  1. Fentanyl: short acting, fast onset. Most commonly used opiate infusion for intubated patients

  2. Morphine: short acting, fast onset. Avoid in renal dysfunction due to accumulation of toxic metabolites.

  3. Hydromorphone (Dilaudid): short acting, fast onset. Seven times stronger than morphine

VI. DELIRIUM IN THE ICU

A. Increases risk of longer hospital stays, death, higher hospital costs, and prolonged cognitive impairment at 1 year

B. CAM-ICU:

   1. Assessment tool for delirium in ICU patients, assessed by nursing

   2. Positive (delirious) or negative (not delirious)

C. Treating Delirium

   1. Frequent reorientation, sleep–wake cycle protection (light during the day, dark at night), familiar surroundings

   2. Medications

     a. Haloperidol (IV, IM): short-acting, fast onset

     b. Quetiapine (PO), Olanzapine (PO, SL): longer-acting, more sedating

     c. Side effects: QTc prolongation, rarely neuroleptic malignant syndrome (NMS), torticollis, extrapyramidal symptoms

D. MIND-USA: Currently enrolling multicenter RCT to determine the role of antipsychotics (haloperidol vs. ziprasidone vs. placebo) in ICU patients at risk for developing delirium.

VII. ASSESSING FOR VENTILATOR DISCONTINUATION POTENTIAL: Patients need to be assessed daily for whether they meet criteria for the discontinuation of mechanical ventilation. Studies indicate that physicians underestimate a patient's readiness for extubation. In a landmark study evaluating methods of spontaneous breathing trials, over 75% of patients who were determined to be ready for mechanical ventilation for the first time went on to be extubated following the first spontaneous breathing trial, supporting the underrecognition by physicians of a patient's readiness for extubation. As a result, clinically guided protocols have been implemented in order to guide clinical decision making.

A. In order to be considered for ventilator discontinuation, the following parameters must be considered:

   1. Underlying pathophysiology: The initial cause for respiratory failure should be either resolved or significantly improving.

   2. Hemodynamics: The patient's blood pressure and heart rate should be stable, with either stable or decreasing vasopressor needs and without serious cardiac instability.

   3. Oxygenation: Generally, an FIO_2 of 0.5 or less and PEEP of ≤ 8 indicate that any remaining hypoxemia will be able to be adequately corrected with supplemental oxygen noninvasively after extubation.

   4. Ventilation: The patient must be able to maintain a pH of 7.3 or higher, with a minute ventilation that they can maintain indefinitely without ventilator assistance.

   5. Miscellaneous parameters: There are several objective measures that assess selected parameters of a patient's readiness for ventilator weaning. At best, they provide marginal support to the above-discussed approach to ventilator weaning. When added to ventilator-weaning protocols, they prolong time to extubation without decreasing reintubation rates. As such, their utility in assessing a patient for extubation readiness is dubious.

     a. RSBI (Rapid Shallow Breathing Index): respiratory rate divided by tidal volume (in liters). RSBI >105 suggests increased risk for exubation failure.

     b. Cuff leak: assessed by the respiratory therapist. The ETT cuff is deflated, and the patient is evaluated for air leaking out of the mouth during inhalation. The presence of a cuff leak suggests that there is space between the ETT and the tracheal wall, implying that there is no airway edema. The lack of an air leak suggests that there may be airway edema. In reality, this parameter has just as much to do with tracheal size as it relates to ETT size. The positive and negative predictive value of a cuff leak are unconvincing.

1. **Caveat**: Patients intubated for angioedema or anaphylaxis will be assessed for a cuff leak prior to extubation. In general, the lack of a cuff leak will delay extubation, as airway edema was the initial reason for intubation.

VIII. **VENTILATOR MODES AND WEANING**: There is no evidence that any method of ventilator weaning is superior, nor is there evidence that gradual, step-wise decrease in ventilatory support leads to more success with ventilator liberation. Commonly used modes of weaning include the following:

A. Gradual weaning of **pressure support ventilation (PSV)**, until the patient is tolerating PSV 5/5

B. Gradually decreasing the respiratory rate for **spontaneous intermittent mandatory ventilation (SIMV)** so that the patient takes more unsupported breaths

C. Direct transition from **assist control ventilation** to PSV 5/5

D. A **daily SBT** of at least 30 minutes was found to be superior to gradual weaning of either SIMV or PSV, and leads to more ventilator-free days.

1. Most patients who tolerate an SBT of 30 minutes will tolerate subsequent extubation, with a few exceptions (see Noninvasive Positive Pressure Ventilation section below).

IX. **TECHNICAL APPROACHES TO THE SBT**: The specifics of SBT performance will depend on institutional practice. Below are some considerations to bear in mind.

A. All sedation should be discontinued. In select patients with agitation, low levels of sedatives may need to continue, but the patient should typically be alert, interactive, and able to follow commands.

B. Older ventilators did not compensate for the resistance of breathing through ventilator tubing, and so **T piece trials** and **tracheostomy collar trials** were often used as SBTs to account for this. Current ventilators have tube compensation programmed, so this is no longer a concern.

C. **Ventilator Settings**

1. **PSV 5/5**—The inspiratory pressure of 5 cmH$_2$O is thought not to alter the results of the SBT and may lead to greater patient comfort for select patients.

2. **PSV 0/0**—the most commonly used setting for SBT. Should be considered when a patient has known or suspected CHF, to ensure that the removal of all positive pressure will not lead to acute pulmonary edema.

D. **Duration of SBT**

1. Most SBTs last 30 minutes. Longer trials will be used for patients who are felt to be more tenuous on the basis of clinical information.

E. **How to Know When an SBT "Fails"**—there is no single marker of a failed SBT. Many clinical details are monitored simultaneously, and it is the constellation of clinical characteristics that leads to the overall assessment. If SBT failure is determined, the patient is returned to their previous ventilator settings and a search for the etiology of the failure is initiated.

1. **Uncontrolled agitation/anxiety**—Anxiety is a natural part of the extubation process, but the patient should be easily calmed and redirectable.

If the patient cannot be refocused, consider whether this is an indication of an underlying process that warrants correction prior to extubation.

2. **Vital sign instability**—The development of tachycardia, hypertension, diaphoresis, dyspnea, and/or tachypnea during an SBT suggests that the patient is not tolerating the additional work of breathing.

3. If a patient is going to fail an SBT, it often occurs within **the first few minutes** of the trial. Therefore, close attention needs to be paid to the patient, especially during this time period.

X. **FACTORS CONTRIBUTING TO A FAILED SBT:** When patients do not tolerate breathing on minimal ventilator support, a search for the contributing factors is initiated. In some instances, the reason for SBT failure may be closely related to the reason for intubation.

A. **Mental Status**—Depressed mental status, anxiety, agitation

1. If anxiety or agitation are the only barrier to extubation, *dexmedetomidine* may be considered as a sedative to facilitate SBT. It is a centrally acting anxiolytic (α_2 agonist) that does not suppress the respiratory drive.

B. **Respiratory Muscle Weakness**—The additional load on the diaphragm and intercostal muscles during an SBT may overwhelm a patient weakened by critical illness.

C. **Volume Status**—Pulmonary edema can cause hypoxemia and respiratory distress when positive pressure is removed.

D. **Tracheostomy Tube Malposition**—In patients for whom a tracheostomy has been placed, the immediate failure of an SBT raises concern for malposition. Obstruction by granulation tissue or the posterior membrane of the trachea may lead to respiratory failure when positive pressure is removed.

E. **Daily SBTs** are as efficacious as SBTs done multiple times daily. Unless the cause for the failed SBT is rapidly resolved, there is no evidence that doing multiple SBTs daily leads to quicker extubation.

XI. **EXTUBATION**—The removal of the endotracheal tube. Extubation is considered once the patient passes a spontaneous breathing trial. Around 10% to 20% of extubations will result in reintubation within the next 24 to 48 hours. Once a patient has passed an SBT as discussed previously, they are considered for extubation.

A. In order to be considered **appropriate for extubation**, the patient should be

1. awake and calm, able to follow simple commands

a. Caveat: In patients who are intubated for respiratory failure related to neurologic conditions, poor mental status has not been shown to predict extubation failure. If mental status is the only concern, the patient may still be considered for extubation.

2. requiring no continuous sedation infusions (or minimal sedation in select cases)

3. show evidence of a cough and gag reflex during suctioning or ETT manipulation

4. have minimal secretions that are easily managed by infrequent suctioning

B. **The Logistics:** The respiratory therapist and ICU nurse should be at the bedside. The patient is positioned upright and thorough suctioning of the oropharynx and through the ETT are completed. The ETT balloon is deflated (which then causes significant coughing), and the ETT is quickly removed. The patient is placed on 100% oxygen via face mask, which is decreased over the next 20 to 30 minutes as dictated by oxygen saturation. The patient is encouraged to cough initially and asked to say something in order to assess vocal cord function.

   1. **A raspy voice** is to be expected for the first day, but if it persists longer the patient will need to be evaluated for vocal cord dysfunction, a known complication of intubation.

 C. **Specific Considerations**
   1. **Upper airway edema:** a situation in which a cuff leak may be part of the assessment for extubation readiness. The lack of a cuff leak implies ongoing airway edema, although it may also relate to the relative size of the ETT and the trachea. It remains a poor predictor of extubation readiness.
      a. **Risk factors**—female gender, children, traumatic intubation, prolonged mechanical ventilation, and trauma
      b. If airway edema is of concern, administer IV steroids 12 hours prior to extubation for possible decreased airway edema.
      c. Consider arranging for an anesthesiologist to be present at bedside at the time of extubation, especially if there is report of a difficult intubation.
      d. If postextubation stridor develops, consider administration of epinephrine nebulizers, HeliOx, and/or an additional dose of IV steroids. CPAP may stent the airway open, allowing time for the above therapies to work, but is not a permanent solution.

XII. **EXTUBATION TO NONINVASIVE POSITIVE PRESSURE VENTILATION (NIPPV)**—In some patients deemed clinically ready for extubation, extubation to NIPPV may decrease rates of reintubation. In general, however, the need to extubate to NIPPV should make one reconsider whether extubation is appropriate.
   A. Consider patients who were intubated for COPD or CHF exacerbations for extubation to NIPPV.
   B. NIPPV should not be used as a rescue technique for patients who develop respiratory distress after extubation, as it delays necessary reintubation, and has been associated with increased mortality.

XIII. **PROLONGED MECHANICAL VENTILATION**
   A. **Definition**—at least 6 hours per day of mechanical ventilation for >21 consecutive days. The etiology of chronic respiratory failure is often multifactorial.
   B. **Outcomes**—In one single-center study of outcomes at 1 year: 74% of time either hospitalized, in postacute care, or receiving home care; <10% functionally independent; 65% either totally functionally dependent or dead.
   C. **Special Considerations**
      1. **Ventilator weaning**—Unless an obviously irreversible disease process is responsible for ventilator dependence (i.e., spinal cord injury, ALS), it can take several months to liberate these patients from mechanical ventilation.
         a. Daily SBTs are unlikely to be successful in this patient population due to the chronicity of disease.
         b. Protocols that focus on gradual decrements in ventilator support are appropriate, with SBTs of increasing duration reinstated once a predetermined amount of ventilatory support has been reached.
      2. **Multidisciplinary team approach**—These patients require close attention to adequate nutritional support, intensive physical therapy

to strengthen and prevent contractures, speech therapy to combat swallowing dysfunction, and palliative care for longer-term goals and discussions.

3. **Long-term weaning units**—Once patients are otherwise hemodynamically stable, specialized care in these units can accomplish all of the above goals. Regular care by physicians, nursing staff, and therapists is provided in a less-intensive manner than the hospital, which often leads to decreased health care costs.

4. Life-long mechanical ventilation may be necessary in some patients, for whom in-home ventilators can be arranged if ventilator settings are stable and they are not otherwise requiring inpatient monitoring.

D. **Tracheostomy**—When a patient fails ventilator weaning or requires reintubation, tracheostomy is considered for longer-term ventilation.

1. **Benefits**—patient comfort, facilitates talking, less sedation required, possibly quicker weaning from mechanical ventilation

2. **Timing**—The optimal timing of tracheostomy placement is debated. Traditionally, patients underwent tracheostomy after 14 days due to concerns over tracheomalacia related to ETT balloon cuff pressures and tracheal wall venous insufficiency. This is no longer a concern due to modern monitoring from respiratory therapists. Early (usually $<$1 week) versus late (usually $>$2 weeks) timing has not been shown to change ICU mortality, ventilator-free days, or length of stay.

XIV. **DECANNULATION**—the removal of the tracheostomy tube once the patient reliably no longer requires mechanical ventilation

A. **Readiness for Decannulation**—A patient should be considered for decannulation when

1. no longer requiring mechanical ventilation for $>$7 days

2. no respiratory distress with a capped tracheostomy and deflated cuff

   a. If respiratory distress prevents capping, the patient should be considered for downsizing of the tracheostomy to a smaller outer diameter. Generally, 7.0 or 8.0 tracheostomies are well tolerated.

   b. If respiratory distress occurs, visual inspection of regions above and below the tracheostomy via bronchoscopy should be conducted to evaluate for granulation tissue, strictures, vocal cord dysfunction, or other anatomic abnormalities that may be preventing independent breathing.

3. effective cough, able to clear secretions

4. no evidence of significant aspiration with a deflated cuff

B. **Approaches to Decannulation**—The stoma will epithelialize 48 to 72 hours after tracheostomy removal, impairing replacement should respiratory distress develop.

1. **Removal of tracheostomy**—can be accomplished for patients in whom chronic respiratory or other medical conditions are not present

2. **Sequential downsizing of tracheostomy**—performed in patients for whom chronic respiratory or other medical conditions raise concern for possible decannulation failure (i.e., COPD, neuromuscular diseases)

3. **Replacement of tracheostomy with a stomal button**—when access to the trachea for continued suctioning is desired

XV. **SUMMARY**—The care of intubated patients in intensive care units has drastically changed over the last 10 years, with improvements leading to decreased days on mechanical ventilation and increased success following extubation. Reducing the duration of mechanical ventilation improves ICU outcomes, which is the goal of all care providers in the intensive care unit.

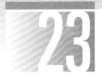

Acute Kidney Injury

William J. Sauer and Andrew L. Lundquist

I. DEFINITION

A. The RIFLE criteria (**R**isk, **I**njury, **F**ailure, **L**oss, and **E**SRD) were developed in 2004 to standardize the definition of acute kidney injury (AKI), formerly called acute renal failure (ARF). Prior to this, no consensus was available on the diagnosis or degree of severity.

1. Several modifications were introduced by the Acute Kidney Injury Network (AKIN) soon after, though the main addition with AKIN was a more inclusive Stage 1 ($\geq$0.3 mg/dL increase in Cr).

2. In 2012, the Kidney Disease Improving Global Outcomes (KDIGO) organization published clinical practice guidelines to create a unified definition with the goal to improve outcome staging and future clinical research (since RIFLE and AKIN did not completely coincide).

3. Although each of these (see Table 23.1) were created to help standardize clinical outcomes research, they are helpful when assessing severity of injury and level of management (Fig. 23.1).

4. **Serum creatinine criteria**: well validated, but discrepancies exist between various definitions (e.g., misclassification of AKI using AKIN with postsurgical ICU patients after cardiopulmonary bypass with significant positive fluid balance resulting in hemodilution).

5. Urine volume criteria are the same for all three (RIFLE/AKIN/KDIGO) but oftentimes it is less accurate (e.g., morbid obesity).

6. Validation studies are currently underway to establish the utility of these guidelines—particularly with regard to diagnosis and outcome.

II. EPIDEMIOLOGY

A. The historical lack of a standardized definition results in variable epidemiological data for AKI. Information bias and residual confounding (e.g., variability in baseline measures, the use of diagnostic code results), as well as ascertainment bias (AKI vs. CKD, which have different pathophysiologic processes and outcome data), results in differences in reported incidence and outcome measurements.

B. Even with the above definitions, studies demonstrate significant differences in the incidence of AKI in the ICU when comparing the same populations.

C. Nonetheless, AKI is common in both hospitalized (5%–20%) and critically ill (30%–40%) patient populations.

D. Higher level of severity in AKI classification (by any of the above definitions) is associated with adverse outcomes, including increased length of stay, progressive kidney disease, and mortality.

E. AKI is an independent risk factor for cardiovascular complications and mortality; AKI requiring renal-replacement therapy reveals an in-hospital mortality of 50% to 75%. Studies have revealed that up to 28% of surviving AKI patients died after discharge from the hospital (i.e., in-hospital mortality likely underestimates the significance of disease).

23.1 Classification of Acute Kidney Injury

	Serum Creatinine Criteria			Urine Output Criteria
	RIFLE	**AKIN**	**KDIGO**	
1—R	>1.5 × baseline or GFR decrease >25%	≥0.3 mg/dL increase or ≥1.5–2 × baseline	1.5–1.9 × baseline or >0.3 mg/dL increase (within 48 h)	<0.5 mL/kg/h for 6–12 h
2—I	>2 × baseline or GFR decrease >50%	>2–3 × baseline	2–2.9 × baseline	<0.5 mL/kg/h for 12 h
3—F	>3 × baseline or Cr >4 mg/dL with an acute rise >0.5 mg/dL	>3 × baseline or ≥4.0 mg/dL with acute increase of ≥0.5 mg/dL or initiation of RRT	3 × baseline or increase in serum Cr ≥4 mg/dL or initiation of RRT	<0.3 mL/kg/h for 24 h or anuria for 12 h
L	Loss of renal function >4 wk			
E	End-stage renal disease	← Outcome classes for RIFLE criteria		

AKI Stage

High risk | 1 | 2 | 3

Discontinue all nephrotoxic agents when possible
Ensure volume status and perfusion pressure
Consider functional hemodynamic monitoring
Monitor serum creatinine and urine output
Avoid hyperglycemia
Consider alternatives to radiocontrast procedures
Noninvasive diagnostic workup
Consider invasive diagnostic workup
Check for changes in drug dosing
Consider renal replacement therapy
Consider ICU admisssion
Avoid subclavian catheters if possible

FIGURE 23.1 Stage-based management of AKI. Shading of boxes indicates priority of action—solid shading indicates actions that are equally appropriate at all stages whereas graded shading indicates increasing priority as intensity increases. AKI, acute kidney injury; ICU, intensive-care unit. (From Kidney Disease: Improving Global Outcomes [KDIGO] Acute Kidney Injury Work Group. KDIGO clinical practice guideline for acute kidney injury. *Kidney Int Suppl* 2012;1(2):1–138.)

F. AKI patients often regain renal function with supportive therapy; however, studies have demonstrated more severe AKI, longer AKI duration, and numerous episodes of AKI are associated with progression to CKD and increasing morality. Future insults are much less well tolerated in these patient populations (e.g., additive effect of renal injuries over time).

III. ETIOLOGY AND PATHOPHYSIOLOGY

AKI is often caused by more than one etiology, but the pathophysiologic processes can be separated into three separate classifications: prerenal, intrinsic (or "renal"), and postrenal injuries. This is helpful both to determine the underlying etiology and for management (Table 23.2).

A. **Prerenal (Kidney Hypoperfusion)**
   1. **Decreased intravascular volume**
      a. Systemic vasodilation (e.g., sepsis). Sepsis is the most common cause of AKI in the ICU (approximately 50% can be attributed) and is associated with a very high mortality.
      b. Hypovolemia (e.g., hemorrhage, GI losses, burns)
      c. Hypotension, decreased cardiac output (CHF, arrhythmias)
      d. Small vessel (renal) vasoconstriction
         1. **Nonsteroidal anti-inflammatory drugs (NSAIDs):** Prostaglandins have important vasodilatory effects on the afferent arteriolar vessels. Cyclooxygenase inhibitors inhibit the production of prostaglandins, resulting in decreased renal blood flow.
         2. **ACEi/ARBs:** Angiotensin-II is a potent efferent arteriolar vasoconstrictor, and the inhibition of its production (ACE inhibitors) or the blockage of angiotensin receptors (ARBs) results in decreased glomerular perfusion pressure. This is of particular concern when the patient has other risk factors (chronic kidney disease, renal artery stenosis, older age) or exposures (diuretics, hypotension, NSAIDs, nephrotoxins).
         3. **Contrast:** IV contrast is both cytotoxic to renal tubular cells and causes intrarenal vasoconstriction.
         4. **Hypercalcemia:** directly causes vasoconstriction
         5. **Calcineurin inhibitors (CNIs):** Both cyclosporine and tacrolimus, which lead to afferent and efferent arteriolar vasoconstriction, are used as immunosuppressants for patients after renal transplant.
         6. **Hepatorenal syndrome (HRS):** Splanchnic and systemic vasodilation causes increased neuroendocrine (angiotensin, vasopressin) tone, resulting in renal vasoconstriction. Prognosis is very poor.
         7. **Intra-abdominal hypertension (IAH; IAP ≥12 mmHg) and abdominal compartment syndrome (ACS; IAP ≥20 mmHg with new organ failure):** The pathophysiology is likely a combination of (initially) intrarenal venous congestion/hypertension (normally a low-pressure system), followed by decreased cardiac output and elevated catecholamines, neurohormones, and cytokines (inflammation). Similar to cerebral perfusion pressure (CPP), abdominal perfusion pressure (APP) is a helpful marker of renal perfusion, where APP = MAP – IAP (typical target APP ≥60 mmHg).
         8. **Cardiorenal syndrome:** In addition to decreased cardiac output (acute CHF) resulting in decreased intravascular volume, other pathophysiological processes are likely involved. Mechanisms likely include a combination of venous congestion (elevated CVP) and visceral edema resulting in decreased abdominal perfusion

TABLE 23.2	Etiologies of Acute Kidney Injury in the Intensive Care Unit	
Prerenal	**Intrinsic Renal**	**Postrenal (Obstructive)**
Intravascular volume depletion • GI fluid loss (e.g., vomiting, diarrhea, EC fistula) • Renal fluid loss (e.g., diuretics) • Burns • Blood loss • Redistribution of fluid (e.g., "third-spacing," pancreatitis, cirrhosis)	Acute tubular necrosis • Ischemic • Toxin-induced • Drugs • IV contrast • Rhabdomyolysis • Massive hemolysis • Tumor lysis syndrome	Upper urinary tract obstruction • Nephrolithiasis • Hematoma • Aortic aneurysm • Neoplasm
Decreased renal perfusion pressure • Shock (e.g., sepsis) • Vasodilatory drugs • Preglomerular (afferent) arteriolar vasoconstriction • Postglomerular (efferent) arteriolar vasodilation	Acute interstitial nephritis • Drug-induced • Infection-related • Systemic diseases (e.g., SLE) • Malignancy	Lower urinary tract obstruction • Urethral stricture • Hematoma • Benign prostatic hypertrophy • Neurogenic bladder • Malpositioned urethral catheter • Neoplasm
Decreased cardiac output • Congestive heart failure • Myocardial ischemia	Acute glomerulonephritis • Postinfectious • Systemic vasculitis • TTP/HUS • Rapidly progressive GN Vascular • Atheroembolic disease • Renal artery or vein thrombosis • Renal artery dissection • Malignant hypertension Hepatorenal syndrome Increased intra-abdominal pressure	

GI, gastrointestinal; EC, enterocutaneous; IV, intravenous; SLE, systemic lupus erythematosus; TTP, thrombotic thrombocytopenic purpura; HUS, hemolytic uremic syndrome; GN, glomerulonephritis. Adapted with permission from Barozzi L, Valentino M et al. Renal ultrasonography in critically ill patients. *Crit Care Med* 2007;35(5 suppl):S198–S205 and Acute renal failure. In: Glassock RJ, ed. Nephrology self-assessment program (NephSAP), Vol. 2. Philadelphia: Lippincott Williams & Wilkins, 2003:42–43.

pressure (APP) and elevated neuroendocrine (angiotensin, vasopressin) hormones, resulting in decreased renal perfusion.

    e. Large-vessel etiologies

        1. Renal artery stenosis (RAS): This usually is in combination with other etiologies (e.g., ACE inhibitors, hypotension).

        2. Aortic or renal artery dissection (or compression)

        3. Thrombosis or embolism of the renal vessels

B. Intrinsic Renal Injury
   1. **Acute tubular necrosis (ATN)**
      a. **Ischemia (prerenal azotemia naturally progresses into ATN)**: This is the most significant cause of ATN in the intensive care unit.
      b. **Pigments (hemoglobin, myoglobin)**: Of note, rhabdomyolysis should be considered with CPK (creatinine phosphokinase) levels >5,000 units/L. This frequently results in hyperkalemia, hyperphosphate-mia, hyperuricemia, hypocalcemia, and acidosis. Injury is second-ary to direct tubular toxicity from cast formation, in addition to intrarenal vasoconstriction and hypovolemia (muscle inflamma-tion and third spacing). It is important to remember that CPK lev-els are a marker for muscle injury, and direct injury is caused by myoglobin.
      c. Warfarin-related nephropathy (WRN) is a recently described en-tity where an elevated INR (>3.0) places patients at risk for he-maturia and erythrocyte occlusion in Bowman's space and renal tubules (erythrocyte casts present on biopsy). Further investiga-tion is underway.
      d. **Drugs**
         1. **Aminoglycosides**, particularly at high doses, are toxic to proximal tubular cells. Once-daily dosing and vigilant dosing of medica-tions can prevent some but not all cases.
         2. **Amphotericin B** can cause AKI due to nephrotoxicity and vasocon-striction. It is also associated with the development of a distal RTA. Liposomal and colloid dispersion may decrease the inci-dence of severe AKI.
         3. **Vancomycin** has been shown to be associated with ATN; however, the incidence has decreased since the preparation has changed. Higher doses/levels may lead to increased incidence.
         4. **Hydroxylethyl starches (HES)** are associated with significant AKI, and increased mortality, when used in the critically ill patients with sepsis as a volume expander. Osmotic nephrosis is seen in the proximal tubules.
         5. **Contrast-induced AKI (CIAKI) or contrast-induced nephropathy (CIN)**: Contrast is both directly cytotoxic and decreases renal blood flow by vasoconstriction. This usually is in combination with hypovolemia/hypotension.
      e. **Proteins (immunoglobulin light chains—multiple myeloma)**: Notably, intravenous immunoglobulin (IVIG) therapy has been associated with proximal tubular osmotic nephrosis and possibly arterial vasoconstriction.
      f. **Crystals** (uric acid, acyclovir, methotrexate)
   2. **Acute interstitial nephritis (AIN)**
      a. **Allergic (drug-induced)**: The most common drugs include β-lactam antibiotics and sulfonamides. Others include NSAIDs, PPIs, fluoro-quinolones, vancomycin, and phenytoin.
      b. **Infection:** Bacterial and viral infections can lead to AIN by direct (py-elonephritis) and indirect (legionella) renal involvement.
      c. **Infiltrative/autoimmune:** Sarcoidosis, lupus, lymphoma/leukemia, and other systemic diseases can lead to interstitial inflammation.
   3. **Glomerulonephritis**
      a. **Intraglomerular inflammation with various timelines of progression and acuity of disease:** Progression can be acute or rapidly progressive and severe requiring early diagnosis. Pulmonary hemorrhage is a

rare but feared complication (can be seen with ANCA or anti-GBM disease). Typically classified on the basis of pathology, that is, pauci-immune (ANCA vasculitis), anti-GBM, and immune complex (postinfectious, IgA, lupus nephritis, membranoproliferative, cryoglobulinemia, etc.).

4. Small vessel disease
   a. Thrombosis: various pathophysiological processes including hemolytic uremic syndrome (HUS), thrombotic thrombocytopenic purpura (TTP), preeclampsia, antiphospholipid antibody syndrome (APLAS), polyarthritis nodosa (PAN), scleroderma, and disseminated intravascular coagulopathy (DIC)
   b. Cholesterol embolism

C. Postrenal (Obstruction and Hydronephrosis)
   1. Bilateral ureteral obstruction
      a. Malignancy (including lymphadenopathy), aneurysmal compression, nephrolithiasis, or retroperitoneal fibrosis or hematoma
   2. Bladder/urethral pathology
      a. Prostate enlargement (from benign prostatic hyperplasia or malignancy), Foley catheter or urethral obstruction, anticholinergic medications, and neurogenic bladder can all contribute to urinary obstruction and postrenal kidney dysfunction.

IV. EVALUATION
   A. History should focus on baseline kidney function, risk factors (see Sections V.A and V.B), including medications, comorbidities, and recent procedures or events.
   B. Physical examination to include vital signs and volume status (intravascular volume), bedside focused ultrasonography (e.g., inferior vena cava diameter), and signs/symptoms of vascular disease
   C. Renal Function Evaluation
      1. BUN (nonspecific; increased with gastrointestinal bleeding, steroids, high-protein tube feeds, hypermetabolism—especially with proteins)
      2. Serum creatinine (Cr; affected by muscle mass, amputation, drugs, and volume status)
      3. 24-hour creatinine clearance (can also check if more rapid results are desired)
      4. Urine output (not sensitive)
      5. Biomarkers of AKI (NGAL, KIM-1, cystatin C, etc.) might provide future early AKI diagnosis; however, prospective trials are necessary before these are clinically applicable.
      6. Urine evaluation (Table 23.3)
         a. Urinalysis and sediment
            1. Prerenal: bland urinalysis and (transparent) hyaline casts
            2. Intrinsic etiologies demonstrate:
               a. Granular (muddy brown) casts (ATN secondary to ischemia or nephrotoxic injuries) can also be seen in the setting of glomerular disease.
               b. Pigmented casts (ATN secondary to hemoglobin or myoglobin or with hyperbilirubinemia)
               c. RBC casts (glomerulonephritis)
               d. WBC casts (pyelonephritis, AIN, or glomerulonephritis)
               e. Urine eosinophils (AIN, cholesterol emboli, though not very sensitive or specific)
            3. Postrenal: bland urinalysis. RBCs with nephrolithiasis

TABLE 23.3 Diagnostic Studies and Indices of Urine

	Prerenal	Renal	Postrenal
Dipstick	0 or trace protein	Mild-moderate protein, hemoglobin, leukocytes	0 or trace protein, red and white cells
Sediment	Few hyaline casts	Granular and cellular casts[a]	Crystals and cellular casts possible
Serum BUN/Cr	20	10	10
Urine osmolality	>500	<350	<350
Urine sodium	<20	>30	
Urine/serum Cr	>40	<20	<20
Urine/serum urea	>8	<3	<3
FENa	<1%	>1%	>1%
FEUr	<35%	>50%	

FENa, fractional excretion of sodium = (urine Na/urine Cr) / (serum Na/serum Cr) %; Cr, creatinine; FEUr, fractional excretion of urea
[a]Composition of casts depends on cause of renal failure.
Adapted with permission from Thadhani R, Pasqual M, Bonventre JV. Acute renal failure. *N Engl J Med* 1996;334:1448–1460.

> **b. Indices** (electrolytes, osmolalities)
> 1. Prerenal injuries preserve renal salt and water balance mechanisms (initially), revealing FeNa <1% and FeUrea <35%; BUN/Cr >20, Uosm >500.
> 2. Intrinsic (e.g., ATN) renal injury disrupts such mechanisms resulting in FeNa >2% and FeUr >50%. Note that diuretic use will prevent FeNa from maintaining utility [FENa = (UNa / PNa) / (UCr / PCr)]; [FEUrea = (UUr / PUr) / (UCr / PCr)]. Note: FeNa may not be accurate in the setting of sepsis, CHF, cirrhosis, or pigment-induced injury.
>
> **7. Serologic testing** (primarily for glomerular etiologies): ANA, C3, C4, ANCA, anti-GBM, cryocrit, HCV, HBV, SPEP, serum-free light chains, urine Bence Jones proteins, PLA2R Ab (membranous nephropathy) (involve nephrology to assist with workup and to assess need for RRT)
> **8. Imaging studies**
> a. **Renal ultrasound:** can assess for hydronephrosis and estimate chronicity of kidney disease (small kidneys <10 cm suggest dysplasia or chronic disease). Color Doppler flow can evaluate perfusion and assess for thrombosis or renal artery stenosis (RAS).
> b. CT scan, pyelography, and angiography have select roles in specific, select circumstances.
> c. **MRI:** Patients with moderate-severe CKD **should not** receive gadolinium due to concern of **nephrogenic systemic fibrosis** (**NSF**), which results in skin and internal organ fibrosis with significant mortality.
> **9. Renal biopsy:** If above workup does not reveal the underlying etiology, biopsy may help evaluate intrinsic AKI.

V. RISK FACTORS: Risk factors can be divided into susceptibilities and exposures; this can be helpful when assessing who is most at risk of developing AKI (susceptible) and what can be minimized or avoided (exposures) to either (1) prevent or (2) minimize injury.

A. Susceptibilities
1. Advanced age (eGFR declines by ~1 mL/min/y/1.73 m^2 after age 30)
2. BMI >30
3. Chronic kidney disease
4. Diabetes mellitus
5. Sepsis/septic shock (very high risk)
6. Liver disease
7. Congestive heart failure
8. Lymphoma/leukemia
9. Low baseline creatinine (less muscle mass—suggested to be a surrogate marker of overall health and age)

B. Exposures
1. Nephrotoxic medications (see drugs listed in Section III)
2. ACEi, ARBs
3. NSAIDs
4. Chronic HTN + shock (see SEPSISPAM study in Section **VI**)
5. Prolonged arterial cross-clamp (aorta, renal artery)
6. Cardiopulmonary bypass
7. Emergent surgery
8. Blood product transfusion
9. IV contrast (CIN)—risk from contrast exposure may be dose dependent. Patients with hypovolemia are more susceptible to CIN.

VI. MANAGEMENT OF AKI (Fig. 23.1)
A. The management of AKI Stage I focuses primarily on (1) assessing and treating the etiology (see evaluation and risk factors), (2) removing and avoiding insults (see exposures above), (3) optimizing hemodynamics, and (4) managing complications. If AKI Stage 2 to 3 develops, (5) check for renal dosing of medications and (6) assess for renal replacement therapy.
B. Assessing and Treating Specific Etiologies
1. **Prerenal**
   a. Optimize hemodynamics and establish appropriate monitoring—including invasive monitors when appropriate.
   b. **Fluid resuscitation:** In general, crystalloid-based resuscitation with balanced salt solutions is preferred initially. In patients with septic shock and hypoalbuminemia, albumin supplementation may have an improved effect on mortality (the ALBIOS trial). Increasing evidence suggests that large volumes of chloride-containing fluids (such as normal saline) may be associated with worse renal outcomes, and perhaps even worse mortality. While these data need confirmation, it seems prudent to avoid the exclusive use of normal saline in most patients. Patients with traumatic brain injuries and other CNS lesions that need hyperosmolar therapy are an exception and will need normal saline-based resuscitation.
   c. **Managing blood pressure:** Clinicians often raise the mean arterial pressure (MAP) target from the conventional 65 to 75–80 mmHg in patients who have a history of chronic hypertension. The recent SEPSISPAM trial compared the use of elevated MAP goals with conventional goals in patients with septic shock and found that in a predefined cohort of patients with chronic hypertension, there was a decreased incidence of AKI and a decreased need for renal replacement therapies (but no mortality benefit) with higher MAPs.

However, targeting a higher MAP was also associated with an increased incidence of atrial fibrillation. The primary methods for increasing MAP (fluids vs. vasoactive drugs) probably effect outcomes and needs to be further investigated.

d. Diuretics, mannitol, and renal-dose dopamine have not demonstrated any outcome benefits (but diuretics may be used to manage volume in the setting of hypervolemia).

e. Hepato-renal syndrome: possible role for midodrine and octreotide as temporizing measures. Liver transplantation is the definitive therapy.

f. Intra-abdominal hypertension/abdominal compartment syndrome: Medical therapy includes deep anesthesia, neuromuscular blockade, paracentesis, nasogastric and rectal decompression, minimizing/correction of positive fluid balance (including ultrafiltration/hemodialysis), vasopressors (for APP >60 mmHg) but surgical decompressive laparotomy may be required.

g. Cardio renal syndrome: Focus should be on (1) optimizing cardiac output/perfusion and (2) decreasing venous congestion (judicious diuresis).

h. Renal artery stenosis: angiography and stent placement in selected circumstances (bilateral RAS with progressive AKI/CKD, refractory HTN, or recurrent pulmonary edema)

2. **Intrinsic renal injury**
   a. Acute tubular necrosis: Remove and avoid possible inciting agent(s)
   b. Acute interstitial nephropathy: Consider steroids if no improvement with removal of the offending agent.
   c. Contrast induced nephropathy
      1. **Prevention**
         a. Minimize number of contrast exposures. Use iso-osmolar and nonionic contrast.
         b. Hydration: Hydration with isotonic crystalloids is likely as efficacious as the use of bicarbonate drips.
         c. N-acetylcysteine (NAC): Some studies suggest the addition of NAC (600 or 1,200 mg PO twice daily for 2 days) plus hydration was superior to hydration alone for the prevention of CIN, while others have not shown a benefit. Given the low-risk profile of NAC, its use may be considered for CIN prophylaxis.
   d. Glomerulonephritis: Steroids and immunosuppressive therapies may have a role. Specialty consultation should be requested for the management of these patients.

3. **Postrenal**
   a. Relieve obstruction (e.g., ureteral stent placement, nephrostomy, Foley manipulation or placement) with close monitoring as complications can occur with rapid decompression (hemorrhagic cystitis) and hypotonic diuresis.

VII. **MANAGING COMPLICATIONS OF AKI:** Renal replacement therapy (RRT) may be required for the management of the complications of AKI (see Section VIII). RRT is usually initiated when more conservative measures have proven ineffective.
   A. Volume Overload
      1. Minimize fluid administration
      2. Diurese (when possible or responsive). Favor intravenous over oral loop diuretics. Use high-dose loop diuretics in the setting of oliguric AKI

(general rule: starting IV lasix dose $= 30 \times$ Cr, i.e., if Cr: 4, use 120 mg IV lasix). The combination of a thiazide diuretic (such as chlorothiazide or metolazone) and a loop diuretic may be used if a loop diuretic alone is ineffective. Diuretics have not been shown to have an outcome benefit in the setting of AKI, but their use may make management of volume status easier.

B. Metabolic Acidosis: Kidney injury can cause a mixed gap and nongap metabolic acidosis (see **Chapter 8**). Acidemia is generally not treated symptomatically unless it is severe (pH <7.15). Sodium bicarbonate infusions may be used for severe metabolic acidemia provided the resulting increase in CO_2 production can be offset by increased minute ventilation. See **Chapter 8** for details of symptomatic management of academia. The use of bicarbonate may be considered therapeutic if the primary reason for acidosis is renal bicarbonate wasting.

C. Electrolyte Abnormalities

1. **Hyperkalemia** (assess for EKG changes, though this is not a sensitive measure to predict subsequent arrhythmias—do not delay treatment of marked hyperkalemia because ECG changes have not yet appeared)

   a. **Antagonism of the effects of potassium (membrane stabilization)**

      1. **Calcium:** Calcium gluconate (or calcium chloride) acts as a physiologic antagonist of potassium at the cell membrane. 10 mL of a 10% calcium gluconate solution should be used initially. If calcium chloride is used instead, remember that it provides about three times the amount of calcium per volume compared with calcium gluconate.

   b. **Promoting an intracellular shift of potassium**

      1. **Insulin:** 10 units of **regular insulin IV** with an ampule of **50% dextrose** (in **normoglycemic** patients) is a typical initial dose. Takes 15 to 20 minutes to begin to take effect

      2. **β-Adrenergic agonists:** High-dose albuterol (10–20 mg, nebulized) has been shown to be effective in the treatment of hyperkalemia. The onset of effect is evident by 30 minutes, and lasts for up to 6 hours. Tachycardia may be dose limiting, although initial studies that used high-dose albuterol did not report significant tachycardia.

      3. **Increasing blood pH:** If pH <7.3, an ampule (50 mEq) of $NaHCO_3$ can be given IV. If possible (within limits of lung-protective ventilation) minute ventilation should be increased.

   c. **Removal of potassium from the body**

      1. **Renal replacement therapy:** See Section VIII.

      2. **Ion-exchange resins:** Kayexalate (sodium polystyrene sulfonate) can effectively remove potassium from the gut. However, it is not effective acutely—may require 12 to 24 hours for effect. In addition, there are multiple reports **of intestinal necrosis** with its use, and it should therefore be used with caution and should be avoided in the setting of altered bowel function. New potassium-binding agents will likely be available soon.

      3. **Loop diuretics** will decrease total body potassium and may be used as adjunctive therapy.

2. **Hyponatremia, hyperphosphatemia, and hypermagnesemia:** See **Chapter 8.**

D. Uremic Encephalopathy: Critically ill patients may have multiple competing reasons for becoming encephalopathic, and the presence of encephalopathy should prompt a detailed evaluation for other metabolic

derangements, infection, or drug toxicity (see **Chapter 29**). Uremic encephalopathy usually improves with RRT.

E. **Coagulation Abnormalities:** usually due to uremic platelet dysfunction. Management is discussed in **Chapter 24**.

F. **Anemia:** multifactorial etiology common. In the absence of active bleeding
or ongoing coronary ischemia, it is recommended that hemoglobin values
as low as 7 g/dL not be treated in critically ill patients (blood transfusion,
erythropoietin supplementation, and iron supplementation are all associated with risks in the critically ill).

G. **Infectious complications** are a major cause of death in patients with AKI.
Both uremia and renal replacement therapy (particularly continuous
RRT) blunt the ability of patients to mount an effective response to infec-
tions, and typical signs (such as fever) may be masked.

H. **Uremic pericarditis** occurs for unknown reasons and can lead to cardiac
tamponade. It is an indication for RRT.

I. **Decreased Drug Elimination:** Assess medications for renal clearance and
adjust doses accordingly. It should be kept in mind that in evolving AKI,
the calculated creatinine clearance may be inaccurate and typically an
overestimate.

J. **Nutritional support** is an important component of the management of critically ill patients with AKI—see **Chapter 11** for details.

VIII. **RENAL REPLACEMENT THERAPY (RRT):** Can be classified into intermittent or
continuous methods. Prototypical examples are intermittent hemodialysis (IHD) or continuous venovenous hemofilteration (CVVH), although
other modalities are occasionally used. IHD is used for hemodynamically
stable patients whereas CVVH may be more appropriate for patients who
are hemodynamically unstable, have intracranial hypertension, or are
encephalopathic secondary to cirrhosis. The choice between intermittent
versus continuous RRT is often based on institutional experience and culture.
Although continuous RRT intuitively seems to be preferable when dealing
with hemodynamically unstable, critically ill patients, the data do not support
a robust benefit for continuous RRT over intermittent modes. Although
several single-center trials revealed possible benefit of high-intensity CVVH,
multicenter RCTs have revealed no such results. In some countries, CVVH is
initiated and managed by critical care physicians, while in the United States
it is much more common for nephrologists to be responsible for managing
patients on CVVH. In either case, close communication between the ICU and
nephrology teams is essential for optimum management.

A. **Indications:** The classic indications for RRT initiation are listed below. Early
initiation of RRT in critically ill patients has been recommended by some
authorities—however, the data do not show improved outcomes for early
CVVH compared with conventional use.

1. **A**cidemia
2. **E**lectrolyte abnormalities (hyperkalemia, tumor lysis)
3. **I**ntoxication (lithium, methanol, salicylates, nephrotoxic medications)
4. **O**verload (volume)
5. **U**remia (if pericarditis, bleeding, or encephalopathy present)

B. **Intermittent Hemodialysis (IHD—Fig. 23.2A)**

1. Semipermeable membrane with countercurrent flow between blood
and a dialysate
2. Fluid removal driven by pressure gradient, solute removal by concentration gradient
3. **Complications:** hypotension, infection, arrhythmias

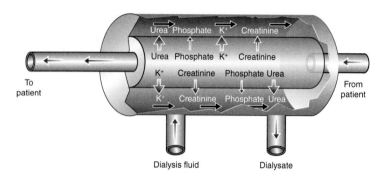

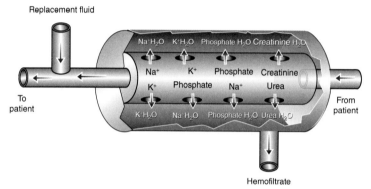

FIGURE 23.2 A: Hemodialysis achieves solute clearance by diffusion across a semipermeable membrane from a higher concentration (in patient's blood) to a lower concentration (in the dialysis fluid). **B:** Hemofiltration (which is the mechanism used in CVVH) achieves solute clearance by convection across a semipermeable membrane from a higher hydrostatic pressure (in a patient's blood) to a lower hydrostatic pressure (in the hemofiltrate). (Modified from Forni LG, Hilton PJ. Continuous hemofiltration in the treatment of acute renal failure. *N Engl J Med* 1997;336:1303–1309.)

C. **Continuous Venovenous Hemofiltration (CVVH—Fig. 23.2B)**
1. Pressurized blood flows next to highly permeable membrane
2. Fluid and solute removal via pressure gradient (convection)
3. Replacement fluid buffer required—either HCO_3 or citrate (provides local anticoagulation by binding calcium in the circuit. Subsequently metabolized by the liver to HCO_3. Use of citrate in patients with significant liver dysfunction can lead to life-threatening acidosis.)
4. Complications: Hypotension (much less common than with IHD), infection, citrate toxicity (in the setting of poor hepatic function), complications associated with anticoagulation (may be required with HCO_3)
D. **Access for RRT:** In the acute setting, double-lumen temporary hemodialysis catheters (14 Fr) are commonly used. The catheters are typically inserted percutaneously using the Seldinger technique and ultrasound guidance. The right internal jugular vein is the most frequent site of cannulation,

often preferred for optimal catheter function. However, a large, randomized study comparing internal jugular with femoral site insertions found that the rate of catheter colonization and bloodstream infection was equivalent between the jugular and femoral sites in **nonobese, bed-bound,** critically ill patients. The subclavian site is often avoided due to concerns for subclavian vein stenosis, which can limit future success of arteriovenous fistulas and grafts.

Selected Readings

Allegretti AS, Steele DJ, David-Kasdan JA, et al. Continuous renal replacement therapy outcomes in acute kidney injury and end-stage renal disease: a cohort study. *Crit Care* 2013;17:R109.

Asfar P, Meziani F, Hamel JF, et al. High versus low blood-pressure target in patients with septic shock. *N Engl J Med* 2014;370(17):1583–1593

Barrett BJ, Parfrey PS. Clinical practice. Preventing nephropathy induced by contrast medium. *N Engl J Med* 2006;354(4):379–386.

Bellomo R, Ronco C, Kellum JA, et al. Acute renal failure—definition, outcome measures, animal models, fluid therapy and information technology needs: the Second International Consensus Conference of the Acute Dialysis Quality Initiative (ADQI) Group. *Crit Care* 8(4):R204–R212.

Bosch X, Poch E, Grau JM. Rhabdomyolysis and acute kidney injury. *N Engl J Med* 2009;361(1):62–72.

Friedrich JO, Adhikari N, Herridge MS, et al. Meta-analysis: low-dose dopamine increases urine output but does not prevent renal dysfunction or death. *Ann Intern Med* 2005;142(7):510–524.

John S, Eckardt KU. Renal replacement strategies in the ICU. *Chest* 2007;132(4):1379–1388.

Kidney Disease: Improving Global Outcomes (KDIGO) Acute Kidney Injury Work Group. KDIGO Clinical Practice Guideline for acute kidney injury. *Kidney Int Suppl* 2012; 1(2):1–138.

Lameire N, Van Biesen W, Vanholder R. Acute renal failure. *Lancet* 2005;365(9457):417–430.

Mohmand H, Goldfarb S. Renal dysfunction associated with intra-abdominal hypertension and the abdominal compartment syndrome. *J Am Soc Nephrol* 2011;22(4):615–621

Okusa MD, Davenport A. Reading between the (guide)lines—the KDIGO practice guideline on acute kidney injury in the individual patient. *Kidney Int* 2014;85(1):39–48.

Parienti JJ, Thirion M, Megarbane B, et al. Femoral vs jugular venous catheterization and risk of nosocomial events in adults requiring acute renal replacement therapy: a randomized controlled trial. *JAMA* 2008;299(20):2413–2422

Pastan S, Bailey J. Dialysis therapy. *N Engl J Med* 1998; 338(20):1428–1437.

Schefold JC, Haehling S, Pschowski R, et al. The effect of continuous versus intermittent renal replacement therapy on the outcome of critically ill patients with acute renal failure (CONVINT): a prospective randomized controlled trial. *Crit Care.* 2014;18:R11.

Singri N, Ahya SN, Levin ML. Acute renal failure. *JAMA* 2003;289(6):747–751.

VA/NIH Acute Renal Failure Trial Network, et al. Intensity of renal support in critically ill patients with acute kidney injury. *N Engl J Med* 2008;359(1):7–20.

Zoungas S, Ninomiya T, Huxley R, et al. Systematic review: sodium bicarbonate treatment regimens for the prevention of contrast-induced nephropathy. *Ann Intern Med* 2009; 151(9):631–638.

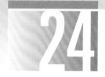

Critical Care of Patients with Liver Disease

Hovig V. Chitilian, Madhukar S. Patel, and Parsia A. Vagefi

I. **CIRRHOSIS**. Annually, more than 26,000 patients with cirrhosis are admitted to an ICU in the United States. Their in-hospital **mortality is more than 50%**. The most common reasons for ICU admission are **variceal hemorrhage, sepsis,** and **encephalopathy**.

   A. **Pathophysiology**. Chronic hepatic **fibrosis** leads to distortion of the hepatic vasculature, increased vascular resistance, and **elevated portal venous pressures**. Impaired hepatic function, coupled with elevated portal venous pressures, lead to end-stage liver disease and the systemic effects of cirrhosis: **encephalopathy, hyperdynamic circulation, renal dysfunction, ascites,** and **variceal hemorrhage**.

   B. **MELD** (Model for End-Stage Liver Disease) is a prognostic scoring system initially developed to predict survival in cirrhotic patients undergoing elective TIPS (transjugular intrahepatic portosystemic shunt) placement. It has been validated as a predictor for survival in patients with liver disease and is the basis for ranking patients on the liver transplantation wait list. **MELD = 9.57*ln[Cr] + 3.78*ln[total bilirubin] + 11.2* ln[INR] + 6.43.** The **Child-Turcotte-Pugh** (CTP) score was originally developed to predict surgical risk in cirrhotic patients. It is based on the concentrations of **total bilirubin** and serum **albumin** as well as the **INR**, degree of **ascites,** and degree of hepatic **encephalopathy**. The subjective components of the score limit its prognostic capacity. General ICU prognostic scores such as the **SOFA** (Sequential Organ Failure Assessment) and **APACHE** (Acute Physiology and Chronic Health Evaluation) scores have been shown to have greater discriminatory power for predicting mortality in cirrhotic patients who are admitted to the ICU.

   C. **Variceal Hemorrhage. Endotracheal intubation** for airway protection, **volume resuscitation,** and the administration of **blood component therapy** should be carried out as needed on the basis of the patient's condition and laboratory values. Standard therapy for acute variceal hemorrhage consists of the administration of a **splanchnic vasoconstrictor** and **prophylactic antibiotic** along with **endoscopic intervention**.

      1. **Splanchnic vasoconstrictors** reduce portal venous pressure and have been shown to be a useful adjunct to endoscopic therapy.

         a. **Octreotide**: 50-mcg IV bolus followed by 50 mcg/h infusion. Administered for 2 to 5 days. Bolus can be repeated in first hour if the hemorrhage remains uncontrolled. **Vasopressin, terlipressin, somatostatin,** and **octreotide** have been shown to be effective.

         b. **Terlipressin**: 2 mg IV every 4 hours for the first 48 hours, followed by 1 mg IV every 4 hours. Administered for 2 to 5 days.

         c. **Somatostatin**: 250-mcg bolus followed by infusion of 250 to 500 mcg/h. Administered for 2 to 5 days.

         d. **Vasopressin**: infusion of 0.2 to 0.4 units/min. Its efficacy is limited by side effects including cardiac and peripheral ischemia. It can only be used continuously at the highest effective dose for 24 hours. It should be accompanied by nitroglycerin administration to minimize the potential harmful effects of vasopressin.

2. **Prophylactic antibiotic** administration reduces the rate of **bacterial peritonitis** and **increases survival** in patients with cirrhosis and variceal hemorrhage.

   a. **Norfloxacin** 400 mg PO BID should be administered for 5 to 7 days. If oral administration is not possible, **ciprofloxacin** may be administered instead.

   b. **Ceftriaxone** 1 g/day IV for 5 to 7 days is recommended in patients with severe cirrhosis or high probability of quinolone-resistant organisms.

3. **Endoscopic variceal ligation.** Esophagogastroduodenoscopy (EGD) should be performed within 12 hours of admission. Variceal ligation is preferred to sclerotherapy.

4. **TIPS** (transjugular intrahepatic portosystemic shunt) is indicated for patients who have uncontrollable or recurrent variceal hemorrhage despite pharmacologic and endoscopic therapy.

D. **Spontaneous Bacterial Peritonitis (SBP)** is an infection of the ascites in the absence of a primary intra-abdominal focus. SBP accounts for 10% to 30% of bacterial infections in hospitalized cirrhotic patients. The in-hospital mortality for the first episode ranges from 10% to 50%.

1. **Diagnosis. As signs and symptoms may be absent,** diagnostic paracentesis should be performed for cirrhotic patients with ascites admitted to the hospital. The diagnosis is made on the basis of the presence of >250 polymorphonuclear cells (PMN)/mm^3 in ascites, in the absence of an intra-abdominal source of infection.

2. **Pathogenesis.** SBP is caused by the **pathologic translocation** of intestinal bacteria due to increased intestinal permeability, impaired immunity, and intestinal bacterial overgrowth in cirrhotic patients. Patients may also develop SBP following gastrointestinal hemorrhage or endoscopic procedures. In the majority of cases, enteric gram-negative bacteria are isolated from the ascites. Less frequently gram-positive cocci or anaerobes may be isolated. **Polymicrobial SBP is rare** and the presence of multiple bacteria in ascites may indicate bowel perforation.

3. **Management.** Empiric antibiotic therapy should be initiated immediately following the establishment of the diagnosis. Treatment consists of **Cefotaxime 2 g every 8 hours.** Alternatively, patients with SBP can be treated with **Ofloxacin 400 mg twice per day** in the absence of (a) prior exposure to quinolones, (b) shock, (c) grade II or more severe hepatic encephalopathy, and (d) serum creatinine >3 mg/dL. **Vancomycin** should be added if **MRSA** is suspected. Antibiotic therapy should be continued for 5 days. If PMN count doesn't decrease by 25% within 48 hours of initiating therapy, the antibiotic should be changed. Patients with a history of SBP or with esophageal hemorrhage should be treated prophylactically with **Norfloxacin.** Adjuvant therapy with **albumin** (1.5 g/kg on day 1 and 1 g/kg on day 3) may prevent worsening of renal function and improve survival in patients with cirrhosis and SBP.

E. **Hepatic Encephalopathy** develops in up to 50% of patients with cirrhosis and is associated with increased mortality. Up to 80% of episodes are precipitated by infection or gastrointestinal bleeding. The **pathophysiology** is thought to be due to the impairment of the hepatic clearance of cerebral toxins by the cirrhotic liver.

1. **Diagnosis** is made on the basis of the patient's symptoms and signs. The severity of symptoms determines the grade of encephalopathy

TABLE 24.1	Grades of Hepatic Encephalopathy

Grades of Encephalopathy

Grade 1: Shortened attention span; mild lack of awareness; impaired addition or subtraction; mild asterixis or tremor

Grade 2: Lethargic; disoriented; inappropriate behavior; obvious asterixis; slurred speech

Grade 3: Somnolent but arousable; gross disorientation; bizarre behavior; clonus; hyper reflexia

Grade 4: Comatose; decerebrate posturing

(see Table 24.1). Serum ammonia levels are elevated but do not correlate with the severity of the disease. Intracranial hypertension (ICH) is rare in patients with hepatic encephalopathy secondary to chronic liver disease unlike in the setting of ALF.

2. **Management** consists of identifying and treating **precipitating causes** and **lowering serum ammonia levels**. Patients who are at risk of aspiration will require intubation.

   a. **Precipitating causes** include GI hemorrhage, infection (SBP, UTI), hypovolemia, renal failure, hypoxia, sedative use, and hypoglycemia.

   b. **Lactulose** (β-galactosidofructose) and **lactitol** (β-galactosidosorbitol) are **first-line** therapeutic agents for hepatic encephalopathy. They are nonabsorbable disaccharides that decrease the absorption of ammonia from the GI tract. Lactulose should be administered at a dose of 20 to 30 g, 2 to 4 times each day, and titrated to achieve 2 to 3 soft stools daily. It can also be administered as an enema. Side effects include dehydration, hypokalemia, and hypernatremia. It is effective in 70% to 80% of patients.

   c. **Rifaximin** 400 mg po tid is added if there is no improvement after 48 hours.

   d. **Neomycin** has been associated with ototoxicity and nephrotoxicity. It is used in patients who are unresponsive to lactulose and intolerant of rifaximin. Oral vancomycin and oral metronidazole have also been used.

F. **Ascites** is the most common complication of cirrhosis leading to hospitalization. The presence of ascites is suspected on the basis of history and physical exam and confirmed by **abdominal ultrasound** (US) and **paracentesis**. Physical exam findings include bulging abdomen and **dullness to percussion** along the flanks. Approximately 1,500 mL of fluid must be present before flank dullness is detected.

1. **Differential diagnosis.** The most common etiology of ascites is cirrhosis and portal hypertension. Other potential causes include heart failure, cancer, nephrotic syndrome, and pancreatitis.

2. **Diagnostic paracentesis** should be performed on all patients presenting with ascites. The fluid should be analyzed for **cell count, differential, total protein,** and **albumin concentration. Serum ascites albumin gradient (SAAG)** is the difference between the serum albumin concentration and the ascites albumin concentration. Patients with **SAAG ≥1.1 g/dL** have ascites secondary to portal hypertension.

3. **Initial treatment** consists of **sodium restriction** (<2,000 mg/day) and **diuretic administration. Spironolactone** is started at 100 mg daily.

Furosemide may be added, starting at 40 mg per day. The doses of both diuretics can be increased every 3 to 5 days if weight loss is inadequate. Daily weight loss of 0.5 kg should be targeted. Plasma and urine electrolytes should be monitored frequently.

4. **Large-volume paracentesis** (>5 L) may be required in patients with tense ascites. The administration of **albumin** at a dose of 6 to 8 g/L is recommended following drainage of greater than 5 L of ascites.

5. **Refractory ascites** is defined as ascites that is unresponsive to a sodium-restricted diet and high-dose diuretic treatment (400 mg/day spironolactone and 160 mg/day furosemide) or which recurs rapidly following therapeutic paracentesis. **Midodrine** 7.5 mg tid may be added to the patient's diuretic regimen. It has been shown to increase urine sodium, mean arterial pressure, and survival. If possible, B-blockers may be discontinued. **Serial paracenteses, TIPS**, and **liver transplantation** are options for patients who remain refractory.

G. **Hepatorenal Syndrome** (HRS)

1. **Diagnostic criteria** are **cirrhosis with ascites, serum creatinine >1.5 mg/dL, no improvement of serum creatinine after** at least 2 days with **diuretic withdrawal** and **volume expansion** with albumin, **absence of shock, no recent exposure to nephrotoxins,** and **absence of parenchymal renal disease. Type I HRS** is rapidly progressive with a 50% reduction of renal function in 2 weeks. **Type II** has a slower course.

2. **Treatment** consists of the infusion of **albumin** (10–20 g/day) along with the administration of **octreotide** (200 mcg subcutaneously tid) and **midodrine** (titrated up to a maximum of 12.5 mg orally tid). Albumin infusion combined with **norepinephrine** infusion may also be used. **Hemodialysis** (HD) or **continuous venovenous hemoconcentration** (CVVH) can be used to maintain volume and electrolyte balance. Ultimately, patients with Type I or Type II HRS will require **liver transplantation**. Patients with HRS who have been **dialyzed for greater than 6 to 8 weeks,** may require a **combined liver–kidney transplantation.**

H. **Hepatic Hydrothorax** is a large pleural effusion that occurs in patients with cirrhosis and ascites. It is usually **right sided. Treatment** consists of **sodium restriction** and **diuretic administration.** Therapeutic **thoracentesis** should be performed for dyspnea. Chest tube insertion is **contraindicated** in patients with hepatic hydrothorax. **TIPS** should be considered for refractory hepatic hydrothorax.

I. **Hepatopulmonary Syndrome** (HPS) can be found in 10% to 30% of patients with cirrhosis. It is due to pulmonary vasodilation and arteriovenous shunting, giving rise to hypoxia.

1. **Signs and symptoms** may include shortness of breath, cyanosis, clubbing, platypnea, and orthodeoxia.

2. **Diagnosis** is based on the presence of **liver disease**, an **A-a gradient ≥15 mmHg** (≥20 mmHg if age is >64), and the demonstration of **intrapulmonary shunting** by contrast echocardiography or radiolabeled macroaggregated albumin.

3. **Management.** In the absence of OLTx, the 5-year survival is 23%. Most patients with PaO_2 <60 mmHg die within 6 months. There is no effective medical therapy for HPS. Intra-arterial coil embolization of pulmonary arteriovenous fistulae has been shown to improve hypoxia. OLTx is the only effective treatment for HPS.

J. **Portopulmonary Hypertension** (PoPH) is found in approximately 6% of candidates for liver transplantation. It is defined as **mean pulmonary artery pressure (mPAP) >25 mmHg** in the setting of a **pulmonary artery occlusion** pressure **(PAOP)** <15 mmHg and **pulmonary vascular resistance (PVR)** >240 dyn·s·cm^{-5} in a patient with portal hypertension.

Liver transplantation in a patient with PoPH and an mPAP >35 mmHg is associated with significant mortality. Screening for PoPH is conducted with TTE. In patients with an estimated right ventricular systolic pressure (RVSP) >40 to 50 mmHg, right heart catheterization (RHC) is conducted to confirm the diagnosis of PoPH. Patients with PoPH are treated with pulmonary vasodilators to reduce the mPAP below 35 mmHg. Therapeutic options include **sildenafil** (phosphodiesterase inhibitor), **bosentan** (endothelin receptor antagonist), and **epoprostenol** (intravenous prostacyclin). **Nitric oxide** may be used in intubated patients. Patients with mPAP <35 mmHg on pulmonary vasodilator therapy are candidates for liver transplantation as long as right ventricular function is preserved and PVR is <400 dyn·s·cm^{-5}.

II. **ACUTE LIVER FAILURE (ALF)** has an incidence of **less than 10 cases per million persons per year.** It most commonly occurs in **previously healthy adults** and presents with hepatic dysfunction, coagulopathy, and encephalopathy. It is associated with a **mortality of up to 50%.** The condition of ALF patients may deteriorate rapidly; thus, early contact with a transplantation center should be made to evaluate for suitability to transfer.

A. **Definition.** ALF is defined as an **INR ≥1.5** and **encephalopathy** in a patient with **no preexisting history of cirrhosis** and an **illness duration of <26 weeks.** Based on the time interval between the onset of jaundice and encephalopathy, ALF can be categorized as **hyperacute** (<1 week), **acute** (1–4 weeks), or **subacute** (4–12 weeks). **Hyperacute** cases are typically due to **acetaminophen toxicity** (in developed countries) or **viral infection** (in developing countries).

B. **Causes.** The most common causes are **drug-induced hepatotoxicity, viral hepatitis, autoimmune hepatitis,** and **shock.** Approximately, 15% of cases have no identifiable cause.

C. **Initial evaluation** should include a **history** focused on potential viral or toxin exposures as well as evidence of prior liver disease. In Western countries, the most common cause is acetaminophen-induced hepatotoxicity. Consumption in excess of 10 g/day or 150 mg/kg is associated with toxicity. Severe liver injury can occur with doses as low as 3 g/day. **Physical examination** should focus on the determination of the degree of encephalopathy as well as the presence of stigmata of chronic liver disease. **Laboratory analysis** should include chemistries, complete blood count, coagulation profiles, and arterial blood gas analysis. Serum glucose should be monitored as patients may develop hypoglycemia. Viral serologies as well as screens for acetaminophen and other toxins should be obtained. Laboratory studies should also be obtained for Wilson's disease and autoantibodies.

D. **Management.** The condition of a patient with ALF can deteriorate rapidly. It is essential to consult a liver transplantation service as soon as possible to determine the appropriateness of listing the patient for transplantation. For most etiologies of ALF, management is supportive (Table 24.2).
1. **Acetaminophen-induced hepatotoxicity**
   a. **Activated charcoal** slurry at a dose of 1 mg/kg should be administered orally if ingestion is suspected to have occurred within a few hours of presentation.
   b. **N-acetylcysteine** is the antidote for acetaminophen poisoning. It should be administered at a dose of 150 mg/kg over 15 min, followed by an infusion or 50 mg/kg over 4 hours, and then 6 mg/kg/h for 16 hours.

| TABLE 24.2 | King's College Criteria for Liver Transplantation |

I. ALF due to acetaminophen toxicity:

   a. pH <7.3 or arterial serum lactate >3.0 mmol/L

OR:

   b. ALL three following conditions occur within a 24-hour period:
      i. Presence of grade 3 or 4 hepatic encephalopathy
      ii. INR >6.5
      iii. Serum creatinine >3.4 mg/dL

II. ALF due to other etiologies

   a. INR >6.5 and encephalopathy present (irrespective of grade)

OR:

   b. ANY three of the following conditions are present:
      i. Age <10 or >40 years
      ii. Jaundice >7 days before development of encephalopathy
      iii. INR ≥3.5
      iv. Serum bilirubin ≥17 mg/dL
      v. Unfavorable etiology such as:
         a. Wilson disease
         b. Idiosyncratic drug reaction
         c. Seronegative hepatitis

2. **Acute Hepatitis B**-associated acute liver failure may respond to **lamivudine**.
3. **Encephalopathy** can be categorized into four grades **(Table 24.1)**. Patients should be monitored for worsening of encephalopathy and signs of intracranial hypertension (ICH) such as changes in pupillary reactivity and posturing. Patients with Grade I or II encephalopathy should be treated with oral or rectal **lactulose** (30–45 mL administered 3–4 times per day to produce 2–3 soft stools daily). Patients with Grade III or IV encephalopathy should be intubated for airway protection.
4. **Cerebral edema and intracranial hypertension** are the most serious complications of ALF. The pathogenesis is not completely understood but involves elevations in the serum ammonia concentration. Intracranial pressure (ICP) monitoring is controversial due to coagulopathy and the risk of intracranial hemorrhage as well as questionable mortality benefit. In the presence of an ICP monitor, ICP should be maintained below 20 mmHg. Cerebral perfusion pressure (CPP) should be maintained above 50 to 60 mmHg. A number of interventions can be used to reduce ICP.
   a. **Mannitol** 0.5–1 g/kg IV gives rise to an osmotic diuresis and reduction in ICP. The dose may be repeated as long as serum osmolality is below 320 mOsm/L.
   b. **Hypertonic saline.** Infusion of hypertonic (3%) saline to maintain a serum sodium of 145 to 155 mEq/L can be used to decrease ICP.
   c. **Hyperventilation** to a $PaCO_2$ of 25 to 30 mmHg can be used to acutely reduce ICP in patients who are unresponsive to mannitol and hypertonic saline. The effect is short lived.

    d. Barbiturate administration may be considered in patients with elevated ICP that is unresponsive to other interventions.

  5. Hypotension in ALF is due to **depleted intravascular volume** coupled with **reduced systemic vascular resistance**. Patients should be volume resuscitated with normal saline. Patients who do not respond to a volume challenge should be treated with vasopressors. **Norepinephrine** is considered a first-line agent. **Vasopressin** may be added in patients who are unresponsive to norepinephrine.

  6. Renal failure is a common complication in patients with ALF. Efforts should be made to maintain mean arterial pressure (MAP) and intravascular blood volume. Nephrotoxic agents should be avoided. **Continuous renal replacement therapy** should be instituted if hemodialysis is required to preserve cardiovascular stability.

  7. Coagulopathy and thrombocytopenia should be corrected only in the presence of hemorrhage or prior to an invasive procedure.

E. Outcomes. The cause of ALF is a significant predictor of mortality. ALF secondary to acetaminophen toxicity, hepatitis A, or shock liver is associated with a >50% transplant-free survival. ALF due to other etiologies is associated with a significantly worse transplant-free survival.

F. Liver Transplantation. Orthotopic liver transplantation (OLTx) may be an option for therapy in ALF. Early consultation with the liver transplant (LT) surgical team should be carried out to determine the suitability of the patient. **The King's College Hospital Criteria** were developed to identify patients with ALF who would benefit from OLTx. They are based on the etiology of ALF as well as clinical characteristics of the patient. They have been found to have a sensitivity and specificity of 69% and 82% to 92%, respectively. A number of studies have shown positive predictive values of 70% to 100% and negative predictive values of 25% to 94%. **OLTx is contraindicated** in patients with hemodynamic instability requiring vasopressors, known malignancy outside of the liver, and advanced age.

III. POSTOPERATIVE MANAGEMENT OF THE LT PATIENT

A. Overview. The success of LT is dependent on a true multidisciplinary effort between all involved in the patient's care. As there can be significant variation between transplant programs in terms of types of donors utilized and the severity of illness within the waitlist candidate population, there are often center-specific practices for postoperative management of an LT recipient. Thus, overall, it is of paramount importance that there be an open line of communication at all times, with a primary point of contact established between the critical care team and the transplant service in advance in order to expedite decision making and care of this patient population.

B. Survival Rates. Current estimates of the 1-year unadjusted survival rate for an LT recipient are nearly 90%.

C. Donor Factors. Consideration must be given to donor factors that influence graft function in the immediate postoperative period. Given the disparity in organ supply and demand, there has been increased application of expanded criteria donors (ECD). Indeed, the use of certain ECD liver grafts may result in slower initial graft function and/or portend a higher risk of primary nonfunction or vascular/biliary complications. Although the definition of these more marginal grafts may vary based on institution, they are generally thought to encompass donors of advanced age (>60 years old), higher degree of steatosis (>30% macrosteatosis), donation after cardiac death (vs. donation after brain death), and split LTs. Additional donor factors to consider as they relate to immediate graft function are donor instability prior to procurement, cold ischemia time, and warm ischemia time.

D. Intraoperative Factors. Sign-out from the anesthesia and surgical team should include occurrence of hypotension, vasopressor use, degree of acidosis, urine output, intraoperative bile production, and technical concerns that may affect outcome.

E. Systems-based Considerations for Postoperative Management. The majority of LT patients are admitted to the Intensive Care Unit (ICU) in the initial postoperative period for a typical 24-to-48-hour stay.

1. Neurological

a. Analgesia. Poor pain control can lead to prolonged recovery and increased pulmonary complications.

1. Delivery route. Patient-controlled analgesia or intravenous drips/boluses are reasonable alternatives until an enteral route can be used. Epidural catheter placement is avoided given risk of bleeding post-LT from resolving coagulopathy.

2. Analgesics. As the majority of analgesics are metabolized and excreted by the liver or the kidney, poor liver graft function or concomitant renal failure may impact clearance of these medications.

a. Paracetamol (acetaminophen) can be used safely at reduced dosing or in combination therapy for mild to moderate postoperative pain.

b. Nonsteroidal anti-inflammatories are typically avoided due to potential effects on coagulation and renal function.

c. Morphine use has been shown to lead to increased sedation in patients undergoing liver surgery.

d. Hydromorphone and fentanyl are alternative opioids that are less affected by renal impairment and are reasonable alternatives to morphine use. Tramadol has also been used safely to provide post-LT analgesia.

b. Mental status. It should be noted that although hepatic synthetic function often recovers quickly following implantation of the liver, encephalopathy can linger in the postoperative period necessitating standard precautions for patients with alterations in mental status. With any change in mental status, in addition to routine workup, attention should be paid to reevaluation of graft function as well as electrolyte and glucose levels, which may be directly affected by hepatic function. Antipsychotics should be avoided if possible as they are often hepatotoxic; however, if needed, low-dose haldol or quetiapine may be used.

2. Cardiovascular

a. Preoperative baseline. Preoperative cardiovascular testing is uniformly used for the waitlisted population, but may vary in type depending on institutional preference. Cardiovascular testing should be reviewed in all patients in whom it was performed. Special consideration should be given to those with known coronary artery disease, a history of nonalcoholic steatohepatitis and diabetes, valvular stenosis or insufficiency, and known portopulmonary hypertension (see I.J. above).

b. Perioperative hypotension may result postoperatively given the risk for bleeding, as well as the fact that vasodilatory and hyperdynamic state of liver failure often takes times to resolve post-LT. Unremitting acidosis or vasopressor requirement should warrant further investigation.

  c. **Venous pressures.** Increased venous pressures may lead to hepatic congestion and graft dysfunction due to outflow obstruction. Invasive monitoring can help distinguish cardiac from vasodilatory hypotension and guide appropriate use of inotropic agents, vasopressors, and fluid administration (see II.E.5.a below).

  d. **Perioperative hypertension** may be seen in the post-LT patient with adequate graft function who may have inadequate analgesia.

  e. **Atrial fibrillation.** Post-LT atrial fibrillation may result due to significant perioperative fluid shifts and electrolyte fluxes. If possible, it should be managed without the use of amiodarone due to this medications potential for hepatotoxicity.

3. **Respiratory**
  a. **Weaning and extubation.** Early weaning and extubation from the ventilator is recommended in post-LT patients in order to decrease risk of infection, deconditioning, and prolonged recovery. Care should be taken for those patients with hepatopulmonary syndrome (HPS), as the hypoxemic state can persist in the postoperative period (see I.I. above and II.E.3.c. below).

  b. **Ventilator management.** In optimizing ventilator settings, given theoretical risks of decreased venous return and hepatic outflow, positive end-expiratory pressure (PEEP) should be limited up to 15 cm of H_2O, which has been shown to not impair overall hemodynamics in the post-LT patient.

  c. **HPS.** The postoperative management of the patient with HPS is difficult, as the timing of resolution of hypoxemia is variable and can take up to 12 months to return to baseline. A lowered expectation of a resting O_2 saturation is needed in the postoperative period. Extubation of the HPS patient postoperatively should be undertaken after careful assessment of the patient. The clinical decompensation of the HPS patient postextubation can be rapid and unexpected. Thus, preparedness for reintubation or noninvasive positive pressure ventilation (NIPPV) is paramount in the management of these complex patients.

  d. **Hypoxemia.** Other etiologies for post-LT hypoxemia include the presence of ascites, atelectasis, and pleural effusion, causing restrictive lung disease. All patients should be optimized with adequate analgesia, rigorous chest physiotherapy, and incentive spirometry. Thoracentesis may be considered for a hydrothorax-limiting extubation, but should be approached with caution given the coagulopathy and thrombocytopenia in the immediate postoperative period. Placement of an indwelling chest tube is avoided given the infectious risk.

4. **Gastrointestinal**
  a. **Liver function tests.** There is a typical rise in transaminase levels due to hepatocellular ischemia/reperfusion injury often peaking within 24 hours. Persistent rise, however, may indicate ongoing ischemia. Laboratory abnormalities should be communicated with the surgeon as they may prompt further investigation with Doppler US. Alkaline phosphatase and bilirubin rise may indicate biliary obstruction.

  b. **Synthetic function laboratory tests.** Platelet count, prothrombin international normalized ratio (INR), fibrinogen level, and activate partial thromboplastin times (aPTT) are markers of coagulation, and abnormalities may reflect insufficient liver synthetic function.

Please see below for additional hematologic considerations (see II.E.7 below).

c. **Graft US with Doppler.** A hepatic graft US with Doppler can evaluate the patency of the vasculature and biliary system.

5. **Genitourinary**

a. **Fluids.** Excessive fluid administration to decrease the pressor requirement, generate urine output, or decrease an elevated creatinine should not be attempted in the setting of a normal CVP and normal cardiac output as this may lead to venous congestion and graft dysfunction. Non–lactate-containing solutions may be beneficial in those patients with rising lactate levels secondary to decreased consumption of lactate due to decreased liver gluconeogenesis in the transplanted graft. Thus, generally, 5% dextrose with 0.45% normal saline is used unless the recipient has a serum sodium of <130 mEq/L at which point 5% dextrose with 0.9% normal saline may be more appropriate. If volume expansion is needed, colloid solutions, or if indicated, packed red blood cells should be considered.

b. **Pretransplant renal dysfunction.** Present in up to 25% of recipients. If renal replacement therapy is needed in the immediate postoperative period, CVVH is the preferred route. Reinstitution of standard hemodialysis posttransplant should not be attempted until the patient has been stabilized. Transplant nephrology is often consulted to aid in the management of dialysis, as well as any electrolyte abnormalities related to renal dysfunction. As fresh LT patients will not metabolize citrate in the setting of liver dysfunction, dialysis replacement fluid should be bicarbonate based in most cases. Even in patients without renal dysfunction prior to LT, some degree of acute kidney injury (AKI) can be observed postoperatively depending on the duration of vena caval clamping, degree of ischemia/reperfusion injury, and presence of hemodynamic instability during the operation. Given the varying degrees of AKI observed with concomitant oliguria or anuria, assessment of intravascular status by CVP measurement will allow avoidance of over- or underresuscitation.

c. **Electrolytes.** Abnormalities should be appropriately addressed promptly.

1. **Hyponatremia**—Sodium should be corrected carefully keeping in consideration that the post-LT patient should be kept euvolemic or marginally hypovolemic in the early postoperative period.

2. **Hypocalcemia**—Calcium should be optimized as it is an important element in the coagulation cascade, which may already be challenged in the early post-LT period.

3. **Hypophosphatemia.** Phosphate is important in cellular energy metabolism, and deficiency can have respiratory, cardiac, neurologic, and endocrine system consequences.

4. **Hypomagnesemia.** Cirrhotic patients often have decreased magnesium, which is often further depleted through operative blood loss as well as certain immunosuppressants (i.e., tacrolimus).

6. **Endocrine**

a. **Glucose levels.** Hyperglycemia may be present due to postsurgical stress and use of steroid therapy for immunosuppression. This should be managed using ICU protocols and may require insulin drips with minimization of dextrose-containing fluids. If hypoglycemia is noted, graft US with Doppler should be performed as this may be indicative of graft dysfunction.

7. **Hematologic**
   a. **Monitoring.** In the early post-LT period (first 24–48 hours), patients should receive serial complete blood count tests and coagulation labs to assess for bleeding and hepatic synthetic function. Any significant changes should prompt notification of the transplant team, and triggers for transfusion should be clarified for each patient.
      1. **General Considerations**
         a. A gradual decline of the INR should be expected with a functioning liver and should not require further fresh frozen plasma (FFP), thus a rising INR should prompt concern for early graft dysfunction and consideration for repeat Doppler US and notification of the transplant team.
         b. More aggressive correction of an INR with FFP should be undertaken in the setting of continued drops in the hematocrit.
         c. Cirrhotic patients can often demonstrate a significant degree of thrombocytopenia due to splenomegaly and sequestration, which is only exacerbated by the immunosuppressive and antiviral/-biotic medications administered. Consideration for administration of platelets should be given for platelet counts <50 for the first 12 hours postoperatively and should be continued beyond 12 hours only if clinical signs of bleeding exist. The latter must be balanced with the understanding that a numerical increase in peripheral platelet counts with continued platelet transfusions will be small and unlikely to be sustained in the setting of splenomegaly.
         d. Consideration for desmopressin acetate (ddAVP) should be given if there is preexisting renal disease.
         e. Cryoprecipitate can be considered for fibrinogen levels <100.
         f. If bleeding persists, consideration for use of ε-aminocaproic acid (amicar) can be considered after discussion with the transplant team, as the management of bleeding must be balanced with the risk of graft thrombosis.

8. **Infectious Disease**
   a. **Bacterial prophylaxis.** Standard perioperative antibacterial prophylaxis is utilized, with consideration for organism-specific antibiotics of longer duration if the recipient has an infectious history or if the donor carries an infectious history.
   b. **Viral prophylaxis.** Herpes simplex virus (HSV) reactivation is the most common opportunistic viral infection in the immediate posttransplant period (first month) and can be reduced by prophylactic antiviral administration. Additional considerations include mismatch of cytomegalovirus (CMV)-seronegative recipients with grafts from CMV-seropositive donors as these patients benefit from antiviral therapy. In patients for lower risk of CMV, antiviral administration can be pursued, or alternatively, monitoring by CMV polymerase change reaction can be done and therapy instituted if the virus is detected.
   c. **Fungal prophylaxis.** *Pneumocystis jirovecii* infection can be prevented by routine use of prophylactic trimethoprim-sulfamethoxazole post-LT. Additional widespread use of antifungal prophylaxis is not standard practice; however, special consideration should be given to patients requiring retransplantation, reoperation, renal replacement therapy pre- or posttransplant, and those receiving transplant for fulminant hepatic failure.

9. **Nutrition.** Enteral nutrition is preferred to the parenteral route as it is associated with a lower incidence of wound infections and complications and should be started as soon as possible postoperatively. Early enteric feeding aids in nourishing enterocytes and thus decreasing bacterial translocation in addition to stimulating enterohepatic circulation. Validated data on the use of probiotics in this patient population is lacking. Special consideration for nasal gastric or nasal jejunal tube feeds should be given for those patients with prolonged intubation or with encephalopathy and at risk for aspiration.

10. **Immunosupression.** Immunosupressive medications will be managed by the transplant team, and typical regimens include triple therapy with a calcineurin inhibitor such as tacrolimus or cyclosporine, an antiproliferative agent such as mycophenolate mofetil, and a steroid such as prednisone.

    a. **Calcineurin inhibitors (tacrolimus or cyclosporine)**—weight based, usually started at a low dose and increased, trough levels needed every morning. Common side effects include nephrotoxicity and mental status changes.

    b. **Antiproliferative agent (mycophenolate mofetil)**—no levels needed. Common side effects include thrombocytopenia and GI upset.

    c. **Steroid (prednisone)**—varying regimens depending on cause of liver disease. Steroids are tapered and no levels checked. Common side effects include altered mental status and hyperglycemia.

11. **Tube/Lines/Drains**

    a. **Surgical intra-abdominal drains.** Decisions on management of surgical drains are made by the surgical team and are dependent on the volume and type of fluid draining. Any significant change in drainage (such as increasing bilious drainage or bloody drainage) should be immediately communicated to the surgical team. Patients with long-standing portal hypertension and ascites prior to transplant will often have high serous output from the surgical drains until the portal hypertension begins to resolve.

    b. **Nasogastric tube (NGT).** The standard LT patient should have NGT removal once they are alert, awake, and able to take their medications orally. Patients with roux-en-y creation for biliary drainage will often have an NGT in the postoperative period.

    c. **Foley catheter.** Although stable patients can have their foley removed on postoperative day 2 in order to decrease the risk of catheter-associated urinary tract infection, complex or debilitated patients or those with renal dysfunction may require bladder drainage for longer periods of time.

    d. **Endotracheal tube (ETT) and invasive vascular lines.** ETT and invasive vascular lines should be removed as soon as clinically indicated in order to decrease risk of ventilator-associated pneumonia (see II.F.4.b) and central line–associated blood stream infection.

12. **Prophylaxis**

    a. **Thromboprophylaxis.** Definitive data on the use of routine prophylactic chemoprophylaxis for deep venous thrombosis or pulmonary embolism is currently lacking; however, mechanical thromboprophylaxis is often employed. Post-LT patients are often thought to be in a hypocoagulable state since coagulation may take time to normalize as it takes the new liver time to make sufficient coagulation factors and for thrombocytopenia to resolve.

    b. **Stress ulcer prophylaxis.** Stress ulcer prophylaxis should be utilized, especially in the setting of high-dose steroid use and should be instituted per ICU protocol.

F. Postoperative Complications after Liver Transplantation

1. **Primary nonfunction (PNF).** PNF is the most devastating complication post-LT and is defined as an aspartate aminotransferase (AST) $\geq$3,000 U/mL and either an INR $\geq$2.5 and/or evidence of acidosis (arterial pH $\leq$7.3 or a venous pH of 7.25 and/or a lactate level $\geq$4 mmol/L) within 7 days of transplantation. The etiology of PNF is often multifactorial, and the only therapy for PNF is retransplantation, with the majority of patients not surviving past 5 days after initial LT.

2. **Vascular complications**

   a. **Hepatic artery thrombosis (HAT) or stenosis.** HAT occurs in approximately 3% of post-LT patients and is the most common technical complication. Early HAT (within 1 week of LT) may clinically result in rapid onset hepatic failure, sepsis, fever, altered mental status, and coagulopathy with laboratory studies suggestive of transaminitis. Delayed diagnosis can result in peritonitis due to biliary necrosis as the bile duct receives its blood supply from the hepatic artery. Hepatic artery stenosis, on the other hand, is often detected incidentally when a graft US is obtained for another indication or upon workup for transaminitis or biliary complications. Diagnostics studies include graft US with Doppler, or either computed tomography angiography (CTA) or magnetic resonance angiography (MRA) if they can be done expeditiously and tolerated from a renal function standpoint. Treatment for both HAT and stenosis in the early post-LT period is often through operative arterial reconstruction in the immediate postoperative period, or alternatively through an interventional approach in select patients. If extensive hepatic necrosis is present at the time of exploration, the patient may need emergent retransplantation.

   b. **Portal vein thrombosis (PVT) or stenosis.** PVT occurs in 1% to 3% of post-LT patients and may clinically result in ascites, sepsis secondary to bacterial translocation due to intestinal congestion, gastrointestinal bleeding, and rapid onset hepatic failure with laboratory studies suggestive of transaminitis. Graft US with Doppler is preferable to CTA or MRA, which have decreased sensitivity. If portal vein stenosis is of concern, percutaneous transhepatic portography may be used to measure pressures across the area of concern (generally considered to be significant if the gradient is >5 mmHg). Treatment of early PVT in the early post-LT period may necessitate operative exploration and vascular reconstruction. Often, portal vein stenosis can initially be managed with angioplasty and stenting.

   c. **Hepatic vein and inferior vena cava (IVC) anastomosis complications.** These complications are relatively uncommon, resulting from kinking, thrombosis, or stenosis and often clinically present with dependent edema and/or ascites due to impeded hepatic outflow. Similar to other vascular complications, diagnostic studies include graft US with Doppler. Depending on the degree of outflow obstruction, hepatic outflow anastomosis complications can often be managed through interventional methods including angioplasty and/or stenting.

3. **Biliary complications**

   a. **Etiology**—typically multifactorial; however, often related to decreased arterial flow (from the hepatic artery)

      1. **Biliary leak.** Defined by the International Study Group of Liver Surgery to be based on drain fluid bilirubin concentration greater than three times the serum concentration on or after postoperative day 3 of surgery or the need for either radiologic or operative

intervention due to bile collection or biliary peritonitis. Clinically, it often presents as increased abdominal pain, nausea, increased ascites, and fever. In addition to checking drain bilirubin levels, graft US with Doppler should be performed to assess for concomitant HAT or stenosis. Endoscopic retrograde cholangiopancreatography (ERCP) can be both diagnostic and therapeutic. CT scan may help localize biloma or other intra-abdominal collections. Treatment options included biliary drainage, biliary stents, possible reconstructive surgery, use of intra-abdominal drains, and possibly antibiotics.

2. **Biliary stricture.** Biliary stricture clinically may present with jaundice, pruritus, or as cholangitis with laboratory studies suggestive of increased serum bilirubin with persistently elevated alkaline phosphatase. In addition to checking drain bilirubin levels, graft US with Doppler should be performed to assess for concomitant HAT or stenosis. ERCP can be both diagnostic and therapeutic. Treatment is similar to that of biliary leak. Surgical conversion from a biliary duct-to-duct anastomosis to roux-en-y drainage can also be considered.

4. **Infectious complications.** These are the most common cause of postoperative morbidity and mortality and include bacteremia, fungemia, pneumonia, wound infection, urinary infection, and *Clostridium difficile* colitis given the immunosuppressed state of the transplant recipient. Prevention (see Infectious Disease section [II.E.8] above regarding antibiotic prophylaxis) as well as source control/treatment form the main principles in management and can be complimented with reductions in immunosuppression when indicated.

   a. **Line- and tube-related infections.** Catheter-associated urinary tract infections, central line–associated blood stream infection, and ventilator-associated pneumonias can be minimized by removal of invasive lines and tubes as expeditiously as possible.

   b. **Pneumonia.** Early onset hospital-acquired pneumonia within 7 days of LT occurs in approximately 15% of patients and is associated with prolonged ventilation (>48 hours). Early diagnostic bronchoscopy is favored over empiric treatment whenever possible.

   c. ***Clostridium difficile* colitis.** *Clostridium difficile* colitis occurs in approximately 19% of liver recipients, compared with 1% of patients without transplants, and is likely due to empiric antibiotic use, immunosuppression, and increased nosocomial exposure. These patients should be managed with close attention given to consequences on allograft function induced by diarrhea and associated hypovolemia and hypotension, as well as electrolyte abnormalities.

5. **Renal Complications**

   a. **Definition.** AKI can be stratified on the basis of the Risk, Injury, Failure, Loss, and End-Stage Kidney Disease (RIFLE) criteria or Acute Kidney Injury Network (AKIN) staging system, both of which use creatinine and urine output as criteria.

      1. In the post-LT patient, AKI has been associated with reduced patient and graft survival in the perioperative and long-term periods.

      2. Baseline creatinine levels in patients with cirrhosis can lead to overestimation of renal function due to lower creatinine production rates secondary to malnutrition and decreased muscle mass in these patients.

   b. **Etiology and risk factors.** Post-LT AKI is often multifactorial and includes intraoperative factors such as hypotension, bleeding, vena cava clamping, increased transfusion requirement, and ischemia/ reperfusion injury.

c. **Management.** Hemodynamic optimization and initiation of renal support may be necessary in the management of post-LT AKI. Consideration for modification of immunosuppression regimen to decrease calcineurin inhibitors as well as decreasing potentially nephrotoxic prophylactic medications should also be performed in patients with post-LT AKI.

6. **Early immunological complications**

   a. **Hyperacute rejection.** Hyperacute rejection, also known as antibody-mediated rejection, is a rare complication that usually occurs within minutes to hours of LT. In this case, rejection is secondary to preformed recipient antibodies that are present at the time of LT depositing in the newly transplanted graft, resulting in activation of the complement and coagulation cascade causing subsequent graft thrombosis and necrosis. This is typically secondary to ABO incompatibility and attempts of plasma exchange, intravenous gamma globulin, B-cell depletion therapy, and splenectomy can be performed, however, if acute hepatic failure ensues, emergent retransplantation may be necessary.

   b. **Acute cellular rejection (ACR).** ACR typically occurs within 6 weeks of LT and is secondary to cytotoxic and helper T-cell activation. The clinical manifestation of ACR is usually nonspecific, but laboratory studies typically manifests with increasing alanine aminotransferase (ALT) followed by elevations in AST and bilirubin. After other etiologies of laboratory abnormalities are ruled out, diagnosis is typically made through biopsy. Management typically involves optimization of immunosuppressive therapy for mild ACR, steroid pulse therapy for moderate ACR, and adjunctive therapy utilizing T-cell depletion therapy for severe ACR.

7. **Bleeding.** Post-LT bleeding may be secondary to insufficient surgical hemostasis or more commonly due to coagulopathy and thrombocytopenia.

   a. Coagulopathy may occur secondary to dilution associated with massive transfusion, inadequate replacement of components, hypothermia, hyperfibrinolysis, or inadequate hepatic synthetic function.

   b. See considerations about management of bleeding post-LT patient above (see II.E.7.1 above).

   c. Ongoing bleeding may require surgical reintervention to assess for surgical hemostasis or in the post-LT patient may be indicative of graft dysfunction.

Selected Readings

Aldenkortt F, Aldenkort M, Caviezel L, et al. Portopulmonary hypertension and hepatopulmonary syndrome. *World J Gastroenterol* 2014;20:8072–8081.

deLemos AS, Vagefi PA. Expanding the donor pool in liver transplantation: extended criteria donors. *Clin Liver Dis* 2013;2(4):156–159.

Diaz GC, Wagener G, Renz JF. Postoperative care/critical care of the transplant patient. *Anesthesiol Clin* 2013;31(4):723–735.

Farid SG, Prasad KR, Morris-Stiff G. Operative terminology and post-operative management approaches applied to hepatic surgery: trainee perspectives. *World J Gastrointest Surg* 2013;5(5):146–155.

Gopal PB, Kapoor D, Raya R, et al. Critical care issues in adult liver transplantation. *Indian J Crit Care Med* 2009;13(3):113–119.

Kamath PS, Kim WR. The model for end-stage liver disease. *Hepatology* 2007;43:797–805.

Kim WR, Stock PG, Smith JM, et al. OPTN/SRTR 2011 Annual data report: liver. *Am J Transplant* 2013;13(suppl 1):73–102.

Mulholland MW, Doherty GM. *Complications in surgery*. Philadelphia: Lippincott Williams & Wilkins, 2011.

Olson JC, Wendon JA, Kramer DJ, et al. Intensive care of the patient with cirrhosis. *Hepatology* 2011;54:1864–1872.

Razonable RR, Findlay JY, O'Riordan A, et al. Critical care issues in patients after liver transplantation. *Liver Transpl* 2011;17(5):511–527.

Saliba F, Ichai P, Levesque E, et al. Cirrhotic patients in the ICU: prognostic markers and outcome. *Curr Opin Crit Care* 2013;19:154–160.

Schuppan D, Afdhal NH. Liver cirrhosis. *Lancet* 2008;371:838–851.

U.S. Department of Health & Human Services. n.d. http://optn.transplant.hrsa.gov/latestData/rptData.asp. Accessed August 7, 2014.

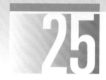

Coagulopathy and Hypercoagulability

Young Ahn and Klaus Goerlinger

Coagulopathy in the critically ill covers a range of abnormal states of coagulation. It is defined as the blood's inability to clot normally.

I. COAGULOPATHIES AND HEMOSTATIC ABNORMALITIES IN THE CRITICALLY ILL

A. Disseminated Intravascular Coagulation (DIC) is defined by the International Society on Thrombosis and Hemostasis as an "acquired syndrome characterized by the intravascular activation of coagulation with loss of localization arising from different causes." There are many potential causes of DIC (Table 25.1).

1. **Pathophysiology** of DIC is based on the following main mechanisms (Fig. 25.1). First, bacterial exo- and endotoxins (LPS) as well as in- flammatory cytokines induce tissue factor-expression on circulation monocytes and endothelial cells. This results in a loss of localiza- tion of thrombin generation to the site of endothelial injury. Tissue factor-expression on monocytes is further enhanced by the surfaces of extracorporeal assist devices such as dialysis, ECMO, and ventricular assist devices (VADs). However, tissue factor-expression on monocytes cannot be detected by standard plasmatic coagulation testing but by

TABLE 25.1	Causes of Disseminated Intravascular Coagulation (DIC)
Acute	**Chronic**
Sepsis	Malignancy (hematologic or solid organ)
Shock	Liver disease
Trauma	Vascular abnormalities
Head injury	Aortic aneurysm
Crush injury	Aortic dissection
Burns (extensive)	Peritoneovenous shunt
Extracorporeal circulation (e.g., ECMO)	Intra-aortic balloon pump
Pregnancy catastrophes	
Placental abruption	
Amniotic fluid embolus	
Septic abortion	
Embolism of fat or cholesterol	
Hepatic failure (severe)	
Toxic/immune reactions (severe)	
Snake bites	
Hemolytic transfusion reactions	

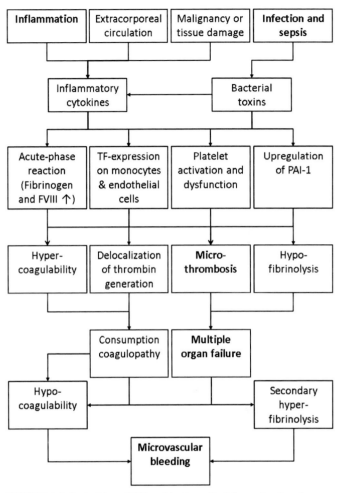

FIGURE 25.1 Pathophysiology of DIC is mainly triggered by inflammation, tissue/organ damage, infection, and sepsis, finally resulting in microthrombosis, multiple organ failure, and microvascular bleeding.

whole-blood viscoelastic testing (ROTEM/TEG). Second, the early phase of DIC is characterized by hypercoagulability (increased clot firmness due to acute phase reaction with high fibrinogen levels and high clot firmness in viscoelastic testing), consumption of physiologic coagulation inhibitors (antithrombin and protein C), platelet dysfunction, and inhibition of fibrinolysis (up-regulation of plasmin activator inhibitor-1 [PAI-1]). This results in thrombosis of the microcirculation and multiple organ failure. Finally, when coagulation factors and fibrinolytic inhibitors are consumed, hypocoagulation and secondary fibrinolysis can result in severe bleeding. Early detection of pathologic thromboelastometric results and platelet dysfunction detected by whole-blood impedance aggregometry on admission at the ICU are associated with worse outcomes.

2. **Clinical features** of DIC include hemorrhage from operative or traumatic wounds, oozing from venipuncture sites, petechiae, and ecchymosis. Micro and macro vascular thrombosis can lead to organ failure.

3. **Diagnosis** includes clinical and laboratory data. Recommendations include the use of a DIC scoring system, of which three exists using different criteria for different types of DIC.

4. **Laboratory tests** such as prolonged PT and INR, reduction of platelet counts, and reduced fibrinogen and antithrombin (AT) levels may overlap with other coagulopathies. Elevation of fibrin-related markers such as D-Dimer, fibrin degradation products, and soluble fibrin are common findings not specific to DIC. Peripheral blood smears can reveal schistocytes (fragmented red blood cells), which are formed as red blood cells flow through fibrin stands in the microvasculature are severed. Point-of-care testing includes thromboelastometry/thromboelastography (ROTEM/TEG) and PTT waveforms to support the diagnosis (Fig. 25.2).

5. **Treatment** of DIC is aimed at correcting the underlying cause, blood product transfusion when indicated, and pharmacologic treatment (Table 25.2). Blood products should be transfused to correct for active bleeding or in preparation for life-saving procedures. Fibrinogen levels should then be corrected to 150 to 200 mg/dL. Platelet transfusion should be considered in patients who are actively bleeding and who have a platelet count of $<$50,000/mm^3. However, platelet transfusion should be considered carefully since it may aggravate multiple organ failure and result in secondary bacterial infections. In nonbleeding patients, the threshold for platelet transfusion should be 10,000–20,000/mm^3. Other blood components such as FFP and PRBC should be transfused only in patients with active bleeding or at high risk of bleeding.

   a. Pharmacologic treatment depends on the type of DIC and includes anticoagulation or antifibrinolytics. The balance of coagulation and fibrinolysis can be further characterized with point-of-care testing (ROTEM/TEG and whole-blood impedance aggregometry) to guide treatment, but hematologic consult should be considered in complicated cases of DIC.

B. **Liver Disease** affects coagulation as the majority of factors, except factor VIII and von Willebrand's factor (vWF), are produced in the liver. In chronic liver disease, coagulation factors (I, II, V, VII, IX, X, and plasminogen) and inhibitors (antithrombin, protein C and S, α_2-antiplasmin, as well as the vWF-cleaving enzyme ADAMTS13) synthesized by the liver are decreased while the vascular endothelium-derived factor VIII, vWF, tPA, and PAI-1 are elevated (Fig. 25.3). Clinically, this results in a rebalanced hemostasis, though standard plasmatic coagulation tests such as PT and PTT may be elevated. In fact, thrombin generation assays containing thrombomodulin and viscoelastic tests (thromboelastography and thromboelastometry) demonstrate that patients with long-standing liver disease tend to be

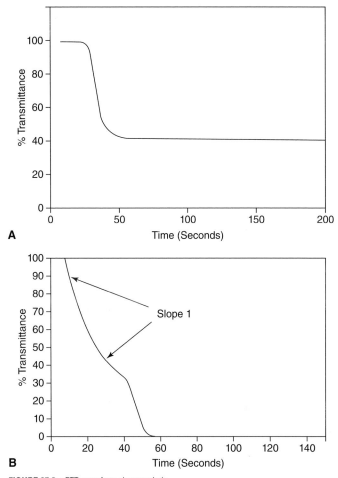

FIGURE 25.2 aPTT waveform characteristic.

hypercoagulable. They should be considered for thromboprophylaxis unless contraindicated. Similarly, in acute liver failure, overt bleeding is less common than would be expected due to a "rebalanced" coagulation dysfunction. Thrombocytopenia frequently occurs as the result of splenic sequestration but may be compensated by high vWF levels.

1. Prophylactic transfusion of FFP and platelets should be avoided, and hemostatic interventions should only be performed in case of clinically relevant bleeding. There is usually response to vitamin K supplementation. Antifibrinolytic drugs or coagulation factor concentrates such as fibrinogen, prothrombin complex concentrate (PCC), or activated recombinant factor VII (rFVIIa) may be appropriate in certain patients.

Treatment	Nonsymptomatic Type	Organ Failure Type	Bleeding Type	Consumptive Type
Underlying conditions	Yes	Yes	Yes	Yes
Blood transfusion	Data lacking	Data lacking	Yes	Yes
Heparin	Yes	Data lacking	No	No
Anti-Xa	Data lacking	Data lacking	No	No
Synthetic protease inhibitor	Data lacking	Data lacking	Yes	Yes
Natural protease inhibitor	Data lacking	Yes	Data lacking	No
Antifibrinolytic treatment	No	No	Yes	Yes

Wada H, Thachil J, Di Nisio M, et al. The Scientific Standardization Committee on DIC of the International Society on Thrombosis Haemostasis. Guidance for diagnosis and treatment of DIC from harmonization of the recommendations from three guidelines. *J Thromb Haemost* 2013;11:761–767.

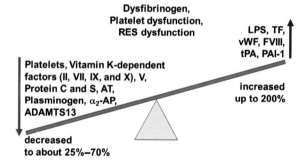

Low-level rebalance →
high risk of bleeding **and** thrombosis!

FIGURE 25.3 Coagulopathy in cirrhosis. In cirrhosis, hemostasis is rebalanced at a low level associated with a high risk of bleeding and thrombosis.

However, the potential benefit of improving hemostasis at the expense of increasing the thrombotic risk should be carefully evaluated in individual patients. Here, viscoelastic testing (ROTEM/TEG) seem to be helpful to guide therapy in bleeding patients. Notably, procoagulant agents such as rFVIIa have been shown to improve laboratory values such as PT, without improving control of bleeding during liver transplant or upper GI hemorrhage.

C. **Vitamin K Deficiency.** Vitamin K, which is produced in the intestinal mucosa, is important in the synthesis of coagulation factors in the liver. These factors include the clotting factors II, VII, IX, and X as well as the anticoagulant factors protein C and protein S. Vitamin K deficiency is common in prolonged illness and can be repleted 2.5 to 25 mg subcutaneously once or 10 mg subcutaneously daily for 3 days. Vitamin K can be given intravenously, though with the risk of anaphylaxis. Oral vitamin K in the critically ill patient depends on ability to have enteric medication and adequate absorption. Furthermore, the activity of vitamin K-dependent coagulation factor is low in patients under oral anticoagulation with coumarins depicted by an increased INR (targeted range 2–3.5). In severe and life-threatening bleeding due to vitamin K-antagonists (VKAs), for example, in intracerebral hemorrhage or GI bleeding, the effect can be reversed rapidly by the administration of four-factor PCCs. Four-factor PCC is FDA-approved for this indication since 2013. Whether four-factor PCCs are useful or not to reverse the effect of new oral anticoagulants (NOACs: dabigatran, rivaroxaban, apivaban, and edoxaban) is still under debate.

D. **Uremia.** Abnormal platelet function in uremia may contribute to significant bleeding in the trauma or perioperative settings. The primary therapy is hemodialysis and should be strongly considered prior to invasive procedures in the event of uremia-related coagulopathy. IV desmopressin as a slow infusion increases multimers of factor VIII: vWf. Cryoprecipitate and treatment of anemia with transfusion of PRBC in the acute setting can be considered, as well. Therapy with less immediate response time includes conjugated estrogens (over the course of 4–7 days) and erythropoietin (over the course of months).

E. **Trauma-Induced Coagulopathy (TIC) or Acute Coagulopathy of Trauma Shock (ACoTS)** is accepted to be a discrete clinical entity different from DIC (Fig. 25.4). In contrast to DIC hypoperfusion-induced activation of protein C with subsequent cleavage of activated factors V and VIII and down-regulation of PAI-1 result in endogenous anticoagulation and primary hyperfibrinolysis. Furthermore, shedding of the endothelial glycocalyx leads to liberation of heparinoids, which intensifies endogenous anticoagulation. In addition, TIC is modulated by hemodilution, hypothermia, and acidosis. TIC is functionally characterized by a reduction in clot strength. With a threshold of clot amplitude at 5 minutes of ≤35 mm, rotational thromboelastometry can identify acute traumatic coagulopathy at 5 minutes and predict the need for massive transfusion. Therefore, early administration of tranexamic acid and fibrinogen replacement is crucial in treatment of TIC. Fibrinogen levels should be corrected to at least 150 to 200 mg/dL. Concepts to treat TIC vary widely between the United States and Europe, using a fixed transfusion ratio of packed red blood cells, FFP, and platelets on the one hand and an individualized goal-directed bleeding management using coagulation factor concentrates (fibrinogen and four-factor PCC) guided by viscoelastic testing (ROTEM/TEG) on the other hand. RCTs are missing to show which approach is superior in severe trauma. In traumatic brain injury (TBI), the risk of bleeding as well as thrombosis is high. A neurointensivist should be involved in the care of a critically ill patient with significant head trauma.

F. **Postoperative Bleeding,** for example, after cardiac surgery or liver transplant, usually is multifactorial. Here, hyperfibrinolysis, fibrinogen deficiency, fibrin polymerization disorders, thrombocytopenia, thrombocytopathy, and impaired thrombin generation can play a major role. Standard plasmatic coagulation tests are limited due to their long turn-around time and their inability for predicting bleeding and guiding hemostatic therapy in the perioperative setting. Here, ROTEM/TEG as well as point-of-care platelet function analysis have been shown to be superior in reducing transfusion

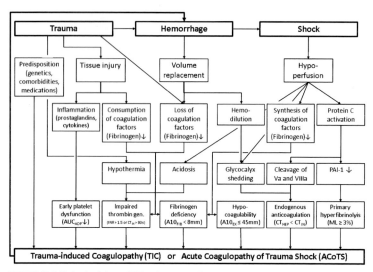

FIGURE 25.4 Pathophysiology of TIC and corresponding triggers of thromboelastometry and whole-blood impedance aggregometry; A10, amplitude of clot firmness 10 minutes after CT; AUC, area under the curve; CT, coagulation time; EX, extrinsic thromboelastometry (EXTEM); FIB, fibrin thromboelastometry (FIBTEM); HEP, heparinase modified thromboelastometry (HEPTEM); IN, intrinsic thromboelastometry (INTEM); INR, International normalized ratio; ML, maximum lysis.

requirements, transfusion-associated adverse events, thromboembolic events, and improving patients' outcomes. The use of perioperative bleeding management algorithms guided by ROTEM/TEG are highly recommended here (Fig. 25.5). Their clinical and cost effectiveness has been proven in several studies and health technology assessments.

G. Clotting

1. **Hypercoagulability abnormalities** include congenital conditions such as factor V Leiden (activated protein C resistance), prothrombin mutation, protein C and S deficiencies, antithrombin deficiency, antiphospholipid antibodies (lupus anticoagulant [LA]), and hyperhomocysteinemia. Evaluation includes thorough history and labs, supported by genetic testing for the patient and family members. However, in the setting of acute illness and elevation of acute-phase reactants, these tests may not be specific. Expert hematologic consultation is recommended in critically ill patients.

   a. Medications such as oral contraceptives and smoking or obesity and diabetes should be taken into consideration when critically ill patients with hypercoagulability are evaluated. Pregnancy, trauma, and surgery predispose and contribute to the multifactorial process of hypercoagulability.

   b. Treatment is individually tailored. Compression stockings, sequential compression devices, and prophylactic and therapeutic anticoagulation are determined on the basis of history and clinical setting.

2. **Heparin-induced thrombocytopenia (HIT)** is classified as nonimmune mediated (HIT type 1) or immune mediated (HIT type 2). HIT type 1 is a benign fall in platelet count, usually within 5 days of initiating heparin.

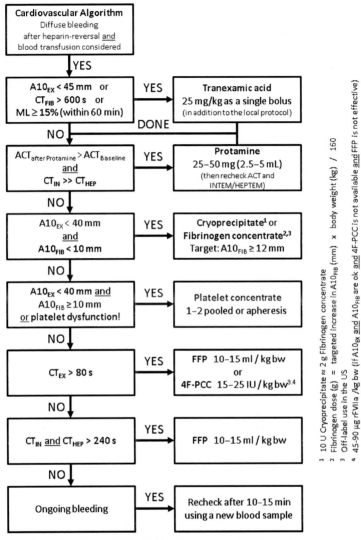

FIGURE 25.5 Point-of-care algorithm for bleeding management in cardiovascular surgery guided by thromboelastometry and whole-blood impedance aggregometry; 4F-PCC, four-factor prothrombin complex concentrate; A10, amplitude of clot firmness 10 minutes after CT; ACT, activated clotting time; bw, body weight; CT, coagulation time; EX, extrinsic thromboelastometry (EXTEM); FIB, fibrin thromboelastometry (FIBTEM); HEP, heparinase modified thromboelastometry (HEPTEM); IN, intrinsic thromboelastometry (INTEM); ML, maximum lysis; rFVIIa, activated recombinant factor VII.

The platelet count usually does not fall below 100,000 mm^3 and heparin does not have to be discontinued or avoided in the future.

a. HIT type 2 is immune mediated. IgG antibodies are formed against heparin-platelet factor 4 (PF-4) complexes. This results in platelet activation and aggregation, leading to pathologic platelet aggregation, thrombocytopenia, and vascular thrombosis. HIT antibodies binding to endothelial cell surfaces may result in tissue factor expression and a prothrombotic state.

b. Up to half of cardiac surgery patients and 15% of orthopedic surgery patients develop HIT type 2 by immunologic assays (ELISA). However, only 1% to 3% of these patients develop clinically significant HIT type 2. This can be significantly reduced by use of low-molecular-weight heparin (LMWH) and eliminated with fondaparinux or direct thrombin inhibitors (DTIs) such as argatroban (Fig. 25.6). Argatroban is approved for prophylaxis and treatment of thrombosis in patients with or at risk of HIT. In patients with hepatic impairment or multiple organ failure, the argatroban dosage should be decreased to 0.1 to 0.2 µg/kg/min in order to avoid bleeding complications. Argatroban therapy can be monitored by aPTT or ecarin clotting time (ECT). Since aPTT reaches a plateau at higher argatroban plasma concentrations, an overdose may not be recognized. Therefore, ecarin-based assays are more reliable for monitoring DTIs.

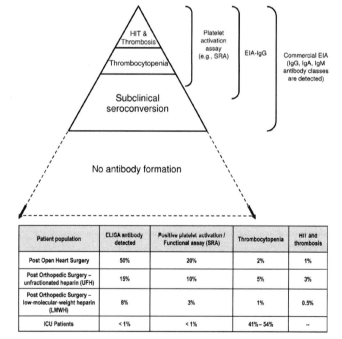

Patient population	ELISA antibody detected	Positive platelet activation / Functional assay (SRA)	Thrombocytopenia	HIT and thrombosis
Post Open Heart Surgery	50%	20%	2%	1%
Post Orthopedic Surgery – unfractionated heparin (UFH)	15%	10%	5%	3%
Post Orthopedic Surgery – low-molecular-weight heparin (LMWH)	8%	3%	1%	0.5%
ICU Patients	< 1%	< 1%	41%– 54%	--

FIGURE 25.6 Iceberg model of HIT.

   c. **Diagnosis** is made by history and physical, as well as a decrease in platelet count by 50% from baseline (but usually not less than 50,000 mm³) within 5 to 14 days of heparin exposure. Previous heparin exposure can lead to a quicker decrease in platelets. Platelet recovery after ceasing exposure to heparin and tachyphylaxis or resistance to heparinization is also suggestive. The clinical 4T-score can be used to estimate the probability of HIT type 2 (Table 25.3). For patients with a 4T-score of less than 4 points, the probability of having immune HIT is less than 5%. Platelet serotonin release assays (SRAs) are more specific than ELISA assays, but take longer to obtain. Whole-blood impedance aggregometry can be used as a functional assay for platelet-activating HIT-antibodies with a similar sensitivity and specificity compared with SRAs but with a shorter turn-around time. A high index of suspicion in the correct clinical setting (4T score ≥4 points) should be treated as positive for HIT type 2.

   d. **Treatment** involves discontinuing all exposure to heparin, including heparin-coated catheters, flushes, hemodialysis, or extracorporeal circuitry. Appropriate anticoagulation is essential as 50% to 75% of patients with HIT type 2 develop thrombotic complications. Appropriate anticoagulation is patient specific and would include direct thrombin inhibitors such as argatroban. Platelet transfusion should be restrictive due to thrombotic concerns. Longer-term anticoagulation (at least 6–8 weeks) will generally be required.

3. **Sickle cell** disease in African Americans are caused by substitution of the amino acid valine for glutamic acid on the β-chain of hemoglobin.

TABLE 25.3 The HIT 4T-Score

4T-Score	2 points	1 point	0 points
Thrombocytopenia	Platelet count fall >50% and platelet nadir ≥20,000/mm³	Platelet count fall 30%–50% or platelet nadir 10–19,000/mm³	Platelet count fall <30% or platelet nadir <10,000/mm³
Timing of platelet count fall	Clear onset between 5–10 d or platelet fall ≤1 d (prior heparin exposure within 30 d)	Consistent with days 5–10 fall, but not clear (e.g. missing platelet counts); onset after day 10 or fall ≤1 d (prior heparin exposure 30–100 d ago)	Platelet count fall <4 d without recent exposure
Thrombosis or other sequela	New thrombosis (confirmed); skin necrosis; acute systemic reaction postintravenous UFH bolus	Progressive or recurrent thrombosis; non-necrotizing (erythematous) skin lesions; suspected thrombosis (not proven)	None
Other causes for Thrombocytopenia	Non apparent	Possible	Definite

For patients with a 4T score of <4 points, the probability of having immune HIT is <5%.

Clinical presentation occurs with homozygotes. Similar presentations can occur for homozygotes of SC or β-thalassemia. Heterozygote carriers usually do not present clinically.

a. Hypoxia, hypothermia, ischemia, acidosis, and hypovolemia can cause a "sickling" deformity of the red blood cell. Resultant microvascular obstruction can cause tissue ischemia and infarction. Sickle cell crisis present with nonspecific signs such as fever, leukocytosis, and tachycardia as well as signs of end-organ dysfunction. Significant anemia can occur due to the shortened lifespan and destruction of the red blood cells. Treatment involves addressing the precipitating causes, providing adequate pain relief, and transfusion only when indicated.

H. Frequent Hematologic Diseases

1. Hemophilia A is a hereditary disorder of factor VIII and hemophilia B is a hereditary disorder of factor IX. History and physical findings are supported by laboratory findings of an elevated intrinsic pathway clotting time (PTT), with a normal PT/INR. Platelet function is normal but the blood clot is unable to be stabilized, so bleeding will recur. Treatment includes factor VIII, factor IX, cryoprecipitate, and desmopressin (DDAVP). rFVIIa and activated PCC (FEIBA = factor eight inhibitor bypassing activity) are indicated in patients with acquired hemophilia due to inhibitors. Expert hematology consultation is recommended in critically ill patients.

2. Von Willebrand's disease is a primarily autosomal-dominant genetic disorder resulting from defects in vWF. vWF normally anchors platelets to collagen while strengthening clotted platelets and stabilizing factor VIII. Treatment includes DDAVP, human factor VIII/vWF complex concentrates, and cryoprecipitate preferably over FFP. In certain patients with acquired von Willebrand's disease, high-dose intravenous gamma globulin has been used successfully. Again, expert hematology consultation is recommended in critically ill patients.

II. DIAGNOSIS

A. Physical Exam and careful history are critical in diagnosing the coagulopathy and cause. Early investigation should include a thorough review and assessment for therapeutic agents contributing to the coagulopathy. Current nutritional status, history of bleeding in the past, and nonmedication causes of coagulopathy should also be assessed. In critically ill patients, concurrent illnesses such as sepsis, multiple organ failure, recent heparin exposure, and mechanical circulatory device requirements are just a few of many contributors to coagulation pathology.

1. The pattern of bleeding helps differentiate between diagnoses that may present with similar laboratory findings. Major vascular sources of bleeding as opposed to petechiae and oozing from vascular catheter sites and mucosal surfaces point to markedly different causes and treatments.

B. Standardized Questionnaire on Bleeding and Drug History

Most of the preexisting hemostatic disorders, resulting in unexpected perioperative bleeding, are impairments of primary hemostasis, for example, von Willebrand's disease or drug-induced platelet dysfunction. Therefore, these patients cannot be identified by standard plasmatic coagulation tests, such as aPTT and PT, but by a standardized questionnaire on bleeding and drug history, complemented by platelet function analysis, if applicable. Notably, not only antiplatelet drugs, such as COX inhibitors, ADP receptor blockers, and glycoprotein IIb/IIa receptor antagonists, can inhibit platelet function but NSAIDs, antibiotics, cardiovascular and lipid-lowering drugs, antidepressants, volume expanders, radiographic contrast agents, as well as chemotherapeutic agents can also result in acquired platelet function disorders. This has to be considered, in particular if standard plasmatic coagulation tests and viscoelastic testing (ROTEM/TEG) show normal results in bleeding patients.

C. **Activated Partial Thromboplastin Time (aPTT)** is performed by adding an activator of the intrinsic pathway, for example, ellagic acid or silica, phospholipids, and calcium to a citrated plasma sample. Normal values of aPTT vary widely depending on the reagent and analyzer used. There is an increasing number of heparin- and lupus anticoagulant–sensitive reagents on the market. The test is sensitive to decreased amounts of coagulation factors of the intrinsic pathway (prekallikrein), factors XII, XI (hemophilia C), IX (hemophilia B), and VIII (hemophilia A), the common pathway (factors X, V, II, and fibrinogen), unfractionated heparin (UFH), direct thrombin inhibitors (DTIs), antibodies to factor VIII or IX (acquired hemophilia), and antiphospholipid antibodies such as lupus anticoagulant (LA), generated in some anti-immune diseases. Antiphospholipid antibodies prolongs aPTT by reducing the availability of phospholipids—required for coagulation—in plasmatic coagulation tests (in vitro). Notably, aPTT prolongation due to an antiphospholipid syndrome (APS) is not associated with bleeding but with thrombosis. In vivo, antiphospholipid antibodies bind to phospholipids and lipoproteins in the cell membrane of platelets, resulting in platelet activation (similar to HIT) and arterial and venous thrombosis. aPTT can be used to guide unfractionated heparin (UFH) therapy but is not sensitive enough to LMWH. Here, anti–factor Xa assays have to be used if monitoring is required. Since aPTT reaches a plateau at higher DTI plasma concentrations, an overdose may not be recognized. The clinician should be aware that the positive and negative predictive value for bleeding is low for aPTT, which means that neither a prolonged aPTT has to be associated with bleeding (e.g., in APS) nor a normal aPTT excludes bleeding. Correction of an abnormal aPTT in surgical patients is not always indicated unless the patient is bleeding. Notably, an abnormal, biphasic aPTT waveform recorded during optical aPTT measurement (**Fig. 25.2**) can be detected in the early phase of sepsis and DIC and is predictive for high mortality. It can be used to discriminate between systemic inflammatory response syndrome (SIRS) and sepsis with a high sensitivity and specificity. Furthermore, thromboelatometric lysis index (LI60) using a cut-off value of ≤3% is superior to blood procalcitonin levels in discriminating between postoperative patients with SIRS and sepsis.

D. **Anti–Factor Xa Assays** are a chromogenic assays that facilitates the measurement of inhibition of factor Xa by UFH, LMWH, fondaparinux, and direct Xa inhibitors (DXaIs), such as rivaroxaban and apixaban. Since LMWH, fondaparinux, and DXaIs do not or even minimally prolong aPTT, anti–factor Xa assays have to be used if therapeutic levels of these drugs have to be monitored. Furthermore, the aPTT cannot be used to monitor UFH in some instances, for example, in the presence of antiphospholipid antibodies or in case of factor XII deficiency. In these cases, monitoring of UFH with anti–factor Xa assays is more appropriate.

E. **Prothrombin Time (PT)** is performed by adding thromboplastin (tissue factor = factor III), as the activator of the extrinsic pathway, phospholipids, and calcium to a citrated plasma sample. The test is sensitive to decreased amounts of coagulation factors of the extrinsic (factor VII) and common pathway (factors X, V, II, and fibrinogen). Since most vitamin K–dependent coagulation factors (II, VII, IX, and X) are involved in the extrinsic and common pathway (except factor IX), PT has been designed for monitoring of VKAs (coumarins), such as warfarin. However, thromboplastin reagents used for PT measurement vary widely regarding their tissue factor activity, in particular between the United States and Europe. Therefore, the **international normalized ratio (INR)** has been instituted in 1983 by the WHO in order to permit comparability of results in warfarin-treated patients between different laboratories. Therefore, warfarin therapy can be guided by a targeted INR value independent from the performing laboratory. The INR is the result of the PT-ratio ($PT_{patient}/PT_{comtrol}$) corrected by a thromboplastin reagent-specific international sensitivity index (ISI). The ISI value of the WHO standard thromboplastin reagent is 1. Most thromboplastin reagents used in Europe have an ISI value close to 1. In contrast, US thromboplastin reagents have an ISI value of 2.0 to 2.6. The majority of PT reagents contain the heparin-neutralizing agent polybrene, a positively charged polymer, in order to eliminate the effect of UFH. This allows for better discrimination between heparin and warfarin effects since heparin prolongs aPTT only, and warfarin prolongs PT and increases INR only. Although the INR is frequently used to assess coagulation impairment in patients with trauma and liver disease (e.g., to verify TIC or to calculate MELD score), it may not be valid here. In liver disease, vitamin K–dependent coagulation factors are low but compensated by high factor VIII levels and a decrease in the activity of the vitamin K–dependent anticoagulants protein C and S. This is not reflected by PT and INR because it is dependent on the presence of thrombomodulin. Accordingly, endogenous thrombin potential (ETP) of plasma samples from patients with cirrhosis is lower compared with plasma from noncirrhotic patients. However, the addition of thrombomodulin, which allows for activation of protein C, results in equalization of ETP between patients with and without cirrhosis, demonstrating a rebalance of hemostasis. Therefore, PT and INR values in patients not treated with warfarin have to be interpreted carefully in the perioperative setting.

F. **Thrombin Time (TT)** is performed by adding thrombin to a citrated plasma sample. The test is sensitive to fibrinogen deficiency, dysfibrinogenemia, fibrin(ogen) degradation products, fibrinolysis, heparin, and direct thrombin inhibitors (DTIs), such as hirudin, argatroban, bivalirudin, and dabigatran. The increasing use of DTIs led to a renaissance of the TT, in particular in its modification as **plasma-diluted TT (dTT)**. For the dTT assay, patient plasma is diluted 1:3 to 1:4 with normal plasma before performing the TT assay, and the results are compared with a DTI-specific calibration curve. Notably, none of the global coagulation tests aPTT, PT, or TT is sensitive to factor XIII deficiency.

G. **Ecarin Clotting Time (ECT)** is performed by adding ecarin to plasma or whole blood. Ecarin converts prothrombin to meizothrombin, an intermediate product of thrombin generation. Meizothrombin has a lower enzymatic activity compared with thrombin but forms 1:1 complexes with hirudin and other DTIs such as argatroban, bivalirudin, and dabigatran (see section III.B.5). ECT is not influenced by heparin and shows a linear correlation to DTI concentration in a wide range. A whole-blood ECT assay (ECATEM) is also available for the ROTEM device but only licensed in Europe, yet.

H. **Fibrinogen** is the first factor dropping down to a critical level in case of severe bleeding. The normal range for fibrinogen is 150 to 400 mg/dL and in the third trimester of pregnancy 450 to 600 mg/dL. In acute-phase reaction, it can rise to about 1,000 mg/dL. In severe bleeding, it is crucial to maintain the plasma fibrinogen level above 150 to 200 mg/dL. Therefore, the historic cutoff value of 100 mg/dL for fibrinogen substitution seems not to be adequate in severe bleeding. FFP is not effective to reach this target. Here, transfusion of cryoprecipitate or fibrinogen concentrate is much more effective. Fibrinogen levels can be measured by several methods. The **Clauss fibrinogen assay** is a modified TT assay using prediluted plasma and high thrombin concentrations. The **PT-derived fibrinogen assay** is using the plateau of the light transmission curve to calculate plasma fibrinogen concentration. All optical methods are influenced by infused colloids resulting in wrong high fibrinogen values by 15% to 90%, depending on the reagent used. In contrast, viscoelastic testing using the **FIBTEM (ROTEM)** or **functional fibrinogen (FF) assay (TEG)** demonstrate impaired fibrin polymerization after colloid infusion, associated with increased blood loss and transfusion requirements. Notably, TEG FF assay result in higher values compared with ROTEM FIBTEM assay since platelets are incompletely blocked in the FF assay. This difference should be considered in interpretation of these functional fibrinogen test results.

I. **Fibrin Monomers (FM)** are produced from the action of thrombin on fibrinogen without cross-linking of the fibrin monomers by factor XIII. FMs are elevated in DIC. Furthermore, increased FM concentration can be a sign of decreased factor XIII availability.

J. **Fibrin(ogen) Degradation Products (FDPs)** are peptides produced from the action of plasmin on fibrinogen or on fibrin monomers. They are measurable by serum assays and may aid the diagnosis of primary fibrinolysis or DIC. Furthermore, FDPs modulate clotting assays by interfering with fibrin monomer polymerization and by impairing platelet function. FDPs are often elevated in cirrhosis due to impaired clearance from circulation.

K. **D-Dimer** is a specific fragment produced when plasmin cleaves cross-linked fibrin and can be measured by a serum assay. Almost all patients with acute venous thromboembolism (VTE) present with an elevated D-dimer level. However, elevated D-dimer is not specific for VTE since it can be associated with several other conditions, including DIC, postsurgical or posttraumatic patients, pregnancy, and malignancy. However, a normal D-dimer test usually excludes the diagnosis of VTE.

L. **Single Factor Assays** are specialized tests quantifying the activity of individual coagulation factors. They can be used to clarify prolonged global plasmatic coagulation tests, such as aPTT, PT, and TT. On the one hand, isolated prolongation of aPTT is suspicious for hemophilia A (factor VIII), B (factor IX), or C (factor XI), but can be prolonged significantly in factor XII deficiency, too, which is not associated with bleeding. On the other hand, isolated prolongation of PT can be a sign of factor VII deficiency. Notably, factor XIII deficiency is not associated with a prolongation of aPTT, PT, or TT, but can be the cause for unexpected postoperative bleeding. Single-factor analyses are usually performed in concert with a clinical pathology or hematology consultation.

M. Activated Clotting Time (ACT) is a clotting test in which kaolin, celite, or glass beads are added to a noncitrated whole-blood sample to activate the intrinsic pathway. ACT usually is performed as a point-of-care test in the acute setting, for example, during cardiopulmonary bypass or ECMO, to monitor high heparin concentrations where aPTT cannot be measured any more (>180 s). Since ACT is a nonspecific whole-blood test, it cannot only be influenced by heparin and protamine but also by a lot of other variables, such as hemodilution, fibrinogen, platelets, aprotinin, and glycoprotein IIb/IIIa receptor antagonists. This is important for a meaningful interpretation of ACT test results. Since normal ACT depends on the test system used, it should be standardized by an institution.

N. Thromboelastometry (ROTEM)/Thromboelastography (TEG) are viscoelastic test devices used most often at the point-of-care in the emergency room (ER), the operating room (OR), or in the ICU. Both devices are assessing the change in viscoelasticity of a small amount of whole-blood activated by different agents in a system where a heated cup and a pin are oscillating against each other. Viscoelastic testing provides real-time, dynamic information about the whole coagulation process, including clot initiation (thrombin generation), clot kinetics, clot strength, and clot stability (lysis). However, it does not detect the effects of antiplatelet drugs, such as aspirin or clopidogrel, since platelets are activated via the thrombin receptor pathway here. Therefore, viscoelastic testing often is combined with point-of-care platelet function analysis if platelet dysfunction is expected (see Section II.P). Both devices differ in some technical points, definition of parameters, and reagents used. Therefore, results are not completely interchangeable between both devices. Due to the use of an automatic pipette, the stabilization of the pin movement by a ball-bearing, and the contact-free detection of the pin movement by a laser light-mirror-system, the ROTEM system is more user friendly, enables even mobile use in military field hospitals, and provides low inter- and intraoperator variability of test results in a multiuser environment, such as in the ER, OR and ICU environment. The definition of ROTEM/TEG parameters and their clinical relevance are displayed in Figure 25.7. Specific patterns of the trace are characteristic for several coagulation abnormalities (e.g., hyperfibrinolysis, fibrinogen deficiency, thrombocytopenia, factor deficiencies of the extrinsic and intrinsic pathway, heparin effects; see Fig. 25.8), assisting the clinician with the diagnosis and appropriate treatment. Here, the use of ROTEM/TEG-guided bleeding management algorithms is highly recommended (**Fig. 25.5**), and their clinical and cost-effectiveness has been proven in several studies and health technology assessments. In ROTEM, decision making is speeded up by using early amplitudes of clot firmness (A5 in Europe, A10 in the United States) to predict final clot firmness. Furthermore, the diagnostic performance can be improved by using test combinations compared with a monotest approach. Both devices

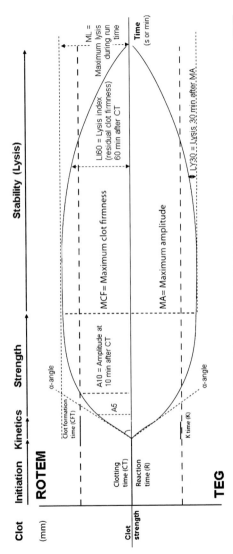

Clot   Initiation   Kinetics   Strength   Stability (Lysis)

(mm)

ROTEM

- α-angle
- Clot formation time (CFT)
- A5
- A10 = Amplitude at 10 min after CT
- MCF = Maximum clot firmness
- LI60 = Lysis index (residual clot firmness) 60 min after CT
- ML = Maximum lysis during run time
- Clotting time (CT)

TEG

- Reaction time (R)
- K time (K)
- α-angle
- MA = Maximum amplitude
- LY30 = Lysis 30 min after MA

Clot strength

Time (s or min)

	ROTEM	TEG	Hemostatic factors
Clot initiation	CT (clotting time) in s	R (reaction time) in min	Enzymatic coagulation factors, anticoagulants, FDPs, tissue factor expression on monocytes
Clot kinetics	CFT (clot formation time) in s α (angle) in degrees	K (kinetic time) in min α (angle) in degrees	Enzymatic coagulation factor, anticoagulants, fibrinogen, platelets
Clot strength	(A5) A10 (amplitude (5) 10 min after CT) in mm MCF (maximum clot firmness) in mm	MA (maximum amplitude) in mm	Platelets, f brinogen, FXII, colloids
Clot stability (lysis)	LI60 (lysis index (residual clot firmness) 60 min after CT) in % of MCF ML (maximum lysis during run time) in % of MCF	LY30 (lysis 30 min after MA) in % of MA	Fibrinolytic enzymes, fibrinolysis inhibitors, FXIII

FIGURE 25.7 ROTEM/TEG parameters.

use different activators and additives in their assays (see Table 25.4). Education is required in perioperative bleeding management and in technical training with these tests as well as test interpretation to obtain the expertise and judgment to improve patient outcomes and decrease transfusion requirements.

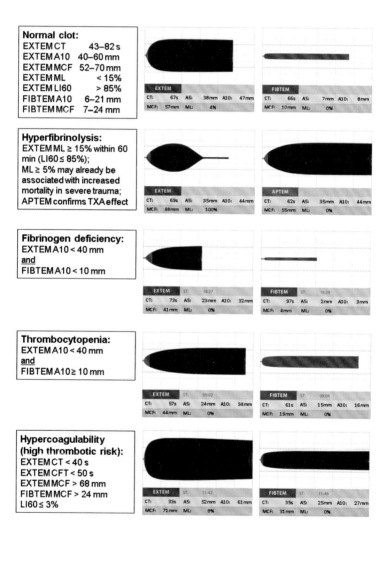

Normal clot:
EXTEM CT   43–82 s
EXTEM A10   40–60 mm
EXTEM MCF   52–70 mm
EXTEM ML   < 15%
EXTEM LI60   > 85%
FIBTEM A10   6–21 mm
FIBTEM MCF   7–24 mm

EXTEM — CT: 67s AS: 38mm A10: 47mm MCF: 57mm ML: 4%
FIBTEM — CT: 66s AS: 7mm A10: 8mm MCF: 10mm ML: 0%

Hyperfibrinolysis:
EXTEM ML ≥ 15% within 60 min (LI60 ≤ 85%);
ML ≥ 5% may already be associated with increased mortality in severe trauma;
APTEM confirms TXA effect

EXTEM — CT: 69s AS: 35mm A10: 44mm MCF: 48mm ML: 100%
APTEM — CT: 62s AS: 35mm A10: 44mm MCF: 55mm ML: 0%

Fibrinogen deficiency:
EXTEM A10 < 40 mm
and
FIBTEM A10 < 10 mm

EXTEM — ST: 18:27 CT: 73s AS: 23mm A10: 32mm MCF: 41mm ML: 0%
FIBTEM — ST: 18:29 CT: 97s AS: 2mm A10: 3mm MCF: 4mm ML: 0%

Thrombocytopenia:
EXTEM A10 < 40 mm
and
FIBTEM A10 ≥ 10 mm

EXTEM — ST: 09:02 CT: 57s AS: 24mm A10: 34mm MCF: 44mm ML: 0%
FIBTEM — ST: 09:04 CT: 61s AS: 15mm A10: 16mm MCF: 19mm ML: 0%

Hypercoagulability (high thrombotic risk):
EXTEM CT < 40 s
EXTEM CFT < 50 s
EXTEM MCF > 68 mm
FIBTEM MCF > 24 mm
LI60 ≤ 3%

EXTEM — ST: 11:42 CT: 33s AS: 52mm A10: 61mm MCF: 71mm ML: 8%
FIBTEM — ST: 11:46 CT: 35s AS: 25mm A10: 27mm MCF: 31mm ML: 0%

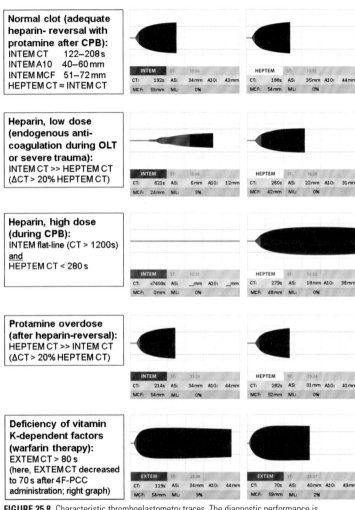

FIGURE 25.8 Characteristic thromboelastometry traces. The diagnostic performance is increased by test combinations, for example, EXTEM and FIBTEM, EXTEM and APTEM, or INTEM and HEPTEM (for assay description, see Table 25.4). 4F-PCC, four factor prothrombin complex concentrate; A10, amplitude of clot firmness 10 minutes after CT; CPB, cardiopulmonary bypass; CT, coagulation time (corresponds to r-time in TEG); LI60, lysis index 60 minutes after CT presented as residual clot firmness in percentage of MCF; MCF, maximum clot firmness (corresponds to MA in TEG); ML, maximum lysis during run time; OLT, orthotopic liver transplantation; TXA, tranexamic acid (or other antifibrinolytic drug).

TABLE 25.4 ROTEM/TEG assays

ROTEM Assay Activators and Additives	TEG Assay Activators and Additives	Clinical Comments
NATEM CaCl$_2$	**Native TEG** (CaCl$_2$)	Tissue factor-expression on monocytes; anticoagulants (e.g., LMWH)
INTEM Ellacic acid + CaCl$_2$	**Kaolin TEG** Kaolin (+ CaCl$_2$)	Deficiency of factors of the intrinsic pathway; heparin and protamine effects (in combination with HEPTEM)
HEPTEM Heparinase + ellacic acid + CaCl$_2$	**Heparinase TEG** Heparinase + Kaolin (+ CaCl$_2$)	Heparin and protamine effects (in combination with INTEM/ Kaolin TEG)
EXTEM Tissue factor + polybrene + CaCl$_2$	**Rapid TEG** Tissue factor + Kaolin (+ CaCl$_2$)	Deficiency of factors of the extrinsic pathway; VKAs (rapid TEG contains activators for both pathways)
FIBTEM Cytochalasin D + tissue factor + polybrene + CaCl$_2$	**TEG functional fibrinogen** Kaolin + monoclonal glycoprotein IIb/IIIa receptor antibody (+ CaCl$_2$)	Fibrin polymerization (TEG FF does not block platelets completely → higher results compared with FIBTEM)
APTEM Aprotinin/tranexamic acid + tissue factor + polybrene + CaCl$_2$	—	Verifying the effect of antifibrinolytic drugs and differential diagnosis to clot retraction and F XIII deficiency
ECATEM Ecarin + CaCl$_2$	—	Direct thrombin inhibitors (argatroban, bivalirudin, dabigatran); only licensed in Europe, yet
ROTEM *platelet* Impedance aggregometry activated with arachidonic acid, ADP, or TRAP-6	**TEG platelet mapping** Reptilase + XIIIa + arachidonic acid or ADP	POC platelet function analysis (COX-inhibitors, ADP-receptor blocker [GP IIb/IIIa receptor antagonists])

- **O. Platelet Count** usually is performed in EDTA blood samples. In case of unexpected thrombocytopenia without any clinical signs, EDTA-dependent pseudothrombocytopenia should be considered since it is a common laboratory phenomenon with a prevalence of up to 2% in hospitalized patients and 17% in outpatients. In these cases, platelet count should be repeated in citrated whole blood. However, a normal platelet count does not exclude severe platelet dysfunction (see Section II.B).
- **P. Platelet Function Analysis** can be performed using several devices and test methods. Light transmission aggregometry (LTA = Born aggregometry) is considered as the gold standard. Here, platelet-rich plasma is used for

analysis and platelet count has to be adjusted to 100,000/mm^3. Therefore, LTA is not applicable for point-of-care testing. Other methods, such as whole-blood impedance aggregometry (Multiplate or ROTEM *platelet*), turbidometric aggregometry (VerifyNow), or platelet mapping (TEG), may be more appropriate to use in the perioperative setting. These systems vary widely in regard to their usability, expenditure of time, ability to detect platelet dysfunction, ability to monitor and guide therapy with antiplatelet drugs, correlation to clinical bleeding and thrombosis, and variability and reproducibility of results.

III. TREATMENT
A. Transfusion

Traditionally transfusion of blood products has been based on conventional laboratory tests such as Hb, platelet count, aPTT, and PT/INR. Most evidence of current transfusion practice is derived from chronic anemia, minor surgical bleeding, or preparation for surgery. However, in massive trauma and hemorrhage, a massive transfusion strategy of transfusing packed red blood cells and fresh frozen plasma in a ratio of 1:1 or 2:1 is widely practiced, since conventional plasmatic coagulation tests are typically not timely available to guide decision making during major hemorrhage. Some data suggest even increased incidence of ARDS, sepsis, and multiple organ dysfunction in patients receiving FFP in nonmassive transfusion, and there is no evidence supporting FFP transfusion in nonmassively transfused patients. Furthermore, ABO-compatible but nonidentical plasma transfusion seems to be associated with a high complication rate of ARDS and sepsis up to 70% and even an increased mortality by 15% compared with transfusion of ABO-identical plasma only. Of note, administration of specific coagulation factor concentrates (fibrinogen and 4F-PCC) guided by rotational thromboelastometry is increasingly used rather than FFP in Europe. However, despite promising results in several clinical studies, efficacy, safety, and cost-effectiveness of this new approach have to be proven in large observational studies and RCTs.

B. Anticoagulation is indicated for underlying medical conditions such as atrial fibrillation with high CHADS scores, pulmonary embolism, DVT, DIC, and underlying hypercoagulable states. Mechanical support devices from intra-aortic balloon pumps to extracorporeal life support and renal replacement circuits may be indications for anticoagulation.

1. **Heparin** is administered subcutaneously or intravenously and acts by binding and accelerating the action of antithrombin (AT). This resultant complex inactivates thrombin and factor X in the coagulation cascade. Therapeutic anticoagulation for DVT or PE requires aPTT of 1.5 to 2 times baseline and should be reached within 24 hours of initiation. Usual dosing includes an IV bolus followed by titration of a continuous infusion. With a half-life of 90 minutes, the therapeutic effects of heparin will be gone by 4 to 6 hours after cessation. Protamine (1 mg/100 units of remaining heparin in circulation) can be slowly administered to reverse heparin sooner if needed.

   a. Resistance to heparin occurs in critically ill patients due to acute-phase reactants that bind heparin, depleted levels of AT, or due to HIT. Increasing the dose of heparin and transfusing AT concentrate or FFP would be appropriate in the first two causes for resistance. Development of HIT requires immediate cessation of heparin and treatment for HIT (see HIT section).

2. **Anti–Factor Xa** includes subcutaneous LMWH such as enoxaparin and dalteparin, which inhibit factor Xa. They do not prolong the aPTT and if therapeutic monitoring is needed, anti-Xa levels must be measured. LMWHs have improved efficacy for prophylaxis of DVT and PE in certain high-risk orthopedic, trauma, and spinal cord injury patients. The therapeutic predictability of LMWH is improved with less binding of acute-phase reactants compared with heparin. Additionally, the incidence of HIT is dramatically reduced with LMWH compared with unfractionated heparin. However, LMWH is more expensive, and if reversal is needed, it has a longer half-life of 4 hours, is incompletely reversed by protamine, and depends on renal clearance.

   a. Fondaparinux selectively inhibits factor Xa and shares many of the advantages and disadvantages of the other LMWH. It is unique in its long half-life of 14 hours and lack of interaction with platelets or platelet factor 4. The combination of renal elimination and long half-life make fondaparinux less suitable for critically ill patients.

   b. Rivaroxaban and apixaban are oral direct factor Xa inhibitors that do not require antithrombin. In the outpatient setting, they are generally considered safe with less drug–drug interactions and do not require monitoring of therapeutic levels, but have less usefulness in critically ill patients. Reversal is more challenging than reversing vitamin K antagonists. Four-factor prothrombin complex concentrate, activated prothrombin complex concentrate (FEIBA), and recombinant factor VIIa have been suggested in emergent situations. Specific antagonists are under development.

3. **Warfarin (vitamin K antagonist; VKAs)** are administered orally and inhibit vitamin K epoxide reductases, effectively. By blocking the epoxide reductases, factors II, VII, IX, X, protein C and protein S cannot be carboxylated to their active forms. The long half-life of warfarin (35 hours) makes it difficult to titrate therapeutic goals rapidly. Since 2013, four-factor PCC is FDA-approved for urgent reversal of VKAs, for example, in intracerebral hemorrhage or GI bleeding. In order to avoid a warfarin-rebound, PCC should be combined with vitamin K. In contrast to FFP, four-factor PCC reverses the effect of VKAs quicker, more effective, and in a smaller volume. If four-factor PCC is not available, FFP can be used for warfarin-reversal; however, it is associated with a higher complication rate, for example, volume overload, and a significant longer time to correct the INR. Vitamin K can be administered, but takes 6 hours or more for reversing the anticoagulation effects of warfarin. Therapeutic goals are monitored with PT and INR levels. Exaggerated effects of warfarin are seen in patients who are nutritionally deficient in vitamin K or are also on amiodarone. In an acute setting with critically ill patients, warfarin is not a first-line agent of anticoagulation.

4. **Platelet inhibitors** such as aspirin and other nonsteroidal anti-inflammatory drugs (NSAIDs) affect the cyclooxygenase (COX) pathway and inhibit platelet aggregation. Due to the irreversible COX inhibition, the effect of aspirin lasts 7 to 10 days, whereas the reversible COX inhibition of other NSAIDs last about 3 days.

   a. In recent multicenter, randomized control trials (POISE-2), aspirin was not shown to decrease perioperative cardiac events in patients undergoing noncardiac surgery compared with placebo. The Food and Drug Administration in the United States removed primary prevention as an indication for daily aspirin use. It is important to note that patients with cardiac or vascular comorbidities such as recent coronary stents or carotid artery stenosis are still recommended to take aspirin for secondary prevention.

   b. Other platelet inhibitors include clopidogrel and ticlopidine, which are potent antiplatelet drugs that inhibit ADP-mediated platelet aggregation. Abciximab and eptifibatide are intravenous glycoprotein IIb/IIIa receptor antagonists. Fibrinogen and von Willebrand's factor are prevented from binding to the platelet and prevents aggregation. The use of glycoprotein IIb/IIIa receptor antagonists are contraindicated within 6 weeks of major surgery or trauma due to an increased incidence of bleeding.

   c. Point-of-care platelet function analysis such as whole-blood impedance aggregometry can help guide the need for platelet transfusion if emergent reversal of antiplatelet therapy is required. Furthermore, updated American and European practice guidelines have issued a Class IIb recommendation (classification of recommendation: IIb = may be considered; benefit ≥ risk; additional studies with broad objectives needed) for platelet function testing to facilitate the choice of P2Y12 receptor inhibitor in selected high-risk patients treated with percutaneous coronary intervention.

5. **Direct thrombin inhibitors (DTIs)** do not require cofactors to inhibit circulating and clot bound thrombin. Laboratory tests include ACT, dilute thrombin time (dTT), ecarin clotting time (ECT), and aPTT to guide therapeutic range. ECT and dTT show the highest sensitivity and a strong linear correlation to drug levels. Since aPTT reaches a plateau at higher DTI plasma concentrations, an overdose may not be recognized. There is no active reversal medication for these potent anticoagulants, but most have short half-lives.

   a. Argatroban has a half-life of 40 minutes and is approved by the FDA for treatment and prophylaxis of HIT. Patients with hepatic dysfunction or multiple organ failure require dose reduction to 0.1 to 0.2 μg/kg/min in order to avoid bleeding complications. Argatroban falsely interferes with the PT/INR values; thus, consideration must be taken when bridging to warfarin anticoagulation. It also crosses the blood–brain barrier and may play a role in the treatment of ischemic or thrombotic stroke.

   b. Bivalirudin has a half-life of 25 minutes and is used for percutaneous coronary interventions. Off-label, it has been used successfully in the treatment of HIT and for cardiopulmonary bypass in patients with HIT.

    c. Lepirudin has a half-life of 80 minutes, but undergoes renal excretion, and thus should be dose-adjusted or avoided in patients with renal failure.

    d. Oral direct thrombin inhibitors include dabigatran etexilate, which requires conversion to dabigatran. It was shown to be as effective as enoxaparin in preventing DVT after total hip replacement, but like most oral agents its usefulness in the critical care setting is limited. Furthermore, dabigatran plasma levels cumulate significantly in patients with renal impairment (creatinine clearance <50 mL/min), which is associated with an increased risk of bleeding. Dabigatran is contraindicated in patients with severe renal impairment (creatinine clearance <30 mL/min). Dabigatran can be eliminated by hemodialysis. Four-factor PCC and activated PCC, but not rFVIIa, seem to be effective in reducing the anticoagulant effect of dabigatran. A specific antidote is under development.

  6. **Thrombolytics** convert plasminogen to plasmin to lyse fibrin clots. These include tissue plasminogen activator (tPA), streptokinase, and urokinase. There is a high risk of bleeding in a perioperative setting due to the hypofibrinogenemic state. In the setting of acute coronary, pulmonary, cerebral, or other major vascular artery occlusion, they can be life or limb saving. Emergent reversal may require administration of aminocaproic acid, tranexamic acid, or transfusion of FPP or cryoprecipitate.

C. Hemostatic Agents

  1. **Desmopressin (DDAVP).** DDAVP increases release of multimer factor VIII: vWf and plasminogen activator from endothelial cells. It is useful in certain coagulopathic states, such as uremia, von Willebrand's deficiency, or hemophilia A, that involves factor VIII deficiency.

  2. **Lysine analogues (aminocaproic acid, tranexamic acid).** Tranexamic acid (TXA) has been proven in a large RCT to reduce mortality from bleeding by one-third if given within 3 hours of injury. Yet the incidence of thrombosis after trauma was not increased. Aminocaproic acid (Amicar) also inhibits fibrinolysis through decreasing plasmin conversion upstream. Its effects have been variable, but has been used in cardiac surgery (10 g IV load over 1 hour followed by 1–2 g/h), prophylaxis for dental procedures in hemophiliac patients, and during liver transplantation surgeries. Thrombotic risks of lysine analogues have been suggested but not proven in randomized controlled trials.

  3. **Coagulation factor concentrates** are available as plasma-derived or recombinant products. In the United States, most of the factor concentrates are FDA-approved for congenital deficiencies only, for example, fibrinogen concentrate for congenital fibrinogen deficiency, factor VIII for hemophilia A, vWF/factor VIII complex concentrates for von Willebrand's disease, factor IX and three-factor prothrombin complex concentrates (3F-PCCs) for hemophilia B, and factor XIII for congenital factor XIII deficiency. Some other coagulation factor concentrates are FDA-approved for acquired coagulation factor deficiencies: four-factor PCCs for urgent reversal of VKAs, such as warfarin, in case of major bleeding, rFVIIa and FEIBA (activated PCC) for acquired hemophilia due to inhibitors, and a solvent detergent-treated pooled plasma product (SD-plasma) for replacement of multiple coagulation factors in patients with acquired deficiencies, for example, due to liver disease, liver transplant, cardiac surgery, or for plasma exchange in TTP. In Europe, most of these co-agulation factor concentrates, in particular fibrinogen concentrate, 4F-PCC, and factor XIII concentrate, are licensed for both congenital and acquired deficiencies and are increasingly used instead of FFP and cryoprecipitate (which is not licensed in several European countries), most often guided by viscoelastic testing (ROTEM/TEG) in severe perioperative or posttraumatic bleeding. The advantages of coagulation factor concentrates is that they can be administered without thawing (no time delay), independent from the blood group (no ABO-mismatch), and in a small volume (no risk of transfusion-associated circulatory overload [TACO]). Furthermore, no case of transfusion-related acute lung injury (TRALI) has been reported related to coagulation factor con-centrates. Pharmaco-economic analyses demonstrated significant cost savings comparing thromboelastometry-guided bleeding management with goal-directed use of coagulation factor concentrates (fibrinogen concentrate and four-factor PCCs) compared with the conventional plasma-based approach. The cost-intensive off-label use of rFVIIa usu-ally is redundant in the goal-directed approach. However, cost analyses have to be done on the basis of the country-specific prices of allogeneic blood products and coagulation factor concentrates, which are both about twice as expensive in the United States compared with Europe. In general, expert hematology consultation is recommended if coagulation factor concentrates are considered to be used in critically ill patients.

IV. FUTURE TRIALS

Upcoming trials include investigating the optimal ratio of red cells to FFP and platelets transfusion practices. This will be studied in the North American Pragmatic, Randomized Optimal Platelets and Plasma Ratios study (NCT01545232). Other multicenter trials are studying the effect of point-of-care testing-guided algorithms or thromboelastometry-guided fibrinogen re-placement on transfusion requirements and patients' outcomes (POC-TACS [NCT02200419], MultiPOC [NCT01826123], and REPLACE [NCT01475669]).

Selected Readings

Adam S, Karger R, Kretschmer V. Photo-optical methods can lead to clinically relevant overestimation of fibrinogen concentration in plasma diluted with hydroxyethyl starch. *Clin Appl Thromb Hemost* 2010;16:461–471.

Adamzik M, Schäfer S, Frey UH, et al. The NFKB1 promoter polymorphism (-94ins/delATTG) alters nuclear translocation of NF-κB1 in monocytes after lipopolysaccha-ride stimulation and is associated with increased mortality in sepsis. *Anesthesiology* 2013;118:123–133.

Adamzik M, Eggmann M, Frey UH, et al. Comparison of thromboelastometry with procal-citonin, interleukin 6, and C-reactive protein as diagnostic tests for severe sepsis in critically ill adults. *Crit Care* 2010;14:R178.

Adamzik M, Görlinger K, Peters J, et al. Whole blood impedance aggregometry as a bio-marker for the diagnosis and prognosis of severe sepsis. *Crit Care* 2012;16:R204.

Adamzik M, Langemeier T, Frey UH, et al. Comparison of thrombelastometry with simpli-fied acute physiology score II and sequential organ failure assessment scores for the prediction of 30-day survival: a cohort study. *Shock* 2011;35:339–342.

Ageno W, Gallus AS, Wittkowsky A, et al; American College of Chest Physicians. Oral anti-coagulant therapy: antithrombotic therapy and prevention of thrombosis, 9th ed: American

College of Chest Physicians Evidence-Based Clinical Practice Guidelines. *Chest* 2012;141(2 suppl):e44S–e88S.

Agren A, Wikman AT, Ostlund A, et al. TEG® functional fibrinogen analysis may overestimate fibrinogen levels. *Anesth Analg* 2014;118:933–935.

Aleshnick M, Orfeo T, Brummel-Ziedins K, et al. Interchangeability of rotational elastographic instruments and reagents. *J Trauma Acute Care Surg* 2014;76:107–113.

Anderson L, Quasim I, Steven M, et al. Inter-operator and intra-operator variability of whole blood coagulation assays: a comparison of thromboelastography and rotational thromboelastometry. *J Cardiothorac Vasc Anesth* 2014;28:1550–1557.

Beiderlinden M, Treschan TA, Görlinger K, et al. Argatroban anticoagulation in critically ill patients. *Ann Pharmacother* 2007;41(5):749–754.

Benson G. Rotational thromboelastometry and its use in directing the management of coagulopathy in the battle injured trauma patient. *J Perioper Pract* 2014;24:25–28.

Bernal W, Wendon J. Acute liver failure. *N Engl J Med* 2013;369:2525–2534.

Berra L, Allain R. Coagulopathy and hypercoagulability. In: Bigatello LM, ed. *Critical care handbook of the Massachusetts general hospital.* 5th ed. Philadelphia: Lippincott Williams & Wilkins, 2009.

Bcynon C, Scherer M, Jakobs M, et al. Initial experiences with Multiplate® for rapid assessment of antiplatelet agent activity in neurosurgical emergencies. *Clin Neurol Neurosurg* 2013;115:2003–2008.

Breuer G, Weiss DR, Ringwald J. "New" direct oral anticoagulants in the perioperative setting. *Curr Opin Anaesthesiol* 2014;27:409–419.

Brohi K, Cohen MJ, Davenport RA. Acute coagulopathy of trauma: mechanism, identification and effect. *Curr Opin Crit Care* 2007;13:680–685.

Chopin N, Floccard B, Sobas F, et al. Activated partial thromboplastin time waveform analysis: a new tool to detect infection? *Crit Care Med* 2006;34:1654–1660.

Collins PW, Solomon C, Sutor K, et al. Theoretical modelling of fibrinogen supplementation with therapeutic plasma, cryoprecipitate, or fibrinogen concentrate. *Br J Anaesth* 2014 Jul 26. doi:10.1093/bja/aeu086.

Craig J, Aguiar-Ibanez R, Downie S, et al. The clinical and cost effectiveness of thromboelastography/thromboelastometry. Health Technology Assessment Report 11, NHS Quality Improvement Scotland 2007. http://www.nhshealthquality.org.

CRASH-2 collaborators, Roberts I, Shakur H, et al. The importance of early treatment with tranexamic acid in bleeding trauma patients: an exploratory analysis of the CRASH-2 randomised controlled trial. *Lancet* 2011;377:1096–1101.

Davenport R, Manson J, De'Ath H, et al. Functional definition and characterization of acute traumatic coagulopathy. *Crit Care Med* 2011;39:2652–2658.

Devereaux PJ, Mrkobrada M, Sessler DI, et al; POISE-2 Investigators. Aspirin in patients undergoing noncardiac surgery. *N Engl J Med* 2014;370:1494–1503.

Edavettal M, Rogers A, Rogers F, et al. Prothrombin complex concentrate accelerates international normalized ratio reversal and diminishes the extension of intracranial hemorrhage in geriatric trauma patients. *Am Surg* 2014;80:372–376.

Eikelboom JW, Weitz JI. Dabigatran monitoring made simple? *Thromb Haemost* 2013;110:393–395.

Escolar G, Fernandez-Gallego V, Arellano-Rodrigo E, et al. Reversal of apixaban induced alterations in hemostasis by different coagulation factor concentrates: significance of studies in vitro with circulating human blood. *PLoS One* 2013;8:e78696.

Fawole A, Daw HA, Crowther MA. Practical management of bleeding due to the anticoagulants dabigatran, rivaroxaban, and apixaban. *Cleve Clin J Med* 2013;80:443–451.

Fenger-Eriksen C, Christiansen K, Laurie J, et al. Fibrinogen concentrate and cryoprecipitate but not fresh frozen plasma correct low fibrinogen concentrations following in vitro haemodilution. *Thromb Res* 2013;131:e210–e213.

Fenger-Eriksen C, Moore GW, Rangarajan S, et al. Fibrinogen estimates are influenced by methods of measurement and hemodilution with colloid plasma expanders. *Transfusion* 2010;50:2571–2576.

Gehrie E, Laposata M. Test of the month: The chromogenic antifactor Xa assay. *Am J Hematol* 2012;87:194–196.

Gerlach R, Krause M, Seifert V, et al. Hemostatic and hemorrhagic problems in neurosurgical patients. *Acta Neurochir* 2009;151:873–900.

Görlinger K, Bergmann L, Dirkmann D. Coagulation management in patients undergoing mechanical circulatory support. *Best Pract Res Clin Anaesthesiol* 2012;26:179–198.

Görlinger K, Schaden E, Saner F. Perioperative hemostasis in hepatic surgery. In: Marcucci CE, Schoettker P, eds. *Perioperative hemostasis: coagulation for anesthesiologists*. Berlin: Springer, 2015.

Görlinger K, Shore-Lesserson L, Dirkmann D, et al. Management of hemorrhage in cardiothoracic surgery. *J Cardiothorac Vasc Anesth* 2013;27(4 suppl):S20–S34.

Görlinger K, Kozek-Langenecker SA. Economic aspects and organisation. In: Marcucci CE, Schoettker P, eds. *Perioperative hemostasis: coagulation for anesthesiologists*. Berlin: Springer, 2015.

Görlinger K, Jambor C, Hanke AA, et al. Perioperative coagulation management and control of platelet transfusion by point-of-care platelet function analysis. *Transfus Med Hemother* 2007;34:396–411.

Görlinger K, Dirkmann D, Solomon C, et al. Fast interpretation of thromboelastometry in non-cardiac surgery: reliability in patients with hypo-, normo-, and hypercoagulability. *Br J Anaesth* 2013;110:222–230.

Greinacher A, Althaus K, Krauel K, et al. Heparin-induced thrombocytopenia. *Hämostaseologie* 2010;30(1):1–50.

Grewal PK, Aziz PV, Uchiyama S, et al. Inducing host protection in pneumococcal sepsis by preactivation of the Ashwell-Morell receptor. *Proc Natl Acad Sci USA* 2013;110:20218–20223.

Grottke O, van Ryn J, Spronk HM, et al. Prothrombin complex concentrates and a specific antidote to dabigatran are effective ex-vivo in reversing the effects of dabigatran in an anticoagulation/liver trauma experimental model. *Crit Care* 2014;18:R27.

Haas T, Görlinger K, Grassetto A, et al. Thromboelastometry for guiding bleeding management of the critically ill patient: a systematic review of the literature. *Minerva Anestesiol* 2014;80:1320–1335.

Hagemo JS, Stanworth S, Juffermans NP, et al. Prevalence, predictors and outcome of hypofibrinogenaemia in trauma: a multicentre observational study. *Crit Care* 2014;18:R52.

Health Policy Advisory Committee on Technology. Rotational thromboelastometry (ROTEM®) – targeted therapy for coagulation management in patients with massive bleeding. HealthPACT, State of Queensland, Australia, 2012. http://www.health.qld.gov.au/healthpact.

Hickey M, Gatien M, Taljaard M, et al. Outcomes of urgent warfarin reversal with frozen plasma versus prothrombin complex concentrate in the emergency department. *Circulation* 2013;128:360–364.

Holbrook A, Schulman S, Witt DM, et al; American College of Chest Physicians. Evidence-based management of anticoagulant therapy: antithrombotic therapy and prevention of thrombosis, 9th ed: American College of Chest Physicians Evidence-Based Clinical Practice Guidelines. *Chest* 2012;141(2 suppl):e152S–e184S.

Holcomb JB, del Junco DJ, Fox EE, et al. The prospective, observational, multicenter, major trauma transfusion (PROMMTT) study: comparative effectiveness of a time-varying treatment with competing risks. *JAMA Surg* 2013;148:127–136.

Holcomb JB, Pati S. Optimal trauma resuscitation with plasma as the primary resuscitative fluid: the surgeon's perspective. *Hematology Am Soc Hematol Educ Program* 2013;2013:656–659.

Holcomb JB, Gumbert S. Potential value of protocols in substantially bleeding trauma patients. *Curr Opin Anaesthesiol* 2013;26:215–220.

Horton S, Augustin S. Activated clotting time (ACT). *Methods Mol Biol* 2013;992:155–167.

Huissoud C, Carrabin N, Benchaib M, et al. Coagulation assessment by rotation thrombelastometry in normal pregnancy. *Thromb Haemost* 2009;101:755–761.

Hunt BJ. Bleeding and coagulopathies in critical care. *N Engl J Med* 2014;370:847–859.

Inaba K, Branco BC, Rhee P, et al. Impact of ABO-identical vs ABO-compatible nonidentical plasma transfusion in trauma patients. *Arch Surg* 2010;145:899–906.

Innerhofer P, Westermann I, Tauber H, et al. The exclusive use of coagulation factor concentrates enables reversal of coagulopathy and decreases transfusion rates in patients with major blunt trauma. *Injury* 2013;44:209–216.

Johansson PI, Sørensen AM, Perner A, et al. Disseminated intravascular coagulation or acute coagulopathy of trauma shock early after trauma? An observational study. *Crit Care* 2011;15:R272.

Juffermans NP, Prins DJ, Vlaar AP, et al. Transfusion-related risk of secondary bacterial infections in sepsis patients: a retrospective cohort study. *Shock* 2011;35:355–359.

Karkouti K, Callum J, Crowther MA, et al. The relationship between fibrinogen levels after cardiopulmonary bypass and large volume red cell transfusion in cardiac surgery: an observational study. *Anesth Analg* 2013;117:14–22.

Khan S, Brohi K, Chana M, et al; International Trauma Research Network (INTRN). Hemostatic resuscitation is neither hemostatic nor resuscitative in trauma hemorrhage. *J Trauma Acute Care Surg* 2014;76:561–568.

Kinard TN, Sarode R. Four factor prothrombin complex concentrate (human): review of the pharmacology and clinical application for vitamin K antagonist reversal. *Expert Rev Cardiovasc Ther* 2014;12:417–427.

Koch CD, Wockenfus AM, Miller RS, et al. Intra-assay precision, inter-assay precision, and reliability of five platelet function methods used to monitor the effect of aspirin and clopidogrel on platelet function. *Clin Chem* 2013;59(suppl):A152.

Konkle BA. Acquired disorders of platelet function. *Hematology Am Soc Hematol Educ Program* 2011;391–396.

Körber MK, Langer E, Ziemer S, et al. Measurement and reversal of prophylactic and therapeutic peak levels of rivaroxaban: an in vitro study. *Clin Appl Thromb Hemost* 2014;20:735–740.

Korte W. F XIII in perioperative coagulation management. *Best Pract Res Clin Anaesthesiol* 2010;24:85–93.

Koscielny J, Rutkauskaite E. Rivaroxaban and hemostasis in emergency care. *Emerg Med Int* 2014;2014:935474.

Koyama K, Madoiwa S, Nunomiya S, et al. Combination of thrombin-antithrombin complex, plasminogen activator inhibitor-1, and protein C activity for early identification of severe coagulopathy in initial phase of sepsis: a prospective observational study. *Crit Care* 2014;18:R13.

Kozek-Langenecker SA, Afshari A, Albaladejo P, et al. Management of severe perioperative bleeding: guidelines from the European Society of Anaesthesiology. *Eur J Anaesthesiol* 2013;30:270–382.

Kutcher ME, Redick BJ, McCreery RC, et al. Characterization of platelet dysfunction after trauma. *J Trauma Acute Care Surg* 2012;73:13–19.

Larsen OH, Fenger-Eriksen C, Christiansen K, et al. Diagnostic performance and therapeutic consequence of thromboelastometry activated by kaolin versus a panel of specific reagents. *Anesthesiology* 2011;115:294–302.

Levi M. Coagulation in sepsis. *Int J Intensive Care* 2013;20:77–81.

Levine GN, Bates ER, Blankenship JC, et al; American College of Cardiology Foundation; American Heart Association Task Force on Practice Guidelines; Society for Cardiovascular Angiography and Interventions. 2011 ACCF/AHA/SCAI Guideline for percutaneous coronary intervention. A report of the American College of Cardiology Foundation/ American Heart Association Task Force on Practice Guidelines and the Society for Cardiovascular Angiography and Interventions. *J Am Coll Cardiol* 2011;58:e44–e122.

Levy JH, Faraoni D, Spring JL, et al. Managing new oral anticoagulants in the perioperative and intensive care unit setting. *Anesthesiology* 2013;18:1466–1474.

Liesenfeld KH, Staab A, Härtter S, et al. Pharmacometric characterization of dabigatran hemodialysis. *Clin Pharmacokinet* 2013;52:453–462.

Lind SE, Boyle ME, Fisher S, et al. Comparison of the aPTT with alternative tests for monitoring direct thrombin inhibitors in patient samples. *Am J Clin Pathol* 2014;141(5):665–674. doi:10.1309/AJCPGTCEX7K4GXQO.

Love JE, Ferrell C, Chandler WL. Monitoring direct thrombin inhibitors with a plasma diluted thrombin time. *Thromb Haemost* 2007;98:234–242.

Maegele M, Schöchl H, Cohen MJ. An update on the coagulopathy of trauma. *Shock* 2014;41(suppl 1):21–25.

Mahla E, Suarez TA, Bliden KP, et al. Platelet function measurement-based strategy to reduce bleeding and waiting time in clopidogrel-treated patients undergoing coronary artery bypass surgery: the timing based on platelet function strategy to reduce clopidogrel-associated bleeding related to CABG (TARGET-CABG) study. *Circ Cardiovasc Interv* 2012;5:261–269.

Mallett SV, Chowdary P, Burroughs AK. Clinical utility of viscoelastic tests of coagulation in patients with liver disease. *Liver Int* 2013;33:961–974.

Mauch J, Spielmann N, Hartnack S, et al. Intrarater and interrater variability of point of care coagulation testing using the ROTEM delta. *Blood Coagul Fibrinolysis* 2011;22:662–666.

Morel-Kopp MC, Tan CW, Brighton TA, et al; ASTH Clinical Trials Group. Validation of whole blood impedance aggregometry as a new diagnostic tool for HIT: results of a large Australian study. *Thromb Haemost* 2012;107(3):575–583.

Müller MC, Meijers JC, Vroom MB, et al. Utility of thromboelastography and/or thromboelastometry in adults with sepsis: a systematic review. *Crit Care* 2014;18:R30.

Mylotte D, Foley D, Kenny D. Platelet function testing: methods of assessment and clinical utility. *Cardiovasc Hematol Agents Med Chem* 2011;9:14–24.

Nascimento B, Callum J, Tien H, et al. Effect of a fixed-ratio (1:1:1) transfusion protocol versus laboratory-results-guided transfusion in patients with severe trauma: a randomized feasibility trial. *CMAJ* 2013;185:E583–E589.

Newland A, Akehurst R, Collinson P, et al. Detecting, managing and monitoring haemostasis: viscoelastometric point-of-care testing (ROTEM, TEG and Sonoclot systems). NICE diagnostics guidance 13. National Institute for Health and Care Excellence (NICE), Manchester, UK, 2014. http://www.nice.org.uk/guidance/DG13.

Orlov D, McCluskey SA, Selby R, et al. Platelet dysfunction as measured by a point-of-care monitor is an independent predictor of high blood loss in cardiac surgery. *Anesth Analg* 2014;118:257–263.

Pötzsch B, Madlener K, Seelig C, et al. Monitoring of r-hirudin anticoagulation during cardiopulmonary bypass—assessment of the whole blood ecarin clotting time. *Thromb Haemost* 1997;77:920–925.

Ranucci M, Baryshnikova E, Soro G, et al; Surgical and Clinical Outcome Research (SCORE) Group. Multiple electrode whole-blood aggregometry and bleeding in cardiac surgery patients receiving thienopyridines. *Ann Thorac Surg* 2011;91:123–129.

Rasmussen KC, Johansson PI, Højskov M, et al. Hydroxyethyl starch reduces coagulation competence and increases blood loss during major surgery: results from a randomized controlled trial. *Ann Surg* 2014;259:249–254.

Sankarankutty A, Nascimento B, Teodoro da Luz L, et al. TEG® and ROTEM® in trauma: similar test but different results? *World J Emerg Surg* 2012;7(suppl 1):S3.

Sarode R, Milling TJ Jr, Refaai MA, et al. Efficacy and safety of a 4-factor prothrombin complex concentrate in patients on vitamin K antagonists presenting with major bleeding: a randomized, plasma-controlled, phase IIIb study. *Circulation* 2013;128:1234–1243.

Schaden E, Saner FH, Goerlinger K. Coagulation pattern in critical liver dysfunction. *Curr Opin Crit Care* 2013;19:142–148.

Schaden E, Schober A, Hacker S, et al. Ecarin modified rotational thrombelastometry: a point-of-care applicable alternative to monitor the direct thrombin inhibitor argatroban. *Wien Klin Wochenschr* 2013;125(5–6):156–159. doi:10.1007/s00508-013-0327-1.

Scharf RE. Drugs that affect platelet function. *Semin Thromb Hemost* 2012;38:865–883.

Schöchl H, Cotton B, Inaba K, et al. FIBTEM provides early prediction of massive transfusion in trauma. *Crit Care* 2011;15(6):R265.

Schöchl H, Maegele M, Solomon C, et al. Early and individualized goal-directed therapy for trauma-induced coagulopathy. *Scand J Trauma Resusc Emerg Med* 2012;20:15.

Shanwell A, Andersson TM, Rostgaard K, et al. Post-transfusion mortality among recipients of ABO-compatible but non-identical plasma. *Vox Sang* 2009;96:316–323.

Skhirtladze K, Base EM, Lassnigg A, et al. Comparison of the effects of albumin 5%, hydroxyethyl starch 130/0.4 6%, and Ringer's lactate on blood loss and coagulation after cardiac surgery. *Br J Anaesth* 2014;112:255–264.

Spahn DR, Bouillon B, Cerny V, et al. Management of bleeding and coagulopathy following major trauma: an updated European guideline. *Crit Care* 2013;17:R76.

Stensballe J, Ostrowski SR, Johansson PI. Viscoelastic guidance of resuscitation. *Curr Opin Anaesthesiol* 2014;27:212–218.

Sucker C, Zotz RB, Görlinger K, et al. Rotational thrombelastometry for the bedside monitoring of recombinant hirudin. *Acta Anaesthesiol Scand* 2008;52:358–362.

Tanaka KA, Bader SO, Görlinger K. Novel approaches in management of perioperative coagulopathy. *Curr Opin Anaesthesiol* 2014;27:72–80.

Tantry US, Bonello L, Aradi D, et al; Working Group on On-Treatment Platelet Reactivity. Consensus and update on the definition of on-treatment platelet reactivity to adenosine diphosphate associated with ischemia and bleeding. *J Am Coll Cardiol* 2013;62:2261–2273.

Tripodi A, Mannucci PM. The coagulopathy of chronic liver disease. *N Engl J Med* 2011;365:147–156.

Tripodi A, Primignani M, Chantarangkul V, et al. Global hemostasis tests in patients with cirrhosis before and after prophylactic platelet transfusion. *Liver Int* 2013;33:362–327.

van Ryn J, Stangier J, Haertter S, et al. Dabigatran etexilate—a novel, reversible, oral direct thrombin inhibitor: interpretation of coagulation assays and reversal of anticoagulant activity. *Thromb Haemost* 2010;103:1116–1127.

Venema LF, Post WJ, Hendriks HG, et al. An assessment of clinical interchangeability of TEG and RoTEM thromboelastographic variables in cardiac surgical patients. *Anesth Analg* 2010;111:339–344.

Villa E, Cammà C, Marietta M, et al. Enoxaparin prevents portal vein thrombosis and liver decompensation in patients with advanced cirrhosis. *Gastroenterology* 2012;143:1253–1260.

Wada H, Thachil J, Di Nisio M, et al. The Scientific Standardization Committee on DIC of the International Society on Thrombosis Haemostasis. Guidance for diagnosis and treatment of DIC from harmonization of the recommendations from three guidelines. *J Thromb Haemost* 2013;11:761–767.

Weber CF, Görlinger K, Meininger D, et al. Point-of-care testing: a prospective, randomized clinical trial of efficacy in coagulopathic cardiac surgery patients. *Anesthesiology* 2012;117:531–547.

Yanamadala V, Walcott BP, Fecci PE, et al. Reversal of warfarin associated coagulopathy with 4-factor prothrombin complex concentrate in traumatic brain injury and intracranial hemorrhage. *J Clin Neurosci* 2014;21:1881–1884.

Zakariah AN, Cozzi SM, Van Nuffelen M, et al. Combination of biphasic transmittance waveform with blood procalcitonin levels for diagnosis of sepsis in acutely ill patients. *Crit Care Med* 2008;36:1507–1512.

Acute Gastrointestinal Diseases

Marc A. de Moya, Jean Kwo, and Eugene Fukudome

I. There are several gastrointestinal (GI) diseases that present in an acute fashion and require critical care, that is, acute pancreatitis, intestinal perforation, ischemic bowel, acute bleeding, or following a major surgical procedure involving the GI tract. In addition, those critically ill may also develop acute GI complications as a result of the systemic inflammatory response. This chapter will focus on the most common GI diseases that may lead to ICU admission and those GI diseases that arise from being critically ill.

II. **EVALUATION OF SUSPECTED GI PATHOLOGY**: The diagnosis of a GI disorder in the critically ill can be challenging as these patients may not be able to articulate their symptoms and often do not present with classic clinical findings. A nonspecific finding such as a change in mental status, fever, leukocytosis, hypotension, or decreased urine output may be the only sign of intra-abdominal pathology. Physical examination may be unreliable, and the patient may be too unstable to leave the ICU to undergo diagnostic studies. Thus, clinicians must maintain a high index of suspicion for an undiagnosed GI problem as a cause of hemodynamic instability.

A. **Signs and Symptoms** that suggest GI pathology are numerous and can include abdominal pain, chest pain, bleeding (hematemesis, melena, rectal bleeding), emesis, change in bowel habits, and tube feed intolerance.

B. **Initial Evaluation** includes assessing for abdominal tenderness and distension, fever, tachycardia, hypotension, and/or change in vasopressor requirement. Correct positioning and function of existing nasogastric tubes and abdominal drains must be confirmed. Laboratory tests such as a complete blood count (CBC), serum chemistries, liver function tests (LFTs), and amylase may be helpful.

C. Increased vigilance is required when caring for solid **organ transplant** recipients or patients with chronic inflammatory or autoimmune disorders treated with immunosuppressive medications. These chronically **immunosuppressed** patients may have no signs or symptoms of ongoing GI pathology.

D. **Further Diagnostic Studies and Procedures** are often necessary to establish a diagnosis and are guided by the initial assessment. Portable plain radiographs can reveal the presence of pneumoperitoneum, intestinal obstruction, or confirm the correct placement of an enteral tube (Fig. 26.1). However, more sophisticated studies are often required to establish a diagnosis. The risks associated with a diagnostic study must be weighed against the expected benefits. Commonly performed tests such as an abdominal CT scan pose a higher risk to the critically ill patient who is at increased risk for contrast-induced nephropathy (see **Chapter 25**), ventilator-associated pneumonia, as well as airway and hemodynamic complications while traveling to the radiology department. Commonly available diagnostic modalities and their advantages and disadvantages in an ICU setting are summarized in Table 26.1.

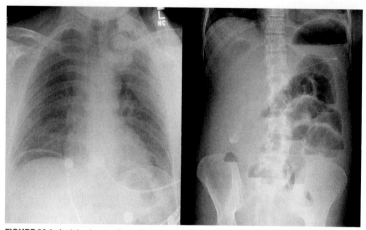

FIGURE 26.1 A plain chest radiograph demonstrating pneumoperitoneum (left) and an abdominal film demonstrating small bowel obstruction and nasogastric tube placement (right) (Courtesy of Hasan Alam, MD).

III. **GI BLEEDING** is commonly seen in an ICU setting (Table 26.2). GI bleeding may originate from the upper (proximal to the ligament of Treitz) or lower GI tract. Risk factors include liver disease, alcoholism, uremia, diverticulosis, peptic ulcer disease, and the intake of a variety of medications, including nonsteroidal anti-inflammatory drugs (NSAIDs), antiplatelet agents, and anticoagulants.
   A. **Signs and Symptoms** include shock, hematemesis, coffee ground emesis, melena, hematochezia, or hematocrit drop with occult blood present in the stool.
   B. **Initial Evaluation** may need to proceed simultaneously, with stabilization depending on the rate of blood loss and hemodynamic stability of the patient.
      1. A **history** focusing on risk factors for GI bleeding, prior abdominal operations, and significant medical comorbidities should be obtained.
      2. **Physical examination** should focus on assessing end-organ perfusion. Certain physical findings such as stigmata of liver disease may suggest an underlying etiology.
      3. **Laboratory studies** including CBC, coagulation studies, and chemistries should be obtained. Initial hemoglobin values will not reflect the degree of acute blood loss.
   C. **Stabilization** is accomplished by ensuring an adequate airway, hemodynamic stability, and adequate monitoring. A patient with an altered level of consciousness and copious hematemesis will likely require endotracheal intubation. Adequate peripheral intravenous access should be secured. Central venous access, an arterial catheter, and a urinary catheter placement may be appropriate for patients in shock. Initial resuscitation with isotonic crystalloid solution is appropriate while preparations for blood transfusions are made. Resuscitation with blood products in a 1:2::FFP:RBC ratio for those who require a massive blood transfusion (>10 units PRBC) is an appropriate goal. There is some

TABLE 26.1	Diagnostic Modalities for Acute Gastrointestinal Diseases in the ICU	
Modality	**Advantages and Usefulness**	**Disadvantages**
Plain radiographs	• Portable and fast • Assess for free air • Confirm tube placement (nasogastric, postpyloric)	• Findings are usually nonspecific • Overlying tubes, monitors, cables, and other ICU equipment often obscure images
Ultrasound	• Portable • Assess gall bladder/biliary tree • Can guide procedures (paracentesis, biliary drains)	• Image quality is operator dependent • Air-filled intestines can obscure images
CT	• Characterizes many forms of intra-abdominal pathology • CT angiography can assess mesenteric vessels	• Patient transport out of the ICU • Optimum study requires IV contrast, which can cause nephropathy and allergic reactions
MRI	• Noninvasive method to assess for choledocholithiasis	• Patient transport out of the ICU • Time-consuming • Requires patient cooperation
Angiography	• Diagnostic and therapeutic in mesenteric ischemia • GI bleeding and intra-abdominal/ pelvic bleeding following trauma	• Patient transport out of the ICU • Requires IV contrast • Risk of vascular injury (arterial injury at the access site, pseudoaneurysms, hematoma, bleeding, arterial dissection, and embolization of vessel plaque)
Radionuclide imaging	• HIDA scan may help characterize suspected biliary pathology such as cholecystitis • Technetium scan can confirm ongoing GI bleeding	• Never an initial diagnostic test • Patient transport out of the ICU • Limited utility in an ICU setting
Endoscopy	• Diagnostic and therapeutic • EGD and colonoscopy can be performed portably • ERCP can be life-saving in cholangitis	• Requires sedation • Colonoscopy requires colonic purge for optimum study • Small risk of intestinal perforation • ERCP can cause pancreatitis
Bedside laparoscopy	• Direct visualization facilitates diagnosis of acalculous cholecystitis and mesenteric ischemia, according to several reports (small case series) • Can potentially avoid nontherapeutic laparotomy	• Invasive • Inability to evaluate some areas (retroperitoneum) • Patient must be mechanically ventilated and sedated • Utility as a diagnostic modality in the ICU has not been rigorously studied

TABLE 26.2	Causes of Gastrointestinal (GI) Bleeding	

Upper GI Source	Lower GI Source
Variceal bleeding	Diverticulum
• Esophageal, gastric, duodenal	• Small bowel, colonic
Mallory–Weiss tears	Inflammatory bowel disease
Peptic ulcers	Mesenteric ischemia, including ischemic colitis
• Gastric, duodenal	Infectious colitis
Gastritis and erosions	Malignancy
Malignancy	Angiodysplasia
Dieulafoy's lesions	• Colonic, small bowel
Arterial-enteric fistula	Hemorrhoids
• Rupture of aneurysm or ulcer	
• Postaortic surgery	
Diverticulum (duodenal)	
Angiodysplasia (duodenal)	
Hemobilia	
Pancreatic bleeding	

controversy regarding the target hemoglobin but overall it appears that having a lower target (7 g/dL), at least in upper GI bleeds, was associated with less bleeding and lower mortality. Severe coagulopathy should be corrected (see **Chapter 27**).

D. Localization of Bleeding

1. **Nasogastric tube lavage** of the stomach is easy to perform and is the first maneuver performed to rule out an upper GI source. A clear lavage of the stomach with some bile staining reassures the clinician that the source is not the upper GI tract.

2. **Endoscopy**

   a. **Esophagogastroduodenoscopy (EGD)** is the diagnostic test of choice for suspected upper GI bleeding and is diagnostic in 90% to 95% of cases. Often, the precise source of bleeding is identified, allowing for immediate endoscopic therapy; however, this can be challenging if a copious amount of blood and clot is present.

   b. **Colonoscopy** for lower GI bleeding is diagnostic in 53% to 97% of cases, depending on the patient population of each study. Colonoscopy is usually undertaken after a colonic purge to increase diagnostic accuracy and visualization. Again, it is possible to perform a therapeutic maneuver as well but these are less successful than the upper GI bleeds. Complications, including perforation, are rare, but the index of suspicion for their occurrence must be high in critically ill, elderly, and immunosuppressed patients.

3. **Angiography** may be required if endoscopy cannot localize bleeding.

   a. Requires ongoing bleeding for successful angiographic detection (0.5–1 mL/min, approximately 3 U of blood per day).

   b. Angiography may direct endoscopic or surgical treatment or may be therapeutic via embolization or selective intra-arterial vasopressin infusion. The risk of significant bowel ischemia as a result of embolization, even in the small or large bowel, is less than 5% but the patient must be monitored for ischemia with serial abdominal exams.

  c. Other complications associated with angiography include contrast-induced nephropathy, distal embolization of vessel wall plaque, and access site complications.
  d. Provocative angiography may be performed if no bleeding is able to be detected by conventional angiography. This technique involves the use of pressors to drive the systolic pressure high (160–180 mmHg), vasodilators to dilate the mesenteric vessels, and heparin. If heparin fails, a low dose of tPA may be considered. By provoking the bleeding, the angiographer may then perform the embolization. If angiographer cannot control the bleeding, the patient must go to the operating room for a resection immediately or if in a hybrid room have the procedure done in the same room. Therefore a multidisciplinary approach with radiology and surgery is key. A provocative angiogram demonstrates the bleeding in approximately 50% of the cases.

4. Radionuclide imaging involves the use of one or two available tracers: technetium-99m–labeled sulfur colloid (^{99m}Tc-SC), and technetium-^{99m}–labeled red blood cells (^{99m}Tc-RBC). ^{99m}Tc-SC can be used immediately, but is taken up by the liver and spleen, which can obscure interpretation of the images when bleeding is located adjacent to these structures. ^{99m}Tc-RBC is not taken up by the liver and spleen, but requires preparation prior to use.
  a. ^{99m}Tc-labeled scans are sensitive and can confirm ongoing bleeding. Their specificity in determining a precise anatomic site of bleeding is debatable.
  b. Their utility in an ICU setting is limited, but may be helpful in hemodynamically stable patients with slow lower GI bleeding not localized by colonoscopy.

5. A **capsule study** can occasionally help identify a bleeding source in the small bowel of hemodynamically stable patients.

E. Specific Therapy for Common Causes of GI Bleeding
 1. Upper GI bleeding
  a. Variceal bleeding may originate in the esophagus, stomach, or duodenum and is usually the result of cirrhosis and portal hypertension. Splenic vein thrombosis can also result in the development of gastric varices.
    1. Prognosis is related mainly to the severity of the patient's underlying liver disease. Mortality following an episode of variceal bleeding ranges from 10% to 70%. The risk of rebleeding is 70% within 6 months.
    2. Early endoscopy is crucial for diagnosis and management. Between 30% and 50% of patients with known varices bleed from other upper GI sources. Endoscopic variceal band ligation and sclerotherapy can control bleeding in 80% to 90% of cases.
    3. Balloon tamponade is indicated when endoscopic interventions cannot control esophageal or gastric variceal bleeding. Because of the risk of pressure necrosis, balloon deflation must occur within 24 to 48 hours and should be followed by another attempt at endoscopy with band ligation or sclerotherapy. *It is important to protect the airway with endotracheal intubation prior to placement of the balloon tube.*
    4. Medical management should occur concurrently with endoscopy or balloon tamponade. **Somatostatin** and its synthetic analog **octreotide,** as well as **vasopressin**, have been used.

5. After the bleeding has stopped and the patient is stabilized, treatment with **nonselective β-blockers** (propranolol or nadolol) should be initiated. These agents decrease the risk of rebleeding and have a proven survival benefit.

6. **Transjugular intrahepatic portosystemic shunting (TIPS)** controls refractory variceal bleeding in up to 90% of cases by reducing the portal pressure gradient to <15 mmHg. Using a trans-jugular approach, a stent is placed in the liver to connect a branch of the portal vein with a hepatic vein. Complications include occlusion, accelerated liver failure, and hepatic encephalopathy.

7. **Surgical therapy** for refractory bleeding includes splenorenal shunt and portacaval shunt and should generally be undertaken after the patient is determined to not be a liver transplant candidate.

8. **Splenectomy** is indicated in patients who are bleeding from gastric varices due to splenic vein thrombosis.

b. **Mallory-Weiss tears** are mucosal lacerations within 2 cm of the gastroesophageal (GE) junction that are likely due to increases in pressure occurring during vomiting. Most of these lesions stop bleeding spontaneously and have less than a 10% chance of rebleeding. However, actively bleeding Mallory-Weiss tears are best addressed endoscopically.

c. **Peptic ulcer disease** can manifest as duodenal or gastric ulcers.

1. **EGD** is the initial diagnostic and therapeutic choice. The **endoscopic appearance** of an ulcer has prognostic significance. Ulcers with a spurting artery or a visible vessel have a high rebleeding risk (50%–100%). Ulcers with adherent clot or a red or black spot are at moderate risk, while ulcers with a clean base are at low risk (<5%) for rebleeding. Repeat EGD may be necessary to control bleeding in some circumstances. In refractory cases, angiographic embolization has been reported to stop bleeding in 80% to 88% of cases. Uncontrolled bleeding in a hemodynamically unstable patient may necessitate surgical intervention.

2. **Acid suppression** with proton pump inhibitors (PPIs) has evolved as a crucial component in the management of ulcer disease. In the acute setting, PPIs are administered intravenously as a continuous infusion or twice-daily boluses. Patients are then transitioned to an oral regimen. PPIs produce more consistent acid suppression than histamine receptor (H2) blockers. Patients with large ulcerations >2 cm have a high risk of failing medical therapy, and surgical resection/acid reduction should be considered.

3. *Helicobacter pylori* **infection** (see **Section IV.B.2**), if present, should be eradicated to decreases the rate of future rebleeding.

4. Mucosal ulcerations may be due to **neoplasm** rather than peptic ulcer disease. The endoscopic appearance in conjunction with a biopsy will help establish the correct diagnosis.

d. **Stress ulceration,** also called stress-related erosive syndrome, erosive gastritis, or hemorrhagic gastritis, leads to upper GI bleeding in 1% to 7% of ICU patients. Mucosal hypoperfusion and increased gastric acidity occurring in critically ill patients are postulated to play a role in pathogenesis.

1. **Endoscopic** findings include mucosal erosions.

2. **Management** is with PPIs as discussed above. *H. pylori* infection should be excluded. Rarely, angiography with selective

embolization (often of the left gastric artery) is necessary. Operative management is reserved for severe refractory hemorrhage.

e. **Aortoenteric fistulae** are communications between the GI tract, most commonly the distal duodenum, and either the native aorta (primary) or an aortic vascular graft (secondary). Secondary fistulas are more common, occurring in 0.6% to 1.5% of patients after open aortic reconstructive surgery. An initial "herald" bleed followed by massive hemorrhage has been described. Patients may also present with graft infection. Accurate and timely diagnosis is facilitated by a high index of suspicion.

   1. **Endoscopy** demonstrating an eroding aortic graft is uncommon. CT scan is the diagnostic study of choice and may demonstrate hematoma or air at the aortic graft. Once the diagnosis is established, emergency operative exploration is indicated.

f. **Dieulafoy's lesion** is an abnormally large artery protruding through the mucosa, most often into the gastric lumen (fundus or body). There is no mucosal ulceration. Bleeding can be massive and can recur in 5% to 15% despite endoscopic therapy. When rebleeding occurs despite endoscopic intervention, surgical ligation or excision of the vessel is indicated.

g. **Duodenal diverticulum** is a rare cause of upper GI bleeding. The diagnosis can be made endoscopically. Bleeding duodenal diverticula are treated with surgical excision.

h. **Angiodysplasia** can be located throughout the entire GI tract and can cause brisk bleeding. Endoscopy can detect and treat these lesions. Surgical excision is indicated when lesions continue to bleed despite medical management.

i. **Pancreatic bleeding** can occur from erosion of a pancreatic pseudocyst into an adjacent vessel, resulting in upper GI bleeding. This is most commonly associated with episodes of pancreatitis.

j. **Hemobilia** can result from trauma, procedures such as liver biopsy, biliary stent placement, malignancy, gallstones, or erosion of blood vessels into the biliary tree. Treatment of choice is angioembolization.

2. **Lower GI bleeding** accounts for approximately 25% of GI bleeding and has a mortality rate of 2% to 4%.

   a. **Intestinal ischemia** can involve either the small bowel or the colon and can present with lower GI bleeding. Intestinal ischemia is discussed later in greater detail (Section IV.F.1).

   b. **Small bowel bleeding** is suspected after two negative EGDs and a negative colonoscopy.

      1. **Angiodysplasia** is the most common cause of GI hemorrhage between the ligament of Treitz and the ileocecal valve. Other causes include tumors, inflammatory bowel disease, Meckel's diverticulum, NSAID-induced ulcers, and Dieulafoy's lesions.

      2. **Diagnosis** is difficult but may be made in approximately 50% to 70% of cases by push enteroscopy (which examines the jejunum) or capsule study. If the bleeding is brisk, radionuclide scans or angiography may be useful. Again, a provocative angiogram (see above) is an option followed by embolization or operative resection. The angiographer may leave the catheter in place and the surgeon may inject the catheter during the laparotomy with methylene blue to visualize the segment of bowel with the bleeding site.

3. **Treatment** of small intestinal sources of bleeding is directed at the underlying disease.

c. **Diverticular bleeding** accounts for 20% of colonic bleeding and is the most common cause of massive lower GI bleeding. Hemorrhage occurs when the *vasa recta* ruptures into an adjacent diverticular lumen. Bleeding is usually self-limited in 85% of cases but can recur in 14% to 53% of patients. Colonoscopy can locate the site of bleeding, but therapeutic maneuvers are difficult. Angiography can also localize the bleeding and is potentially therapeutic. Urgent operative resection is indicated when bleeding and hemodynamic instability persists. Elective colectomy is considered after multiple episodes of diverticular bleeding.

d. **Colonic angiodysplasias** are more frequent in patients above the age of 60. Most lesions are found in the ascending colon, and most patients have multiple lesions. Colonoscopy and angiography are very successful for diagnosis and treatment, and colon resection is reserved for failures of these modalities.

e. **Colorectal neoplasm** (adenocarcinoma as well as polyps) can present with acute lower GI bleeding, although chronic or occult blood loss and microcytic anemia is a more common presentation. Treatment is multidisciplinary, including surgical resection. Postpolypectomy bleeding can be treated with colonoscopy and coagulation.

f. **Hemorrhoids and other benign anorectal diseases** make up nearly 10% of acute hematochezia. In patients with portal hypertension, hemorrhoidal bleeding can be life threatening, and treatment must be aggressive and may involve a portosystemic shunting procedure.

g. **Colitis** may be ischemic, infectious, or a result of inflammatory bowel disease (**Crohn's disease** or **ulcerative colitis**) and can present with bloody diarrhea, hematochezia, or melena. Colonoscopy usually reveals diffuse mucosal inflammation. Management of inflammatory bowel disease is best directed by a gastroenterologist and consists of hydration, bowel rest, and steroids. Ischemic and infectious colitis are discussed in **Sections IV.F.1** and **IV.F.4**.

IV. SPECIFIC GI PROBLEMS BY ORGAN
A. Esophagus

1. **Esophageal perforation** is often iatrogenic and may follow upper endoscopy procedures, NG tube placement, balloon tamponade of bleeding varices, endotracheal tube placement, or transesophageal echocardiography. Abnormal anatomy such as a Zenker's diverticulum may predispose the patient to this complication. Perforation can occur in the cervical, thoracic, or abdominal esophagus, leading to cervical abscess, mediastinitis, empyema, or peritonitis.

a. **Diagnosis.** Patients may have pain, fever, subcutaneous crepitus, leukocytosis, pneumomediastinum, or a pleural effusion. A contrast swallow study, CT scan, or esophagoscopy can confirm and localize esophageal perforations.

b. **Treatment** is urgent and includes broad-spectrum antibiotics, drainage, and gastric acid suppression. Some patients may be candidates for primary repair at the time of drainage. Most patients will remain npo for a prolonged period and will require nutritional support via a feeding tube.

2. **Boerhaave's syndrome** refers to spontaneous esophageal perforation, which may have no obvious precipitant or may be related to retching/

vomiting, blunt trauma, weightlifting, or childbirth. Predisposing factors include reflux esophagitis, esophageal infections, peptic ulcer disease, and alcoholism.

3. **Ingestion** of foreign bodies and caustic substances can cause significant esophageal injury.

   a. Ingested **foreign bodies,** most commonly food boluses, can present with dysphagia, odynophagia, chest pain, or airway obstruction. Blunt objects less than 2 cm in size traverse the GI tract uneventfully, while objects larger than 6 cm will obstruct within the duodenum if not in the esophagus. Most objects that do not pass spontaneously may be removed endoscopically—this should be done early to minimize the risk of perforation from pressure-induced necrosis of the esophageal wall.

   b. **Acids** (pH <2) and **alkalis** (pH >12) cause severe burns when ingested. Vomiting after the ingestion exposes the esophagus to the caustic substance a second time.

      1. **Initial management** includes a careful assessment of the airway. Intraoral burns, edema of the uvula, and inability to swallow saliva may suggest impending airway compromise. Assessment of the airway should be ongoing as the injury evolves. Patients may also require significant **resuscitation** due to inflammation of the mediastinal tissues. Radiographs of the chest and abdomen are helpful to evaluate for perforation. There is no role for gastric lavage, induced emesis, or activated charcoal.

      2. **Endoscopy** early in the patient's course is controversial but can be helpful to assess the degree of injury. Endoscopy is helpful in evaluating and managing esophageal strictures that develop later on as a complication of caustic ingestions.

B. **Stomach**

   1. **Stress ulceration** is discussed in **Section III.E.1.**

   2. Peptic ulcer disease (PUD) refers to gastric and duodenal ulcers. Risk factors include *H. pylori* infection, NSAIDs, and aspirin use. Patient can present with pain, upper GI bleeding, obstruction, or peritonitis from perforation.

      a. The **diagnosis** of active *H. pylori* infection can be made during endoscopy utilizing the biopsy specimen and include histology, culture, urease testing, and polymerase chain reaction.

      b. **Treatment** of *H. pylori* is indicated in most patients on the basis of its association with peptic ulcers, gastric carcinoma, and gastric lymphoma. First-line regimens consist of a PPI plus two antibiotics such as amoxicillin + clarithromycin (first-line therapy), amoxicillin + metronidazole (for macrolide allergy), or metronidazole + clarithromycin (for penicillin allergy).

      c. **Complications** of PUD include upper GI bleeding (**Section III.E.1**), perforation, and obstruction. Perforation requires an operation with either a laparoscopic or an open approach.

C. **Pancreas**

   1. **Acute pancreatitis**

      a. Most common **etiologies** are alcohol and gallstones (70%–80% of cases). Other causes include biliary reflux, contrast reflux, hypercalcemia, hyperlipidemia, trauma, and so on.

      b. The **pathogenesis** of acute pancreatitis is related to the release of activated pancreatic enzymes that autodigest the pancreatic parenchyma and cause inflammation, microvascular injury, and necrosis. Activated enzymes may also circulate to distant organs, causing

activation of the complement and coagulation cascades, vasodilatation, and endothelial injury. Systemic consequences may include
shock, acute lung injury and acute respiratory distress syndrome
(ALI/ARDS), and acute renal failure.

c. **Symptoms** of acute pancreatitis include severe epigastric pain radiating to the back, nausea and vomiting, and fever.

d. The **diagnosis** is established with a consistent history and physical
examination and increased serum amylase or lipase levels. An abdominal CT scan demonstrating pancreatic inflammation, edema,
or necrosis is not necessary for the initial diagnosis (Fig. 26.2).

e. The **prognosis** for the majority of patients is good and they experience mild, self-limiting disease. Severe acute pancreatitis, defined as
acute pancreatitis with organ dysfunction, develops in 10% to 20%
of patients, necessitating admission to the ICU. Various tools have
been developed to assess the severity of acute pancreatitis—the
most commonly used is Ranson's criteria (Table 26.3).

f. **Clinical course**

1. **The early phase** is characterized by local inflammation, significant
retroperitoneal fluid sequestration, and a systemic inflammatory
response that can be robust and may lead to **multiple organ system
failure.**

a. **Initial treatment** is largely supportive. Aggressive fluid resuscitation and electrolyte repletion should be undertaken. Nasogastric tube decompression can be helpful to alleviate nausea
but does not shorten the clinical course. Pain relief, supplemental oxygen, invasive monitoring, mechanical ventilation,
and inotropic support may be necessary.

b. **Prophylactic antibiotics** are not indicated in severe pancreatitis
without overt signs of sepsis with a positive culture or aspiration. Even in patients with a large amount of necrosis (30% or
more), routine use of antibiotics have been associated with no
improvement in outcomes.

c. **Nutrition** should be provided. Several trials support the use
of early enteral feeding via a nasogastric or nasojejunal tube
within the first 48 hours. Total parenteral nutrition (TPN)
should only be considered for patients who cannot tolerate
adequate enteral nutrition.

d. Patients with mild gallstone pancreatitis should undergo **cholecystectomy during the index hospitalization** to prevent recurrence. The type of intervention and timing for patients with
severe gallstone pancreatitis must be individualized. Patients
who are too sick to undergo cholecystectomy may be treated
with ERCP and sphincterotomy.

2. **The later phase** of severe acute pancreatitis is characterized by local complications and can carry on for weeks or months.

a. **Pancreatic necrosis (Fig. 26.2)** should be suspected in patients
who fail to improve or suffer clinical deterioration. Necrosis is
not present in the first 2 to 3 days of symptoms. The extent of
pancreatic necrosis correlates well with the amount of devas-
cularized pancreas as demonstrated by a contrast-enhanced
CT scan. By the end of the second week, infection of the necrosis may occur. New organ failure, new fever, or an increasing
leukocytosis should prompt CT-guided aspiration of necrotic
tissue. Gram stain and culture aid in establishing the diagnosis

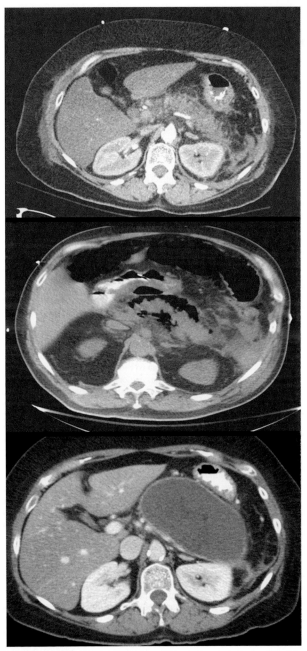

FIGURE 26.2 Acute pancreatitis. Axial CT images demonstrating: acute pancreatitis with prominent pancreatic inflammation (top), pancreatic necrosis with air around the pancreas (middle), and a giant pancreatic pseudocyst that developed several weeks after the acute episode (bottom) (Courtesy of Hasan Alam, MD).

TABLE 26.3	Ranson's Criteria for Prognosis of Acute Pancreatitis

At admission
- Age >55 y
- WBC count >16,000/μL
- Blood glucose >200 mg/dL
- Serum lactate dehydrogenase (LDH) >350 IU/L
- Serum glutamic oxaloacetic transaminase (SGOT, AST) >250 IU/L

During initial 48 h
- Hematocrit decrease of >10%
- Blood urea nitrogen (BUN) increase of >5 mg/dL
- Serum calcium <8 mg/dL
- Arterial Pao_2 <60 mmHg
- Base deficit >4 mEq/L
- Estimated fluid sequestration >6 L

Number of Criteria Met	Expected Mortality (%)
Less than 3	Less than 1
3 or 4	15
5 or 6	40
7 or 8	90

of infected pancreatic necrosis. Patients with infected pancreatic necrosis should be treated with antibiotics and drainage. There has been evidence to suggest that percutaneous treatment as a bridge to definitive drainage is an option. The use of either transgastric endoscopic debridement or video-assisted retroperitoneal debridement are newer modalities that may be considered if debridement is needed. The morbidity is significantly less than a laparotomy. Early debridement may result in incomplete debridement and the need for a second operation. The ideal timing for debridement appears to be between 21 and 27 days but the later the better.

b. **Pancreatic pseudocysts** (**Fig. 26.2**) are encapsulated fluid collections, rich in pancreatic enzymes, which form 4 to 6 weeks after an episode of acute pancreatitis. Typically, they communicate with the pancreatic duct. Collections that are observed earlier are referred to as acute fluid collections and may spontaneously regress. Small, asymptomatic pseudocysts can be observed safely.

   i. Large (>6 cm) or symptomatic pseudocysts can be drained either endoscopically or surgically.

   ii. **Complications** associated with pseudocysts include rupture into the peritoneal cavity (resulting in pancreatic ascites), rupture into the pleural space (resulting in pancreaticopleural fistula), erosion into an adjacent vessel (resulting in upper GI bleeding), compression of intra-abdominal structures, and infection (resulting in abscess formation).

c. **Pseudoaneurysms** occur most commonly in the **splenic artery** due to the proximity of this structure to the inflamed pancreas. Splenic artery pseudoaneurysms have a 75% bleeding rate and may rupture into a pseudocyst or intraperitoneally. Hemorrhage requires immediate intervention, either angiographically or surgically.

d. **Splenic vein thrombosis** may occur and lead to the later development of portal hypertension. Patients may require splenectomy if variceal bleeding develops. Thrombosis of the mesenteric vessels leading to gut ischemia is rare.

D. Biliary Tree

1. **Acute acalculous cholecystitis (AAC)** is an inflammatory disease of the gallbladder occurring in the absence of gallstones. Predisposing factors include critical illness, trauma, sepsis, burns, hypotension, TPN, atherosclerosis, and diabetes.

   a. The **pathogenesis** of AAC is multifactorial and appears to be related to chemical and ischemic injury of the gallbladder. Pathology specimens reveal an occluded or impaired gallbladder microcirculation, possibly due to inflammation or inappropriate activation of the coagulation cascade.

   b. **Diagnosis** requires a high index of suspicion, as fever may be the only symptom. Other signs and symptoms can include right upper quadrant or epigastric pain, nausea/vomiting, and new intolerance of enteral feeding. Laboratory findings may be limited to leukocytosis and LFT abnormalities, which may already be present in the critically ill ICU patient. Ultrasound and CT scans are used to confirm the diagnosis.

      1. **Ultrasound** can be performed at the bedside. Diagnostic findings include gallbladder wall thickness >3.5 mm, gallbladder distension >5 cm, sludge or gas in the gallbladder, pericholecystic fluid, mucosal sloughing, and intramural gas or edema. However, the sensitivity of ultrasound in diagnosing AAC may be as low as 30%.

      2. **CT** scan (Fig. 26.3) may be helpful when the diagnosis is uncertain and other intra-abdominal pathology needs to be excluded.

      3. **HIDA** scan is another option to establish the diagnosis. A nonfilling gallbladder confirms the diagnosis.

   c. **Treatment** involves antibiotics and cholecystectomy if the patient can tolerate an operation, or more commonly in the critically ill placement of a percutaneous cholecystostomy tube for drainage.

2. **Cholangitis** is an infection of the biliary tract, often associated with septic shock and is described in **Chapter 30**.

E. Spleen: Patients may be admitted to the ICU for management of a splenic laceration or rupture following blunt abdominal trauma. Other splenic pathology encountered in the ICU includes splenomegaly, infarction, or abscess. Splenic infarct usually occurs in patients with preexisting splenomegaly due to portal hypertension or hematologic disorders such as leukemia, sickle cell disease, polycythemia, or hypercoagulable states. **Splenic abscess** usually requires splenectomy or percutaneous drainage and can be due to direct extension of infection or hematogenous seeding. Thus, the possibility of endocarditis should be entertained. Patients who undergo splenectomy should receive vaccination against *Streptococcus pneumoniae*, *Haemophilus influenzae*, and *Neisseria meningitides* and should be counseled about their immunocompromised state and the need for revaccination.

F. Intestines

1. **Intestinal ischemia** may be acute or chronic and may affect the small or large intestine.

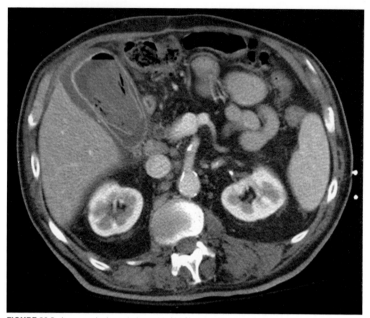

FIGURE 26.3 Acute acalculous cholecystitis (AAC). Axial CT image demonstrating several common findings of AAC, including an enhancing gallbladder wall, distended gallbladder, pericholecystic fluid, and air within the gallbladder (Courtesy of Hasan Alam, MD).

    a. Acute mesenteric ischemia (AMI) occurs as a result of arterial obstruction (embolic, thrombotic, or due to aortic dissection) or venous obstruction. AMI can also be nonocclusive and result from hypoperfusion, vasoconstriction, or vasospasm.

        1. AMI typically presents with severe abdominal pain out of proportion to physical examination findings. Other signs include sudden intolerance of enteral feeding, nausea, vomiting, fever, intestinal bleeding, abdominal distension, and altered mental status.

        2. Leukocytosis and **metabolic acidosis** are common early laboratory abnormalities, while elevated serum lactate and amylase are late findings.

        3. Abdominal radiograph may show an ileus. **CT scan** may show thickened bowel. Portal venous gas and *pneumatosis intestinalis* are late findings of intestinal ischemia and suggest infarction. **CT angiography** may reveal the site of arterial occlusion. **Conventional angiography** can also be used to establish the diagnosis and may be therapeutic. **Duplex ultrasound** can be used to assess proximal celiac and superior mesenteric artery (SMA) flow. However, overlying edematous bowel can make ultrasonography nondiagnostic.

        4. Treatment of acute mesenteric ischemia should be prompt and is aimed at restoring intestinal blood flow to avoid intestinal infarction. Patients should be given volume resuscitation, correction of hypotension, broad-spectrum antibiotics, and nasogastric drainage. Systemic anticoagulation is appropriate after aortic dissection is ruled out as a cause of mesenteric ischemia. Depending on the cause of ischemia, patients may require surgical or endovascular revascularization or observation. A second-look laparotomy may be necessary in 12 to 24 hours to reassess bowel viability.

   a. **SMA emboli** cause 50% of AMI. Emboli typically originate from the left atrium, left ventricle, and cardiac valves. The SMA is susceptible due to its anatomy (large caliber, nonacute angle off aorta). Vasoconstriction of surrounding nonobstructed arteries further exacerbates intestinal hypoperfusion. Treatment involves aggressive resuscitation and anticoagulation. Intra-arterial administration of **papaverine** may improve bowel viability. Laparotomy and embolectomy is performed prior to evaluating bowel viability.

   b. **SMA thrombosis** generally occurs acutely in patients with chronic mesenteric ischemia from atherosclerosis. Blunt trauma to the abdomen is also a risk factor, presumably from endothelial disruption. As with SMA embolism, intra-arterial **papaverine** can improve bowel viability. Surgical revascularization usually requires thrombectomy, a bypass graft, or an endovascular stent.

   c. **Nonocclusive mesenteric ischemia** results from mesenteric arterial vasospasm and accounts for 20% to 30% of AMI. Vasopressors, diuretics, cocaine, arrhythmia, and shock predispose patients to this condition. Therapy involves resuscitation, anticoagulation, administration of vasodilator agents, and discontinuation of the offending agent.

   d. **Mesenteric venous thrombosis** is a less common cause of intestinal ischemia. Risk factors include inherited or acquired hypercoagulable states, abdominal trauma, portal hypertension, pancreatitis, and splenectomy. Diagnosis is by CT scan. Treatment is with systemic **anticoagulation** (heparin followed by warfarin). Laparotomy is indicated only in cases of suspected bowel infarction.

b. **Ischemic colitis** is a common form of mesenteric ischemia typically affecting the "watershed" areas (splenic flexure and rectosigmoid junction) of the colon. It is usually caused by underlying atherosclerotic disease in the setting of hypotension, although embolism, vasculitis, hypercoagulable states, vasospasm, and inferior mesenteric artery (IMA) ligation during aortic surgery are other causes.

   1. The **diagnosis** of ischemic colitis is suspected in patients with left-sided crampy abdominal pain, often associated with mild lower GI bleeding, diarrhea, abdominal distension, nausea, and vomiting. Other signs and symptoms include fever, leukocytosis, and abdominal tenderness to palpation. The diagnosis is confirmed by CT scan or by endoscopy.

   2. Most cases resolve within days to weeks with **supportive care** including bowel rest, fluid resuscitation, and broad-spectrum antibiotics. Fifteen percent of patient will develop transmural necrosis. Indications for colon resection include peritonitis, colonic perforation, and clinical deterioration despite adequate medical therapy. Long-term complications include chronic colitis and colonic strictures.

2. **Adynamic or paralytic ileus** refers to an alteration in GI motility that leads to failure of intestinal contents to pass. Ileus can affect the entire GI tract or a localized segment.

   a. Ileus may be related to a number of predisposing factors. After an uncomplicated abdominal operation, small bowel motility generally returns within 24 hours. Gastric motility follows within 48 hours and colonic motility returns in 3 to 5 days. Early feeding decreases the incidence of ileus.

   b. **Diagnosis** is clinical and radiologic. Patients may present with nausea/vomiting, abdominal distension, intolerance of enteral feeding, and diffuse abdominal discomfort. Abdominal radiographs show distension of the affected part of the GI tract with intraluminal air throughout. Contrast studies are sometimes needed to exclude mechanical obstruction.

   c. **Complications** of ileus depend on the portion of the GI tract involved. A severe ileus can lead to increased intra-abdominal pressure and even abdominal compartment syndrome. Ileus can also lead to bacterial overgrowth, and reflux of bowel contents into the stomach can predispose to aspiration. **Fluid sequestration** due to intestinal wall edema can compromise the gut's microcirculation. **Colonic dilation** can lead to ischemia, necrosis, and perforation. Patients with a cecal diameter more than 12 cm are at higher risk for perforation, although perforations have been reported with smaller cecal diameters. Patients with chronic colonic dilation may tolerate much larger diameters.

   d. **Treatment** begins with **supportive care,** which consists of fluid and electrolyte repletion and nasogastric tube drainage. Potential causes of ileus should be reviewed and corrected (Table 26.4). If tolerated, fiber-containing enteral diets or minimal enteral nutrition can promote GI motility. Patients should be encouraged to ambulate. Medications such as metoclopramide, erythromycin, and neostigmine have been used with mixed results.

      1. **Neostigmine** (2–2.5 mg IV given over 3 minutes) can successfully treat Ogilvie syndrome (colonic pseudo-obstruction) in approximately 80% of cases. Close monitoring for bradycardia is required. Atropine should be readily available at the bedside if needed during the administration.

      2. If conservative measures fail or if perforation appears imminent, **colonoscopic** or **operative decompression** is indicated.

3. **Bowel obstruction** presents with signs and symptoms similar to ileus. As with ileus, plain x-rays (**Fig. 26.1**) and CT scan (Fig. 26.4) can confirm the diagnosis.

   a. **Small bowel obstruction (SBO)** is most often due to adhesions. Other causes include abdominal wall and internal hernias, tumors, foreign bodies, and gallstones. Patients with partial SBO often respond to nonoperative management, which consists of fluid and electrolyte repletion and nasogastric tube drainage. Fevers, leukocytosis, persistent pain, and tenderness on examination are indications to proceed with exploratory laparotomy. Complete SBO should be managed surgically due to high risk for bowel ischemia, necrosis, and perforation.

   b. **Large bowel obstruction** (LBO) is commonly due to malignancy and develops insidiously over time. Other causes include sigmoid or cecal volvulus (Fig. 26.5), diverticular strictures, and fecal impaction.

TABLE 26.4	Causes of Ileus

Postoperative
Intraperitoneal or retroperitoneal pathology:
- Inflammation, infection
- Hemorrhage
- Intestinal ischemia
- Bowel wall edema (may be due to massive fluid resuscitation)
- Ascites

Systemic sepsis
Trauma
Uremia
Sympathetic hyperactivity
Electrolyte derangements
Drugs:
- Catecholamines
- Calcium channel blockers
- Narcotics
- Anticholinergics
- Phenothiazines
- β-blockers

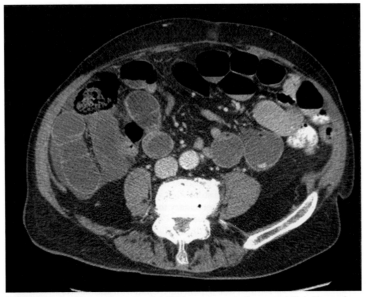

FIGURE 26.4 Small bowel obstruction. Axial CT image demonstrating several dilated loops of small bowel, consistent with small bowel obstruction.

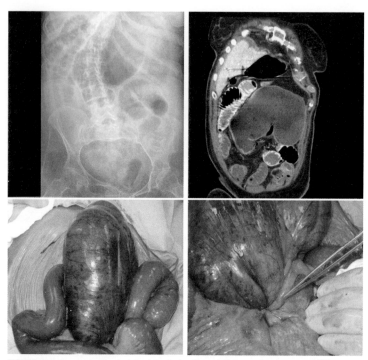

FIGURE 26.5 Cecal volvulus. A plain abdominal radiograph (left upper) and a coronal CT image (right upper) demonstrating cecal volvulus. Intraoperative photographs reveal a dilated and ischemic cecum (left lower), as well as the site of torsion (right lower) (Courtesy of Hasan Alam, MD).

Treatment of large bowel obstruction is usually operative. Sigmoid volvulus may respond to decompression via contrast enema or colonoscopy.

4. **Diarrhea** occurs when fluid intake into the gut lumen does not match fluid absorption from the GI tract.

   a. Under normal conditions, 9 to 10 L of fluid enters the bowel lumen each day from oral intake and intestinal secretions. The majority is absorbed in the small bowel, leaving the remaining 1 to 1.5 L to be absorbed in the proximal half of the colon, with approximately 100 mL lost daily in stool.

   b. Water is absorbed secondary to osmotic flow as well as active and passive transport of sodium. Changes in GI motility and epithelial mucosal integrity can drastically affect fluid absorption.

   c. Common **etiologies** of diarrhea in the critically ill patient include infections, enteral nutrition, medications, ischemic colitis, fecal impaction, intestinal fistula, pancreatic insufficiency, and hypoalbuminemia.

      1. **Infectious diarrhea** in the ICU setting is usually due to *Clostridium difficile* infection in patients treated with antibiotics.

         a. **Clinical presentation** varies from asymptomatic leukocytosis to severe colitis and toxic megacolon.

b. Because the sensitivity of the toxin assay for *C. difficile* is no greater than 90%, testing three separate stool samples is the standard for diagnosis if the clinical suspicion is there, unless PCR is available. PCR has a sensitivity nearing 100%. Treatment is with metronidazole or oral vancomycin, as described in **Chapter 28.**

c. Indications for operative management, subtotal colectomy, are failure of medical therapy in the face of escalating cardiopulmonary support. The mortality approaches 80% for those who need a subtotal colectomy; however, earlier intervention seems to be associated with a mortality closer to 30%.

2. **Enteral nutrition** causing diarrhea is a diagnosis of exclusion. Osmotic diarrhea is secondary to malabsorption of nutrients and usually stops with fasting. Malnutrition and hypoalbuminemia can also cause malabsorption.

a. An **osmolar gap** in the stool of >70 mOsm suggests an osmotic diarrhea. The osmolar gap is the difference between the measured stool osmolarity and the predicted osmolarity, which is $2 \times ([Na^+] + [K^+])$, based on serum electrolyte measurements.

b. **Treatment** of enteral nutrition–related diarrhea involves slowing the rate of feeding, diluting the tube feeds, changing the formula, or temporarily stopping enteral nutrition. Enteral nutrition should be lactose free. In some patients, peptide-based, fiber-rich, or elemental diets with reduced fat and residue may be helpful.

3. **Fecal impaction** can paradoxically lead to diarrhea as a result of decreased fecal tone, mucus secretion, and impaired anorectal sensation.

4. An **altered enterohepatic circulation,** leading to increased bile acid in the colon, can induce net fluid secretion. This is seen in diseases of the ileum, fatty acid malabsorption, and altered bowel flora.

d. **Management** of diarrhea consists of replacement of lost fluids and electrolytes and treatment of the underlying cause. After excluding infectious etiologies, diarrhea can be treated symptomatically with agents such as **diphenoxylate with atropine** (Lomotil 5 mg/dose, 4 doses/d, reduce dose once controlled), **loperamide** (Imodium 4–16 mg/d), **bismuth subsalicylate** (Pepto-Bismol 262 mg/dose up to 8 doses/d), and **deodorized or camphorated opium tincture** (0.3–1 mL/dose every 2–6 hours up to 6 mL/d).

5. **Constipation** may affect up to 83% of ICU patients and has been associated with prolonged ICU length of stay, infectious complications, pulmonary complications, and increased mortality in some studies.

a. The **etiology** of constipation in the ICU is incompletely understood. Proinflammatory mediators, poor perfusion, dehydration, immobilization, and medications (vasopressors and opiates) likely contribute to the problem.

b. A **bowel regimen** should be initiated and titrated to avoid constipation and can include **stool softeners** (Colace), **bulking agents** (methylcellulose, psyllium), **stimulants** (castor oil, senna), **lubricants** (mineral oil), or **osmotic agents** (lactulose, magnesium).

Selected Readings

Batke M, Cappell MS. Adynamic ileus and acute colonic pseudo-obstruction. *Med Clin North Am* 2008;92:649–670.

Cheatham ML, Malbrain ML, Kirkpatrick A, et al. Results from the International Conference of Experts on intra-abdominal hypertension and abdominal compartment syndrome. II. Recommendations. *Intensive Care Med* 2007;33:951–962.

Chey WD, Wong BC; Practice Parameters Committee of the American College of Gastroenterology. American College of Gastroenterology guideline on the management of *Helicobacter pylori* infection. *Am J Gastroenterol* 2007;102:1808–1825.

Crandall M, West MA. Evaluation of the abdomen in the critically ill patient: opening the black box. *Curr Opin Crit Care* 2006;12:333–339.

Dellinger EP, Tellado JM, Soto NE, et al. Early antibiotic treatment for severe acute necrotizing pancreatitis. A randomized, double blind, placebo-controlled study. *Ann Surg* 2007;245:674–683.

Haney JC, Pappas TN. Necrotizing pancreatitis: diagnosis and management. *Surg Clin North Am* 2007;87:1431–1446.

Heinrich S, Schafer M, Rousson V, et al. Evidence-based treatment of acute pancreatitis. *Ann Surg* 2006;243:154–168.

Jaramillo EJ, Treviño JM, Berghoff KR, et al. Bedside diagnostic laparoscopy in the intensive care unit: a 13-year experience. *JSLS* 2006;10:155–159.

Maerz L, Kaplan LJ. Abdominal compartment syndrome. *Crit Care Med* 2008;36:S212–S215.

Proctor DD. Critical issues in digestive diseases. *Clin Chest Med* 2003;24:623–632.

Raju GS, Gerson L, Das A, et al; American Gastroenterological Association. American Gastroenterological Association (AGA) Institute technical review on obscure gastrointestinal bleeding. *Gastroenterology* 2007;133:1697–1717.

Ramasamy K, Gumaste VV. Corrosive ingestion in adults. *J Clin Gastroenterol* 2003;37:119–124.

Stewart D, Waxman K. Management of postoperative ileus. *Am J Ther* 2007;14:561–566.

Villanueva C, Colomo A, Bosch A., et al. Transfusion strategies for acute upper gastrointestinal bleeding. *NEJM* 2013;368:11–21.

Villatoro E, Bassi C, Larvin M. Antibiotic therapy for prophylaxis against infection of pancreatic necrosis in acute pancreatitis. *Cochrane Database Syst Rev* 2006;(4):CD002941.

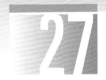

Endocrine Disorders and Glucose Management

Kevin H. Zhao and Elizabeth Cox Williams

I. GLUCOSE HOMEOSTASIS, INSULIN RESISTANCE, AND INSULIN DEFICIENCY

A. **Normal Blood Glucose Dynamics.** In the normal fasting state, blood glucose (BG) is regulated between **70 and 110 mg/dL** and does not increase to more than 200 mg/dL despite significant fluxes of glucose into the bloodstream after meals. Absorption of a typical meal may require 150 g of glucose (a 30-fold excess of the steady-state amount in the blood) to move through the circulation and into storage within a few hours. A rise in BG of twofold (more than 200 mg/dL) during this movement is abnormal and is sufficient to diagnose **diabetes mellitus (DM)** in the outpatient setting. Glycated hemoglobin (HbA1c) can be used to evaluate average plasma glucose concentration over an interval of several months.

B. **Endocrine Control of Blood Glucose.** Pancreatic β-cells secrete **insulin** directly into the portal circulation in response to the BG level. Glucose is converted to glycogen for storage in the liver and muscle and to triglycerides for storage in the adipose tissue. During fasting, pancreatic β-cells secrete **glucagon** to promote breakdown of glycogen stores and release of glucose into the blood. Glucagon is also the first line of defense against hypoglycemia.

C. **Insulin Resistance and Deficiency.** Insulin stimulates glucose uptake and promotes cell growth and survival. In states of insulin resistance, such as type 2 DM and critical illness, much higher levels of insulin can be required for the same degree of glucose uptake. Postreceptor signaling events can be inhibited by the **counterregulatory hormones** glucagon, epinephrine, norepinephrine, cortisol, and growth hormone, as well as inflammatory cytokines and intracellular free fatty acids. These same counterregulatory hormones can stimulate glycogen breakdown, glucose production from amino acids, and release of fatty acids from lipids. If pancreatic β-cells cannot sufficiently increase insulin production in response to insulin resistance, relative insulin deficiency leads to hyperglycemia. Toxicity of cytokines and hyperglycemia itself can lead to β-cell failure and absolute insulin deficiency superimposed on insulin resistance.

II. HYPERGLYCEMIA OF CRITICAL ILLNESS

A. **Pathophysiology.** Critically ill patients without preexisting DM frequently become insulin resistant and hyperglycemic due to elevated levels of cytokines such as IL-1, IL-6, and TNF and stress hormones such as cortisol, glucagon, and adrenergic hormones. Treatment with glucocorticoids and sympathomimetic drugs, increased nutrition to compensate for a catabolic state, and administration of intravenous (IV) dextrose all contribute to hyperglycemia. Patients with preexisting DM have insulin resistance and almost always need higher levels of insulin to maintain normal glucose levels when they are critically ill.

B. **Hyperglycemia and Outcomes.** Hyperglycemia appears to be a **marker for severity of illness** and is **associated with poor outcomes** including increased infarct volume after stroke, decreased cardiac function after myocardial infarction, increased wound complications after heart surgery, and increased mortality.

1. While hyperglycemia attributed to critical illness is associated with worse outcomes, hyperglycemia attributed to preexisting diabetes is also associated with increased mortality. In one study, preoperative hyperglycemia (>200 g/dL) was associated with a twofold increase in 30-day mortality and a fourfold increase in 30-day cardiovascular mortality. Studies also suggest that diabetic patients in particular have an increased risk of wound infections, renal failure, and rehospitalization following heart surgery.

C. **Intensive Insulin Therapy (IIT).** A series of clinical trials that started in 2001 have tested the efficacy of using **IV insulin to tightly regulate BG to normal or near normal,** a much narrower range than had been customary in the ICU. The trial led by Van den Berghe targeted a blood-glucose level of 80 to 110 g/dL and reduced in-hospital mortality of surgical ICU patients by as much as 34%, as well as reducing the incidence of acute renal failure, bloodstream infections, critical illness polyneuropathy, and the duration of mechanical ventilation and of ICU stay. However, follow-up studies noted the increased risk of severe hypoglycemia and some studies even required early termination due to increased risks in the IIT group. The GluControl and VISEP trials both noted no difference in mortality between tight versus conventional glucose control. In 2009, the NICE-SUGAR trial randomized medical and surgical ICU patients to glucose ranges of 80 to 110 versus 140 to 180 and found a small increase in mortality with intensive glucose control with a number needed to harm of 38. Furthermore, there was no difference in median number of ICU days, duration of mechanical ventilation, or need for renal replacement therapy. Retrospective analysis seems to suggest that the mortality difference could be attributed to whether a patient has preexisting diabetes. Nondiabetics who develop hyperglycemia in the acute setting seem to be at greater mortality risk, although it is unclear whether intensive glucose control seems to favor one population over another.

1. The reason for such wide discrepancy among large, controlled clinical trials is not entirely clear. Confounding factors may include methodology, the different ranges of BG goals tested, preexisting diabetes, the proportions of medical versus surgical patients, and the different provision of total calories as well as their source (enteral vs. parenteral). Although not proven, it may also be that the benefits of IIT derive not only from glucose control, but also from the anabolic effects of insulin. Insulin has been shown to improve protein synthesis, stimulate anti-inflammatory effects, and modulate energy usage.

D. **Risks of IIT.** The primary risk of IIT is **hypoglycemia.** Throughout the various IIT trials, severe hypoglycemia (BG <40 mg/dL) occurred in 5% to 19% of study patients and was in some cases identified as an independent risk factor for death in patients treated with IIT. Severe hypoglycemia may cause neurologic damage because the brain depends on glucose. The risk of hypoglycemia to other organs systems is not as well defined, but hypoglycemia due to excess insulin is also associated with low blood levels of free fatty acids, the preferred fuel for the heart. This may be particularly problematic because of increased cardiac demand during critical illness. Intensive glucose control in poorly controlled diabetics may stimulate the body to cause a hypoglycemic stress response.

1. The consequences of hypoglycemia may counteract some or all of the benefits of IIT. In the ICU, the most common cause of hypoglycemia

is **interruption of nutrition** without stopping the insulin infusion. This can occur due to occlusion of feeding tubes, depletion of TPN or IV glucose bags, or accidental removal of tubes or lines. The BG level can fall very rapidly when feeding is interrupted, requiring a **high degree of vigilance** from staff. If enteral feeding or TPN is interrupted, a D10 infusion should be started immediately and the rate of insulin infusion decreased to prevent a precipitous fall in blood glucose (see **Chapter 11**).

E. **Implementation of Insulin Therapy.** To reduce the risk of hypoglycemia and achieve adequate BG control, most ICU protocols specify point-of-care testing of BG every 1 to 2 hours, although this approach requires up to 2 hours of nursing time each day. Given the lack of uniformity of the results of the IIT trials, a wider target range for blood glucose control may confer most of the potential benefit with less risk of hypoglycemia. The 2012 international guidelines from the **Surviving Sepsis Campaign** sponsored by a number of critical care societies suggest a few main points in implementing IIT:

1. Following initial stabilization, hyperglycemia (BG >180 mg/dL) should be treated with insulin.
2. All patients receiving IV insulin should have BG monitored as frequently as every 1 to 2 hours until BG values are stable, then every 4 hours.
3. Low BG levels obtained from capillary blood by point-of-care testing should be confirmed with a full blood or plasma sample, as the former may not be accurate.
   a. As a result, while glucose control in the ICU remains a priority, intensive glucose control to normoglycemic levels is no longer advised. Based on current evidence, targeting a glucose level of <180 mg/dL seems advisable.

F. **Dosing Algorithms for Insulin.** No consensus has emerged on the best algorithms to use for control of BG with IV insulin, and many forms of paper-based algorithms have been used. There has been interest in developing automated "closed-loop" systems for glucose regulation in the ICU to improve quality of BG control and safety. When such a system becomes available, it will be much easier to conduct the studies required to resolve the many remaining uncertainties about IIT. Very high doses of insulin may be required to control BG in critically ill patients. Insulin infusion rates of greater than 10 U/h are not uncommon and some patients require rates in excess of 50 U/h.

G. **Appropriate Use of Insulin Dosing Algorithms.** Protocols are not appropriate for all hyperglycemic patients. They are not appropriate for treatment of patients with type 1 DM who need a basal rate of insulin administration to prevent lipolysis and ketone body formation. Protocols for critical illness are also not appropriate for treatment of diabetic ketoacidosis (DKA) and hyperosmolar hyperglycemic states (HHSs) where the primarily goals are closure of the anion gap and normalization of the serum osmolarity, respectively (see below).

H. **Transition from IV to Subcutaneous (SC) Insulin.** The transition from IV to SC insulin injections requires careful attention. The first dose of a long-acting analog of insulin (usually **NPH insulin, twice daily**) should be given at least **2 hours prior to discontinuation of the infusion.** The total daily dose of long-acting insulin (divided into two daily doses if using NPH insulin) should be at least half of the total insulin dose administered IV over the last 24 hours. The remainder of the insulin requirement may be provided with a sliding scale of **regular** or **rapid-acting** formulation (insulin aspart, lispro, or glulisine). A sliding scale order alone, without any standing insulin, is not sufficient and will result in recurrent hyperglycemia. The dose of long-acting insulin should be reevaluated every day. A useful rule of thumb is to add at least half of the sliding scale given on the previous day to the basal insulin dosing for the upcoming day and repeat the process until all or most of the blood glucose values are in the desired range. Conversely, hypoglycemia should usually prompt reduction in the basal insulin dose unless it occurred after a large sliding scale bolus to treat hyperglycemia. **All type 1 diabetic patients require basal insulin,** whether or not they are eating, to prevent development of DKA. A modest reduction from the home basal insulin dose may be appropriate upon hospital admission depending on the form of basal insulin and tightness of control.

III. DIABETIC KETOACIDOSIS

A. Pathophysiology. DKA occurs due to a lack of insulin or severe insulin deficiency. Clinical states often involve extreme stress, such as infection, myocardial infarction, or postoperative inflammation. In addition to insulin deficiency, DKA is also characterized by an excess of counterregulatory hormones or inflammatory cytokines. The downstream effects include hyperglycemia, lipolysis, ketogenesis, and hyperosmolarity. Hyperkalemia is common despite whole-body potassium depletion because insulin in an important mediator of potassium uptake into cells. Glucosuria results in an osmotic diuresis with prominent potassium and phosphate wasting. There is loss of water in excess of sodium resulting in dehydration and volume depletion. Decreased peripheral vascular resistance, nausea, vomiting, and abdominal pain are likely due to elevated levels of prostaglandins.

B. Symptoms of DKA. Symptoms may include polyuria, polydipsia, polyphagia, weight loss, vomiting, abdominal pain, dehydration, weakness, confusion, or coma. The examination may find poor skin turgor, ileus, Kussmaul respirations (very deep breaths without tachypnea), tachycardia, hypotension, the fruity aroma of ketones on the breath, coffee-ground emesis (hemorrhagic gastritis), altered mental status, shock, and coma. The patient may have a warm and well-perfused periphery despite severe volume depletion. Full-blown DKA can evolve in less than 24 hours.

C. Causes of DKA. DKA occurs when **insulin is mistakenly withheld or reduced,** when insulin is inactive, or when an **acute illness** increases insulin requirements. Patients with type 1 DM are most at risk but patients with type 2 DM can also develop DKA in the setting of a catastrophic illness or as the initial presentation of the disease. Newly diagnosed type 1 diabetics account for 15% of DKA. The possibility of DKA should be considered in any patient with diabetes and critical illness. Drugs can uncommonly precipitate DKA. A partial list of causes for DKA is shown in Table 27.1.

D. Diagnosis of DKA. Diagnosis requires the presence of serum ketones and is supported by anion gap >12 mEq/L (AG = Na $-$ [Cl + HCO$_3$]), plasma glucose >250 mg/dL, pH <7.3, serum bicarbonate <18 mEq/L, and moderate to large ketones in the urine. Patients who have been able to keep up with volume and water losses by drinking may have been able to excrete enough ketones as sodium salts with retention of chloride so that they present with a hyperchloremic nonanion gap metabolic acidosis. Treatment of DKA with extra insulin by the patient or another provider can decrease BG to <200 mg/dL without clearing ketones to produce "normoglycemic DKA." See Table 27.2 for the differential diagnosis of anion gap acidosis. See Figure 27.1 for summary of diagnosis and management of hyperglycemic emergencies.

Causes of Diabetic Ketoacidosis

- Omission of insulin, inappropriate reduction in dose, inadvertent use of denatured insulin (insulin exposed to heat)
- Infection/sepsis
- Infarction
  - MI, bowel ischemia, stroke
- Endocrine abnormalities:
  - Pheochromocytoma
  - Acromegaly
  - Thyrotoxicosis
  - Glucagonoma
  - Pancreatectomy
- Medications/drugs:
  - Ethanol abuse (DKA can be confused with alcoholic ketosis)
  - Atypical antipsychotics—olanzapine, clozapine, risperidone
  - Anticalcineurin drugs—FK506
  - HIV protease inhibitors
  - α-Interferon/ribavirin therapy
  - Corticosteroids
  - Sympathomimetics (cocaine, terbutaline, dobutamine)
  - Pentamidine
  - Thiazides
- Other conditions that may predispose to DKA:
  - Pancreatitis (reduced insulin secretion and insulin resistance)
  - Surgery
  - Trauma
  - Pregnancy
  - Eating disorder

 Differential Diagnosis of Anion Gap Acidosis

- Starvation ketosis—bicarbonate rarely <18, no hyperglycemia
- Alcoholic ketoacidosis—glucose usually <250, may be hypoglycemic
- Lactic acidosis—serum lactate
- Renal failure—BUN, Cr (note that the measured Cr can be artifactually elevated by acetoacetate depending on the assay used)
- Salicylate intoxication—salicylate level
- Methanol—methanol level
- Ethylene glycol—calcium oxalate and hippurate crystals in urine
- Paraldehyde ingestion—usually hyperchloremic, strong odor on breath

---

E. **Measurement of Serum Ketones.** Measurement of serum ketones with traditional methods such as the nitroprusside test may initially underestimate or overestimate ketone levels. Treatment may increase the apparent levels of ketones in the blood by converting a poorly detected form (β-hydroxybutyrate) to a more easily detected form (acetoacetate). Therefore, ketone levels should be used to make the diagnosis, but not to follow the progress of therapy.

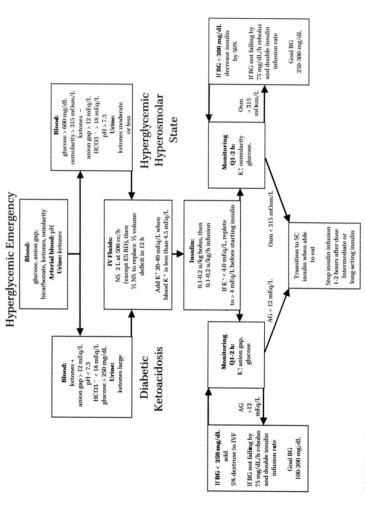

FIGURE 27.1 Diagnosis and management of hyperglycemic emergencies. Not all elements are required for diagnosis—key elements for DKA are blood ketones and anion gap >12, for HHS BG >600 and Osm >315 mOsm/L.

F. **Goals of Therapy and Search for the Cause of DKA.** Normalization of glucose is not sufficient treatment of DKA. The **primary goals of therapy are to treat hypovolemia, to normalize blood potassium concentration and replete potassium stores, to close the anion gap, and to identify and treat the underlying cause of DKA**. Even if insulin omission is suspected, a full workup for other causes is mandatory. Initial evaluation should include a comprehensive set of serum electrolytes, but strong consideration should also be given to cultures to rule out infection. CXR, ECG, and CT should be considered to find a precipitating cause. Certain laboratory anomalies are common in DKA, which may obscure the underlying cause. Amylase and lipase elevations of less than threefold are not sufficient to diagnose pancreatitis in DKA. Leukocytosis with elevated PMNs may be due to stress and proportional to ketonemia, or secondary to underlying infection. Creatinine is often elevated due to hypovolemia (with elevated BUN/Cr ratio), but ketone bodies may also interfere with the creatinine assay. Liver enzymes may be elevated. All of these abnormalities should resolve with treatment of DKA if there is not another underlying cause.

G. **Volume Repletion.** Typical volume deficits in DKA are 10% of body mass. Fluid repletion should **begin with approximately 2 L of NS** administered at a rate of 1,000 mL/h. After the initial hydration, fluids should change to $\frac{1}{2}$ NS, assuming the corrected serum sodium (taking serum glucose into account) is normal or high. The rate should be reduced with a goal of correcting half of the volume deficit in the first 12 hours and the remainder in the next 12 hours. More rapid administration of fluid may delay resolution of acidemia by diluting bicarbonate. In children, too rapid repletion of volume has been associated with cerebral edema, which can be fatal. In adults, excess administration of NS can delay resolution of the **hyperchloremic metabolic acidosis,** which may underlie or follow treatment of the anion gap acidosis. End-stage renal failure patients who are anuric are a special case and are likely to need little or no IV fluid, as they are not capable of osmotic diuresis in response to hyperglycemia.

H. **Potassium Repletion.** Potassium (K^+) depletion is almost universal in DKA (with the exception of oliguric or anuric patients) with a typical deficit of 3 to 5 mEq K^+ per kilogram body weight that requires aggressive repletion. Glucosuria can result in the loss of 70 mEq of potassium for each liter of volume lost. The initial serum K is often elevated despite severe total body depletion due to shifts from within cells to the extracellular fluid. Insulin administration will lower the potassium concentration in the blood. Potassium should be added at 20 to 40 mEq/L to the IVF when the serum K^+ is 4.5 or less. The serum K^+ should be followed closely and repleted aggressively with cardiac monitoring to a level of 4 to 5 mEq/L. If the patient is hypokalemic on presentation, potassium should be repleted to the lower limit of normal before insulin is given to avoid severe hypokalemia and life-threatening arrhythmias.

I. **Insulin Therapy.** Insulin is given IV with an initial bolus of 0.1 to 0.2 U/kg (or **10 U**) followed by a **continuous IV infusion of approximately 0.1 U/kg/h (or 10 U/h).** Insulin is typically mixed at 1 U/mL. Lower concentrations may lead to proportionally large losses by adherence to the infusion bag or IV tubing. In-line filters may bind and deplete insulin. The combined effect of insulin effect and fluid repletion will usually lead to a decrease in the blood glucose of 75 to 100 mg/dL/h. If the decrease in BG is less than 75 mg/

dL/h, the insulin dose may be doubled. If the decline is still too slow, a new bottle of insulin should be used.

J. Closure of the Anion Gap. The endpoint of therapy should be closure of the anion gap ($<$12 mEq/L) **and resolution of the acidosis** (pH $>$7.3, bicarbonate $>$18 mEq/L). If glucose falls to less than 250 mg/dL but the anion gap is not closed, 5% dextrose should be added to the IV fluids (e.g., D5 $\frac{1}{2}$ NS at 100 cm³/h) and the insulin dose should be decreased to 0.05 to 0.1 U/kg/h (or 5 U/h). The insulin dose should then be adjusted as needed to hold the glucose at 100 to 200 mg/dL until the anion gap is closed. Measurement of ketones should not be used to determine the endpoint of therapy. It is not necessary to eliminate ketonemia and ketonuria as long as the anion gap is closed. A hyperchloremic, nonanion gap acidosis is a very common consequence of aggressive hydration with saline. It does not need to be treated and will correct itself over several days by renal excretion of ammonium chloride if renal function is adequate.

K. Phosphorus and Bicarbonate. Phosphate is often normal to high in DKA, but falls with treatment. Phosphorus repletion is only indicated in patients with phosphorous less than 1.0 mEq/L and with a clinical syndrome consistent with hypophosphatemia, which may include hemolytic anemia, platelet dysfunction with petechial hemorrhage, rhabdomyolysis, encephalopathy, seizure, heart failure, and weakness of respiratory or skeletal muscles. There is **no benefit of bicarbonate treatment in patients with pH greater than 6.9.** Administration of insulin will result in utilization of ketones in the TCA cycle and regeneration of bicarbonate. Extra bicarbonate can increase potassium requirements, may increase hepatic production of ketones, and may delay resolution of cerebral acidosis.

L. Complications of DKA. The most feared complication of DKA is **cerebral edema,** which occurs in up to 1% of children with DKA, but rarely in adults. However, the mortality in cerebral edema can be as high as 24%. Cerebral edema as a complication of DKA is a diagnosis of exclusion in adults, and other causes of depressed mental status should be carefully investigated.

M. Transition from IV to SC insulin (see **Section II.H**) should begin when the patient is able to eat. A dose of the long-acting insulin (NPH, glargine, or detemir) should be given or continuous SC infusion should be started 1 to 2 hours before the insulin infusion is stopped. In cases of uncomplicated DKA (i.e., due to insulin omission), the patient's home regimen can be restarted if home control (as judged by the HgbA1c) was adequate. Making the transition to SC insulin in the morning or evening is strongly preferred so that there is a smooth transition to the patient's usual insulin schedule.

IV. HYPEROSMOLAR HYPERGLYCEMIC STATE

A. Pathophysiology. Insulin is able to suppress lipolysis and ketogenesis at much lower concentrations than is required to stimulate glucose uptake. In contrast to patients with type 1 DM, patients with type 2 DM usually have sufficient insulin production to prevent the excessive production of ketones. When **severe hyperglycemia occurs in the absence of ketosis,** the syndrome is called **HHS** or hyperosmolar nonketotic coma (**HONKC**). BG may rise to levels that are unusual in DKA, often greater than 1,000 mg/dL. The blood pH and bicarbonate levels are typically normal and tests for ketones are negative. Both HHS and DKA are associated with hyperosmolarity, polyuria, polydipsia, volume depletion, and whole-body potassium depletion, although the serum potassium is usually normal or elevated before treatment. The two syndromes are part of a spectrum and approximately one-third of patients have some aspects of both syndromes.

Altered mental status, including obtundation and coma, are more common in HHS because the degree of hyperglycemia and hyperosmolarity are higher. Patients with HHS may also develop seizures or focal neurologic signs, and up to 50% of patients present with coma. As in DKA, patients with oliguric renal failure have a different presentation. Although glucose levels are high, the serum sodium is reduced to compensate so that there is minimal hyperosmolarity and few neurologic symptoms.

B. **Diagnosis.** The diagnosis of HHS requires **severe hyperglycemia** (>600 mg/dL, often >1,000 mg/dL) and **hyperosmolarity without an anion gap acidosis**. The American Diabetes Association categorizes HHS with a serum osm of >320 mOsm/kg and a pH >7.3. HHS exists on a spectrum with DKA and some patients with HHS may have modest ketonemia, while some patients with DKA may have more severe hyperosmolarity than is typical of DKA. See **Figure 27.1** for summary of diagnosis and management of hyperglycemic emergencies.

C. **Treatment. IV fluid replacement and insulin therapy** are the mainstays of treatment for HHS, just as they are for DKA, but the goals of insulin therapy differ. Fluid replacement in HHS is similar to that in DKA, although the fluid requirement may be greater due to the more extreme hyperosmolarity. By lowering plasma osmolality, IV fluid also improves insulin responsiveness and stress hormone levels. Sodium levels may need to be corrected in cases of extreme hyperosmolality. **Insulin therapy starts** similarly **with an initial bolus of 0.1 to 0.2 U/kg and an infusion rate of approximately 0.1 to 0.2 U/kg/h.** Instead of closing the anion gap, **the goal is to bring the glucose into a reasonable range and then to normalize the osmolarity.** While most patients with DKA are insulin sensitive, **many patients with HHS are very insulin resistant.** Much higher doses of insulin may be required. Once the BG falls to less than 300 mg/dL, the insulin infusion rate should be reduced by 50%. The serum glucose should be maintained between 250 and 300 mg/dL by adjusting the insulin infusion rate until the plasma osmolality is less than 315 mOsm/L. **Potassium repletion** is similar to that in DKA with $\frac{1}{2}$ NS being used for fluid repletion with 20 to 40 mEq/L of supplemental potassium.

V. **NORMAL ADRENAL PHYSIOLOGY AND PATHOPHYSIOLOGY OF ADRENAL INSUFFICIENCY**

A. **Adrenal Functional Anatomy.** Each adrenal gland is made up of a **cortex**, which produces sex steroids, such as aldosterone and glucocorticoids, and a **medulla**, which produces adrenergic hormones such as epinephrine. The term "adrenal insufficiency" is commonly used to describe deficiency of both **cortisol** (which may be isolated) and **aldosterone** (which is almost always associated with cortisol deficiency).

B. **Regulation of Adrenal Hormone Production** (Fig. 27.2). Cortisol production by the adrenal glands is dependent on **adrenocorticotrophic hormone (ACTH)**, which is produced by the pituitary gland. ACTH is regulated by corticotropin-releasing hormone (CRH), which is produced in the hypothalamus. Cortisol feeds back to inhibit CRH and ACTH release, closing the control loop. Cortisol deficiency may be caused by injury either to the adrenal cortex (primary adrenal insufficiency with elevated ACTH) or to the pituitary or hypothalamus (secondary or central adrenal insufficiency with low or "inappropriately normal" ACTH). Primary adrenal insufficiency is often associated with aldosterone deficiency, but central forms of adrenal insufficiency are limited to a deficit in cortisol production because aldosterone production is not dependent on ACTH.

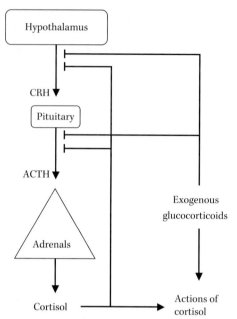

FIGURE 27.2 Regulation of adrenal hormone secretion. Arrows indicate positive action, production, or conversion. Lines ending in cross-bars indicate inhibition.

C. **Categorization of Adrenal Insufficiency.** Adrenal insufficiency can be defined on the basis of the origin of the disease.
   1. **Primary:** The adrenal gland is unable to produce steroid hormones despite adequate corticotropin from the pituitary gland (e.g., Addison's disease, autoimmune diseases).
   2. **Secondary:** A lack of ACTH from the pituitary or CRH from the hypothalamus to stimulate the adrenal gland (brain tumors, infarction, granulomatous disease)
   3. **Tertiary:** Adrenal deficiency due to the withdrawal of exogenous glucocorticoids (chronic steroid use)
D. **Signs of Adrenal Insufficiency. The adrenal gland is activated in states of stress, activating the release of catecholamines, glucocorticoids, mineralocorticoids, and factors of the renin–angiotensin–aldosterine axis.** Cortisol deficiency is acutely dangerous and causes **circulatory collapse** with **refractory hypotension** that may be fatal within hours to days without glucocorticoid replacement. Symptoms and signs of glucocorticoid deficiency including nausea, vomiting, anorexia, weight loss and wasting, weakness, hyponatremia, and eosinophilia. Suspicion of glucocorticoid deficiency is sufficient cause to begin treatment immediately; treatment can be discontinued if adequate adrenal function is demonstrated.
E. **Causes of Adrenal Insufficiency.** A "functional" or "relative" deficiency in cortisol secretion **may occur in critical illness,** but this is controversial and there are no universally accepted criteria for diagnosis of this condition.

Adrenal insufficiency may be caused by drugs that inhibit cortisol production, notably ketoconazole and etomidate. Drugs that accelerate the metabolism of cortisol, such as phenytoin, barbiturates, and rifampin, can contribute to the development of adrenal insufficiency in patients with limited reserve. The **most common cause of adrenal insufficiency is exogenous glucocorticoids** (or drugs with glucocorticoid activity such as megestrol acetate) that cause feedback inhibition of ACTH production, which in turn causes atrophy of the cortisol-producing cells in the adrenal gland. Iatrogenic adrenal insufficiency should be considered in all patients with significant history of glucocorticoid use (e.g., more than 5 mg prednisone daily for more than 3 weeks the previous year). **Complete recovery** from iatrogenic adrenal insufficiency **may take months or even years.** Causes of adrenal insufficiency are listed in Table 27.3.

F. **Aldosterone Deficiency.** Aldosterone production is regulated by the **renin–angiotensin system.** The most important action of aldosterone is to promote sodium retention by the kidney. Deficiency of aldosterone causes sodium wasting, hypovolemia, and hypotension. Aldosterone deficiency can be managed in the short term with sufficient sodium and fluid intake, but long-term deficiency is managed with medications having aldosterone receptor agonist activity, such as fludrocortisone. The most common

Primary Adrenal Insufficiency	Central Adrenal Insufficiency
• Hemorrhagic infarction	• Iatrogenic
• Sepsis	• Glucocorticoids
• Adrenal vein thrombosis	• Megestrol acetate
• Anticoagulation	(glucocorticoid activity)
• Coagulopathy	• Tumor or other mass lesion
• Thrombocytopenia	• Pituitary adenoma
• Hypercoagulable state	• Metastasis
• Trauma	• Lymphoma
• Postoperative	• Primary tumor of brain or meninges
• Severe stress	• Rathke's cleft cyst
• Cancer metastasis/lymphoma	• Empty sella
• Autoimmune	• Pituitary apoplexy
• Addison's disease	• Sheehan's syndrome (postpartum
• Polyglandular autoimmune syndromes	hemorrhage)
I and II	• Infiltrative process
• Infectious process	• Hemachromatosis
• Disseminated fungal infections	• Histiocytosis
(histoplasmosis)	• Tuberculosis
• Tuberculosis	
• HIV (CMV, MAI, Cryptococcus)	
• Infiltrative process	
• Iatrogenic	
• Ketoconazole	
• Etomidate	
• Metyrapone	
• Suramin	

TABLE 27.3 Differential Diagnosis of Adrenal Insufficiency

cause of aldosterone deficiency is injury to the adrenal gland itself, which is typically also associated with glucocorticoid deficiency. Isolated aldosterone deficiency is unusual except as a consequence of medications that affect the renin–aldosterone axis.

VI. DIAGNOSTIC TESTING AND TREATMENT FOR ADRENAL INSUFFICIENCY

A. Diagnosis of Adrenal Insufficiency in Critical Illness. The diagnosis of cortisol deficiency in the setting of critical illness is much more challenging than in the outpatient setting. Cortisol is secreted diurnally, which is lost during critical illness. Cortisol secretion is naturally increased during times of physiologic stress, which can result in unmasking of preexisting subclinical adrenal insufficiency. Critical illness may also cause a functional deficiency in cortisol production or responsiveness. Improvement of critical illness in response to glucocorticoids does not necessarily imply that the patient had diminished adrenal function. It is important to make a conceptual distinction between treatment of adrenal insufficiency and pharmacological treatment with glucocorticoids, which may improve clinical outcomes independent of adrenal functional status. These two concepts are sometimes confused in literature on this topic.

B. Total versus Free Cortisol. Widely available assays for cortisol measure total cortisol, but free cortisol is responsible for the physiological effects of the hormone. Cortisol is bound to cortisol-binding globulin (CBG) in the blood. Critical illness is often associated with reductions in the level of CBG, so total cortisol may be reduced without reduction of free cortisol, leading to overdiagnosis of adrenal insufficiency. As a result of the wide variance in total cortisol levels in septic shock, it is not a useful test for adrenal insufficiency. Studies to date have also not demonstrated the utility of free cortisol in sepsis.

C. ACTH Stimulation Test. The main test for cortisol deficiency is the ACTH stimulation test. A blood sample for cortisol and ACTH is obtained, and synthetic ACTH (cosyntropin) is administered IV or IM. A blood sample for a second cortisol measurement is obtained 30 to 60 minutes after cosyntropin administration. The amount of cosyntropin used in the stimulation test is a matter of debate.

1. High-dose ACTH stimulation test: This test uses an IV dose of 250 μg cosyntropin. One prospective study suggested that a high baseline serum cortisol (>34 μg/dL) level coupled with a diminished cortisol increase (<9 μg/dL) to a high-dose stimulation test is predictive of increased mortality.

2. Low-dose ACTH stimulation test: This test uses 1 μg of cosyntropin for stimulation. Advocates of the low-dose stimulation test have argued that the 250-μg cosyntropin stimulation test would stimulate cortisol release even in adrenally insufficient patients. The low-dose ACTH stimulation test identifies more patients with adrenal insufficiency. In a study comparing the low-dose-versus-high-dose cosyntropin test, it was found that a cortisol response to the high-dose, but not low-dose, cosyntropin test was predictive of increased mortality risk.

3. Diagnostic criteria for adrenal insufficiency. Glucocorticoid levels are normally elevated in response to stress, so a very low baseline plasma cortisol ($<$**3 μg/dL**) in the setting of critical illness is diagnostic of adrenal insufficiency. Moderate levels of baseline cortisol ($<$**10 μg/dL**) suggest adrenal insufficiency but may be misleading in the setting of a low CBG where free cortisol may be appropriately elevated. A **baseline (nonstimulated) cortisol of** $>$**18 μg/dL** effectively rules out adrenal insufficiency in most patients. In between, **a rise from baseline of less than 9 μg/dL has been proposed to identify patients who would benefit from glucocorticoid therapy while a peak level of 18 to 20 μg/dL excludes primary adrenal insufficiency.** CBG can be elevated in response to oral estrogen and liver inflammation so cortisol more than 18 μg/dL cannot rule out adrenal insufficiency in these settings.

4. **Limitations:** The utility of the ACTH stimulation test and the appropriate stimulation dose remains unresolved. The ACTH stimulation test does not determine whether sufficient cortisol is being produced by the hypothalamic–pituitary–adrenal axis; it measures only the ability of the adrenal cortex to respond to exogenous ACTH. As a result, it should not be used to diagnose secondary adrenal insufficiency. It may also be altered in the case of etomidate administration due to pharmacologic suppression. In the case of recent-onset central adrenal insufficiency, the adrenal cortex may not yet have atrophied and the stimulated cortisol response may be normal.

D. **Therapy. Therapy should be directed at addressing the cause of the adrenal insufficiency and steroid replacement.** Ideally, cortisol and ACTH levels should be drawn before any empiric therapy is begun. Empiric therapy with dexamethasone (1 mg q6h) does not interfere with the ACTH stimulation test. Once the postcosyntropin cortisol sample has been drawn, **hydrocortisone,** which provides complete glucocorticoid and mineralocorticoid replacement, should be used at a total daily dose of **300 mg daily, divided every 6 or 8 hours or given via continuous infusion at 10 mg/h.** Dexamethasone, while not offering mineralocorticoid replacement, can be used as well in an adrenal crisis since it is glucocorticoid deficiency that is causing the hemodynamic instability. It should be noted that the appropriate "stress" dose of glucocorticoids is a matter of controversy. Commonly used doses may provide glucocorticoid activity in excess of that produced by the normal adrenal gland during critical illness. There is no reliable test to determine the appropriateness of the replacement dose, so the dosing must be adjusted empirically. Doses of hydrocortisone should not be reduced below a replacement dose for a hospitalized patient with known adrenal insufficiency (50–60 mg orally divided in two doses) until follow-up testing demonstrates adequate adrenal function. An equivalent minimal dose of prednisone is 10 to 15 mg every morning or dexamethasone 1.5 to 2.5 mg daily. Doses of hydrocortisone less than 50 mg daily do not provide sufficient mineralocorticoid activity for patients with primary adrenal insufficiency, and prednisone and dexamethasone have essentially no mineralocorticoid activity. Patients requiring mineralocorticoid replacement should be treated with fludrocortisone at doses of 0.1 to 0.2 mg orally daily. As the clinical situation improves, the glucocorticoid dose should be tapered due to the risks of hyperglycemia, weight gain, congestive heart failure, and hypertension.

E. **Identifying the Cause of Adrenal Insufficiency.** An adrenocorticotropin (ACTH) sample drawn before initiation of empiric glucocorticoid therapy can help to localize the cause of adrenal insufficiency. An elevated ACTH suggests primary adrenal insufficiency and a low or (inappropriately, in this case) "normal" ACTH is consistent with central adrenal insufficiency. If the test suggests primary cortisol insufficiency (elevated ACTH levels), the evaluation should include imaging of the adrenal glands (usually with CT) to evaluate for metastatic, inflammatory, or infiltrative processes. In the setting of central cortisol deficiency, imaging of the pituitary and hypothalamus is indicated. Pituitary protocol MRI is the most appropriate test, but CT can rule out large tumors or gross hemorrhage. See **Table 27.3** for differential diagnosis of adrenal insufficiency.

F. **Pituitary Apoplexy.** Pituitary apoplexy, also referred to as Sheehan's syndrome, is a clinical syndrome caused by hemorrhage or infarct within a preexisting pituitary mass lesion. It is a rare cause of adrenal insufficiency but it deserves special mention in the ICU because it is one of the true **endocrine emergencies**. Pituitary apoplexy can lead to abrupt and severe adrenal insufficiency in the setting of severe physiologic stress, a combination that may prove fatal if not treated promptly. In addition, mass effect on surrounding structures, including the optic nerve and cranial nerves III and VI, can lead to permanent visual deficits or blindness. Therefore, pituitary apoplexy should always be considered in the differential diagnosis of adrenal insufficiency. Unfortunately, the signs and symptoms of apoplexy (headache, visual disturbance) may be masked in critically ill patients, so imaging must be the mainstay of diagnosis. A noncontrast head CT does not reliably allow detection of hemorrhage or infarction in pituitary tumor, but is sensitive for pituitary masses larger than 1 cm, the substrate for most cases of apoplexy. MRI can be used to identify hemorrhage or infarction if a mass is found. High-dose glucocorticoids and rapid surgical decompression are the therapies of choice for pituitary apoplexy.

VII. ADRENAL INSUFFICIENCY IN SEPTIC SHOCK

A. **Sepsis and the Hypothalamic–Pituitary Axis (HPA):** The HPA is activated in states of physiological stress. The normal physiologic response includes reduced cortisol metabolism, decreased cortisol protein binding, and increased free cortisol levels. Critical illness can impair the ability of the HPA to generate an adequate stress response. Studies have demonstrated increased mortality in septic patients who do not respond to a cosyntropin stimulation test. Unfortunately, there is no clear consensus for what constitutes adrenal insufficiency in sepsis.

B. **Steroid Supplementation:** The usage of steroids in septic shock is based on their anti-inflammatory properties, such as its inhibition of endothelial cell activation, capillary leak, complement activation, and free radical formation.

1. In clinical trials, glucocorticoid use has decreased vasopressor requirements and improved systemic vascular resistance in septic shock. Multiple studies have demonstrated quicker withdrawal of pressors following supplemental steroid initiation. A randomized control trial in 2002 by Annane et al. showed a reduction in all-cause mortality by 10% among nonresponders to a cosyntropin stimulation test to supplemental steroids, while there was no mortality difference in the cosyntropin responders. However, the Corticosteroid Therapy of Septic Shock (CORTICUS) trial, a multicenter, randomized, controlled trial of 499 patients in 2008 found no benefit to stress dose hydrocortisone in both responders and nonresponders to a stimulation test. The two trials are notable for several methodological differences, including the Annane study using both hydrocortisone and fludrocortisone, while the CORTICUS used only hydrocortisone. The Annane study also initiated steroids closer to the time of onset of shock.

2. The Surviving Sepsis Campaign observational study found that patients who received systemic corticosteroids (50 mg q6h or 100 mg q8h of hydrocortisone) had a 6% statistically significant increase in hospital

mortality. In the 2012 Surviving Sepsis Guidelines, steroids are recommended only if IV fluids and vasopressors are inadequate to restore hemodynamic stability. An ACTH stimulation test, due to a reported lack of utility in sepsis, is not advised to determine steroid eligibility. There is no clear consensus on when to discontinue steroids in sepsis, although a rapid taper has been recommended when patients clinically improve and have substantially reduced vasopressor requirements.

VIII. CUSHING'S SYNDROME
   A. Diagnosis. Cushing's syndrome is defined by excessive production of cortisol and loss of the normal diurnal rhythm of cortisol production. Since the normal response to critical illness is to dramatically increase cortisol production, the usual screening tests for Cushing's syndrome cannot be used in the ICU. Suspicion of Cushing's syndrome may arise in the setting of a typical body habitus, but the most specific signs are the presence of enlarged supraclavicular and dorsal cervical fat pads, wide ($>$1 cm) violaceous (not pink) striae, and proximal weakness.
   B. Treatment. Definitive treatment of Cushing's syndrome is usually surgical, involving removal of an ACTH-secreting pituitary tumor, an adrenal tumor, or, in rare cases, an ectopic ACTH-secreting tumor. Temporizing treatment options include adrenal enzyme inhibitors, adrenolytic agents, and glucocorticoid antagonists.

IX. THYROID FUNCTION AND DISEASE
   A. Physiology (Fig. 27.3). There are two forms of thyroid hormone, **T4 (levothyroxine),** which contains four iodine atoms, and **T3 (triiodothyronine),** which contains three iodine atoms. Both T4 and T3 are produced in the thyroid gland and are stored in the form of thyroglobulin. The production and release of thyroid hormone is controlled by **thyroid-stimulating hormone (TSH)** secreted by the pituitary gland. TSH stimulates the breakdown of thyroglobulin to release T3 and T4 and promotes the conversion of some T4 to T3 prior to release into the bloodstream. TSH secretion is regulated by thyrotropin-regulating hormone (TRH), which is secreted by the hypothalamus. TRH and TSH secretion are under negative regulation by thyroid hormone, thereby completing a feedback regulatory loop.
      1. Thyroid hormone acts through receptors for T3 while T4 is essentially a prohormone. Approximately 10% of T3 is directly released by the thyroid, but 80% of T3 is produced in other tissues by conversion of T4 to T3 by deiodinase enzymes. Production of T3 outside of the thyroid gland by deiodinase activity is suppressed by conditions common to the ICU, including poor nutrition, diabetes (insulin resistance or relative insulin deficiency), high levels of free fatty acids, inflammatory cytokines, illness in general, and drugs including β-blockers and amiodarone. The production of active T3 is increased by high calorie intake and glucose plus insulin.
   B. Functions of Thyroid Hormone and Symptoms and Signs of Thyroid Dysfunction. Thyroid hormone is an important modulator of metabolic rate and the rate of protein synthesis and turnover. Thyroid hormone increases both cardiac contractility and heart rate and promotes relaxation of arteries, reducing systemic vascular resistance. **Hyperthyroidism** is associated with tachycardia, systolic hypertension, widened pulse pressure, high-output heart failure, atrial fibrillation, and myocardial ischemia. **Hypothyroidism** is associated with bradycardia and hypertension and can precipitate

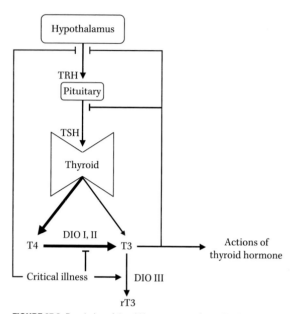

FIGURE 27.3 Regulation of thyroid hormone secretion and activity. Arrows indicate positive action, production, or conversion. Lines ending in cross-bars indicate inhibition. TRH, thyrotropin-releasing hormone; TSH, thyroid-stimulating hormone; T4, levothyroxine (prohormone, minimal activity); T3, triiodothyronine (active thyroid hormone); rT3, reverse T3 (inactive); DIO I, II, III, deiodinase types I, II, and III.

congestive heart failure in those with underlying cardiac disease. Myopathy associated with hypothyroidism and hyperthyroidism can cause respiratory muscles to become weak in both conditions, which can cause inadequate ventilation. Poor ventilation can be especially problematic in hyperthyroidism, in which oxygen consumption and CO_2 production are increased. Thyroid hormone promotes gut motility; hypothyroidism is associated with constipation, and hyperthyroidism with frequent stools or diarrhea, which may be associated with malabsorption. Thyroid hormone is important for free water clearance, and hypothyroidism is associated with hyponatremia. The metabolism of many drugs and endogenous hormones is regulated by thyroid hormone. Drug dosages may need to be reduced in hypothyroidism due to slow clearance or increased with hyperthyroidism due to increased clearance. Cortisol clearance is promoted by thyroid hormone so that treatment of hypothyroidism with thyroid hormone can precipitate adrenal crisis in individuals with adrenal insufficiency. Hypothyroidism is associated with accumulation of matrix glycosaminoglycans in many tissues, which can lead to coarse skin and hair, enlargement of the tongue, hoarseness, and nonpitting edema. Graves' disease, the most common cause of hyperthyroidism, can also cause autoimmune infiltration of the fatty tissue of the orbit and autoimmune attack on the eyes, which can cause ocular inflammation and protrusion of the eyes from the orbits.

X. THYROID FUNCTION IN CRITICAL ILLNESS

A. Sick Euthyroid Syndrome. In contrast to the outpatient setting, TSH levels in hospitalized patients can be misleading, and particularly so in patients with critical illness. Low TSH levels as well as low T4 and T3 levels are very common in critical illness so that normal thyroid studies are the exception rather than the rule. **In sick euthyroid syndrome, patients have low T3 levels from the inhibition of type 1 deiodinase that converts T4 to T3.** The weight of evidence suggests that **treatment of critically ill patients with sick euthyroid syndrome is not beneficial** and may be harmful, perhaps because relative hypothyroidism reduces catabolism and is therefore protective.

1. In patients receiving therapy with T4 before hospitalization, the dose of T4 should generally not be changed. If gut absorption is compromised, orally administered levothyroxine should be replaced with IV levothyroxine, reducing the dose by 20% to account for increased bioavailability by the IV route. In patients on therapy for hyperthyroidism prior to their critical illness, the dose of medications should not be changed unless there is evidence of new toxicity.

B. Lab Testing

1. **Thyroid testing in the ICU.** Because sick euthyroid syndrome is so common in critical illness, **thyroid studies should not be sent unless there is a strong suspicion of thyroid dysfunction**. In this setting, the TSH alone is of little use. TSH is typically normal or suppressed in sick euthyroid syndrome, although TSH levels can be elevated during the recovery as well. A full panel of thyroid function studies including TSH, total T4, free T4 (or free thyroxine index), and T3 should be ordered. The TSH must be interpreted not only in light of the T4 and T3 values, but also in the clinical context. It is important to decide *a priori* what kind of thyroid dysfunction (hyperthyroidism or hypothyroidism) is suspected on clinical grounds before thyroid laboratories are ordered.

2. **Interpretation of a low TSH.** A normal or low TSH is an expected component of critical illness. If the TSH is low and hyperthyroidism is suspected on clinical grounds, the **serum T3** may be helpful. Patients with sick euthyroid syndrome should have low or low-normal T3 values, while those with hyperthyroidism should have high or high-normal T3 values. A patient with an **undetectable TSH** using a modern high-sensitivity assay is likely to have hyperthyroidism, and this diagnosis can be supported by an elevated or high-normal T3.

3. **Interpretation of an elevated TSH.** An elevated TSH can be seen in patients recovering from sick euthyroid syndrome, although the TSH rarely rises to more than 20 mU/L. In a patient who is still critically ill, an elevated TSH is suggestive of **primary hypothyroidism** due to a defect in thyroid hormone synthesis or release by the thyroid gland. A diagnosis of hypothyroidism can be supported by a low or low-normal T3.

4. **Interpretation of T4 levels.** T4 is highly bound by serum proteins, primarily by thyroid-binding globulin, but also transthyretin, albumin, and lipoproteins—only a tiny fraction of T4 is unbound. Reductions of binding proteins, which is common in critical illness, will reduce T4 binding and total T4 levels. Therefore, **total T4 levels are low in up to half of ICU patients.** "Direct" free T4 assays are variably affected by drugs and

circulating substances such as free fatty acids. A total T4, free thyroxine index, or direct free **T4 measurement that is elevated** in a critically ill patient **can support a diagnosis of hyperthyroidism.** If a direct free T4 is obtained in a critically ill patient, a total T4 measurement should also be obtained to increase the likelihood that an artifactual elevated free T4 measurement can be recognized as such. **Low or normal values for total T4, free thyroxine index, or direct free T4 are generally not helpful.**

C. **Treatment of Thyroid Dysfunction in ICU Patients**
   1. **Treatment of Hypothyroidism.** Although sick euthyroid syndrome is probably a state of relative hypothyroidism, **treatment with thyroid hormone does not improve outcomes in patients with critical illness** or in postsurgical patients. This may be because a mild degree of hypothyroidism is protective in the face of a catabolic state. Patients with preexisting hypothyroidism should not have their usual dose of thyroid hormone adjusted. Treatment of newly diagnosed hypothyroidism should be with T4, and initial dosing should be weight based. A **replacement dose of T4 by the enteral route** is approximately **1.6 µg/kg daily,** although individual patients may require substantially more or less. A somewhat lower initial dose is appropriate for patients who are elderly and frail or if there is concern for precipitating cardiac ischemia or atrial fibrillation. **T4 should be given separately from all other medications, and enteral feeds should be paused** until there is minimal gastric residual before the thyroid hormone is given and should not be started for 30 minutes afterward. **In cases where this is not practical** (such as in patients receiving insulin therapy) or when enteral feeds are not tolerated, **IV administration is preferred.** In this case, the **dose should be reduced by 20%** to account for improved bioavailability. It takes at least 6 weeks after a change in dose before the T4 and TSH to reach a new equilibrium, so dosage changes based on measurements made earlier than this should be made with caution. Treatment of hypothyroidism with T3 is generally not indicated except in cases of myxedema coma.
   2. **Treatment of hyperthyroidism.** Patients under active treatment for hyperthyroidism before developing critical illness should be monitored by an endocrine consultant because antithyroid medications can have significant toxicities, and because large iodine loads from medications (such as amiodarone) or from imaging contrast can change the thyroid state and may necessitate changes in therapy. If a new diagnosis of hyperthyroidism is suspected, endocrine consultation should be obtained to confirm the diagnosis and to monitor treatment. Thyroid hormone action **increases the number of α-adrenergic receptors** in many tissues, explaining many of the symptoms of hyperthyroidism. Therapy for hyperthyroidism typically includes treatment with an α-blocker to counteract the increased α-adrenergic action. **Propranolol and metoprolol** both can be given IV and have the additional advantage of inhibiting T4 to T3 conversion by deiodinase. Other therapies should be initiated in consultation with an endocrinologist. A typical course of therapy includes treatment with thionamide antithyroid drugs such as **methimazole** (more potent) and **propylthiouracil (PTU,** less potent). These drugs **block new production of thyroid hormone but do not prevent release of thyroid hormone** that has already been synthesized, so thionamide drugs have little immediate effect on their own. However, once the thionamide has blocked new thyroid hormone synthesis, large doses of **iodine may be given to block release of T3 and T4** from the thyroid. If

new synthesis of thyroid hormone is not first blocked by a thionamide, the iodine will be converted into new thyroid hormone, so the order of administration is critical.

XI. SPECIAL CONSIDERATIONS IN THYROID DISORDERS
A. Myxedema Coma
1. **The clinical syndrome.** Myxedema coma is a medical emergency and is associated with a high mortality rate. Due to long-standing severe hypothyroidism, patients with myxedema coma present with altered mental status (usually lethargy but occasionally psychosis; actual coma is rare), hypothermia, bradycardia, hypotension, hypoventilation, hyponatremia, and hypoglycemia. **Myxedema coma can occur acutely** in persons with preexisting untreated or inadequately treated hypothyroidism who are exposed to the stress of an illness, cold ambient temperatures, dehydration, or sedative drugs. Due to the loss of thermoregulation, patients can be profoundly hypothermic with temperatures less than 30°C. Myxedema coma will not occur quickly after **discontinuation of thyroid hormone** even in a patient with severe hypothyroidism because the **half-life of thyroid hormone is long** (approximately 1 week).
2. **Diagnosis and treatment.** The severity of hypothyroidism required to produce this clinical syndrome is extreme, so high levels of TSH are to be expected. Due to a high mortality rate as high as 60%, myxedema coma should be immediately treated without waiting for the laboratory testing if suspicion is high. Treatment of the precipitating illness is essential. Supportive care, including rewarming, ventilatory support, hemodynamic support, and electrolyte correction are paramount. Passive warming should be immediately initiated—active rewarming should be avoided since it could precipitate rapid vasodilation and circulatory collapse. Myxedema coma can be associated with adrenal insufficiency. **Administration of thyroid hormone** to a patient with adrenal insufficiency can acutely **precipitate an adrenal crisis.** Therefore, a cosyntropin test should be performed at the time thyroid tests are obtained and **stress-dose glucocorticoid therapy** must be started before initiation of thyroid hormone therapy. Glucocorticoids can be discontinued if the cosyntropin stimulation test demonstrates sufficient adrenal reserves. The appropriate treatment for myxedema coma is controversial, with different authorities preferring T3 alone, T4 alone, or both hormones together.

B. Thyroid Storm
1. **The clinical syndrome:** Thyroid storm is a life-threatening condition of severe hyperthyroidism with exaggerated symptoms and signs, usually occurring as an acute exacerbating of preexisting hyperthyroidism. Because the thyroid hormone concentrations are similar to those observed in uncomplicated thyrotoxicosis, the diagnosis of thyroid storm is made clinically. TSH is often undetectable, but it is not sufficient to make the diagnosis. Signs and symptoms include fever, tachycardia, mental status changes, delirium, tremor, congestive heart failure, nausea, diarrhea, sweating, dehydration, and abdominal pain. Although thyroid surgery was previously a more common trigger for thyroid storm, it is now less common due to routine treatment of hyperthyroidism. Possible triggers include infection, stress, and trauma.
2. **Treatment** consists of supportive therapy and medications targeted specifically at the excessive action, production, and release of thyroid

hormone. Initial therapy should include an **IV β-blocker**, such as esmo-lol or propranolol, titrated to control tachycardia. Stress-dose **glucocor-ticoids** (100 mg hydrocortisone IV every 8 hours) are administered to reduce T4-to-T3 conversion by deiodinase and to ensure thyroid storm is not complicated by adrenal insufficiency due to rapid glucocorticoid metabolism. Thionamide medications, such as propylthiouracil or methimazole, are used to reduce the production of thyroid hormone. Iodides, while useful, should not be given first since they may increase the synthesis of new thyroid hormones. Supportive care includes aggressive treatment of hyperpyrexia, fluid resuscitation, rate control in atrial fibrillation, and the diagnosis and treatment of any precipitating conditions.

XII. REGULATION OF CALCIUM HOMEOSTASIS

A. Calcium Uptake from the Gut and Secretion by the Kidney. Calcium is essential for a variety of functions, including neural transmission, intracellular signaling, blood coagulation, skeletal structure, and myocardial contractility. Under ordinary circumstances, the intake and excretion of calcium are balanced. From a typical daily intake of 1,000 mg, there may be 200 mg net absorption from the gut and a similar amount excreted in the urine. Calcium is filtered by the glomerulus and must be actively reabsorbed so that only a few percentage of the filtered load is actually excreted. Both the absorption of calcium (along with phosphate) from the gut and liberation of calcium and phosphorus from bone are promoted by **parathyroid hormone (PTH)**. In addition to direct effects on the gut, PTH promotes the activation of vitamin D to **1,25-dihydroxyvitamin D,** which also promotes calcium and phosphorus absorption from the gut. In the kidney, PTH promotes calcium reabsorption but phosphate excretion. The net effect of increasing PTH is to raise the serum calcium and reduce serum phosphorus. Calcitonin opposes the action of PTH and inhibits bone and renal resorption of calcium. Most of the **calcium reabsorption** by the kidney occurs in the proximal tubule and **is associated with sodium absorption**. Calcium absorption is promoted in sodium-avid states (dehydration) and calcium excretion is promoted by saline infusion.

B. Calcium Equilibrium between the Blood and Bone. A small fraction (approximately 1%) of the total body calcium is found within cells and in the extracellular fluid. Approximately half the serum calcium concentration is protein bound while the other half is ionized. The calcium value should be adjusted as well for albumin, with a calcium decrease of 0.8 mg/dL for every 1 g/dL decrease in albumin. The remainder is found along with phosphorus in hydroxyapatite crystals within the bone. If bone reabsorption is increased out of proportion of bone mineralization, quite large amounts of calcium can be released into the blood. Equilibrium between the blood and the bone is primarily regulated by PTH, but mechanical stress also promotes bone formation.

C. Causes of Hypercalcemia

1. Primary hyperparathyroidism. This syndrome is typically caused by **benign parathyroid tumors.** It is the most common cause of hypercalcemia in the outpatient setting, typically occurring in the third to fifth decade of life. The sensitivity of parathyroid tumors to the ambient calcium levels is reduced so that higher levels of calcium are required to fully suppress PTH production. A new equilibrium is reached in which serum calcium levels are elevated, yet PTH levels are not fully suppressed. **PTH levels**

are not usually elevated, but are not appropriately suppressed to undetectable levels in the setting of elevated calcium levels.

2. **Secondary hyperparathyroidism (renal osteodystrophy).** Renal insufficiency reduces the ability to excrete phosphorus. **Elevated phosphorus,** like low calcium, is a **stimulus to PTH secretion.** PTH promotes phosphorus excretion and the absorption of calcium from the gut and liberation of calcium from the bone. The elevation of calcium may be exacerbated by administration of calcium-containing phosphate binders. PTH is usually not elevated, but is inappropriately high ("normal") in the setting of hypercalcemia.

3. **Tertiary hyperparathyroidism.** Long-standing secondary hyperparathyroidism may lead to a degree of **parathyroid autonomy** from calcium feedback regulation. Once this occurs, PTH production is not appropriately suppressed even if phosphate levels are controlled by dialysis or phosphate binders. The consequence is inappropriately high ("inappropriately normal") PTH levels in the setting of hypercalcemia.

4. **Hypercalcemia of malignancy.** This syndrome may develop in the setting of large lytic lesions of bone, but more commonly is associated with secretion of **PTH-related protein (PTHrP)** from tumors, which circulates systemically and acts similarly to PTH. PTHrP is classically associated with multiple myeloma and breast, lung, and squamous cell cancer, but may be found with tumors of many types. PTH production from the parathyroid glands is suppressed by the elevated calcium, and PTH is typically undetectable.

5. **Paget's disease of bone.** Localized patches of increased bone resorption and disorganized reformation are the hallmark of Paget's disease. By itself, Paget's disease usually does not cause hypercalcemia because bone resorption is balanced by bone formation. However, immobilization can lead to the abrupt development of hypercalcemia. Paget's disease is present in up to 3% of individuals older than 50 years.

6. **Drugs and ingestions.** Excess ingestion of vitamin D or vitamin D metabolites such as 1,25-hydroxyvitamin D can cause hypercalcemia. Other drugs that may cause hypercalcemia include vitamin A (increased bone turnover), lithium (increasing PTH secretion), theophylline (increased bone turnover), and thiazide diuretics (reduced calcium excretion).

7. **Endocrinopathies.** Nonparathyroid endocrinopathies that may cause hypercalcemia include hyperthyroidism (increased bone turnover), adrenal insufficiency (decreased calcium excretion), and pheochromocytoma (PTHrP secretion).

XIII. DIAGNOSIS AND TREATMENT OF HYPERCALCEMIA
A. Diagnosis
1. **Signs and symptoms associated with severe hypercalcemia** include polyuria, abdominal pain, nausea, vomiting, constipation, headache, altered mental status, lethargy, weakness, and depression. Hyporeflexia, hypertension, and bradycardia may occur. In the critical care setting, hypercalcemia is primarily diagnosed by laboratory studies.
2. **Measurement of serum calcium.** Approximately 50% of serum calcium is found as free, ionized calcium, while approximately 40% is bound to albumin and 10% is complexed with anions. Total serum calcium levels can be corrected for the serum albumin level (corrected Ca^{2+} = total Ca^{2+} + 0.8 × [normal albumin − patient albumin]), but this correction is not entirely reliable. It is preferable to directly

measure the ionized calcium and make diagnostic and therapeutic decisions on this basis.

3. **PTH-dependent hypercalcemia.** Serum PTH is not usually elevated even when PTH is the cause of hypercalcemia. Rather, PTH is "inappropriately normal" in the setting of hypercalcemia. A frankly elevated PTH may also be found, but extreme elevations of PTH are rare and suggest the diagnosis of parathyroid carcinoma. In the setting of hypercalcemia, any detectable PTH suggests hyperparathyroidism as the cause. Primary hyperparathyroidism can be distinguished from secondary and tertiary hyperparathyroidism by renal function studies and history.

4. **PTH-independent hypercalcemia.** If PTH is undetectable, past medical history and medication history will provide important clues. Additional laboratory workup should include PTHrP (for hypercalcemia of malignancy), 25-hydroxyvitamin D (if ingestion is suspected), 1,25-dihydroxyvitamin D (for granulomatous disease), and thyroid studies (TSH, free T4, T3). Alkaline phosphatase is usually strikingly elevated in Paget's disease and less so in other causes of increased bone turnover.

B. Treatment

1. **Promotion of renal calcium excretion.** Calcium is freely filtered into the urine and most of it is actively reabsorbed along with sodium. Delivery of sodium in the form of **saline hydration** can be very effective in lowering serum calcium in volume-depleted patients. The goal in most cases should be to adequately hydrate the patient, although saline therapy may be limited by development of volume overload and edema. In such cases, a loop diuretic such as furosemide may be required and may further promote calcium excretion. Loop diuretics should not be used without saline treatment, as dehydration may worsen hypercalcemia. The combination of saline and furosemide for **forced diuresis has fallen out of favor** as the first-line therapy for hypercalcemia. In the setting of renal failure, renal replacement therapy with dialysis or continuous hemofiltration with a low calcium dialysate is usually necessary to treat hypercalcemia. **Dialysis** may also be used for emergency treatment of severe hypercalcemia in patients with normal or only modestly impaired renal function.

2. **Inhibiting calcium release from bone. Calcitonin** inhibits bone resorption as well as renal calcium resorption. Treatment with calcitonin, at 4 to 8 U/kg subcutaneously every 6 hours, can be very effective in **rapidly lowering serum calcium,** often within hours. The combination of calcitonin and saline hydration is probably the most appropriate **first-line therapy** for hypercalcemia. **Tachyphylaxis** to the effects of calcitonin usually occurs after a few days of treatment, so it is usually used in the acute phase of treatment only. Rebound hypercalcemia can occur upon development of tachyphylaxis when calcitonin is the sole therapy. Either the underlying cause should be treated or **bisphosphonates** should be given concurrently with calcitonin and saline hydration. Bisphosphonates are deposited in the mineral matrix of bone and inhibit the release of calcium from bone. Pamidronate and zoledronic acid can be administered IV. **Pamidronate is given at 60 to 90 mg IV over 4 hours, zoledronic acid at 4 mg IV over 15 minutes.** The peak effect of both drugs occurs after 48 to 72 hours. These drugs are clearly indicated for treatment of **hypercalcemia of malignancy,** but should be used cautiously in other settings because their effects may last for years. They inhibit bone loss in high-turnover states, but also delay bone formation when conditions would otherwise favor it. Bisphosphonates

may cause **hypocalcemia** in certain clinical situations, such as patients with **vitamin D deficiency.** These drugs should be used when the ultimate cause of the hypercalcemia cannot be reversed in the short-to-medium term (malignancy) or when they directly address the pathophysiology of the hypercalcemia (Paget's disease of bone). Bisphosphonates are relatively contraindicated in the setting of renal failure. Glucocorticoids may also provide benefit in combination with bisphosphonates for hypercalcemia of malignancy due to osteolytic lesions.

3. **Inhibition of PTH and active vitamin D production. Cinacalcet** is a drug that increases the sensitivity of the **calcium-sensing receptor,** found on parathyroid cells, to extracellular calcium. It is useful in PTH-dependent hypercalcemia by decreasing PTH secretion and serum calcium levels. Cinacalcet is approved for the treatment of secondary hyperparathyroidism and parathyroid carcinoma. It is also clinically used for treatment of primary hyperparathyroidism. It has no role in the treatment of PTH-independent hypercalcemia. **Glucocorticoids** are the treatment of choice for treatment for hypercalcemia due to granulomatous disease, but may obscure a pathological diagnosis if used prior to a biopsy.

XIV. CARCINOID SYNDROME

A. **Carcinoid Tumor Physiology.** Carcinoid tumors are slowly growing neoplasms most frequently found in the **bronchi (20%)** and in the **gastrointestinal (GI) tract (70%).** The liver inactivates most of the products of carcinoid tumors, so GI tumors typically do not cause symptoms without metastasis to the liver. Lung tumors can cause symptoms without metastasis because the carcinoid products are secreted directly into the systemic circulation. When metastases reach the heart, they can cause significant cardiac valvular diseases at the tricuspid and pulmonic valve. Since carcinoid tumors originate from neuroendocrine cells, they can secrete a wide variety of products, including serotonin, histamine, tachykinins, kallikrein, and prostaglandins. Less common products include norepinephrine, dopamine, gastrin, glucagon, ACTH, and growth hormone. Almost all carcinoid tumors take up and metabolize tryptophan, resulting in hypoproteinemia due to the depletion of a key amino acid. In most cases, they convert it to **serotonin,** which is then metabolized to 5-hydroxyindoleacetic (5-HIAA) acid, but in some cases no serotonin is produced and the primary metabolites are 5-HIAA and **histamine.** 5-HIAA can be measured in the blood and urine to diagnose carcinoid syndrome.

B. **Features of Carcinoid Syndrome.** Secretory diarrhea, flushing, and itching of the skin are the most common manifestations caused by excess of serotonin, histamine, and kinins. The diarrhea can be explosive and result in substantial fluid loss and malabsorption. Peripheral vasodilation may lead to hypotension and tachycardia. Episodes are usually spontaneous and last less than 30 minutes. However, serotonin can also cause vasoconstriction, resulting in hypertension. Flushing episodes can be precipitated by drugs, especially anesthesia, or palpation of the tumor, and this "carcinoid crisis" can last for hours and be associated with severe hypotension, bronchoconstriction, arrhythmias, and death. Flushing may be associated with bronchospasm, particularly when associated with bronchial carcinoids. High levels of serotonin may lead to cardiac valvular abnormalities, typically involving fibrous thickening of the right heart valves and leading most commonly to tricuspid regurgitation and/or pulmonic stenosis or regurgitation. Depletion of tryptophan (by conversion to serotonin and 5-HIAA) may lead to muscle wasting due to poor protein synthesis and nicotinic acid deficiency, which may result in overt pellagra (rough skin, glossitis, angular stomatitis, and altered mental status). Serotonin can also cause increased drowsiness and delayed emergence from anesthesia. In nonfunctional tumors, patients do not develop the hormonal effects, but rather present with abdominal pain, GI obstruction, or bleeding.

C. **Diagnosis.** In patients with the carcinoid syndrome, typical levels of 5-HIAA in urine are more than 10-fold above the upper limit of normal. Serotonin levels greater than 25 mg/24 h are considered diagnostic for carcinoid. However, the sensitivity of the test is only 80%. Many drugs and foods can give falsely elevated levels of 5-HIAA including acetaminophen, phenobarbital, and ephedrine. Bronchial and gastric carcinoids may have normal urinary 5-HIAA levels even in the absence of interfering substances. In such cases, blood measurements of chromogranin A and serotonin may be helpful. In the ICU, the provocation of paradoxical flushing and hypotension by epinephrine should prompt consideration of carcinoid syndrome. Multiple imaging modalities, including endoscopy, ultrasound, CT, MRI, and barium radiography can be used to locate the tumor. Radiolabeled somatostatin analog scintigraphy is the gold standard for location confirmation. Echocardiography is useful if cardiac lesions are suspected.

D. **Treatment.** Definitive treatment of carcinoid syndrome involves surgical removal of the tumor. However, most patients who develop the classic syndrome have gut carcinoids with metastasis to the liver, so definitive surgical management is not possible. **Flushing and diarrhea are treated primarily with octreotide,** which is highly effective. Octreotide is also used to prevent progression of carcinoid cardiac valvular disease. Octreotide can be used prophylactically to prevent carcinoid crisis during anesthesia and surgery. Levels of urinary 5-HIAA can be followed to monitor the effectiveness of treatment. Wheezing can be treated with albuterol. The treatment of hypotension in carcinoid crisis is unusual because **catecholamines can worsen the crises** and further lower blood pressure. Hypotension should be treated with intravenous octreotide (IV bolus of 300 μg followed by an infusion of up to 150 μg/h) and fluid resuscitation. **Somatostatin** is a GI peptide that can reduce serotonin release. However, due to a half-life of less than 3 minutes, it must be given by continuous infusion.

XV. PHEOCHROMOCYTOMA AND PARAGANGLIOMA

A. **Diagnosis.** These are tumors of neural crest origin that secrete catecholamines (norepinephrine, epinephrine, and/or dopamine) in an unpredictable manner. They are found arising from the medulla of the adrenal gland or from the sympathetic ganglia along the aorta up to the carotid bifurcation. The classical history is one of "spells" of palpitations, headache, and pallor, classically associated with **hypertension,** but tonic hypertension without spells is an equally likely presentation. No "normal" ranges for these hormones exist for hospital inpatients, much less ICU patients. Therefore, the appropriate strategy in most cases of suspected pheochromocytoma is to wait until the patient has recovered from their acute illness to perform diagnostic testing. Tests typically include urinary and plasma-fractionated metanephrines and catecholamines. Approximately 5% of all incidentally discovered adrenal masses are pheochromocytomas. Characteristics of the mass on MRI imaging and specialized tests such as meta-iodobenzylguanidine (MIBG) scintiscanning can be used to support the diagnosis in patients for whom biochemical testing is not appropriate.

B. Treatment. All patients with catecholamine-secreting tumors require **preparation for surgery.** Even external palpation of these masses may provoke a crisis, so no manipulations should be done without careful thought and appropriate medication availability. Definitive treatment of pheochromocytoma involves surgical resection, but the same methods used for surgery preparation can be used as temporizing measures until a definitive diagnosis can be made or until other medical issues are resolved. The usual regimen includes loading with **phenoxybenzamine,** an irreversible α-blocker, and treating tachyarrhythmias with β-blockade. It is important to not β-block prior to α-blockade to avoid an uncontrolled α-adrenergic response. Pheochromocytomas are often associated with tonic vasoconstriction and volume contraction, so patients may be hypovolemic despite being hypertensive. Therefore, administration of phenoxybenzamine must be accompanied by volume repletion. Optimal blockade occurs when the patient has nasal congestion, orthostatic hypotension (but BP no less than 80/45), an ECG free of ST changes, and no more than one PVC every 5 minutes. In the operating room, vigilance is essential as hemodynamic lability can be extreme while surgeons manipulate and remove the tumor.

C. Postoperative Management of Pheochromocytoma. Patients can be either hypertensive or hypotensive postoperatively following resection. If residual tumor exists, catecholamine levels may remain elevated and require antihypertensive treatment. In addition to phenoxybenzamine, doxazosin is shorter-acting option for α-blockade. However, patients can also be hypotensive as the body adjusts to the sudden decrease in catecholamine levels. In such a scenario, vasopressors and IV fluids may be needed to maintain hemodynamics. Phenoxybenzamine can be discontinued. Hypoglycemia can complicate the immediate postoperative period, so glucose monitoring should occur at regular intervals in the first postoperative day.

Selected Readings

Abdelmalak BB, Lansang MC. Revisiting tight glycemic control in perioperative and critically ill patients: when one size may not fit all. *J Clin Anesthes* 2013;25:499–507.

Annane D, Sebille V, Charpentier C, et al. Effect of treatment with low doses of hydrocortisone and fludrocortisone on mortality in patients with septic shock. *JAMA* 2002;288:862–871.

Annane D, Sebille V, Troche G, et al. A 3-level prognostic classification in septic shock based on cortisol levels and cortisol response to corticotropin. *JAMA* 2000;283:1038–1045.

Arafah BM. Hypothalamic pituitary adrenal function during critical illness: limitations of current assessment methods. *J Clin Endocrinol Metab* 2006;91:3725–3745.

Baird TA, Parsons MW, Phanh T, et al. Persistent poststroke hyperglycemia is independently associated with infarct expansion and worse clinical outcome. *Stroke* 2003;34:2208–2214.

Beall DP, Henslee HB, Webb HR, et al. Milk-alkali syndrome: a historical review and description of the modern version of the syndrome. *Am J Med Sci* 2006;331:233–242.

Bendelow J, Apps E, Jones LE, et al. Carcinoid syndrome. *Eur J Surg Oncol* 2008;34:289–296.

Brunkhorst FM, Engel C, Bloos F, et al. Intensive insulin therapy and pentastarch resuscitation in severe sepsis. *N Engl J Med* 2008;358:125–139.

Casserly B, Gerlach H, Phillips GS, et al. Low-dose steroids in adult septic shock: results of the surviving sepsis campaign. *Intensive Care Med* 2012;38:1946–1954.

Dellinger RP, Levy MM, Rhodes A. Surviving sepsis campaign: international guidelines for management of severe sepsis and septic shock: 2012. *Crit Car Med* 2013;41:580–637.

Devos P, Preiser J, Melot C. Impact of tight glucose control by intensive insulin therapy on ICU mortality and the rate of hypoglycaemia: final results of the Glucontrol study. *Intensive Care Med* 2007;33:S189.

Dickstein G. On the term "relative adrenal insufficiency"—or what do we really measure with adrenal stimulation tests? *J Clin Endocrinol Metab* 2005;90:4973–4974.

Egi M, Bellomo R, Stachowski E, et al. The interaction of chronic and acute glycemia with mortality in critically ill patients with diabetes. *Crit Care Med* 2011;39:105–111.

Fietsam R Jr, Bassett J, Glover JL. Complications of coronary artery surgery in diabetic patients. *Am Surg* 1991;57:551–557.

Hamrahian AH, Oseni TS, Arafah BM. Measurements of serum free cortisol in critically ill patients. *N Engl J Med* 2004;350:1629–1638.

Ilias I, Pacak K. Current approaches and recommended algorithm for the diagnostic localization of pheochromocytoma. *J Clin Endocrinol Metab* 2004;89:479–491.

Jacobs TP, Bilezikian JP. Clinical review: rare causes of hypercalcemia. *J Clin Endocrinol Metab* 2005;90:6316–6322.

Kohl BA, Schwartz S. How to manage perioperative endocrine insufficiency. *Anesthesiology Clinics* 2010;28:139–155.

Krinsley JS, Grover A. Severe hypoglycemia in critically ill patients: risk factors and outcomes. *Crit Care Med* 2007;35:2262–2267.

Kwaku MP, Burman KD. Myxedema coma. *J Intensive Care Med* 2007;22:224–231.

LeGrand SB, Leskuski D, Zama I. Narrative review: furosemide for hypercalcemia: an unproven yet common practice. *Ann Intern Med* 2008;149:259–263.

Lumachi F, Brunello A, Roma A, et al. Medical treatment of malignancy-associated hypercalcemia. *Curr Med Chem* 2008;15:415–421.

Maletkovic J, Drexler A. Diabetic ketoacidosis and hyperglycemic hyperosmolar state. *Endocrinol Metab Clin North Am* 2013;42:677–695.

Mancuso K, Kaye AD, Boudreaux JP. Carcinoid syndrome and perioperative anesthetic considerations. *J Clin Anesth* 2011;23:329–341.

Mebis L, Debaveye Y, Visser TJ, et al. Changes within the thyroid axis during the course of critical illness. *Endocrinol Metab Clin North Am* 2006;35:807–821.

Meijering S, Corstjens AM, Tulleken JE, et al. Towards a feasible algorithm for tight glycaemic control in critically ill patients: a systematic review of the literature. *Crit Care* 2006;10:R19.

Mesotten D, Vanhorebeek I, Van den Berghe G. The altered adrenal axis and treatment with glucocorticoids during critical illness. *Nat Clin Pract Endocrinol Metab* 2008;4:496–505.

Mundy GR, Edwards JR. PTH-related peptide (PTHrP) in hypercalcemia. *J Am Soc Nephrol* 2008;19:672–675.

Nayak B, Burman K. Thyrotoxicosis and thyroid storm. *Endocrinol Metab Clin North Am* 2006;35:663–686.

Nayak B, Hodak SP. Hyperthyroidism. *Endocrinol Metab Clin North Am* 2007;36:617–656.

NICE-SUGAR Study Investigators. Intensive versus conventional glucose control in critically ill patients. *N Engl J Med* 2009;360:1283–1297.

Noordzij PG, Boersma E, Schreiner F. Increased preoperative glucose levels are associated with perioperative mortality in patients undergoing noncardiac, nonvascular surgery. *Eur J Endocrinol* 2007;156:137–142.

Pacak K. Preoperative management of the pheochromocytoma patient. *J Clin Endocrinol Metab* 2007;92:4069–4079.

Shepard MM, Smith JW III. Hypercalcemia. *Am J Med Sci* 2007;334:381–385.

Siraux V, De Backer D, Yalavatti G, et al. Relative adrenal insufficiency in patients with septic shock: comparison of low-dose and conventional corticotropin tests. *Critical Care Med* 2005;33:2479–2486.

Van den Berghe G, Wilmer A, Hermans G, et al. Intensive insulin therapy in the medical ICU. *N Engl J Med* 2006;354:449–461.

Van den Berghe G, Wouters P, Weekers F, et al. Intensive insulin therapy in critically ill patients. *N Engl J Med* 2001;345:1359–1367.

Vincent JL, Abraham E, Moore FA, et al. *Textbook of critical care.* 6th ed. Philadelphia: Elsevier, 2011:1205–1233.

Wiener RS, Wiener DC, Larson RJ. Benefits and risks of tight glucose control in critically ill adults: a meta-analysis. *JAMA* 2008;300:933–944.

Wilson M, Weinreb J, Hoo GW. Intensive insulin therapy in critical care: a review of 12 protocols. *Diabetes Care* 2007;30:1005–1011.

Wisneski LA. Salmon calcitonin in the acute management of hypercalcemia. *Calcif Tissue Int* 1990;46(suppl):S26–S30.

Young WF Jr. Adrenal causes of hypertension: pheochromocytoma and primary aldosteronism. *Rev Endocr Metab Disord* 2007;8:309–320.

Infectious Diseases—Empiric and Emergency Treatment

Alexander R. Levine and Sameer S. Kadri

Infectious disease specialists are often consulted for infections in the critically ill given the degree of diagnostic and therapeutic complexity. That being said, the "first-responder" provider needs to familiarize him-/herself with fundamental management principles. This chapter emphasizes the fundamentals of clinical presentation, microbiology, and diagnostic and therapeutic approaches for infections in the critically ill.

Chapter 29 provides a review on the sepsis syndrome and has not been separately discussed here. Infection prophylaxis is beyond the scope of this chapter and likewise has not been included. Unless otherwise indicated, the potential antibiotic regimens mentioned represent initial empiric therapy. Subsequent therapy should be tailored to culture and susceptibility data as they become available.

I. **THORACIC INFECTIONS:** This section focuses on infections of the lungs, pleura, and thoracic cavity that may either be the presenting diagnosis or discovered during the ICU stay.
   A. **Community-Acquired Pneumonia** (CAP) is an infection of the lower respiratory tract that is acquired in the community. While most cases can be managed in the outpatient setting with oral antibiotics, a subset of severe cases requires critical care and often even mechanical ventilation and is associated with significant morbidity and mortality. Advanced age, multiple comorbidities, and immune suppression are common host factors, whereas high virulence and large organism load are agent-related factors associated with severe CAP. While fever, chills, cough, expectoration, and chest pain are common, symptoms of air hunger, confusion, and signs of tachypnea, accessory muscle use, hypoxemia despite oxygen supplementation, hypotension, and evidence of high leukocytosis, bandemia, and lactic acidosis should arouse suspicion for severe CAP and lower the threshold for ICU admission.
      1. **Microbiology.** The distribution of organisms varies slightly between CAP and severe CAP. The most frequent pathogen in both categories is *Streptococcus pneumoniae.* The other common causes of CAP that often require ICU care are nontypeable *Hemophilus influenza, Pseudomonas aeruginosa, Staphylococcus aureus* (including community-acquired methicillin-resistant strains), *Legionella pneumophila, Chlamydia pneumoniae,* and respiratory viruses, namely, influenza. *Moraxella catarrhalis* and *P. aeruginosa* usually cause CAP in patients with bronchiectasis or chronic bronchitis. Certain fungi like *Histoplasma capsulatum, Coccidioides immitis,* and *Mycobacteria (M. tuberculosis)* may cause CAP in regions where they are endemic, and some like *Pneumocystis jirovecii* cause CAP in specific immune-suppressed populations (e.g., AIDS).
      2. **Diagnosis.** Findings on chest radiography (CXR) may be variable depending on the pathogen and the underlying condition of the host. Depending on the etiological agent, infiltrates may be interstitial or

parenchymal, which may be unilobar or multilobar. Infiltrates may not be apparent on initial CXR in the setting of hypovolemia and "blossom" following rehydration on subsequent films. Despite all efforts, the causative microorganism will not be identified in close to 40% cases of severe CAP. Yet, a specific microbial etiology is desirable and must be searched for through sputum sampling or bronchoalveolar lavage (BAL), serological testing (e.g., *Mycoplasma pneumoniae*, *C. immitis*), sputum sampling for immunoassays or PCR (respiratory viruses), and urine for specific antigens (*S. pneumoniae*, *L. pneumophila* Serotype I and Histoplasma). Gram stain of sputum or BAL fluid may provide important clues regarding the potential causative organism early on based on abundance, morphology, and presence of neutrophils, which findings can be subsequently confirmed on culture. Blood cultures may also be positive in severe CAP with certain bacterial etiologies. If a significant pleural effusion accompanies pneumonia, the pleural fluid should be analyzed with gram stain and culture, pH, lactate dehydrogenase, glucose, and protein concentration. These tests allow ruling out empyema, which if present, warrants drainage or decortication.

3. **Triage.** Several well-validated severity scores have been developed to triage patients with CAP such as the Pneumonia Severity Index, which is complex and uses up to 20 variables, or the CURB-65, which is a simpler score that is easier to apply in practice (see Fig. 28.1) (American Thoracic Society; Infectious Diseases Society of America, 2005). While a CURB-65 score of 4 or 5 should prompt ICU admission in most cases, scores such as these should only supplement clinical gestalt.

4. **Treatment.** Initial management of CAP is based on established guidelines coupled with acknowledgement of host and epidemiological factors and Gram-stain results, when available. Outcome is improved with early administration of antibiotics, especially in severe CAP. Clinical presentation does not reliably predict the pathogens involved. The potential for antibiotic resistance should influence the choice of antibiotics (e.g., *S. pneumoniae* may be penicillin resistant). Early empiric antibiotic regimens should include coverage of typical as well as atypical microorganisms. Patient-specific risk factors for pseudomonas should be considered, which include structural lung diseases, frequent severe COPD exacerbations, recent antibiotic use, and chronic alcoholism. Therapy should be subsequently tailored on the basis of results of cultures, susceptibility, and serology where applicable.

Potential empiric regimens for severe CAP (in the ICU) include the following:

a. A β-lactam third- or fourth-generation cephalosporin such as cefotaxime, ceftriaxone, cefepime, or ampicillin/sulbactam plus an intravenous (IV) macrolide such as azithromycin.

b. A third- or fourth-generation cephalosporin plus a fluoroquinolone such as levofloxacin.

c. A β-lactam/β-lactamase inhibitor such as ampicillin/sulbactam plus IV macrolide or fluoroquinolone.

d. If pseudomonas is a possibility, an antipseudomonal and antipneumococcal β-lactam/β-lactamase inhibitor such as piperacillin/tazobactam, or a carbapenem such as imipenem or meropenem should be used along with either azithromycin, levofloxacin or ciprofloxacin.

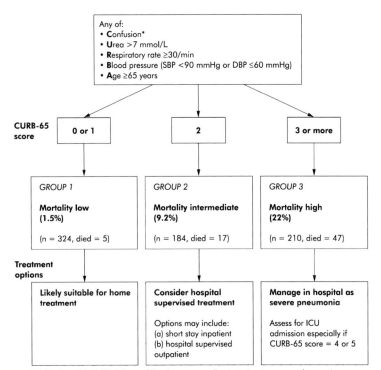

*defined as a Mental Test Score of 8 or less, or new disorientation in person, place or time

FIGURE 28.1 Severity assessment in a hospital setting: the CURB-65 score. One-step strategy for stratifying patients with CAP into risk groups according to risk of mortality at 30 days when the results of blood urea are available. (From Lim WS, van der Eerden MM, Laing R, et al. Defining community acquired pneumonia severity on presentation to hospital: an international derivation and validation study. *Thorax* 2003 May;58(5):377–382.)

      e. Ciprofloxacin should only be used in combination with an antipneumococcal β-lactam/β-lactamase inhibitor because it does not have antipneumococcal coverage.

      f. If methicillin-resistant *Staphylococcus aureus* (MRSA) is a possibility, add vancomycin or linezolid.

  B. Hospital-acquired pneumonia (HAP) is defined as pneumonia that occurs at least 48 hours after admission to the hospital and did not appear to be incubating at the time of admission. It carries the highest risk of mortality among nosocomial infections. Health care–associated pneumonia (HCAP) is a broader term that encompasses pneumonias acquired in a health setting and not limited to the hospital—a definition that is less specific and diminishing fast in its appeal. Ventilator-associated pneumonia (VAP) is a subset of HAP that occurs more than 48 to 72 hours after intubation. VAP affects between 9% and 27% of intubated patients and is associated with high attributable mortality. Bacteria enter the lungs through various routes, including aspiration of oropharyngeal secretions or gastric contents, inhalation of droplets or aerosolized microorganisms from health care surroundings, hematogenous seeding, direct inoculation from colonized hospital personnel and contaminated equipment or devices.

1. **Microbiology.** The microorganisms causing nosocomial pneumonia differ substantially from those causing CAP. Infections can be polymicrobial. Common pathogens include gram-negative bacilli, such as *P. aeruginosa, Escherichia coli, Klebsiella pneumoniae, Acinetobacter baumannii*, and less commonly *Serratia marcescens, Enterobacter cloacae, Stenotrophomonas maltophilia*, and *Burkholderia cepacia* or gram-positive cocci such as *S. aureus*. Antimicrobial resistance is on the rise among these organisms, which may be preexisting or may develop *de novo* under selective pressure of antibiotics. MRSA is a common cause of hospital acquired pneumonia, particularly in patients with diabetes mellitus and those colonized with the microorganism. Risk factors for multidrug-resistant (MDR) infections include being hospitalized for >5 days, use of antibiotics during the preceding 90 days, a high frequency of antibiotic resistance in the specific hospital/unit, and immune-suppressive disease or therapy.

2. Diagnosis of VAP can be difficult because many conditions (e.g., sepsis, ARDS, CHF, atelectasis, thromboembolic disease, pulmonary hemorrhage, etc.) that are common in critically ill patients demonstrate similar clinical signs. The clinical criteria to diagnose VAP include the presence of new or progressive radiographic infiltrates in addition to one or more of the following: fever, purulent secretions, leukocytosis, tachypnea, diminished tidal volume, and hypoxemia. Radiographic signs alone are too nonspecific (see Fig. 28.2) (Bratzler, 2013). Acknowledging the difficulties in making the diagnosis of VAP using the existing definition of VAP, a new three-tier approach of ventilator-associated condition (VAC), infection-related ventilator-associated complication (IVAC), and possible or probable VAP has been proposed by the CDC but are currently limited to epidemiological surveillance and performance and quality assessments (Centers for Disease Control and Prevention, 2013).

   a. Lower respiratory tract sampling is the cornerstone of VAP management. This is achieved by any of the following:

      1. **Deep tracheal aspiration:** Deep suction using a catheter introduced through the ET tube or tracheostomy
      2. **Bronchoalveolar lavage (BAL):** Wedging the tip of the bronchoscope in a segmental bronchial orifice and infusion of sterile saline followed by aspiration of the infusate-secretion mixture
      3. **Protected specimen brush (PSB):** Introduction of a sampling brush via the bronchoscope that is covered by a protective sheath to minimize trans-bronchoscopic contamination

         a. Results must be interpreted in light of time of antibiotic administration relative to sampling. Whenever possible, empiric antibiotics must be administered postsampling to maximize culture yield.
         b. While BAL and PSB sampling were shown not to provide a survival benefit over deep tracheal aspiration, they do provide greater microbiological specificity, which potentially allows early antibiotic de-escalation and diminishes *de novo* resistance development and should be attempted whenever possible, if the risk is low and trained personnel are available.

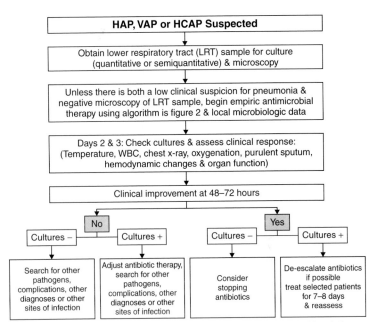

HAP, VAP or HCAP Suspected

Obtain lower respiratory tract (LRT) sample for culture (quantitative or semiquantitative) & microscopy

Unless there is both a low clinical suspicion for pneumonia & negative microscopy of LRT sample, begin empiric antimicrobial therapy using algorithm is figure 2 & local microbiologic data

Days 2 & 3: Check cultures & assess clinical response: (Temperature, WBC, chest x-ray, oxygenation, purulent sputum, hemodynamic changes & organ function)

Clinical improvement at 48–72 hours

No   Yes

Cultures –   Cultures +   Cultures –   Cultures +

Search for other pathogens, complications, other diagnoses or other sites of infection

Adjust antibiotic therapy, search for other pathogens, complications, other diagnoses or other sites of infection

Consider stopping antibiotics

De-escalate antibiotics if possible treat selected patients for 7–8 days & reassess

FIGURE 28.2 Summary of the management strategies for a patient with suspected hospital-acquired pneumonia (HAP), ventilator-associated pneumonia (VAP), or health care–associated pneumonia (HCAP). The decision about antibiotic discontinuation may differ depending on the type of sample collected (PSB, BAL, or endotracheal aspirate), and whether the results are reported in quantitative or semiquantitative terms (see text for details). (From American Thoracic Society; Infectious Diseases Society of America. Guidelines for the management of adults with hospital-acquired, ventilator-associated, and healthcare-associated pneumonia. *Am J Respir Crit Care Med* 2005;171:388–416.)

b. **Gram stain:** This is a valuable tool especially if empiric antibiotics may have sterilized respiratory samples. In these situations, morphological identification of bacterial "carcasses" may be the only available hint while making decisions for targeted therapy. Abundance of neutrophils on gram stain increases the likelihood of VAP.

c. **Semiquantitative cultures:** These are reported as none, mild, moderate, or abundant bacterial growth. The latter two strata are suggestive of VAP, but discrimination between colonization and infection using such ordinal strata is challenging.

d. **Quantitative cultures:** Bacterial growth of >100,000 CFU/mL in cultures from deep tracheal aspirate, >10,000 CFU/mL from BAL cultures, and >1,000 CFU/mL from PSB cultures are considered reasonable cutoffs for discriminating between VAP and colonization. Severely ill cases may warrant treatment despite failure to meet these cutoffs for VAP. While they may minimize resistance development by limiting inadvertent antimicrobial use, quantitative cultures have not shown to improve clinical outcomes. Severely ill cases warrant treatment despite failure to meet these cutoffs for VAP.

3. **Treatment.** Principles for managing VAP include use of early, appropriate empiric antibiotics in adequate doses, de-escalation of initial antibiotic therapy based on lower respiratory tract culture data and patient response, and avoiding unduly long durations of therapy. Use of a unit-specific broad-spectrum antibiotic regimen can reduce the incidence of inappropriate initial therapy to <10%.

   a. Uncomplicated mild to moderate disease (i.e., without respiratory failure, hemodynamic instability, or signs of injury to other organs) occurring early during hospitalization (<5 days) is often treated with a single antibiotic; such as a third- or fourth-generation cephalosporin, a carbapenem, or a fluoroquinolone in patients who are allergic to penicillin. Numerous studies suggest that monotherapy is safe and effective when used properly and may decrease the likelihood of infection due to antibiotic-resistant microorganisms. If anaerobes are a possibility, a β-lactam/β-lactamase inhibitor combination such as ampicillin/sulbactam, piperacillin/tazobactam, or ticarcillin/clavulanate can be used as monotherapy. Alternatively, clindamycin or metronidazole may be added to a β-lactam or fluoroquinolone for adequate anaerobic coverage.

   b. Severe HAP (i.e., respiratory failure, hemodynamic instability, extrapulmonary organ damage) is treated with combination therapy. Combination therapy should also be considered when mild to moderate pneumonia occurs later in the hospitalization, occurs in patients with significant comorbidities, or occurs in patients with recent antibiotic exposure. These situations increase the likelihood that pneumonia is caused by *P. aeruginosa*, other multidrug-resistant enteric gram-negative bacilli such as *Acinetobacter* spp., *Enterobacter* spp., *Klebsiella* spp., and/or MRSA. Generally, combination therapy includes any empiric monotherapy agent mentioned previously along with a fluoroquinolone or an aminoglycoside. Linezolid or vancomycin should be added if there is a possibility of MRSA pneumonia. Linezolid may be favorable in patients who have an MRSA infection with an MIC >1 mcg/mL as these infections have been associated with slower clinical response and higher rates of vancomycin failure. Daptomycin is inactivated by surfactant and should not be used to cover MRSA in suspected or confirmed cases of VAP. Aerosolized aminoglycoside or polymyxin antibiotics treatment may be considered as an adjunct to IV therapy in MDR gram-negative pneumonias in patients who are not improving with systemic therapy alone. However, adjunctive aerosolized antibiotics have so far only shown to provide improved microbiological eradication, not clinical outcomes necessarily.

C. Lung abscess results from focal necrosis of the pulmonary parenchyma leading to a fluid-filled cavity. The most frequent predisposing factor for lung abscess is aspiration, followed by periodontal disease and gingivitis. Bronchiectasis, pulmonary infarction, septic embolization from bacteremia, right-sided endocarditis, or septic venous thrombosis (e.g., Lemierre's syndrome) also predispose to lung abscess.

   1. **Microbiology.** Bacteria causing aspiration pneumonia and subsequent abscess formation differ depending on whether aspiration occurs in the community or health care setting. Anaerobic organisms appear to be key players. Community-acquired aspiration pneumonia is typically caused by *S. pneumoniae*, *H. influenzae*, community-acquired *S. aureus*, and *Enterobacteriaceae*, and the health care–associated variety

is caused by gram-negative bacteria flora. Abscesses resulting from hematogenous spread of infection are usually peripheral, multifocal, and monomicrobial, most commonly caused by *S. aureus*. *Mycobacterium tuberculosis*, Nocardia, parasites (e.g., amebae and paragonimus spp.), and fungi are less frequent causes of lung abscess.

2. Diagnosis of lung abscess may be made on the basis of chest radiograph or chest computed tomography (CT). The distinction between pleural and peripheral parenchymal-based collections is clearer using CT. Cultures of expectorated sputum are unreliable. While transtracheal and transthoracic aspiration are ways to sample lung abscesses, these are rarely performed.

3. **Treatment.** With some exceptions, witnessed aspiration rarely requires antibiotics. Exceptions include patients whose stomachs are colonized with enteric flora (such as patients with small bowel obstruction), severely immune compromised, or continue to remain severely ill after the aspiration episode. Lung abscesses require prolonged (2–4 months) antibiotic therapy. Antibiotic choices will depend on culture isolates. Historically, antibiotics with anaerobic coverage were used to treat aspiration pneumonia. However, more recent studies that used protected-brush bronchoscopy to obtain samples failed to isolate pathogenic anaerobes. Postural drainage is an important aspect of the management, and bronchoscopy can be helpful in facilitating drainage or removing foreign bodies. Occasionally, a lung abscess is treated with surgical resection; however, this is not a first-line therapy. Complications of lung abscess include empyema, bronchopleural fistula formation, and bronchiectasis.

D. Empyema usually originates from intrapulmonary infection such as lung abscess or pneumonia, but pathogens also can be introduced into the pleural space from extrapulmonary sites as in trauma or thoracic surgery.

1. **Microbiology.** The most common bacterial cause of empyema is *S. aureus*. Enteric and nonenteric gram-negative bacteria (including *Legionella pneumophila*), gram-positive bacteria, anaerobic bacteria, fungi, and *M. tuberculosis* also can cause empyema.

2. Diagnosis requires direct analysis of pleural fluid for pH, total protein, red blood cells (RBC), and leukocyte (WBC) count and differential, Gram stain and bacterial cultures (anaerobic and aerobic), and possibly fungal and mycobacterial smear and culture in the right setting. Pleural fluid with pus or pH <7.2 and/or Gram-stain evidence of bacteria on pleural fluid sampling is highly suggestive of an empyema.

3. **Treatment.** An empyema is refractory to medical therapy alone. It must be treated with a combination of antibiotics and drainage via a thoracostomy tube. Occasionally, open drainage or decortication by video-assisted thoracoscopic surgery (VATS) of the empyema sac may be required.

E. **Mediastinitis.** The commonest presentation of mediastinitis in the modern day is as a postoperative complication of cardiac or thoracic surgery. Some cases may be associated with bacteremia, penetrating chest trauma, retropharyngeal abscess extension, and viscus rupture (e.g., Boerhaave syndrome).

1. **Microbiology.** Mediastinitis following cardiothoracic surgery that does not involve the esophagus is generally monomicrobial and is most often due to *S. Aureus*. Mediastinitis from disruption of the esophagus is usually polymicrobial and is caused by mixed anaerobic bacteria (*Peptococcus* spp., *Peptostreptococcus* spp., *Fusobacterium* spp.,

and *Bacteroides* spp.), gram-positive bacteria, enteric and nonenteric gram-negative bacteria, and fungi (*C. albicans, C. glabrata*). Other rare etiologies include *Legionella, Mycoplasma, Histoplasma*, and *M. tuberculosis*.

2. **Diagnosis.** Clinical signs and symptoms commonly include fever, leukocytosis, and chest pain. It is often difficult to differentiate superficial postoperative wound infection from wound infection with mediastinitis that is usually accompanied with signs of toxicity. Wound crepitus and sternal dehiscence are more specific but not always present. Chest CT may reveal widening of the mediastinum, complicated pleural effusions, and subcutaneous or mediastinal emphysema. However, most findings are difficult to distinguish from postoperative changes in the early postoperative period and results must be interpreted in light of clinical findings.

3. **Treatment.** In most cases, a combination of antibiotics and surgical intervention, including drainage, debridement, and removal or repair of the infected material and tissue must be initiated rapidly. In some situations, contained rupture or small perforations of the esophagus can be treated conservatively with careful monitoring. Broad empiric antibiotic coverage should be employed initially. Antibiotics should then be adjusted on the basis of results of intraoperative cultures. Coverage for head and neck sources (including esophageal disruption) should include antibiotics against gram-positive and gram-negative aerobes, as well as obligate and facultative anaerobes. Combination therapy with penicillin G or clindamycin plus agents against gram-negatives (such as a third-generation cephalosporin or a fluoroquinolone) is effective. Metronidazole will also provide adequate anaerobic coverage. Broadly active β-lactams such as ticarcillin/clavulanate, piperacillin/tazobactam, imipenem/cilastatin, or meropenem also offer reasonable early coverage. Empiric coverage for postsurgical mediastinitis should include an antistaphylococcal agent such as nafcillin or vancomycin (for MRSA or for patients who are allergic to β-lactams).

II. **INTRA-ABDOMINAL INFECTIONS:** These arise either from sources within the gastrointestinal (GI) tract, through contiguous spread from the urogenital/reproductive tract, through hematogenous or lymphatic seeding, or introduced from the outside (as occurs with trauma or surgery). Infections are predominantly polymicrobial. They include enteric gram-negative rods (*E. coli, Klebsiella, Enterobacter*, and *Proteus* spp.), *P. aeruginosa*, aerobic gram-positive cocci (*Enterococcus* and *Streptococcus* spp.), and anaerobes (*Clostridium, Bacteroides, Fusobacterium*, and *Peptostreptococcus* spp.).

Management of intra-abdominal infections depends on the cause and extent of involvement.

A. **Microflora of Abdomen and Pelvis**

1. **GI tract.** Normally, concentrations of bacteria increase progressively from the stomach through the small bowel and colon. Bacteria in the stomach and proximal small bowel include *Streptococcus* spp. and *Lactobacillus* spp. as well as anaerobes such as *Peptostreptococcus* spp. The concentrations of enteric gram-negative rods such as *E. coli* and anaerobic gram-negatives such as *Bacteroides* spp. increase progressively as one moves distally toward the colon. Colonic bacteria include enteric gram-negative rods, *Enterococcus* spp., *Lactobacillus* spp., and anaerobes such as *Bacteroides* spp., *Clostridium* spp., and *Peptostreptococcus* spp.

Factors that influence the quantity or quality of the GI microflora include the following:
  a. pH (antacids, histamine-2 blockers, proton-pump inhibitors)
  b. Antimicrobial use
  c. GI dysmotility
  d. Small-bowel obstruction, ileus, or regional enteritis
  e. Bowel resection or intestinal diversion procedures
  f. Hospitalization or residence in a chronic care facility prior to developing infection
  2. Genital tract microflora include gram-positive aerobic bacteria such as *Streptococcus* spp., *Lactobacillus* spp., and *Staphylococcus* spp. as well as anaerobic bacteria such as *Peptostreptococcus* spp., *Clostridium* spp., and *Bacteroides* spp.

B. Peritonitis. Peritoneal infections can occur following penetrating abdominal trauma, contamination of peritoneal dialysis catheters, perforation of abdominal viscus, or even without a surgically correctable cause in specific populations.
  1. Spontaneous bacterial peritonitis (SBP) is defined as peritonitis due to bacteria without a surgically correctable cause. It almost exclusively occurs in patients with end-stage liver disease (ESLD) from cirrhosis. The pathogenesis is postulated to translocation of gut bacteria across edematous intestinal mucosa and lymphatic or hematogenous seeding in the milieu of third spacing of fluid into the peritoneal cavity under high portal pressures. Infection of ascitic fluid that has accumulated as a result of congestive heart failure, malignancy, or hypoproteinemia in the absence of liver disease is exceedingly rare. Fever, abdominal pain, and confusion are the commonest symptoms. However, patients with SBP may be asymptomatic or have only minor symptoms.
    a. Microorganisms. SBP is predominantly a monomicrobial condition. Enteric gram-negative bacteria are the commonest cause, followed by streptococci. Anaerobes rarely cause SBP. The presence of anaerobic bacteria or mixed flora suggests the possibility of secondary peritonitis.
    b. Diagnosis. Early diagnosis is key; in the absence of treatment, most cases will progress to septic shock, which carries a dismal prognosis in the ESLD population. A diagnostic paracentesis must be performed prior to the administration of antibiotics if SBP is suspected. Ascites fluid should, at minimum, be sent for cell counts, Gram stain, and culture. A polymorphonuclear leukocyte (PMN) count of more than 250 or positive ascitic fluid cultures is highly suggestive of SBP. However, cultures of ascites fluid are often negative despite a cell count that is consistent with SBP. Use of blood culture bottles (anaerobic and aerobic) to culture ascites fluid may increase the likelihood of detecting the bacteria. Blood cultures should also be obtained.
    c. Treatment. Empiric antibiotic therapy should be initiated prior to obtaining the results of cultures if the ascites fluid PMN counts are greater than 250 cells/mm^3. Antibiotics should be modified appropriately when culture and sensitivity data become available. Potential empiric regimens include the following:
      1. Cefotaxime is the primary agent for SBP. High doses (2 g IV every 4 hours) are used for life-threatening SBP.
      2. A β-lactam/β-lactamase inhibitor combination, such as piperacillin/tazobactam or ticarcillin/clavulanate.

   3. Ceftriaxone
   4. Fluoroquinolone (use an alternative agent in patients taking flu-oroquinolones for SBP prophylaxis or at high risk of fluoroquino-lone resistance)
   5. Ertapenem
   6. If resistant enteric gram-negatives are a possibility, imipenem or meropenem should be considered.

2. Secondary peritonitis usually results from perforation or necrosis of a solid viscus (ruptured appendix, diverticulitis, duodenal ulcer), anas-tomotic leaks following bowel surgery or suppurative infections of the biliary and female reproductive tracts.

   a. Diagnosis is often made with assistance of upright plain abdominal radiograph films that may show free air under the diaphragm. A CT scan with oral contrast usually identified the area of perforated vis-cus from extravasation of contrast material. Exploratory laparotomy may be necessary to diagnose and treat the source of peritonitis.

   b. Treatment usually involves a combination of surgery and place-ment of drainage catheters and broad-spectrum antibiotics that are active against gram-negative and gram-positive bacteria and anaerobes. Conservative management may be attempted in cases of a small walled-off perforation or when operative mortality obviates any chance of a benefit. Knowledge of local resistance patterns and known colonization by drug-resistant microorganisms should influence empiric antibiotic choices. Antibiotic choices differ on the basis of severity and setting in which infection occurs.

      1. Mild to moderate community-acquired peritonitis. This occurs very early in the hospitalization and without recent antibiotic therapy in patients who are not in chronic care facilities and is unlikely to result from antibiotic-resistant bacteria. Potential reg-imens include the following:

         i. A third-generation cephalosporin (ceftriaxone, cefotaxime) or fluoroquinolone plus an agent against anaerobes (clinda-mycin or metronidazole). Ampicillin-sulbactam is not rec-ommended for empiric treatment because of high rates of community-acquired *E. coli* resistance).

         ii. Monotherapy with a carbapenem

         iii. Fluoroquinolone plus an agent against anaerobes such as metronidazole

         iv. Severe, high-risk, community-acquired or health care–associ-ated peritonitis.

      2. Peritonitis that develops during hospitalization, in a chronic nursing facility, or in the context of recent therapy with antibac-terial agents may be caused by antibiotic-resistant microorgan-isms. Potential regimens include the following:

         i. Monotherapy with a carbapenem (imipenem/cilastatin or meropenem)

         ii. A third- or fourth-generation cephalosporin (ceftazidime or cefepime) or fluoroquinolone plus metronidazole. Although, fluoroquinolones as the only gram-negative coverage should be avoided in this setting and reserved for hospitals that demonstrate >90% sensitivity to *E. coli*. If ceftazidime is used, an additional agent with gram-positive coverage should be considered as ceftazidime has but modest activity against gram-positive bacteria. The regimen should include agents effective against enterococci such as ampicillin or vancomycin (in setting of β-lactam allergy or high rates of penicillin resistance). Linezolid or daptomycin should be used instead of ampicillin or vancomycin if infection with vancomycin-resistant enterococci (VRE) is a possibility.

C. Intra-abdominal abscesses may result from persistence of bacteria after secondary peritonitis or hematogenous spread of extra-abdominal infection. Locally, these may originate from the GI, upper urinary, or female genital tract. Abscesses should be suspected in the setting of focal abdominal pain and tenderness with high fevers, chills, and/or high leukocytosis that persist despite coverage with empiric antibiotics. Untreated, they may rupture, cause peritonitis, septic shock, and multiple-organ dysfunction syndrome.

   1. Microorganisms commonly cultured from abscesses include *Bacteroides* spp. (especially *B. fragilis*), enteric gram-negative bacteria, gram-positive bacteria such as *Enterococcus* spp. and *S. aureus*, as well as candida.

   2. Diagnosis. CT is useful for diagnosing and localizing abscesses. Ultrasonography can be done at the bedside and can be particularly useful in diagnosis of right-upper-quadrant (RUQ), renal, and pelvic abscesses. Low specificity of indium-labeled WBC and gallium scans limit their utility. Rarely, exploratory laparotomy must be performed in cases of high clinical probability with low yield on imaging.

   3. Treatment of intra-abdominal abscess includes drainage and antibiotics. The method of drainage (percutaneous under CT or ultrasound guidance vs. operative) depends on a variety of factors including the abscess location, whether the abscess is associated with perforation or gangrene, and the presence of loculations when it makes drainage even with multiple catheters unlikely. Often culture data are available to guide antibiotic selection. For initial empiric coverage, it is reasonable to use one of the combinations suggested previously for treating secondary peritonitis in hospitalized patients. Enterococcus spp. discovered in abscesses as part of a polymicrobial process is usually considered relatively avirulent (in immune-competent individuals) and it is acceptable to hold off on providing specific coverage for the same. Serial imaging can be used to monitor treatment, and in cases where a drain is in place, an abscessogram may be performed (imaging following retrograde instillation of contrast into the drain).

D. Infections of the Hepatobiliary System

   1. Acute cholecystitis results from cystic duct obstruction. When this is due to a stone it is called calculous cholecystitis. This can be encountered in the ICU when severe sepsis and septic shock related to gangrene or perforation occur. Acalculous cholecystitis (accounting for a tenth of all acute cholecystitis cases, but more commonly seen in the ICU) occurs in the setting of critical illness, endothelial injury, gall bladder hypoperfusion, stasis edema, and cystic duct luminal narrowing. Complications such as gangrene and perforation as well as untreated mortality are higher in the acalculous variety.

   a. Complications include GB gangrene and perforation with subsequent peritonitis, emphysematous cholecystitis, and empyema of the GB, all of which can lead to septic shock if left untreated.

   b. Microbiology. Bacteria include enteric gram-negative bacteria such as *E. coli*, *Klebsiella*, *Proteus*, and *Enterobacter* spp., gram-positive bacteria such as *Enterococcus* spp., and anaerobes such as *Clostridium* and *Bacteroides* spp. Emphysematous cholecystitis is caused by *Clostridium* spp. and gram-negative bacteria like *E. coli* and *Klebsiella* spp.

c. **Diagnosis.** Acute cholecystitis produces more continuous pain and usually manifests with peritoneal signs like rebound tenderness and Murphy's sign not seen with biliary colic that is accompanied by pain-free intervals and an absence of systemic toxicity and peritoneal signs. Abdominal ultrasonography has reasonable sensitivity and specificity. It may reveal gallstones, GB wall thickening, a dilated gallbladder, or a pericholecystic fluid collection. In ambiguous cases, cholescintigraphy (HIDA scan) can demonstrate nonfilling of the GB. Morphine administered prior to the test may result in a false-negative HIDA scan.

d. Treatment of acute calculous cholecystitis includes antibiotics and surgery. The timing of surgery depends on a number of factors. Surgery is often performed on an urgent basis when the more severe complications of acute cholecystitis as just described occur. Surgery may be delayed for stabilization of the patient or for optimizing the patient with serious medical conditions. Cholecystitis can be treated with the antibiotic regimens previously described for secondary peritonitis. For acalculous cholecystitis, the treatment of choice is percutaneous cholecystostomy tube and antibiotics. These usually cause rapid improvement in clinical and laboratory parameters. In the absence of such improvement, gangrene and/or perforation must be suspected and cholecystectomy is indicated, especially if the risk of untreated complicated acalculous cholecystitis outweighs the surgical risk in these critically ill patients.

2. Acute cholangitis is usually caused by partial or complete common bile duct (CBD) obstruction. This obstruction may be due to calculus, strictures, or an obstruction or extrinsic compression by malignant neoplasms of the biliary tract or pancreas.

a. **Diagnosis.** The classic presentation is Charcot's triad of jaundice, fevers, chills, and RUQ pain. Blood cultures are often positive. No further diagnostic tests are needed if this triad is present and one can move directly to treatment. In the absence of all features of the classic presentation, a RUQ ultrasound may reveal biliary duct dilatation and CBD stone. In early cases, not much time may have lapsed to cause discernible CBD dilatation or the stones may be too small to be seen on ultrasound, in which case magnetic resonance cholangiopancreatography (MRCP) is helpful.

b. Treatment differs depending on whether there is partial or complete CBD obstruction. Nonsuppurative cholangitis, which results from partial CBD obstruction, will often respond to antibiotic therapy alone. Suppurative cholangitis, which is due to complete CBD obstruction causing pus under pressure, bacteremia, and septic shock, must be treated as early as possible, with a combination of antibiotics and decompression. Cholangitis can be treated with the antibiotic regimens described previously for secondary peritonitis. Decompression may be achieved endoscopically (endoscopic retrograde cholangiopancreatography), via a naso-biliary tube or percutaneously using a T-tube (esp. among poor surgical candidates).

3. **Liver abscess.** Abscesses can be solitary or multiple. Manifestations range from fever, leukocytosis, and RUQ pain to sepsis. Liver abscesses

can result from seeding from the blood stream and portal pyemia or from local extension of biliary tract infection.

    a. Microbiology. There is a wide spectrum of microbial etiologies that are difficult to predict beforehand and underscore the importance of sampling. Infections are monomicrobial or polymicrobial, which may include mixed aerobic, anaerobic, enteric bacteria and candida. Multiple monomicrobial abscesses with *S. aureus* or *Streptococcus anginosus* group are indicative of hematogenous spread and potential sources must be investigated. A large number of liver abscess are accompanied with bacteremia and blood cultures must be drawn in each case prior to empiric antibiotics. Patients with a liver abscess from or with recent travel to regions where amebiasis is endemic should raise suspicion of this etiology.

    b. Diagnosis of liver abscess is generally made by CT scan or ultrasonography, and a microbiological diagnosis is obtained by percutaneous aspiration or concurrently positive blood cultures.

    c. Treatment includes drainage and antibiotics. Drainage yields diagnostic and therapeutic benefits. For smaller abscesses, this can be done by needle aspiration but larger ones may require placement of a drain. Abscess arising from the biliary tract or peritoneum should be treated with antibiotics directed against the organisms involved in the initial infection. Abscess suspected to be of hematogenous origin should be treated empirically with regimens that include agents active against gram-positive bacteria or the specific organism when this is known. In most other cases, empiric broad-spectrum therapy with coverage of at least enteric gram-negative organisms and anaerobes should be used such as ampicillin-sulbactam or amoxicillin-clavulanate monotherapy or even levofloxacin plus metronidazole. Anaerobes are difficult to grow, and, given their high prevalence in liver abscesses, many recommend presumptive therapy with a regimen that includes anaerobic coverage even if they are not cultured.

E. Splenic abscess is rare, but has high mortality if left untreated. It usually results from hematogenous spread, but can result from splenic trauma or contiguous spread. The diagnosis of splenic abscess should prompt a search for bacterial endocarditis as the source.

    1. Microbiology. The most common organisms isolated on culture are *Streptococcus* spp. followed by *S. aureus. Salmonella* spp. and, rarely, anaerobic bacteria also cause splenic abscess.

    2. Left-upper-quadrant pain, fever, leukocytosis, and a left-sided pleural effusion suggest the diagnosis. A splenic abscess can often be mistaken for splenic infarcts on imaging, which has important therapeutic implications. These can often coexist.

    3. Treatment. Splenic abscess is usually treated with antibiotics and with splenectomy rather than percutaneous drainage. The duration of antibiotic therapy is extended to 4 to 6 weeks when concurrent endocarditis is discovered.

F. *Clostridium difficile*–**Associated Diarrhea (CDAD):** One in every five patients admitted to a US hospital acquires *C. difficile*, a toxigenic sporeforming, gram-positive bacillus, as part of their colonic flora. While only a fraction develop clinical disease, they form a sizable reservoir and contribute to propagation of CDAD. While most cases are acquired in the health care setting, severe CDAD cases acquired in the community are on the rise. One must not rule out CDAD when evaluating a patient with consistent clinical features and an absence of antibiotic and health care exposure. That being said, the commonest modifiable risk factor remains antibiotic exposure, especially clindamycin, fluoroquinolones, broad-spectrum penicillins, and cephalosporins. Advanced age, comorbidities, immune suppression, gastric acid suppression, and health care exposure are other important risk factors. In the recent years, a hypervirulent strain (NAP1) has been implicated in epidemics of severe CDAD in the United States and other parts of the world. Interestingly, the same strain does not typically cause severe disease outside of epidemics. Antibiotics alter the normal flora, providing an environment for the conversion of *C. difficile* spores to vegetative forms leading to rapid replication and toxin production.

1. **Clinical features:** Nosocomial diarrhea (as frequent as 15 bouts of watery stool) occurring more than 3 days after hospitalization in patients that are receiving antibiotics should be assumed to be CDAD until proven otherwise. Other features may include bloody diarrhea, abdominal cramps and tenderness, toxic megacolon, bowel perforation, and peritonitis. Leukocytosis can be marked, sometimes in excess of 50,000 cells/μL.

2. **Diagnosis.** Although the *C. difficile* cytotoxicity assay is still considered the gold standard for diagnosis of CDAD, it is labor intensive, time-consuming, and not practical for wide clinical use. The commercially available enzyme immunoassay (EIA) on liquid/semisolid stool samples for *C. difficile* glutamate dehydrogenase (GDH) is highly sensitive and is a good screening tool. The stool EIA to detect toxin A and toxin B are more specific and used commonly in diagnostic algorithms.

   a. Recently, the role of *C. difficile* PCR on stool samples has expanded across hospitals nationwide. While some solely rely on PCR for its high sensitivity, specificity, and rapid turnover (as early as 1 hour), others consider routine use of *C. difficile* PCR to be cost-prohibitive and restrict its use for confirmation when two EIA tests yield discordant results. As a large proportion of hospitalized individuals are colonized with *C. difficile*, testing on formed stool produces high rates of false-positive results and is discouraged.

   b. CT imaging in fulminant CDAD may show diffuse colonic thickening and pericolic stranding. Flexible sigmoidoscopy with visualization of "pseudomembranes" can be helpful in making the diagnosis if serologic tests are inconclusive or an urgent diagnosis of fulminant disease is warranted.

3. **Treatment.** Timely discontinuation of causative antibiotics is a common therapeutic dictum for *C. difficile*, regardless of severity. Therapeutic options, otherwise, vary with disease severity and frequency. Criteria for severe disease are still based on expert opinion (Cohen, 2010). However, features considered as indicative of severe disease include WBC count >15,000, presence of shock despite fluid resuscitation, severe lactic acidosis, acute kidney injury (Cr >1.5 times premorbid level), and toxic mega colon.

   a. Metronidazole (500 mg oral or IV; 3 times a day) is comparable to oral vancomycin (125 mg every 6 hours) for initial therapy for nonsevere disease. Higher doses of PO vancomycin provided no additional benefit.

   b. Initial recurrences of nonsevere CDAD can be treated with PO vancomycin; although fidaxomicin was shown to lower further recurrences and may be a preferred choice for that reason. Some suggest adjunctive rifaximin for recurrences but evidence is limited to a few case series.

   c. For initial severe CDAD, vancomycin PO 125 mg every 6 hours is the drug of choice. The dose may be pushed to 500 every 6 hours in severe cases. The drug usually concentrates well in the colon; however, in the setting of profound ileus or inability to tolerate PO medication, vancomycin 500 mg 4 times a day may be administered in the form of an enema. Colonic perforation is a rare but serious adverse effect of this route of administration. Treatment is usually continued for 10 to 14 days. Surgical consultation is indicated in patients who have signs of shock or organ failure, or who have not responded to 24 to 72 hours of maximal medical therapy. The surgical treatment of choice is a total abdominal colectomy with an end ileostomy.

   d. Experimental therapies include the nitazoxanide, IV immunoglobulin, and monoclonal antibodies against toxins A and B, but sufficient evidence is lacking. Replenishment of GI flora with probiotics (*Lactobacillus* spp., *Saccharomyces boulardii*) for prevention or treatment of CDAD are also not routinely recommended due to limited data and an increased risk of bloodstream infections, especially in the immune compromised. There is growing evidence to support fecal microbiota (stool) transplants from healthy subjects for recurrent, refractory, or severe CDAD. Attempts are being made at standardization of sample storage, delivery media, and administration protocols that will hopefully allow more robust inferences of efficacy in the near future.

III. SKIN AND SOFT TISSUE INFECTIONS

  A. Postoperative wound infections. Multiple factors influence the development and severity of wound infections. The incidence of postoperative wound infection due to antibiotic-resistant bacteria increases with the length of hospitalization prior to surgery.

    1. Microbiology. Microorganisms often reflect the site of origin and are altered by recent treatment with antibiotics, prolonged preoperative hospitalization, and coexisting diseases. Clean surgical wound infections are most often caused by *S. aureus*, coagulase-negative *Staphylococcus*, and *Streptococcus* spp. Severe wound infections that occur in the first 48 hours after surgery may be caused by Clostridium or group A streptococcus (*Streptococcus pyogenes*). The distributions of microorganisms in contaminated wounds can often reflect the origin of contamination (respiratory, GI, or genitourinary [GU] tract).

    2. Clinical Presentation and Diagnosis. Wound infections vary in severity from superficial infections of the skin and subcutaneous tissues to deep and severe infections involving the underlying fascia and/or muscles. Superficial wound infections are most frequently manifested by erythema, warmth, and swelling. Fever and purulence are variably present. Diagnosis is essentially clinical. Surface wound swabs are not entirely helpful. They may grow skin flora in culture. Deeper sampling (such as during debridement in the OR) provides greater specificity for the offending microorganism.

    3. Prevention. Detection and treatment of infection at other sites, limiting the duration of hospitalization before surgery, proper surgical technique, and proper preoperative scrubbing of the patient and the surgical team are important measures. While recommendations vary for clean procedures that do not involve placement of foreign material, prophylactic antibiotics are routinely administered for clean procedures involving placement of foreign material and for all procedures that enter, or are complicated by spillage from internal organs. Prophylactic antibiotics that can be rapidly infused should be given within the 30 minutes prior to incision, and for clean or clean-contaminated operations should be discontinued within 24 hours of surgery to minimize the risk of colonization with antibiotic-resistant organisms. Antibiotics such as vancomycin and ciprofloxacin require a longer time for infusion and should be started at least 120 minutes prior to incision to ensure that a maximum amount of drug is infused. Longer courses of antibiotics are generally given for contaminated or dirty wounds. Choices of prophylactic antibiotics are guided by site and type of surgery, duration of hospitalization prior to surgery, and recent use of antibiotics. Many institutions have established specific guidelines for prophylactic antibiotics.

B. Treatment
1. Mild superficial wound infections may be treated with removal of sutures or staples and opening of the wound to drain fluid collections.
2. Severe wound infections are usually treated with a combination of parenteral antibiotics and surgical debridement. As stated earlier, cultures of fluid or tissue collected in a sterile fashion should be used to guide antimicrobial therapy. Initial empiric antibiotic coverage will be dictated by the clinical setting. First-generation cephalosporins offer reasonable coverage for uncomplicated postoperative wound infections. Clindamycin is an alternative in patients allergic to β-lactams. Vancomycin, linezolid, daptomycin, or ceftaroline should be reserved for cases where there is a reasonable possibility that the infection is caused by MRSA. Gram-negative coverage should be considered for infections originating in the GI, GU, and respiratory tracts.

C. Necrotizing soft tissue infections: These can be classified on the basis of microbial etiology as polymicrobial (also referred to as Type I) or monomicrobial (Type 2). They are also classified on the basis of the tissue plane involved as necrotizing fasciitis or myonecrosis or both. These life-threatening infections have the propensity to spread rapidly and cause severe systemic toxicity early in the course of infection. The mortality due to necrotizing soft tissue infections approaches 100% in the absence of timely surgical control or if unresectable portions of the body are involved. Timely administration of appropriate antimicrobial therapy, while essential, is not able to arrest the process without debridement due to poor antibiotic delivery to necrotic tissue.
1. **Microbiology**
   a. **Necrotizing fasciitis.** *Streptococcus* spp. are most commonly isolated from wound cultures. Polymicrobial infections with anaerobes, enteric gram-negatives, and *Streptococcus* spp. also occur.
   b. **Myonecrosis.** Clostridial myonecrosis (gas gangrene) is a severe, fulminant skeletal muscle infection caused by *Clostridium* spp. Exotoxins released by bacteria are important in the pathogenesis of clostridial myonecrosis. Nonclostridial myonecrosis is generally polymicrobial due to *Streptococcus* spp., enteric gram-negative rods (*E. coli, K. pneumoniae, Enterobacter* spp., etc.), and anaerobic bacteria.
2. **Diagnosis.** Early features include pain out of proportion to the local external findings and systemic toxicity. Crepitus may be present due to gas in soft tissues.

3. Treatment

a. **Debridement.** Immediate recognition and prompt surgical exploration and debridement are critical. Frequent surveillance of the wound is essential and repeated surgical debridement is often necessary.

b. Antibiotics are chosen on the basis of the presentation and the likely source of infection. Gram stain of intraoperative wound samples can guide initial therapy. Empiric therapy should be broad and include coverage of *Streptococcus* spp. and *Staphylococcus* spp., enteric gram-negative bacteria, and anaerobes. Clindamycin is included in regimens for treatment of suspected exotoxin producing necrotizing soft-tissue infections because it acts as a bacterial protein synthesis inhibitor.

c. The role of hyperbaric oxygen in necrotizing fasciitis and that of intravenous immune globulin in superantigen-mediated toxic shock like syndrome from necrotizing fasciitis are still unclear.

IV. URINARY TRACT INFECTIONS

Urinary tract infections (UTIs) in the ICU either present as the reason for admission in the form of urosepsis from community- or hospital-acquired pathogen or as cystitis/urethritis that develops during the ICU stay among patients with indwelling urinary catheters. They are responsible for 40% of nosocomial infections and cause up to 30% cases of gram-negative bacteremia in hospitalized patients. Fungal UTIs are discussed in Section VIII.

A. **Predisposing Factors:** Indwelling urinary catheters remain the leading cause in the ICU. Other factors include neurologic or structural abnormalities of the urinary tract and nephrolithiasis.

B. **Microbiology:** In most cases, the infection is of the ascending variety. In these cases, the organisms most commonly encountered are gram-negative rods including *E. coli, Klebsiella, Proteus*, and *Enterobacter* spp. or gram-positive cocci like Enterococci and *S. saprophyticus*. *Serratia* and *Pseudomonas* spp. are additional causes of catheter-related infections. Bacteriuria from *S. aureus* should raise suspicion of hematogenous seeding and prompt a search for bacteremia. Contiguous peritoneal infection can predispose to perinephric and renal abscesses. Urethritis can also be caused by *Chlamydia trachomatis, Neisseria gonorrhoeae*, Trichomonas, *Candida* spp., and herpes simplex virus (HSV).

C. **Diagnosis.** Analysis of the urinary sediment for leukocytes in conjunction with urine cultures and clinical features can be useful in distinguishing colonization from true infection. Urinary sediment that contains WBC casts suggests that the infection involves the kidneys or tubules.

D. **Specific UTIs**

1. Cystitis is infection of the bladder characterized by dysuria and frequency, cloudy or bloody urine, and localized tenderness of the urethra and suprapubic regions. More severe symptoms such as high fever, nausea, and vomiting suggest upper urinary tract involvement.

2. Acute pyelonephritis is a pyogenic infection of the renal parenchyma and pelvis. It is characterized by costophrenic angle tenderness, high fevers, shaking chills, nausea, vomiting, and diarrhea. Laboratory analysis reveals leukocytosis, pyuria with leukocyte casts, and occasional hematuria. Bacteria are often visible on Gram stain of unspun urine. Evaluation of the urinary tract should be considered because a significant proportion of pyelonephritis is associated with structural abnormalities. Treatment includes antibiotics and removal or correction of

the source. Complications include papillary necrosis, urinary obstruction causing hydro or pyonephrosis, and frank sepsis/septic shock.

3. Renal and perinephric abscesses are uncommon and usually are due to ascending infection from the bladder and ureters. Major risk factors include nephrolithiasis, structural urinary tract abnormalities, urologic trauma or surgery, and diabetes mellitus. Most abscesses in the urinary tract are usually bacterial but may be caused by *Candida* spp. in some cases. Renal and perinephric abscesses may present nonspecifically with fever, leukocytosis, and pain over the flank, groin, or abdomen). Urine cultures may be negative, particularly if the patient has already received appropriate antibiotics. Diagnosis can be confirmed by abdominal ultrasound or CT scan. Treatment is drainage and antibiotics.

4. Prostatitis is an infrequent infection in the ICU that can occur as a result of bladder catheterization. Symptoms and signs include fevers, chills, dysuria, and an enlarged, tender, and boggy prostate on per rectal examination.

E. **Treatment of UTIs.** Prior to receiving culture results, empiric broad therapy should be initiated that cover likely organisms. Fluoroquinolones or third- or fourth-generation cephalosporins are a reasonable empiric choice for most patients. However, fluoroquinolones should be avoided in patients with recent fluoroquinolone use, admitted from long-term care facilities, or use in institutions with high rates of resistance. Antimicrobial therapy must be tailored to species and susceptibility data when they become available. Duration of treatment is uncertain; however, 7 to 14 days is an accepted range. Often those with resistant organisms are treated for 14 days.

V. **INTRAVASCULAR CATHETER-RELATED INFECTIONS** can be localized to the site of insertion (exit-site infections) or can be systemic (catheter-related bloodstream infections or CRBSI). Important risk factors for CRBSI include total parenteral nutrition (TPN), prolonged central line use, and femoral location. Fever is the most common presenting feature, and localized signs of infection at the insertion site are often absent. Inflamed exit site or unexplained fever among patients with central lines should prompt assessment for CRBSI.

A. **Microbiology.** The most common pathogens are coagulase-negative Staphylococcus (CoNS) followed by *S. aureus*. Since CoNS are also the commonest organisms to contaminate blood cultures, CRBSIs caused by them are often difficult to diagnose. A variety of gram-negative and other gram-positive bacteria are less frequent causes. *Candida* spp. account for close to 10% of CRBSI and are commonly associated with TPN administration.

B. **Management**
1. Depending on the type and extent of infection and microorganism involved, treatment options may range between systemic, topical or no antibiotic therapy, antibiotic lock therapy, and removal of the catheter.
2. Indications for catheter removal:
   a. Septic shock
   b. CRBSI due to *S. aureus, P. aeruginosa, Candida*, or *Mycobacterium* spp.
   c. CRBSI with persistent bacteremia despite 3 days of appropriate antibiotic therapy
3. In general, there is a lower threshold to removing temporary catheters. It is considered safe to insert a new catheter (including peripherally

inserted or tunneled varieties) if blood cultures remain negative 72 hours after catheter removal.

4. The choice of antibiotics is dictated by the clinical situation and culture data. Empiric therapy is often started with vancomycin if there are systemic signs of infection or if preliminary blood culture results indicate gram-positive bacteremia. Sometimes an additional agent is added to cover gram-negatives or *Candida* spp. when suspicion for these is high. Further therapy should be tailored to the specific organism identified.

5. Duration of systemic antibiotics upon removal of catheter: 7 to 10 days (14 days minimum in cases of *S. aureus*). One may wait to start antibiotic therapy in CRBSI where only blood cultures drawn from the line grow a microorganism that is not *S. aureus*, *P. aeruginosa*, or *Candida* spp. Longer duration of antibiotics may be necessary if there is evidence of endocarditis, venous thrombosis, or presence of an implanted device.

6. When central-line salvage is attempted, antibiotics may be administered systemically for 1 to 2 weeks with or without antibiotic lock therapy. The latter strategy targets microorganisms within the biofilm by allowing the antibiotic to dwell within a long-term catheter since removal of these often presents management problems. Isolated exit-site infection may be treated with appropriate topic antimicrobials. However, a 7-day course of targeted systemic antibiotic therapy is recommended if purulence is observed at the exit site.

7. Catheter exchange over a guide wire in response to CRBSI is not routinely recommended. If an exchange is performed and catheter tip cultures are positive, the rewired catheter should be removed and a new line placed at a fresh site. A strong suspicion that the catheter is the source of fever or septic complications should prompt a change in site and, at a minimum, blood cultures.

VI. **INFECTIVE ENDOCARDITIS (IE).** IE is caused by microbial invasion of the endocardium. It most commonly involves the cardiac valves, but can also occur in the septal or mural myocardium. IE is classified on the basis of course, as acute or subacute, or type of valve affected, as native valve (NVE) or prosthetic valve endocarditis (PVE).

PVE that occurs within 2 months of valve replacement (early PVE) results from colonization of the valve by microbes at the time of surgery and most commonly is caused by *Staphylococcus* spp. Late PVE is similar to NVE. Microorganisms gain entry into the bloodstream via direct inoculation during airway, GU, GI, and dental procedures or from an existing focus of infection such as pneumonia or dental abscess.

A. Predisposing factors for IE include IV drug use, previous IE, cicatricial complications of rheumatic heart disease, and congenital heart disease. However, endocarditis can occur in previously normal hearts as well. Intravascular devices such as central venous catheters, pacemaker wires, hemodialysis shunts, and prosthetic valves are additional risk factors.

B. **Microbiology:** IE is most commonly caused by bacteria, but can be caused by fungi, viruses, and rickettsiae.

1. **Gram-positive bacteria.** *Streptococcus* spp. are common, particularly the viridans group (such as *S. sanguis*, *S. mutans*, and *S. intermedius*). *Enterococcus* spp. also causes endocarditis, particularly in elderly patients who have undergone GU procedures. *Staphylococcus* spp., particularly *S. aureus*, is a common cause of NVE in drug users. *S. aureus* endocarditis is usually severe and commonly complicated by inflammatory

damage to valvular and perivalvular structures, myocardial and valve ring abscesses, emboli, and metastatic lesions (e.g., lung, central nervous system [CNS], and splenic abscess). Identification of *Streptococcus bovis* as the causative organism should prompt a workup for a GI source such as colon cancer. Contrary to their reputation as blood culture contaminants, coagulase-negative staphylococci often cause PVE that is accompanied by significant valvular destruction.

2. **Gram-negative bacteria infrequently cause IE.** It is often severe, with an abrupt onset and high mortality. A characteristic NVE affecting structurally abnormal valves is caused by a group of bacteria collectively called HACEK (*Haemophilus, Actinobacillus, Cardiobacterium, Eikenella,* and *Kingella* spp.) and is characterized by a delayed growth in blood cultures, subacute course, large vegetations, and frequent embolic events. *Brucella* spp. is a common cause in areas where it is endemic.

C. **Diagnosis.** A severe systemic illness with high fevers and chills along with a new heart murmur should raise suspicion for acute endocarditis. The subacute variety may be less evident and is difficult to diagnose clinically.

1. Physical examination commonly includes a heart murmur, petechiae, and splinter hemorrhages in the nail beds. More specific but less common findings include retinal hemorrhages (Roth's spots), painful red or purple nodules on digital pads (Osler's nodes), and painless red macules on the palms or soles (Janeway lesions). Often complications may be discovered before IE is diagnosed, such as stroke, osteomyelitis, or metastatic abscesses.

2. **Blood cultures:** Three or more sets of blood cultures should be obtained within the first 24 hours if IE is suspected. Rarely, blood cultures are negative, particularly when IE is due to intracellular organisms such as rickettsiae, anaerobic bacteria, the HACEK group of bacteria, and fungi. Special media may be necessary to isolate the responsible microorganism underscoring the need to inform the laboratory when these pathogens are suspected.

3. Echocardiography is an important tool for diagnosing and managing IE. While transthoracic echocardiography (TTE) is less sensitive than transesophageal echocardiography (TEE) for detecting vegetations, it is a reasonable first choice, especially for NVE in nonobese patients that are not mechanically ventilated. Echocardiography can be used to follow the progression of vegetations and to identify and follow complications such as valvular insufficiency, valve ring or myocardial abscesses, pericardial effusions, and heart failure.

   The Modified Duke Criteria is a helpful guide to make a diagnosis in less obvious cases of IE (Tables 28.1 and 28.2).

D. **Treatment:** Patients with acute IE are often critically ill and in addition to usual supportive care, early empiric antibiotics and prompt management of complications form the cornerstones of treatment of acute IE. Initial blood cultures must be obtained prior to the first dose of antibiotics.

1. **Antibiotics**

   a. **NVE:** Vancomycin is a reasonable empirical choice, as it would cover streptococci, staphylococci, and most strains of enterococci. Gentamicin may be added if streptococci or enterococci are clinically suspected.

   b. **PVE:** Empirical therapy usually includes vancomycin, gentamicin, and either a fourth-generation cephalosporin or a carbapenem. Rifampin is added subsequently when staphylococcal PVE is identified.

| **TABLE 28.1** | **Definition of Infective Endocarditis According to the Proposed Modified Duke Criteria, with Modifications Shown in Boldface** |

Definite infective endocarditis
Pathologic criteria
1. Microorganisms demonstrated by culture or histologic examination of a vegetation, a vegetation that has embolized, or an intracardiac abscess specimen; or
2. Pathologic lesions; vegetation or intracardiac abscess confirmed by histologic examination showing active endocarditis
Clinical criteria[a]
1. Two major criteria; or
2. One major criterion and three minor criteria; or
3. Five minor criteria
Possible infective endocarditis
1. **One major criterion and one minor criterion;** or
2. **Three minor criteria**
Rejected
1. Firm alternate diagnosis explaining evidence of infective endocarditis; or
2. Resolution of infective endocarditis syndrome with antibiotic therapy for >4 d; or
3. No pathologic evidence of infective endocarditis at surgery or autopsy, with antibiotic therapy for >4 d; or
4. Does not meet criteria for possible infective endocarditis, as above

[a]See Table 28.2 for definitions of major and minor criteria.
From Li JS, Sexton DJ, Mick N, et al. Proposed modifications to the Duke criteria for the diagnosis of infective endocarditis. *Clin Infect Dis* 2000;30(4):633–638.

Determinations of minimum inhibitory and bactericidal concentrations (MIC and MBC, respectively) are extremely important in deciding the optimal regimen. Blood cultures should be obtained during therapy to verify clearance of bacteremia. Failure to clear bacteremia may indicate an abscess. The duration of targeted antibiotic therapy depends on microbial strain, MICs, location of IE, and presence of complications. Some cases of right-sided NVE can be successfully treated with 2 weeks of parenteral antibiotics but most other cases must receive 4 to 6 weeks of parenteral therapy.

2. **Surgery.** Most cases of PVE and some cases of NVE required valve replacement or repair. Indications for surgery vary depending on the valve location and include severe and refractory heart failure, acute severe valvular regurgitation or valve obstruction, IE due to fungi or resistant bacteria, and failure to clear bacteremia despite appropriate antibiotic therapy. Surgery also may be indicated for recurrent IE, extension to the myocardium or paravalvular region, two or more embolic events, or prosthetic valve instability or periprosthetic leaks.

E. **Complications of Infective Endocarditis**
   1. **Cardiac**
      a. Valvular insufficiency and heart failure. Heart failure is the most common cause of death in patients with IE.
      b. Myocardial and paravalvular abscess
      c. Heart block may result from extension of a paravalvular abscess.
      d. Obstruction. Rarely, large vegetations (usually caused by fungi) may cause obstruction.
      e. Purulent pericarditis occurs most commonly with IE due to *Staphylococcus* spp.

Definition of Terms Used in the Proposed Modified Duke Criteria for the Diagnosis of Infective Endocarditis (IE), with Modifications Shown in Boldface

Major Criteria

Blood culture positive for IE

Typical microorganisms consistent with IE from two separate blood cultures:

   Viridans streptococci. *Streptococcus bovis,* **HACEK** group, *Staphylococcus aureus;* or

   Community-acquired enterococci, in the absence of a primary focus; or

   Microorganisms consistent with IE from persistently positive blood cultures, defined as follows:

      At least two positive cultures of blood samples drawn >12 h apart; or

      All of three or a majority of ≥4 separate cultures of blood (with first and last sample drawn at least 1 h apart)

Single positive blood culture for Coxiella burnetii or antiphase I IgG antibody titer >1:800

Evidence of endocardial involvement

Echocardiogram positive for IE **(TEE recommended in patients with prosthetic valves, rated at least "possible IE" by clinical criteria, or complicated IE [paravalvular abscess]: TTE as first test in other patients),** defined as follows:

      Oscillating intracardiac mass on valve or supporting structures, in the path of regurgitant jets, or on implanted material in the absence of an alternative anatomic explanation; or

      Abscess; or

      New partial dehiscence of prosthetic valve

New valvular regurgitation (worsening or changing of preexisting murmur not sufficient)

Minor Criteria

Predisposition, predisposing heart condition, or injection drug use

Fever, temperature >38°C

Vascular phenomena, major arterial emboli, septic pulmonary infarcts, mycotic aneurysm, intracranial hemorrhage, conjunctival hemorrhages, and Janeway's lesions

Immunologic phenomena: glomerulonephritis, Osler's nodes, Roth's spots, and rheumatoid factor

Microbiological evidence: positive blood culture but does not meet a major criterion as noted above[a] or serological evidence of active infection with organism consistent with IE

Echocardiographic minor criteria eliminated

---

[a]Excludes single positive cultures for coagulase-negative staphylococci and organisms that do not cause endocarditis.

TEE, transesophageal echocardiography; TTE, transthoracic echocardiography.

From Li JS, Sexton DJ, Mick N, et al. Proposed modifications to the Duke criteria for the diagnosis of infective endocarditis. *Clin Infect Dis* 2000;30(4):633–638.

   2. **Extracardiac**
      a. Immune complex disease such as glomerulonephritis
      b. Embolization causing ischemia and infarction and subsequent abscesses formation is common. Left-sided vegetations can embolize to kidneys, brain, spleen, and heart, while right-sided ones can cause pulmonary embolization.
      c. Mycotic aneurysms complicate bacterial endocarditis and result from focal inflammatory dilatation of a blood vessel. Mycotic

aneurysms are friable and when in the CNS vasculature can result in catastrophic subarachnoid or intracerebral hemorrhage.

    d. Neurologic complications include meningitis, cerebritis, brain abscess, stroke (infarction or hemorrhage), subarachnoid, or intracerebral hemorrhage.

    e. Renal failure

    f. Osteomyelitis

    g. Sepsis

VII. MISCELLANEOUS INFECTIONS

  A. Sinusitis: Sinusitis is a cause of fever in the ICU that is often overlooked. Nosocomial bacterial sinusitis may be encountered in the ICU following trauma or burns involving the facial structures and following prolonged use of nasogastric or nasotracheal tubes. Invasive fungal sinusitis may be seen among patients with prolonged neutropenia or poorly controlled diabetes.

    1. Microbiology. Gram-negative bacteria or *S. aureus* usually causes nosocomial bacterial sinusitis. Common causes of invasive fungal sinusitis (IFS) include *Mucor*, *Rhizopus*, *Aspergillus*, and *Fusarium* spp.

    2. Diagnosis can be difficult. Many experts recommend CT scans of the face and sinuses. Needle aspiration of the sinuses may provide helpful bacteriologic data, particularly in patients who have been hospitalized for prolonged periods and may be infected with antibiotic-resistant organisms.

    3. Treatment is often initiated on the basis of the presence of fever without an alternative etiological explanation, presence of nasal tubes, history of head and neck trauma, and purulent nasal discharge. Treatment includes removal of nasal tubes to allow drainage of the obstructed sinus outflow tract, nasal humidification and decongestants, and antibacterial or antifungal agents that target likely pathogens. Surgical drainage is rarely indicated for nosocomial bacterial sinusitis, but debridement and surgical reduction and restoration of immune function are key components of therapy for IFS.

  B. CNS Infections

    1. Meningitis. Most cases of acute bacterial meningitis (ABM) are admitted to the ICU through the emergency room. A few health care–associated cases may occur after neurosurgical intervention, skull base fractures, and following introduction of hardware in the CNS. The meninges are infected either by contiguous or hematogenous seeding, direct invasion, or extension following rupture of an abscess into the subarachnoid space.

      a. Microbiology. Many organisms cause meningitis. Community-acquired pathogens include *S. pneumoniae, H. influenzae, Neisseria meningitidis*, and *Listeria monocytogenes*. Meningitis caused by enteric and nonenteric gram-negative bacteria and *S. aureus* may result from trauma, neurosurgery, or bacteremia. *S. aureus* meningitis may originate from infections at other sites such as pneumonia, sinusitis, and endocarditis. Meningitis associated with CSF shunts is most often caused by *S. epidermidis.*

      b. Diagnosis. While the classic triad of fever, neck stiffness, and altered mental status is present in less than half of all ABM cases (even less so in meningococcal cases), if none of these is present, ABM can be ruled out with 99% certainty. Stroke, cranial nerve palsies, papilledema, seizures, and, in cases of meningococcal ABM, palpable purpura may be accompanying clinical features. Clinical tests such as Kernig's and Brudzinski's signs, while specific, are highly insensitive. Cerebrospinal fluid must be tested for cell counts, glucose, protein, Gram stain, bacterial culture, AFB smears, and mycobacterial and fungal cultures. Other tests on CSF, including cryptococcal antigen, the Venereal Disease Research Laboratory (VDRL), and herpes simplex virus antigen may be indicated depending on the clinical presentation and host factors. In patients suspected of having cerebral edema, a CT scan of the brain should be performed prior to the lumbar puncture. Blood cultures should be obtained prior to starting antibiotics, although the lumbar puncture must not delay the timely administration of antibiotics. Presence of high opening pressures, low glucose, raised protein, and high WBC count should raise suspicion for ABM.

   c. Treatment. Intravenous antibiotics covering the broad spectrum of expected microbial etiologies must be administered within 1 hour of presentation with suspected ABM. Emergence of penicillin-resistant community-acquired pathogens has resulted in a shift in treatment to third-generation nonantipseudomonal cephalosporins such as ceftriaxone, which penetrates the CNS well. Vancomycin is often added to cover third-generation-cephalosporin-resistant pneumococci and this may be discontinued once susceptibility results rule this out. When meningitis from *Listeria* spp. is a possibility, empiric ABM therapy must include ampicillin (or trimethoprim/sulfamethoxazole in penicillin-allergic patients). An aminoglycoside is usually added to ampicillin for synergy when *Listeria* meningitis is confirmed. If nosocomial pathogens are suspected, in addition to vancomycin to cover MRSA, ceftazidime, cefepime, or meropenem should replace ceftriaxone to cover pseudomonas and other resistant gram-negative bacteria. The recommended duration of treatment of ABM is 2 to 3 weeks. Dexamethasone when administered early (before or at the time of administration of antibiotics) has shown to reduce neurological complications such as hearing loss following pneumococcal meningitis. All cases of suspected ABM should receive dexamethasone initially, but this must only be continued upon microbiological evidence of pneumococcus. Close contacts of patients with meningococcal meningitis must receive chemoprophylaxis with ciprofloxacin or rifampin.

2. **Epidural abscesses:** Most epidural abscesses occur in the vertebral column, and only a few are found to be intracranial. They result from hematogenous seeding, trauma, neurosurgery, epidural catheter placement, or contiguous extension from infected paranasal sinuses and paravertebral spaces. Spinal epidural abscesses are notorious for rapid progression and risk major neurological damage that is usually irreversible without prompt diagnosis, antimicrobial therapy, and drainage of the abscess.

   a. Microbiology. *S. aureus* is the most common cause of epidural abscess. Enteric gram-negatives also cause epidural abscesses, particularly in patients with bacteremia from urosepsis.

   b. Diagnosis. Severe localized spinal pain is the most common presenting symptom of epidural abscess. Magnetic resonance imaging is the diagnostic test of choice for spinal epidural abscesses.

   c. Treatment includes antibiotics and drainage. Empiric therapy is broad spectrum and usually includes vancomycin, third-generation cephalosporin, and metronidazole. Therapy is narrowed on the basis of drainage culture results and generally continued for 6 to 8 weeks, contingent on resolution on interval MRI.

VIII. **FUNGAL INFECTIONS**. Fungi cause a wide spectrum of clinical disease in critically ill patients; the severity and extent of which is highly dependent on host immune factors. They range from minor skin and mucosal involvement to disseminated and invasive disease causing multiorgan failure.

A. **Candida**

1. *Candida* spp. are the most common cause of opportunistic fungal infections in surgical and medical ICUs. The increased incidence of nosocomial candidal infections in the recent years is related to candidal overgrowth following elimination of bacterial flora with increased use of antibacterial agents, higher use of indwelling vascular, urinary and peritoneal catheters, total parenteral nutrition, and an increase in the immune-compromised proportion of hospitalized patients.

2. **Clinical manifestations**

   a. Candiduria due to colonization or infection of the urinary tract are difficult to distinguish. Quantification of candida burden or pyuria is not helpful. Persistent candiduria in asymptomatic individuals may be ignored but further evaluation with an ultrasound or CT is recommended in patients with diabetes mellitus, structural abnormalities of the urinary tract, and, in some cases, renal allograft recipients.

   b. Mucocutaneous infections include oropharyngeal candidiasis, esophagitis, GI candidiasis, vulvovaginitis, and intertrigo.

   c. Candidemia is a serious condition, which may or may not be associated with dissemination to visceral organs such as the eyes, cardiac valves, and indwelling devices, but must be searched for the same. All indwelling urinary and vascular catheters in patients with candidemia should be removed. Depending on need, these may be replaced at new sites.

   d. Disseminated or invasive candidiasis. Deep-organ infections can result from hematogenous spread, by direct extension from contiguous sites, or by local inoculation. Diagnosis can be difficult because blood cultures are frequently negative. Positive superficial cultures (e.g., urine, sputum, wounds) may represent colonization or contamination, and diagnostic serologic tests are not available. A high level of suspicion must be maintained in patients with the risk factors described previously. Definitive criteria for disseminated infection include positive cultures from otherwise sterile sites (e.g., peritoneal fluid), actual invasion (histologically) of burn wounds, and endophthalmitis.

      1. Hepatosplenic candidiasis is a rare entity that almost exclusively occurs in neutropenic patients with hematologic malignancies. This is a difficult diagnosis to make and is suggested by RUQ pain, fevers, and elevated alkaline phosphatase, with or without characteristic findings on CT scan. Diagnosis can be confirmed by liver biopsy.

      2. Candidal peritonitis results from perforation of the intestines or stomach or infection of a peritoneal dialysis catheter.

      3. Cardiac candidiasis includes myocarditis, pericarditis, and endocarditis. Valvular vegetations can be quite large, and major embolic events are common and devastating.

4. Renal candidiasis arises from ascending infection from the bladder, resulting in fungus balls and papillary necrosis, or from hematogenous seeding, in which case bilateral abscesses are usually found.

5. Ocular candidiasis can cause blindness.

6. Other sites of disseminated candidiasis include the CNS and the musculoskeletal system.

3. **Treatment of candidal infections.** The choice of antifungal agent is dependent on candida species, penetration, and concentration at infection site and relative toxicity. *In vitro* susceptibility testing is not as reliable for antifungals as it is for antibacterial agents.

   a. Candiduria is only treated in the presence of neutropenia, involvement of upper tract, or peri-procedurally for interventions on the urinary tract. This can be achieved with a few days of oral fluconazole or IV amphotericin. Amphotericin bladder washes clear candiduria but do not treat cystitis and certainly not upper urinary tract involvement. Echinocandins and lipid formulations of amphotericin do not achieve adequate levels in the urinary tract. Voriconazole and posaconazole have not been sufficiently studied for this indication. Replacement of indwelling urinary catheters is always recommended.

   b. Mucocutaneous candidiasis is initially treated with a topical agent such as nystatin, clotrimazole, or miconazole. Systemic therapy with oral fluconazole may be indicated when patients do not respond to topical therapy or in cases where mucosal involvement is deep and not easily accessible.

   c. Candidemia is treated with systemic antifungal therapy. All blood isolates should be treated and not considered contaminants. Venous and arterial catheters should be replaced at new sites. Tunneled central venous lines may be preserved in the setting of uncomplicated infection unless there is failure to clear fungemia with antifungal agents. Nonneutropenic patients that are clinically well may be treated with fluconazole or echinocandins (caspofungin, micafungin, or anidulafungin). Neutropenic patients are usually treated with liposomal amphotericin or an echinocandin. *Candida glabrata* and *Candida krusei* are often resistant to fluconazole.

   d. Disseminated candidiasis requires a combination of systemic antifungal therapy, drainage or debridement of infected areas, removal of intravascular catheters, and sometimes removal and replacement of infected valves and other foreign bodies. Although there is general consensus that *Candida* spp. grown from the peritoneal cavity (i.e., not just peritoneal drains) should be treated, opinions differ with respect to whether amphotericin, echinocandins (caspofungin and micafungin), or fluconazole should be used. The same is true for hepatosplenic candidiasis. Lack of response to fluconazole is an indication to change the antifungal coverage. Chorioretinitis is treated with systemic therapy alone but may need to be supplanted with intravitreal antifungal therapy and sometimes vitrectomy in the presence of significant vitreal involvement.

B. Aspergillus-related illness in the ICU is encountered in invasive (usually pulmonary or sinus) or disseminated forms in the immune compromised. Angioinvasion and hemorrhage in cavitatory disease are important causes of major hemoptysis that require ICU support. Distinguishing colonization, indolent infection, and invasive aspergillosis (IA) can be difficult. Sputum cultures are neither sensitive nor specific for invasive aspergillosis. Histopathology or a combination of radiological, culture, and serum or BAL galactomannan assay is needed to establish a high probability of invasive disease.

1. **Clinical manifestations**
   a. Invasive pulmonary disease presents with fever and pulmonary infiltrates in an immune-compromised host. Pathologic analysis reveals infarction and hemorrhage and direct invasion of vessel walls by acute angle (45°) branching septate hyphae.
   b. Dissemination to a variety of organs occurs due to vascular invasion and is associated with a very poor prognosis. Abscesses occur in the CNS, lung, liver, and myocardium. Budd-Chiari syndrome and myocardial infarction may occur.
   c. **Other pulmonary manifestations**
      1. Aspergillomas are fungus balls that occur in cavities usually in the upper lobes of the lungs, especially in bullae and occasionally in preexisting cavities. Patients present with cough, hemoptysis (which can be life threatening), fever, and dyspnea.
      2. Allergic bronchopulmonary aspergillosis causes episodic bronchospasm and usually occurs in patients with chronic asthma or cystic fibrosis. Radiographic findings range from segmental infiltrates to transient nonsegmental infiltrates. Eosinophilia may be present in the sputum and blood.

2. **Treatment of aspergillosis**
   a. **Voriconazole** is the treatment of choice in confirmed invasive aspergillosis. In cases with intolerance to or failure of voriconazole, it may be replaced with liposomal amphotericin or an echinocandin. Data favoring voriconazole plus an echinocandin as potential first-line combination therapy are emerging but have not made it to guidelines yet. Although *A. fumigatus* is the commonest species identified in cases of IA, *A. terreus* is less susceptible to amphotericin. Radiologic embolization may be necessary for cases of IA with massive hemoptysis. Surgical resection may be indicated in such cases when embolization fails or upon failure of systemic antifungal therapy in other cases of IA.
   b. **Localized pulmonary manifestations**
      1. **Aspergilloma**. Asymptomatic cases in immune-competent patients may be observed. Antifungal therapy is not usually adequate for eradication, and surgical excision is indicated in patients with recurrent hemoptysis.
      2. **Allergic bronchopulmonary aspergillosis**. Systemic glucocorticoids (aerosolized steroids are not of benefit) are the mainstay of therapy and are usually administered as a taper during flares. Concomitant antifungal therapy with itraconazole or voriconazole has been found to improve outcomes and reduce the amount of steroid required.

IX. VIRAL INFECTIONS

A. **Cytomegalovirus** (CMV) infection and disease are not synonymous. Infection only requires serological evidence, and disease usually requires histopathological evidence of inclusion bodies or immunohistochemical evidence of CMV in an end organ. CMV infection can either be primary infection or more frequently secondary, either as reactivation or infection with a new strain of CMV. Reactivation is common in critically ill patients, but the significance of the same is not clearly defined. CMV infection is common in immunocompromised patients and in fact the commonest infection among solid-organ and hematopoietic cell-transplant recipients. Among immunocompetent hosts, CMV infection is usually asymptomatic or produces a self-limiting mononucleosis-like syndrome. Diagnosis of CMV infection requires detection of CMV antigen, high viral DNA, or an increase in the same. Diagnosis of CMV disease usually requires evidence of cytopathogenic effect (characteristic inclusion bodies) in infected tissue or high titres of viral DNA in CSF or in bronchoalveolar lavage of lung-transplant recipients. Quantitative cultures, however, are not helpful.

1. Manifestations of CMV disease in immune-compromised patients:
   a. Pneumonitis
   b. Hepatitis
   c. Colitis
   d. Retinitis and CNS involvement
2. **Treatment.** CMV infection (viremia) in organ and hematopoietic cell–transplant patients is preemptively treated with oral valganciclovir or IV ganciclovir to prevent transformation to CMV disease, which can be devastating in this population. Ganciclovir is the treatment of choice for CMV disease in organ-transplant recipients. Foscarnet is used in cases of intolerance or resistance to ganciclovir. Life-threatening CMV infection (such as CMV pneumonitis) may be treated with the combination of ganciclovir and high-dose IV CMV immunoglobulin. CMV immunoglobulin may also be used as prophylaxis of CMV disease in CMV+ organ transplanted into CMV- recipients. Ganciclovir and foscarnet are both used to treat CMV retinitis in AIDS patients. Neutropenia is a common adverse effect of ganciclovir, and renal failure can occur with use of foscarnet.

B. Herpes Simplex Virus (HSV) I and II
1. Manifestations of HSV infection include the following:
   a. Mucocutaneous and genital disease
   b. Respiratory tract infection
      1. Tracheobronchitis
      2. HSV pneumonia generally occurring in immune-compromised patients
   c. Ocular infection such as blepharitis, conjunctivitis, keratitis, corneal ulceration, and blindness
   d. Esophagitis
   e. Encephalitis and meningitis
2. Disseminated HSV usually occurs in patients who are highly immune compromised. Manifestations include necrotizing hepatitis, pneumonitis, cutaneous lesions from hematogenous spread, fever, hypotension, disseminated intravascular coagulation, and CNS involvement.
3. **Diagnosis.** Tzanck smear of material scraped from lesions is insensitive and cannot distinguish between HSV and varicella zoster virus (VZV) infection. Viral culture, histologic examination of tissue or skin biopsy, and DNA or immunostaining of viral antigens are other diagnostic tests. Herpes simplex virus DNA testing on CSF helps rule out HSV encephalitis.
4. **Treatment**
   a. Severe HSV infections, including encephalitis, pneumonitis, and disseminated HSV, are treated with IV acyclovir. Foscarnet may be used to treat acyclovir-resistant HSV.

   b. Mucosal, cutaneous, and genital infections may be treated with acyclovir, famciclovir, or valacyclovir. Although normal hosts do not always require treatment, consideration should be given to treating critically ill or debilitated patients even if they do not fit classic criteria for immune compromise.

   c. Ocular infection may be treated with topical agents such as acyclovir and should be managed in consultation with an ophthalmologist.

C. Varicella zoster virus (VZV) infection may be encountered in the ICU as a primary infection (chicken pox) or reactivation infection (herpes zoster or shingles) and can cause mild to life-threatening disease.

   1. Primary VZV infection in adults may have severe systemic effects and pulmonary involvement that causes respiratory failure. Immune-compromised patients are prone to severe systemic disease with involvement of lungs, kidneys, CNS, and liver.

   2. Herpes zoster usually manifests as a dermatomal cutaneous infection from reactivation of VZV that has been dormant in the sensory ganglia. The same can be multidermatomal and cross the midline in severely immune-compromised patients (e.g., AIDS). Rarely, reactivated herpes zoster causes CNS disease such as encephalitis and cerebral vasculitis.

   3. Treatment. IV acyclovir is used for serious VZV infection (pneumonia, encephalitis) in immunocompromised or immunocompetent hosts. The role of adjunctive steroids in these cases is unclear.

D. Severe Influenza: Influenza A and B viruses are responsible for a spectrum of respiratory illnesses that manifest as large pandemics or seasonal outbreaks, especially in the winter months. Major rearrangements of genetic material (that code for hemagglutinin and neuraminidase) that may or may not include gene components from other species (e.g., poultry, swine) are called antigenic shifts. These are responsible for pandemics, while minor rearrangements are called antigenic drifts, which can cause local outbreaks. The earliest evidence of a pandemic from influenza based on retrospective serological assessments dates back to 1898. The major pandemic in 1918 to 1919 due to an H1N1 strain claimed 5% of the world's population. Nearly a century later in 2009, a human–swine–avian reassortant H1N1 strain caused the most recent pandemic. Several seasonal outbreaks have also occurred due to a variety of strains over the last century, the epidemiology of which is beyond the scope of this chapter.

   1. In the ICU, a high suspicion for severe influenza is raised in all cases of acute respiratory failure in the right seasonal or pandemic setting; although sporadic cases may be rarely seen all year round. The virus can cause a primary viral pneumonia with a high incidence of ARDS or be complicated by severe secondary bacterial CAP. Contrary to popular belief, *S. pneumoniae* is still the commonest cause of postinfluenza CAP, but in the recent years there has been a rise in the proportion of cases due to community-acquired *S. aureus.* Nonpulmonary manifestations are rare and include encephalitis, transverse myelitis, Guillain-Barré Syndrome, rhabdomyolysis, and myopericarditis.

   2. The factors associated with a high risk of complications from influenza among adults as reported by the CDC include the following:

   a. Age 65 years and older
   b. Pregnancy
   c. Asthma
   d. Heart disease
   e. Stroke
   f. Diabetes

    g. HIV/AIDS

    h. Cancer

3. **Diagnosis:** Rapid antigen detection in nasal smears using enzyme-linked immune assay (EIA) has a low sensitivity but costs less and is an acceptable initial screening modality. They cannot be used to rule out disease. Detection is higher in peak season and when there is high clinical probability. Immunofluorescence testing has a higher sensitivity but with RT-PCR is the highest and is coupled with very high specificity as well and must be used for diagnosis whenever possible.

4. **Treatment:** The general principles of treatment of acute respiratory failure and ARDS apply here. Please refer to Chapter 19 for the management of ARDS.

    a. Antiviral therapy: While in nonsevere cases, the recommendation is to only start antiviral therapy in cases that present within 48 hours of symptom onset, for severe and complicated cases (ICU patients) of confirmed or suspected influenza, antiviral therapy should be instituted regardless of duration of symptoms.

    b. Oral oseltamivir 75 mg twice a day or inhaled zanamivir 10 mg twice a day are the regimens of choice. Duration of treatment is typically 5 days but can be extended in severely ill and immune-compromised patients. Recently, oseltamivir-resistant cases of the H1N1 variety have emerged that can be treated with IV zanamivir, which can be obtained on a compassionate basis.

X. MISCELLANEOUS INFECTIONS

A. Drug-Resistant Bacterial Infections: This crisis has predominantly emanated from our own practices of widespread global and, until recently, unchecked use of antimicrobial agents. Drug-resistance is on the rise among both gram-positive and gram-negative bacteria. Depending on the organism and methods used, isolates are usually categorized on the basis of susceptibility to certain key antimicrobial agents based on certain prespecified cutoffs of minimum inhibitory concentration (MIC) or disk-diffusion diameters and sometimes molecular testing that identifies genes that code for enzymes that confer resistance (e.g., carbapenemase). Descriptions of mechanisms of resistance or details of resistance testing are beyond the scope of this chapter.

    The clinically relevant drug-resistant bacterial isolates encountered in the ICU may include MRSA, vancomycin-intermediate *S. aureus* (VISA), vancomycin-resistant *S. aureus* (VRSA), and vancomycin-resistant enterococci (VRE) among gram-positive isolates and extended-spectrum β-lactamase (ESBL)–producing *Enterobacteriaceae*, and carbapenem-resistant gram-negative infections. The latter is thought to be the most serious threat to ICUs today and is described in further detail below.

1. **Carbapenem-Resistant Gram-Negative (CRGN) Infections:** These infections have emerged in the last decade. Carbapenems are broad-spectrum β-lactam agents, and resistance to these is usually due to carbapenem-hydrolyzing β-lactamase enzymes, also called *carbapenemases*. Carbapenem-resistance (CR) is usually coupled with resistance to lower classes of gram-negative active agents conferring either multidrug-resistance (MDR; nonsusceptible to at least one agent in three or more antimicrobial categories), extensively drug-resistance (XDR; nonsusceptible to at least one agent limited to all but two or fewer antimicrobial categories), or, much to everyone's horror, pan drug-resistance (PDR, nonsusceptible to all agents in all antimicrobial categories)

(Lim, 2003), leaving very few or no therapeutic options, respectively. Moreover, the gram-negative active antimicrobial pipeline is slim and highly effective agents are not expected in the immediate future. Incidence continues to rise, posing a major public health-threat to ICUs worldwide.

a. The organisms most commonly encountered as carbapenem-resistant include carbapenem-resistant *Enterobacteriaceae (CRE)*, the commonest of which is *Klebsiella pneumoniae* carbapenemase-producing *Klebsiella pneumoniae (KPC-Kp)*. The *KPC* gene can be horizontally transferred via plasmids among other Enterobacteriaceae and even *Pseudomonas* and *Acinetobacter* spp. The New Delhi Metallo-beta-lactamase-1 (NDM-1) is another popular carbapenem-hydrolyzing enzyme that confers multidrug resistance and has been identified in a few returning travelers and immigrants from South Asia (India, Pakistan).

b. Until recently, the Modified Hodge Test (MHT) was used at many centers to detect the presence of carbapenemases on an agar plate by specific inhibition around an imipenem disc. However, the test is poorly sensitive and some cases with the KPC or *metallo-beta-lactamase* gene are found to be MHT negative. Most laboratories now use automated systems dilution, and some use genotypic testing using PCR.

c. Treatment: The presence of carbapenem-resistance in a cultured isolate may not be known until 3 days or longer after the culture is drawn and critically ill patients with severe sepsis and septic shock may not receive appropriate empiric therapy as agents active against CR organisms are not part of routine empiric therapy, even for septic shock. The agents that are usually effective against CRGN organisms usually carry a risk of significant systemic toxicity. These include IV Colistin, Polymixin-B, Tigecycline, and in some cases aminoglycosides, and it may be reasonable to add these agents to a patient with presumed septic shock that is decompensating despite hours of routine empiric agents and source control. Antibiotic choices must be based on susceptibility results and one may have to request additional susceptibility testing against agents like colistin, fosfomycin, and tigecycline. For targeted therapy, there is some evidence that combination therapy with two or more of these agents may be preferred, but this could increase the risk of toxicity. The comparative effectiveness of various therapeutic modalities against CRGN infections has not yet been evaluated in head-to-head randomized controlled trials. The role of inhaled antibiotics such as colistin or aminoglycosides for CR respiratory infections is being explored as a means to avoid nephrotoxicity.

B. Bioterror Agents: These represent a group of bacterial and viral pathogens that can cause life-threatening syndromes in large populations. Known or suspected agents that cause acute pneumonias in this category include inhalational anthrax, tularemia pneumonia, and pneumonic plague.

Selected Readings

American Thoracic Society; Infectious Diseases Society of America. Guidelines for the management of adults with hospital-acquired, ventilator-associated, and healthcare-associated pneumonia. *Am J Respir Crit Care Med* 2005;171(4):388–416.

Bratzler DW, Dellinger EP, Olsen KM, et al. Clinical practice guidelines for antimicrobial prophylaxis in surgery. *Am J Health Syst Pharm* 2013;70(3):195–283.

Centers for Disease Control and Prevention (CDC). Prevention and control of seasonal influenza with vaccines. Recommendations of the Advisory Committee on Immunization Practices—United States, 2013–2014. *MMWR Recomm Rep* 2013;62(RR-07):1–43.

Cohen SH, Gerding DN, Johnson S, et al. Clinical practice guidelines for *Clostridium difficile* infection in adults: 2010 update by the Society for Healthcare Epidemiology of America (SHEA) and the Infectious Diseases Society of America (IDSA). *Infect Control Hosp Epidemiol* 2010;31(5):431–455.

Klompas M. Complications of mechanical ventilation—the CDC's new surveillance paradigm. *N Engl J Med* 2013;368(16):1472–1475.

Li JS, Sexton DJ, Mick N, et al. Proposed modifications to the Duke criteria for the diagnosis of infective endocarditis. *Clin Infect Dis* 2000;30(4):633–638.

Lim WS, van der Eerden MM, Laing R, et al. Defining community acquired pneumonia severity on presentation to hospital: an international derivation and validation study. *Thorax* 2003;58(5):377–382.

Magiorakos AP, Srinivasan A, Carey RB, et al. Multidrug-resistant, extensively drug-resistant and pandrug-resistant bacteria: an international expert proposal for interim standard definitions for acquired resistance. *Clin Microbiol Infect* 2012;18(3):268–281.

Solomkin JS, Mazuski JE, Bradley JS, et al. Diagnosis and management of complicated intra-abdominal infection in adults and children: guidelines by the Surgical Infection Society and the Infectious Diseases Society of America. *Clin Infect Dis* 2010;50(2):133–164.

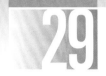

Advances and Challenges in Sepsis

Aranya Bagchi and J. Perren Cobb

Sepsis and its complications continue to impose a significant public heath burden in terms of their high morbidity and mortality, reduced quality of life in survivors, and overall financial burden to the health care system. Although the last 15 years have been characterized by significant progress in combating sepsis, many challenges remain. Notwithstanding the significant advances in sepsis biology over the last three decades, major impediments to improving the care of patients with sepsis include (1) a relatively poor understanding of the pathophysiology of sepsis, (2) lack of accurate diagnostics, and (3) the failure of all studies to date to identify a therapeutic molecular target. This chapter focuses on the state of the art in the clinical management of sepsis and its complications, while also highlighting innovative diagnostic and therapeutic approaches to this complex problem.

I. **DEFINITIONS:** Sepsis traditionally has been defined as the host's systemic response to an infection or, as defined by the International Sepsis Forum (2010), is "a life-threatening condition that arises when the body's response to an infection injures its own tissues and organs." In 1991, a North American consensus conference introduced criteria for sepsis phenotypes, including systemic inflammatory response syndrome (SIRS), sepsis, severe sepsis, septic shock, and multiple organ dysfunction syndrome that continue to be used today (Table 29.1). A second consensus conference in 2001 attempted to improve upon these definitions, but without notable success, and the 1991 definitions continue to be used by most clinicians. These definitions have a number of drawbacks. They are extremely sensitive (a common viral illness would satisfy the definition of sepsis if it causes fever and tachycardia), a "host response" is one of the characteristics of any infection (the absence of a host response in an immunocompetent individual suggests colonization, not infection) and these definitions do not clarify the role of infection in the pathogenesis of SIRS, since sterile inflammation (such as trauma, acute pancreatitis, burns, etc.) can present with clinical features identical to severe sepsis. In fact, the use of two or more SIRS criteria to define severe sepsis in a recent study failed to identify one in eight otherwise similar patients and failed to define a transition point in the risk of death (mortality increased linearly with each additional SIRS criterion).

II. **EPIDEMIOLOGY:** Recent data suggest that the incidence of sepsis and the number of sepsis-related deaths are increasing, although the overall mortality rate among patients with sepsis is declining. The declining mortality rate is related, at least in part, to increased awareness and early effective management of patients with sepsis, but may also reflect an increase in the overall number of reported cases of sepsis with the inclusion of more patients with less severe disease. While the precise incidence of sepsis in the United States is unclear, studies suggest a steady increase in incidence (between 8.7% and 13% per year) over the last few decades. As mentioned above, in-hospital

TABLE 29.1	1991 ACCP/SCCM Consensus Definitions of Sepsis and Its Complications

Infection: Microbial phenomenon characterized by an inflammatory response to the presence of microorganisms or the invasion of normally sterile host tissue by those organisms

Bacteremia: The presence of viable bacteria in the blood

Systemic inflammatory response syndrome: The systemic inflammatory response to a variety of severe clinical insults. The response is manifested by two or more of the following conditions:

Temperature $>38°C$ or $<36°C$

Heart rate >90 beats/min

Respiratory rate >20 breaths/min or $Paco_2$ <32 torr (<4.3 kPa)

WBC $>12,000$ cells/mm^3, $<4,000$ cells/mm^3, or $>10\%$ immature (band) forms

Sepsis: Systemic inflammatory response syndrome caused by a suspected or proven infection. This systemic response is manifested by two or more of the following conditions as a result of infection:

Temperature $>38°C$ or $<36°C$

Heart rate >90 beats/min

Respiratory rate >20 breaths/min or $Paco_2$ <32 torr (<4.3 kPa)

WBC $>12,000$ cells/mm^3, $<4,000$ cells/mm^3, or $>10\%$ immature (band) forms

Severe sepsis: Sepsis associated with organ dysfunction, hypoperfusion, or hypotension. Hypoperfusion and perfusion abnormalities may include, but are not limited to, lactic acidosis, oliguria, or an acute alteration in mental status

Septic shock: Sepsis with hypotension, despite adequate fluid resuscitation, along with the presence of perfusion abnormalities that may include, but are not limited to, lactic acidosis, oliguria, or an acute alteration in mental status. Patients who are on inotropic or vasopressor agents may not be hypotensive at the time that perfusion abnormalities are measured

Hypotension: A systolic BP of <90 mmHg or a reduction of >40 mmHg from baseline in the absence of other causes for hypotension

Multiple organ dysfunction syndrome: Presence of altered organ function in an acutely ill patient such that homeostasis cannot be maintained without intervention

Adapted from Bone RC, Balk RA, Cerra FB, et al. American College of Chest Physicians/Society of Critical Care Medicine Consensus Conference: definitions for sepsis and organ failure and guidelines for the use of innovative therapies in sepsis. *Crit Care Med* 1992;20:864–74, with permission.

mortality has declined (from 35% in 2004 to 26% in 2009), although patients with severe sepsis and septic shock have significantly higher mortality rates. Estimates of the economic impact of sepsis on the U.S. health care system range from $17 to $26 billion per year.

III. PATHOPHYSIOLOGY

A. Host–Pathogen–Microbiome–Hospital Interactions: Humans harbor an extraordinarily diverse microbial ecosystem that has coevolved with our species and that has increasingly being recognized as essential for health. This "extended genome" of millions of microbial genes is referred to as the microbiome. As we learn more about the microbiome, it is becoming evident that pathogenic bacteria, physiologic derangements associated with critical illness, as well as therapeutic agents common to health care environments (such as antibiotics) can all significantly influence the microbiome, with important consequences for critical illness. For example, alterations in the composition and function of the gut microbiome (e.g., increasing colonization of *C. difficile*) may influence the course of critical illness and validate the decade-old hypothesis that "the gut is the driver of multiple organ dysfunction." In addition to genetic factors, age, comorbid medical conditions, and current medications may substantially affect the severity of illness (e.g., gut decontamination contributing to multidrug-resistant organisms). While host genetic diversity and gene–environment interactions are no doubt critical to the sepsis response, we should not underestimate the impact of the health care environment. Infection control measures (including measures as simple as hand hygiene) have been shown to dramatically impact infectious disease transmission rates within health care environments and can achieve lasting improvement in patient outcomes. Sometimes, the best defense against complex diseases is to rigorously enforce simple practices that reduce the likelihood of initiating the infectious–inflammatory cascade.

B. **Initiation of the Acute Inflammatory Response:**
   1. **PAMPs and DAMPs: Pathogen-associated molecular patterns (PAMPs)** refer to evolutionarily conserved components of microorganisms that are recognized by the host innate immune system, such as **lipopolysaccharide (LPS,** or **endotoxin)** that is a component of the cell membranes of gram-negative bacteria. Gram-positive and gram-negative bacteria, fungi, viruses, and protozoa have multiple PAMPs that come into contact with the host immune system and initiate a "preprogrammed" inflammatory response. Likewise, tissue or cellular damage provokes the release of endogenous molecules (such as **mitochondrial DNA** or **High Mobility Group Box 1 [HMGB1]** protein) that are also highly effective at binding to molecular patterns that trigger an innate immune response. These molecules are known as **damage-associated molecular patterns (DAMPs)** or **alarmins.** The fact that multiple pathogens, as well as sterile tissue injury, can activate a strikingly similar immune response partly accounts for the fact that the initial presentation of severe sepsis as well as severe noninfectious insults produces similar clinical manifestations (a.k.a., SIRS).
   2. **The host innate immune system:** The last two decades have seen an explosion in our understanding of the innate immune system. Unlike the adaptive immune system, the innate immune system does not require prior exposure to a pathogen to be able to respond to it. The innate immune system consists principally of four receptor systems: the **toll-like receptors** (TLRs), **C-type lectin receptors, retinoic acid inducible gene-1-like receptors,** and **nucleotide-binding oligomerization domain–like receptors** (NLRs). A diverse group of cells express these receptors, including macrophages, neutrophils, epithelial cells, and endothelial cells, making these cells the "first responders" of the immune system. The innate immune system also has extensive cross talk with the acquired immune system and plays a critical role in modulating the adaptive immune system's more specific response to the pathogens.
   3. **Effector molecules:** Activation of the host response results in the production of multiple species of molecules such as cytokines, proteases, reactive oxygen species, complement products, and altered coagulation proteases. Depending on the specific molecules and the temporal sequence of their production, the host may experience what has been called a hyperinflammatory SIRS response or a hypoinflammatory

CARS (compensatory anti-inflammatory response syndrome) phenotype. For many years, the prevailing view was that the initial sepsis response was hyperinflammatory, followed by a period of immune suppression (hypoinflammation), the so-called "two-hit" phenomenon. However, recent data have shown that severe sepsis and trauma induce a so-called "genomic storm" that affects about 80% of the leukocyte transcriptome. In this situation, pro- and anti-inflammatory genes are activated simultaneously rather than sequentially and differences in syndrome severity are associated not with the relative balance of "hyper" versus "hypo" responses, but rather the magnitude of the abnormality and length of time to return to genomic homeostasis.

4. **End-organ damage:** An intriguing fact about severe sepsis and septic shock is the discordance between the severity of organ dysfunction and relatively minor cell death seen in autopsy studies. This suggests a level of functional rather than irreversible structural injury. Common findings seen in patients with severe sepsis/septic shock include activation of the coagulation cascade with deposition of microvascular thrombi, loss of endothelial barrier function (the "leaky capillaries" of sepsis) resulting in excess extravascular fluid, and mitochondrial damage, resulting in ineffective oxygen utilization at the cellular level. The aggregate result of these changes is nonspecific organ dysfunction—the cells are alive but dysfunctional—often culminating in multiple organ dysfunction syndromes or MODS.

C. **Clinical Features:** The manifestations of severe sepsis and septic shock can vary considerably depending on host and pathogen characteristics, site of infection, and time to appropriate treatment. Early signs include tachycardia, hyperventilation, fever, and disorientation/delirium. Later signs reflect the degree of organ system impairment. While earlier literature emphasized "warm" and "cold" shock phases (early and late, respectively), it appears that most appropriately resuscitated patients with septic shock have features consistent with a distributive shock (high cardiac output, low systemic vascular resistance). Of note, recent literature suggests that cardiac diastolic dysfunction is more common in severe sepsis than systolic dysfunction and is associated with a worse outcome. Unsurprisingly, the degree of organ failure is closely tied to mortality in severe sepsis.

IV. DIAGNOSIS AND MANAGEMENT

A. **Diagnosis:** Conventional culture-based systems for the detection of bacteremia or fungemia remain the gold standard but are not sensitive. Blood cultures are positive in only 30% to 40% of patients with septic shock. Ninety percent of positive blood cultures are detected with 24 hours of incubation, 95% after 48 hours, and 99% after 72 hours. As immediate, appropriate antimicrobial therapy in patients with a new diagnosis of sepsis is associated with improved survival, more rapid identification of bacteremia or fungemia using molecular techniques has the potential to improve outcomes significantly by identification of specific pathogens and antibiotic susceptibility patterns. Current techniques employ genomic testing (typically some form of polymerase chain reaction, or PCR) or proteomic methods (mass spectrometric methods, used for the identification of organisms growing from conventional culture techniques). Genomic methods hold promise for rapid detection of pathogens directly from blood, potentially decreasing detection times to a few hours. However, there remain issues with suboptimum sensitivities and specificities for many molecular assays, and they are not yet in general clinical use.

B. Biomarkers: The search for biomarkers that discriminate between inflammation and infection has been a major goal of translational sepsis research. An ideal sepsis biomarker would be a molecule that has fast kinetics, is highly sensitive and specific for sepsis, has a short turnaround time, and is inexpensive. Given the complexity of the sepsis syndrome and its poorly defined phenotype, it seems unrealistic to expect a single biomarker to be useful in all cases of sepsis (and indeed, these types of studies have largely proven negative). It is our expectation that systems biology approaches (the "Omics") will eventually lead to identification of a suite of informative biomarkers that in turn generate a "biomarker score" analogous to an APACHE score. Proving this hypothesis, however, has been difficult. Currently, the biomarker used most widely is procalcitonin to guide discontinuation of antibiotic therapy for bacterial disease (e.g., community-acquired pneumonia). Even here, the recommendation is weak with low-quality evidence behind it (see Surviving Sepsis Campaign, below).

C. Treatment: In 2002, the Society of Critical Care Medicine, the International Sepsis Forum, and The European Society of Intensive Care Medicine started the **Surviving Sepsis Campaign** (SSC) to improve the diagnosis, treatment, and outcomes of sepsis. A recent review of hospital mortality data from over 200 hospitals in three continents showed that compliance with the SSC "bundles" was associated with improved patient outcomes. The three foundations are fluid resuscitation; early, appropriate antibiotic therapy; and elimination ("control") of the septic source. The recommendations given here follow the latest, 2012 iteration of the SSC guidelines, modified by the authors to take into account more recent evidence.

1. **Initial resuscitation:** The landmark Early Goal-Directed Therapy (EGDT) trial established the importance of early, aggressive, and protocolized resuscitation in the management of patients with severe sepsis. While the principles underlying EGDT remain valid (i.e., resuscitate patients in septic shock), a number of recent trials have cast doubts on the specific metrics derived from the EGDT trial (i.e., the use of CVP, $Scvo_2$, and lactate levels as endpoints) and the use of blood transfusions and dobutamine to increase $Scvo_2$. The recent **ARISE, ProCESS,** and **ProMISE** trials each demonstrated that "usual care" or nonprotocolized care is equivalent to EGDT-derived protocols. One caveat is that the baseline mortality in these later trials was significantly lower than in the original EGDT trial and that a substantial percentage of patients in each of the three recent trials did get central lines, arterial lines, and required vasopressor agents as promulgated by EGDT. The new trials support an aggressive, individualized approach to the initial resuscitation of patients with septic shock without being dogmatically tied to specific end points. The SSC guidelines have been recently modified, taking the above trials into account. At our institution, it is typical practice to use a combination of focused bedside ultrasonography, base deficit, and lactate while addressing the adequacy of fluid resuscitation and to interpret the information in the context of the clinical situation rather than aim for fixed numbers.

2. **Cultures and broad-spectrum antibiotics:** The use of effective intravenous antimicrobial treatment within an hour of the recognition of septic shock remains one of the cornerstones in the management of these patients. Typical empiric therapy often begins using a combination of

antibiotics that can be expected to be active against all likely pathogens in a specific clinical situation. Adequate dosing is as important as prompt initiation of antibiotics, particularly for frequently underdosed antibiotics such as vancomycin. A number of studies have shown that every hour of delay in the appropriate initiation of antibiotics increases the risk of death in patients with septic shock. Blood and other relevant cultures form the bedrock of the diagnosis of sepsis. Cultures should be drawn prior to starting antibiotics whenever possible but should not delay initiation of antibiotic therapy.

3. **Source control:** If a *nidus* of infection is identified, surgical or percutaneous intervention should be considered as soon as possible. The choice of intervention is based on patient stability, resources available, and the source of the infection and should target the least invasive option that will provide adequate source control (e.g., choosing percutaneous drainage for intra-abdominal abscess when possible rather than open surgery).

4. **Hemodynamic support:**
   a. **Fluids:**
      1. **Volume:** We prefer **not** to give a predetermined amount of fluid, but to titrate volume resuscitation with fluid boluses of 250 to 1,000 mL, followed by frequent reassessment of volume status (often using point-of-care ultrasound). Since no assessment method of volume status is foolproof, we often combine information from two or more complementary methods (such as bedside echocardiography and a passive leg raise test) to determine ongoing fluid requirements. Recent data suggest an association between increasingly positive fluid balance and mortality, further underlining the need to individualize fluid therapy.
      2. **Type of fluid: Crystalloids** are the initial fluids of choice in most patients. Of note, **Chloride**-containing fluids (such as **normal saline**) may be associated with worse renal function, and perhaps worse mortality. Large volume resuscitation with normal saline also causes a hyperchloremic acidosis that makes it, paradoxically, an inferior choice compared with Ringer's lactate in patients with impaired renal function. **Hydroxyethyl starch solutions** should **not be used** in patients with septic shock as multiple trials (VISEP, 6S, and CHEST) have shown worse renal function and mortality with their use in patients with septic shock. **Albumin** has been proven to be safe (and perhaps beneficial) in patients with septic shock. The ALBIOS trial showed that using 20% albumin to keep serum albumin levels >3 g% in patients with septic shock had a mortality benefit (albeit in a *post hoc* analysis). It is reasonable to use albumin in hypoalbuminemic patients with septic shock, although the relatively high cost of albumin should temper its indiscriminate use.
   b. **Vasopressors and ionotropes: Norepinephrine** is the initial vasopressor agent of choice in septic shock. **Vasopressin** is often added to norepinephrine in an effort to limit norepinephrine dosage, although the VASST study shown no survival benefit. **Epinephrine** can be used if additional hemodynamic support is required, especially chronotropy. Norepinephrine has been shown to be superior to dopamine as a primary agent in cardiogenic shock as well as septic shock (SOAP II trial), particularly in the presence of hypotension. **Dobutamine** can be added to increase cardiac output, provided there is no significant

hypotension and the cardiac output is low. Recent studies have shown that there is no benefit to raising cardiac output to supranormal levels.

c. **Corticosteroids**: There is wide variance globally on the use of steroids in refractory septic shock, as the two most widely quoted trials in the field were different enough (one showed benefit, the other did not) that it is difficult to compare them directly (Annane's 2002 trial and CORTICUS in 2008). Proponents of steroids will recommend using them as early as possible after the development of septic shock. A subgroup analysis of the VASST trial suggested a beneficial interaction between patients on vasopressin and hydrocortisone, but this effect requires confirmation. If steroids are used, hydrocortisone should be used at a dose of 200 mg/day (as a continuous infusion or repeated boluses). Higher doses are not indicated, and there is no need for the addition of fludrocortisone. Steroids should be used for the shortest time possible—it is unclear if there is a need for tapering the dose.

d. **Blood transfusion**: Multiple large randomized controlled trials have shown no advantage of liberal transfusion goals (usually defined as a target Hb >10 g%) over more restrictive approaches (targeting Hb between 7 and 9 g%), most recently in the Transfusion Requirements in Septic Shock (TRISS) trial. In the absence of ongoing bleeding or **active** myocardial ischemia (during current admission), it seems to be very safe to adopt restrictive transfusion practices.

e. **Other supportive therapies**:
   1. **Mechanical ventilation**: Twenty to forty percent of patients with severe sepsis will develop acute respiratory distress syndrome. They should be ventilated with the principles of lung-protective ventilation described in Chapters 8 and 21.
   2. **Glycemic control**: Hyperglycemia in septic shock is associated with worse outcomes, as are large swings in blood glucose. Glucose should be maintained between 140 and 180 mg/dL for patients with severe sepsis. Patients who are on a regular insulin infusion should have hourly glucose checks and be on a glucose source to avoid hypoglycemia.

V. **INNOVATIVE/EXPERIMENTAL THERAPIES**: Several new therapeutic approaches may be more widely available in the near future. They are described briefly below.

A. **Immunomodulation**: Most patients with severe sepsis and organ dysfunction are immune suppressed, such as selective depletion of $CD4^+$ T cells or low HLA-DR expression on monocytes. Rather than treat patients broadly with anti-inflammatory agents (steroids or anticytokine molecules), patients will be tested to define their immunophenotype and, depending on the results, be treated with specific immune-enhancing therapies. An example is a recent study that used GM-CSF in patients with severe sepsis who were also immune suppressed as determined by circulating monocyte HLA-DR quantification.

B. **Stem Cells**: Mesenchymal stromal cells (MSCs) are nonhematopoietic precursor cells derived from a variety of sources including bone marrow, adipose tissue, and the placenta. MSCs are easily harvested and rapidly expanded in culture. Prominent features of MSCs that are of value to the treatment of severe sepsis include their ability to "home in" on injured tissue, versatile paracrine signaling effects, immunomodulatory capacity, and potential for direct antimicrobial effects. MSCs have shown very encouraging results in preclinical studies and are in human phase I and II trials for patients with acute respiratory distress syndrome. The results of these trials may inform the use of MSC therapy in severe sepsis as well.

C. Polymyxin B Hemoperfusion: LPS or endotoxin (see section III B) is a potent proinflammatory molecule that is found in the circulation of almost 50% of patients with septic shock. Polymyxin B (PmB) hemoperfusion has the ability to remove endotoxin from blood and is widely used in Japan. Currently, a randomized controlled trial of PmB hemoperfusion (EUPHRATES) is underway in the United States that randomizes patients in septic shock **and** detectable endotoxin levels to PmB hemoperfusion or a "façade" of hemoperfusion. The results should be available in 2016 and have the potential to significantly impact the standard of care for septic shock.

D. Sepsis Trials and the Future: In spite of significant advances in our understanding of sepsis biology over the past four decades, the history of "disease-modifying agents" in the field has been one of repeated failure, with more than a hundred randomized clinical trials failing to improve outcomes. The one (transient) exception was activated protein C, which was the first drug to be approved for septic shock before it too was discontinued in 2012 on the basis of the negative results of a follow-up study. When it comes to sepsis, our continued use of arguably crude classification systems like the one outlined in Table 29.1 do not permit sufficiently exact diagnostic phenotypes of sepsis to drive therapy. With the advent of "precision medicine," an individualized approach to disease that leverages molecular diagnostics and genomics has become a major focus of both researchers and funding agencies. We expect that discoveries in the near future will be successful in the creation of better stratification systems to identify patients who would be most likely to benefit from a given intervention.

Selected Readings

Angus DC, van der Poll T. Severe sepsis and septic shock. *N Engl J Med* 2013;369:2063.

Caironi P, Tognoni G, Masson S, et al. Albumin replacement in patients with severe sepsis or septic shock. *N Engl J Med* 2014;370:1412–1421.

Cohen J, Vincent JL, Adhikari NK, et al. Sepsis: a roadmap for future research. *Lancet Infect Dis* 2015;15:581–614.

De Backer D, Biston P, Devriendt J, et al. Comparison of dopamine and norepinephrine in the treatment of shock. *N Engl J Med* 2010;362:779–789.

Holst LB, Haase N, Wetterslev J, et al. Lower versus higher hemoglobin threshold for transfusion in septic shock. *N Engl J Med* 2014;371:1381–1391.

Kaukonen KM, Bailey M, Pilcher D, et al. Systemic inflammatory response syndrome criteria in defining severe sepsis. *N Engl J Med* 2015;372:1629–1638.

Martin GS, Mannino DM, Eaton S, et al. The epidemiology of sepsis in the United States from 1979 through 2000. *N Engl J Med* 2003;348:1546–1554.

Mouncey PR, Osborn TM, Power GS, et al. Trial of early, goal-directed resuscitation for septic shock. *N Engl J Med* 2015;372:1301–1311.

Peake SL, Delaney A, Bailey M, et al. Goal-directed resuscitation for patients with early septic shock. *N Engl J Med* 2014;371:1496–1506.

Perner A, Haase N, Guttormsen AB, et al. Hydroxyethyl starch 130/0.42 versus Ringer's acetate in severe sepsis. *N Engl J Med* 2012;367:124–134.

Russell JA, Walley KR, Singer J, et al. Vasopressin versus norepinephrine infusion in patients with septic shock. *N Engl J Med* 2008;358:877–887.

Yealy DM, Kellum JA, Huang DT, et al. A randomized trial of protocol-based care for early septic shock. *N Engl J Med* 2014;370:1683–1693.

Stroke, Seizures, and Encephalopathy

Alice D. Lam, M. Brandon Westover, and Pratik V. Patel

Acute cerebral dysfunction is often the initial reason for presentation to the hospital and frequently develops as a complication of medical or perioperative care. The majority of causes require specific and urgent intervention, and understanding acute dysfunction of the brain is of paramount importance in leading the rapid and focused workup and guided therapies. Common disorders include ischemic stroke, intracerebral hemorrhage (ICH), subdural hemorrhage, subarachnoid hemorrhage (SAH), seizures, and encephalopathy (of infectious, inflammatory, hypo- or hypertensive, or toxic/metabolic origin). A timely and focused neurologic examination is critical in distinguishing focal versus generalized processes and can help to identify the likely etiology.

I. **STROKE** is the acute onset of a focal neurologic deficit or disturbance in the level of arousal due to cerebral ischemia, hemorrhage, or venous occlusion. Therapy is aimed at maintaining or acutely restoring adequate cerebral blood flow and preventing secondary brain injury.

   A. **Acute Ischemic Stroke** is due to acute vascular occlusion. Symptoms often include sudden onset of visual loss, weakness or numbness on one side of the body, ataxia, unexplained falling, dysarthria, or aphasia. Thrombosis in situ may occur in diseased segments of small penetrating vessels (e.g., lacunar stroke) or larger arteries (e.g., atherosclerotic stenosis, arterial dissection), and emboli may be dislodged from proximal sites (e.g., heart, aorta, carotid artery) to lodge in otherwise normal major cerebral arteries or their distal branches.

      1. **Lacunar strokes** tend to occur in patients with diabetes and chronic hypertension and may be clinically silent, but most often present (in descending order of frequency) as pure motor hemiparesis, sensory-motor stroke, ataxic-hemiparesis, pure sensory stroke, dysarthria-clumsy hand syndrome, or a variety of well-defined syndromes (e.g., hemichorea-hemiballism). As symptomatic lacunar stroke typically occurs in regions that interrupt major white matter tracts or brainstem nuclei, their initial presentation can be quite striking. However, the prognosis for recovery with lacunar stroke is better than with large-artery territory stroke. Nevertheless, because the risk of hemorrhagic transformation in these patients is low, many centers favor the use of intravenous (IV) **thrombolysis** in all but the most clinically mild lacunar strokes. Because initial small-vessel clinical syndromes may sometimes be due to large-artery thrombosis affecting end vessels, all patients presenting with acute ischemic symptoms should undergo some form of acute neurovascular imaging to establish large-vessel patency (e.g., computed tomographic angiography [CTA], magnetic resonance angiography [MRA], ultrasound, or conventional catheter angiography). Obtaining this imaging should not delay IV thrombolysis using recombinant **tissue plasminogen activator** (**tPA,** alteplase) in appropriate patients.

2. **Large-artery occlusion** is divided into disorders of the anterior (internal carotid artery and branches) and posterior (vertebrobasilar arteries and branches) circulations. These strokes carry a risk of swelling and hemorrhagic transformation. The "ischemic penumbra" refers to a region of brain with inadequate blood supply that still may be salvaged with rapid restoration of normal blood flow. Although the center of an ischemic zone (the core) may be irreversibly injured before the patient obtains medical attention, the surrounding ischemic penumbra may be saved by rapid intervention.

   a. **Middle cerebral artery (MCA) occlusion** is characterized by weakness of the contralateral face and arm with hemianopia and a gaze preference toward the side of the involved hemisphere ("eyes looking toward the lesion"). Additional findings include aphasia in dominant-hemisphere strokes (the left hemisphere in the large majority of individuals), dense hemineglect in nondominant-hemisphere strokes (i.e., patient "ignores" the left side of the body, the surroundings, or the presence of the deficit itself; this is most often seen in lesion involving the R parietal lobe), and a variable degree of leg weakness depending on how much of the deep territory of the MCA is involved (and thus how much of the underlying white matter or basal ganglia is affected). Occlusion limited to branches of the MCA may produce partial versions of the MCA syndrome and are more likely to spare leg strength.

   b. **Anterior cerebral artery (ACA) occlusion in isolation** is rare and causes isolated weakness of the lower limb. If both ACAs are affected, a generalized decrease in initiative (abulia) may also occur.

   c. **Border zone** or "watershed" infarction is the result of insufficient blood flow to parts of the brain supplied by the distal territories of the major cerebral vessels. This develops most commonly in the setting of severe, sustained hypotension (e.g., cardiac arrest, profound shock prior to resuscitation) or in the presence of severe atherosclerotic narrowing of one or both carotid arteries. Because the region most commonly affected is the white matter underneath the motor areas (the ACA/MCA border zone), the classic presentation is that of proximal arm/leg weakness with preservation of distal strength, the so-called "man-in-a-barrel syndrome."

   d. Posterior circulation infarction involves the brainstem, cerebellum, thalamus, and occipital and mesial temporal lobes. As a result, patients can present with bilateral limb weakness or sensory disturbance, sensory and/or motor cranial nerve deficits, ataxia, nausea and vomiting, visual field deficits, or decreased level of consciousness, including coma. The full-blown syndrome results from occlusion of the majority of the basilar artery with fragments of the syndrome produced by occlusions of branches of the vertebrobasilar system. Edema and mass effect from cerebellar stroke may be life threatening due to confined space of the posterior fossa, with resulting upward or downward transtentorial herniation (see section on cerebellar hemorrhage).

3. Conditions mimicking stroke include seizure, migraine, toxic-metabolic derangement, and amyloid spells. Diffusion-weighted MR imaging helps to distinguish cerebral infarction from stroke mimics by identifying areas of intracellular swelling (i.e., cytotoxic edema) associated with ischemia and frank infarction.

   a. While complex partial **seizures** may mimic stroke, especially if speech is impaired, postictal neurologic deficits (Todd's phenomena) may masquerade as any focal neurologic deficit, including weakness, sensory loss, or aphasia lasting hours to days after a seizure.

b. The aura associated with a **migraine** headache may include focal neurologic deficits such as weakness, numbness, or aphasia and may occur in the absence of headache ("typical aura without headache"). Patients with recurrent migraine headaches are at a somewhat increased risk for true ischemic stroke. Patients who present with persistent symptoms similar in quality to their typical migrainous aura or who present with a new focal deficit accompanied by their typical aura should be evaluated for stroke.

c. **Toxic-metabolic states** such as hypo- or hyperglycemia, hyponatremia, hypoxia, or intoxication may produce focal or global neurologic deficits. Laboratory evaluation including rapid glucose evaluation (i.e., point-of-care glucose) and electrolytes should be performed in all cases. Occult infections can also exacerbate deficits from old strokes and brain injury and masquerade as new or recurrent stroke.

d. Patients with **cerebral amyloid angiopathy** may have transient neurologic dysfunction associated with microscopic hemorrhages that are suggestive of transient ischemic attacks (TIAs). Brain MR imaging with sequences sensitive to blood and blood breakdown products (i.e., gradient-echo or susceptibility-weighted imaging) may suggest a diagnosis of cerebral amyloid angiopathy.

4. **Important etiologies of ischemic stroke** include **cardiac or arterial thromboembolism,** intracranial and extracranial **atherosclerosis,** endocarditis, paradoxical emboli, arterial dissection, vasculitis, and inherited and acquired hypercoagulable disorders. Carotid or vertebral artery **dissection** may occur spontaneously, after trauma, or in connective tissue disease (e.g., fibromuscular dysplasia). Dissection can be recognized on axial T1 fat-suppression MR imaging or CTA or conventional angiography. **Vasculitis** may occur in primary central nervous system (CNS) disease or as part of a systemic syndrome such as systemic lupus erythematosus (SLE) or polyarteritis nodosa. **Hypercoagulability** may be due to clotting factor imbalance (e.g., protein C, protein S, or antithrombin III deficiency), autoimmunity (e.g., antiphospholipid antibodies), or inherited hypercoagulable states (e.g., prothrombin gene mutation). Sickle cell disease can also lead to focal cerebral arterial occlusion. In young patients with stroke, special attention should be given to the possibility of arterial dissection, hypercoagulable states, autoimmune syndromes, and hemoglobinopathies.

5. **Acute evaluation** for IV **thrombolysis** should be performed in all patients presenting within 4.5 hours of symptom onset to an appropriate facility. The only drug approved for use in acute ischemic stroke remains IV **tPA.** This includes accurate neurologic assessment, emergent CT (or MRI at some specialized centers) to exclude hemorrhage and early ischemic changes, laboratory exclusion of stroke mimics, hemostatic laboratories (platelets, prothrombin time [PT], activated partial thromboplastin time [aPTT]), electrocardiogram [ECG], and historical/imaging findings consistent with acute ischemia. Acute CT angiography (or if rapidly available MRA) of the head and neck can be very useful in selecting patients for catheter-directed thrombectomy. Specialized centers may offer endovascular approaches to reperfusion, including intra-arterial thrombolysis, mechanical thrombectomy, or angioplasty. These approaches may provide benefit beyond the 4.5-hour window of IV tPA, extending the window for acute intervention up to 6 to 8 hours in the anterior circulation, and perhaps up to 12 to 24 hours in the posterior circulation. Many therapeutic efforts to extend the window for acute intervention in ischemic stroke focuses upon the ischemic penumbra, that is, the region critically hypoperfused but potentially viable tissue around an irreversibly damaged core region of infarction. The penumbra can be imaged as a mismatch between perfusion-weighted magnetic resonance imaging (MRI) (PWI) and diffusion-weighted MRI (DWI) and is present in up to 80% of patients within 3 hours of symptom onset, although it diminishes rapidly with time. See http://www.acutestroke.com for the Massachusetts General Hospital Acute Stroke Service protocols and http://www.stroke-center.org for completed and active clinical trials in cerebrovascular disease.

6. **Subacute evaluation** should identify the cause and help define the risk for recurrent stroke. **Transthoracic echocardiography (TTE)** should be performed to exclude intracardiac thrombus and to assess left ventricular size and function, left atrial size, mitral and aortic valvular disease, and right-to-left shunt. In patients with suspected paradoxical embolism, agitated-saline contrast echocardiography should be performed to increase the sensitivity for the detection of shunt. **Transesophageal** studies are more sensitive to left atrial thrombus and atheromatous disease of the aortic arch. A 24-hour Holter monitor may identify paroxysmal atrial fibrillation, and if negative a 30-day event monitor increases the sensitivity for detecting atrial fibrillation. Particularly in young patients, the cause of the stroke should be vigorously pursued, including evaluation for inherited or acquired hypercoagulable syndromes.

7. **TIAs** are traditionally considered to be sudden, focal neurologic deficits that last less than 24 hours and are believed to be of vascular origin (Fig. 30.2). This definition is falling out of favor because ischemic symptoms lasting more than several hours almost always are associated with evidence of infarction on advanced imaging techniques (diffusion-weighted imaging [DWI]), and occasionally symptoms lasting only a few minutes also have imaging that demonstrates infarction. Therefore, even transient symptoms consistent with ischemic injury should be evaluated as potential ischemic stroke, and the newest American Heart/American Stroke Association guidelines recognize that similar principles apply in the workup and secondary prevention of TIA and ischemic stroke. The ABCD2 risk factor stratification score after acute TIA has been developed to estimate the risk for stroke within 2 days after TIA, and some centers have developed a "TIA clinic" allowing for expedited neurological evaluation and workup of patients with TIA.

8. **Acute treatment.** If the time of onset is clearly established to be less than 4.5 hours and cranial CT excludes intracranial hemorrhage or well-established stroke, all patients with a significant persistent deficit and the clinical diagnosis of ischemic stroke are potential candidates for **IV tPA.** A 0.9-mg/kg (maximum 90 mg) dose is infused over 60 minutes with 10% of the total dose administered as an initial IV bolus over 1 minute. Contraindications to IV tPA are summarized in Table 30.1. In 2009, the AHA/ASA issued a science advisory about the use of IV tPA in the 3-to-4.5-hour time window; they are essentially similar to those in the standard 3-hour time window but have the following additional exclusion criteria: older than 80 years, any history of recent oral anticoagulant use, NIHSS >25, or those patients with a concomitant history of stroke and diabetes. Following IV tPA, no aspirin, heparin, or warfarin

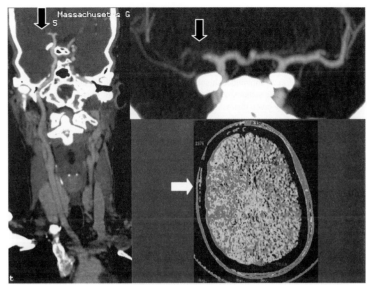

FIGURE 30.1 CT angiography three-dimensional formatted images in a 28-year-old female, demonstrating complete right MCA occlusion due to paradoxical embolism through a patent foramen ovale. The initial image shows a curved reformat from the aortic arch to the distal ICA bifurcation. The second image is a magnified view of the MCA stem occlusion. The third is a CT perfusion image showing abnormal perfusion to the right hemisphere in the territory of the occluded artery.

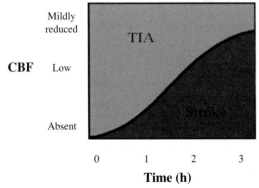

FIGURE 30.2 Graphic representation of cerebral ischemia as a function of both the degree of cerebral blood flow reduction and the duration of ischemia. Relatively mild reductions in blood flow can be tolerated for hours without progression to infarction, whereas steep reductions are poorly tolerated even for less than 1 hour.

TABLE 30.1	MGH Inclusion and Exclusion Criteria for Administering Intravenous Tissue Plasminogen Activator to Adult Patients with Acute Ischemic Stroke

Inclusion Criteria
- A significant neurologic deficit expected to result in long-term disability
- Noncontrast CT scan showing no hemorrhage or well-established new infarct
- Acute ischemic stroke symptoms with the patient last known well, clearly defined, <3 h before rt-PA will be given (Note: For additional warnings for the 3–4.5 h time period, see text.)

Contraindications
- SBP >185 or DBP >110 mmHg (despite measures to reduce it)
- CT findings (intracranial hemorrhage, subarachnoid hemorrhage, or major infarct signs)
- Platelets <100,000, PTT >40 s after heparin use, or PT >15 or INR >1.7, or known bleeding diathesis
- Recent major surgery or trauma (<15 d)
- Seizure at onset (if residual deficits are postictal impairments)
- Active internal bleeding (within prior 21 d)
- Recent intracranial or spinal surgery, head trauma, or stroke (<3 mo)
- History of intracranial hemorrhage or brain aneurysm or vascular malformation or brain tumor (may consider in patients with CNS lesions with very low likelihood of hemorrhage)
- Suspicion of subarachnoid hemorrhage (by imaging or clinical presentation)
- Current use of novel oral anticoagulants (NOACs) within 48 h, or with abnormal coagulation labs if >48 h since last dose

Warnings (conditions that might lead to unfavorable outcomes but not necessarily contraindications)
- Stroke severity too mild
- Rapid improvement
- Stroke severity—too severe (e.g., NIHSS >22; many centers do not exclude patients on the basis of an increased NIHSS alone)
- Glucose <50 or >400 mg/dL
- Life expectancy <1 y or severe comorbid illness or CMO on admission
- Increased risk of bleeding
  - Subacute bacterial endocarditis
  - Hemostatic defects including those secondary to severe hepatic or renal disease
  - Diabetic hemorrhage retinopathy, or other hemorrhagic ophthalmic conditions
  - Septic thrombophlebitis or occluded AV cannula at seriously infected site
  - Patients currently receiving oral anticoagulants, e.g., warfarin sodium with INR >1.7
- Increased risk of bleeding due to pregnancy
- Advanced age (increased risk of bleeding)
- Documented left heart thrombus or recent MI (within 3 mo)

CT, computed tomography; NIHSS, National Institutes of Health Stroke Scale; INR, International Normalized Ratio; tPA, tissue plasminogen activator; CMO, comfort measures only.
From the Massachusetts General Hospital Acute Stroke Services (www.acutestroke.com).

should be given for 24 hours. Patients with severe strokes (National Institutes of Health Stroke Scale [NIHSS] >20; Table 30.2) have a higher rate of hemorrhage after tPA; however, many centers favor treatment of these patients, given their otherwise unfavorable prognosis. Proximal artery occlusions are less likely to recanalize with IV tPA and are more likely to produce severe clinical deficits.

TABLE 30.2 National Institutes of Health Stroke Scale (NIHSS)

NIH Stroke Scale Item (with Abbreviated Scoring Instructions)	Scoring Definitions	Score (0–42)
1a. **Loss of consciousness**	0 = Alert and responsive 1 = Arousable to minor stimulation 2 = Arousable only to painful stimuli 3 = Reflex responses or unarousable	
1b. **Questions**—Ask patient's age and month. Must be exact	0 = Both correct 1 = One correct (or dysarthria, intubated, foreign language) 2 = Neither correct	
1c. **Commands**—Open/close eyes, grip and release nonparetic hand (other 1-step commands or mimic OK)	0 = Both correct (OK if impaired by weakness) 1 = One correct 2 = Neither correct	
2. **Best gaze**—Horizontal eye movement by voluntary or Doll's eyes	0 = Normal 1 = Partial gaze palsy, abnl gaze in one or both eyes 2 = Forced eye deviation or total paresis, which cannot be overcome by Doll's	
3. **Visual field**—Use visual threat if necessary. If monocular, score field of good eye	0 = Normal 1 = Partial hemianopia, quadrantonopia, extinction 2 = Complete hemianopia 3 = Bilateral hemianopia or blindness	
4. **Facial palsy**—If stuporous, check symmetry of grimace to pain	0 = Normal 1 = Minor paralysis, flat NLF, asymm smile 2 = Partial paralysis (lower face) 3 = Complete paralysis (upper & lower face)	
5. **Motor arm**—Arms outstretched 90° (sitting) or 45° (supine) for 10 s. Encourage best effort. Score both arms separately	0 = No drift × 10 s 1 = Drift but doesn't hit bed 2 = Some antigravity effort, but can't sustain 3 = No antigravity effort, but even minimal mvt counts 4 = No movement at all X = Unable to assess due to amputation, fusion, fracture, etc.	L R
6. **Motor leg**—Raise leg to 30° supine × 5 s. Score both legs separately	0 = No drift × 5 s 1 = Drift but doesn't hit bed 2 = Some antigravity effort, but can't sustain 3 = No antigravity effort, but even minimal mvt counts 4 = No movement at all X = unable to assess due to amputation, fusion, fracture, etc.	L R

(Continued)

National Institutes of Health Stroke Scale (NIHSS) (Continued)

NIH Stroke Scale Item (with Abbreviated Scoring Instructions)	Scoring Definitions	Score (0–42)
7. **Limb ataxia**—Check finger–nose–finger, heel–shin–knee, and score only if out of proportion to paralysis	0 = No ataxia (or aphasic, hemiplegic) 1 = Ataxia in upper or lower extremity 2 = Ataxia in upper *and* lower extremity X = Unable to assess due to amputation, fusion, fracture, etc.	L R
8. **Sensory**—Use safety pin. Check grimace or withdrawal if stuporous. Score only stroke-related losses	0 = Normal 1 = Mild-mod unilateral loss but pt aware of touch (or aphasic, confused) 2 = Total loss, pt unaware of touch. Coma, bilateral loss	
9. **Best language**—Describe picture, name objects, read sentences. May use repeating, writing, stereognosis	0 = Normal 1 = Mild-mod aphasia (difficult but partly comprehensible) 2 = Severe aphasia (almost no info exchanged) 3 = Mute, global aphasia, coma. No 1-step commands	
10. **Dysarthria**—Read list of words	0 = Normal 1 = Mild-mod; slurred but intelligible 2 = Severe; unintelligible or mute X = Intubation or mech barrier	
11. **Extinction/neglect**—Simultaneously touch patient on both hands, show fingers in both visual fields, ask about deficit, left hand	0 = Normal (visual loss alone) 1 = Neglects or extinguishes to double simult stimulation in any modality (visual, auditory, sensory, spatial, body parts) 2 = Profound neglect in more than one modality	

Adapted NIHSS scoring instructions from www.ninds.nih.gov/doctors/NIH_Stroke_Scale.pdf; Brott T, Adams HP Jr, Olinger CP, et al. Measurements of acute cerebral infarction: a clinical examination scale. *Stroke* 1989;20:864–870.

a. **Mechanical clot retrieval** has achieved renewed interest in the field since the publication of a number of randomized trials in late 2014–early 2015 with a newer generation of thrombectomy devices in conjunction with IV tPA and improved and timely patient selection with intracranial vascular imaging demonstrating a large artery anterior circulation thrombus. The first generation of devices was fed through the clot and meant to pull the clot out (Fig. 30.3). The newer devices used in these recent trials include temporary intra-arterial stents that are deployed into the clot and then retrieved or suction-aspirator devices that can break up and aspirate a clot in situ. There are multiple retrospective studies that demonstrate an association with worse neurologic outcomes in patient receiving general anesthesia for acute stroke therapies, and thus many centers are

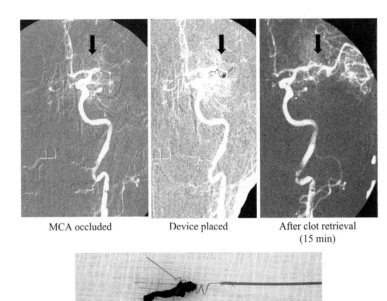

MCA occluded   Device placed   After clot retrieval
                                                            (15 min)

FIGURE 30.3 Serial angiographic images showing occlusion of the left middle cerebral artery, deployment of a clot retrieval device, and restoration of vessel patency. An example of residual thrombus is displayed below. The patient made a full recovery and was discharged several days later.

now preferring to treat patients with monitored anesthesia care or "conscious sedation" whenever feasible.

b. Continuous IV **unfractionated heparin,** although without proven benefit in acute stroke, is sometimes used in patients ineligible for thrombolysis and can be considered in patients with basilar stenosis, internal carotid or extradural vertebral artery dissection, fluctuating deficits, or symptomatic critical carotid stenosis without large MCA infarct. This use must be balanced against the risks of hemorrhagic complications. The aPTT should be monitored every 6 hours and the heparin dose adjusted accordingly. Because of high variability in individual heparin and aPTT assays, the aPTT should be maintained in the desired numerical range on the basis of the levels associated with achieving therapeutic anticoagulation (equivalent to 0.3–0.7 IU/mL by factor Xa inhibition), rather than a simple ratio of 1.5 to 2.5 times control. Initial heparin bolus may raise the risk of hemorrhage and is deferred except in fluctuating deficits or acute basilar thrombosis. While chronic anticoagulation reduces the risk of recurrent stroke in patients with atrial fibrillation, in patients with large infarcts, initiation is often deferred for days to weeks to minimize the risk of hemorrhagic transformation. Any patient who experiences a clinical deterioration on heparin must be imaged immediately to rule out **hemorrhagic transformation.**

    c. **Antiplatelet therapy** should be considered for patients who do not qualify for thrombolytic therapy. **Aspirin** in doses ranging from 160 to 1,300 mg daily may benefit patients with **acute stroke** for whom thrombolytics or anticoagulants are not indicated, the AHA/ASA guideline recommends oral administration of aspirin 325 mg within 24 to 48 hours after stroke onset. Other antiplatelet agents such as IV **glycoprotein IIb/IIIa inhibitors** continue to be studied in acute ischemic stroke. Daily doses of aspirin commonly prescribed for secondary stroke prophylaxis range from 50 to 325 mg, with guidelines for coronary event prevention recommending a minimum dose of 75 mg daily. Combination aspirin (25 mg) plus extended-release **dipyridamole** (200 mg) has been shown to be superior to aspirin alone for secondary prophylaxis. **Clopidogrel,** another antiplatelet agent, is also useful for reducing the risk of recurrent vascular events and appears to be associated with less major bleeding than combination aspirin/dipyridamole in secondary stroke prevention. Dual antiplatelet therapy with the combination of aspirin and clopidogrel might be superior to aspirin alone when initiated within 24 hours of minor ischemic stroke or TIA for secondary stroke prophylaxis for the first 21 days, but because of increased risk of major bleeding complications it is not recommended for long-term secondary stroke prevention.

    d. Urgent **carotid revascularization** may be indicated in cases of stroke in which there is a critical degree of carotid stenosis, a small distal infarction, and a large territory of vulnerable brain. Revascularization of larger strokes may be associated with acute reperfusion injury and should be delayed by weeks to months.

    e. In some patients with stenosis of major vessels, **pharmacologically induced hypertension** with **phenylephrine or other vasopressors** may improve neurologic function acutely and rescue viable brain tissue, perhaps due to penumbral salvage. Early studies suggest that induced hypertension is safe in patients without cardiac comorbidities, such as angina or congestive heart failure. It is not clear which population will benefit from induced hypertension, and thus if it is attempted, a short period (30–60 minutes) of a modest (10%–20%) pharmacologic elevation with repeated neurologic exam should assess for potential improvement. If improvement is observed, it may be reasonable to continue modest induced hypertension with repeated neurologic evaluation and frequent (i.e., at least daily) to see if the patient continues to have a neurologic improvement with induced hypertension.

9. Subacute treatment. Hypovolemia and hyponatremia should be avoided, and intravascular volume should be maintained with isotonic solutions. **Fever** should be aggressively controlled because even mild hyperthermia worsens outcome. Swelling is maximal at 2 to 5 days after stroke onset, and standard increased intracranial pressure (ICP) management should be initiated (see **Chapters 10** and **37**). In massive hemispheric or cerebellar infarction, decompressive surgery can be lifesaving and may improve outcome.

B. Primary Intracerebral Hemorrhage (ICH). The broad differential diagnosis for intracranial bleeding includes ICH, epidural and subdural hemorrhage, SAH (described subsequently), venous sinus thrombosis (also described subsequently), and, rarely, isolated intraventricular hemorrhage. These can often be distinguished initially by noncontrast CT scan, though more advanced imaging (to be discussed) may be required. The most common locations for ICH are basal ganglia, thalamus, cerebral white matter, pons, cortical lobar surface, and the cerebellum. **Long-standing hypertension** is the most common cause (up to 75% of cases), although other etiologies are recognized, such as aneurysm, trauma, vascular malformations, cerebral amyloid angiopathy, coagulopathies, neoplasms, sympathomimetic drugs, septic emboli, and vasculitis. Metastases, especially adenocarcinoma and melanoma, may present with ICH or swelling. ICH as a primary process should be differentiated from hemorrhagic transformation of ischemic infarction, in which a bland ischemic stroke develops petechial bleeding or turns into a space-occupying hematoma.

1. **Clinical syndromes.** ICH often presents with headache, nausea, vomiting, and focal neurologic signs similar to those seen in ischemic strokes. The evolution of symptoms may occur more slowly than in ischemic stroke or may present as an acute and devastating condition. As a rule, patients with ICH present with systolic hypertension. In patients who were normotensive at baseline, this usually resolves over the first week; in chronic hypertensive patients, aggressive, multiple-drug treatment is often required to control blood pressure. In contrast to most cortical hemorrhages, the progression to death from cerebellar hemorrhage may be rapid.

   a. **Supratentorial** ICH presents with symptoms referable to the site of bleeding. With rebleeding or development of vasogenic edema or hydrocephalus, there is often worsening of symptoms with decline in arousal. Transtentorial herniation is the mode of death in fatal massive lobar and basal ganglia hemorrhage.

   b. **Midline infratentorial** hemorrhage produces only dysequilibrium on standing, walking, and sometimes sitting. Romberg sign cannot be assessed because balance is already impaired with eyes open. If gait is not tested, this lesion may not be detected until other cerebellar signs emerge secondary to brain swelling. **Lateral cerebellar hemispheric** lesions produce symptoms ipsilateral to the lesion. Patients complain of limb incoordination and demonstrate ataxia with falling toward the side of lesion, dysmetria (overshoot) on finger–nose–finger testing, dysdiadochokinesia (inaccuracy on rapid alternating movements), intention tremor (exaggerated on approaching the target), and nystagmus (worse looking toward lesion). Speech may be dysarthric (slurred), scanning, or explosive.

2. **Acute evaluation** of patients with suspected ICH consists of brain imaging; both CT and MR are very sensitive. In addition, toxicology screen, PT, aPTT, and platelets should be checked. Signs of occult malignancy should be excluded especially in patients without a history of hypertension. Hemorrhage volume correlates with outcome and can be estimated easily in cubic centimeters on unenhanced head CT using the "ABC/2" method, where A is the greatest diameter of the hemorrhage on a single slice, B is the hemorrhage diameter perpendicular to A on the same slice, and C is the approximate number of axial CT slices revealing hemorrhage multiplied by slice thickness in centimeters. The Intracerebral Hemorrhage Score was described over a decade ago and demonstrated that thirty-day mortality for patients with a parenchymal hemorrhage volume of greater than 60 cm^3 on their initial CT and a Glasgow Coma Scale (GCS) score of 8 or less is 90%, and for those with a volume of less than 30 cm^3 and a GCS score of 9 or greater it is 20%. The FUNC score is a recently validated clinical assessment tool

that predicts, at hospital admission, functional independence at 90 days, and is available for use to clinicians (http://www.massgeneral. org/stopstroke/funcCalculator.aspx). **Subacute evaluation** should identify the etiology by imaging and history. MRI with gradient-echo or susceptibility-weighted imaging may identify areas of prior occult cortical hemorrhage and suggest a diagnosis of amyloid angiopathy in patients with lobar ICH. Repeat MR in 3 to 6 weeks may also detect lesions (e.g., tumor) masked by acute hemorrhage. Rarely, aneurysmal hemorrhage may result in primarily parenchymal hematoma, mimicking ICH. Conventional catheter angiography or CTA is indicated in any suspicious case. Prognosis is based on clinical presentation and imaging findings. Patients with cerebellar lesions less than 2 cm in diameter or with self-limited cerebellar signs usually do well, those with 3-cm lesions or progressive drowsiness do poorly without intervention, and 20% have lesions greater than 3 cm and a poor prognosis regardless of treatment. Prognosis in patients with cortical ICH is also related to hematoma size. It should be noted, however, that the most common cause of death in large ICH is withdrawal of supportive care, and the prognosis for large ICH with extended rehabilitation is less clear. Patients treated at hospitals that have a high rate of institution of DNR orders have higher mortality rates, and a recent trial of early full-aggressive medical care in patients with intracerebral hemorrhage demonstrated consistently lower mortality rates compared with the predicted mortality based on that predicted from prior ICH cohorts.

3. **Acute treatment** consists largely of supportive care, acute blood pressure control, reversal of coagulopathy, and ICP monitoring or surgical intervention in selected cases. To correct elevated PT, **vitamin K,** 10 mg infused at 1 mg/min, should be given IV, accompanied by rapid administration of prothrombin complex concentrate or transfusion of fresh frozen plasma (FFP); **protamine** is used for elevated aPTT associated with unfractionated heparin or low-molecular-weight heparin. Platelets should be provided to patients with platelet counts less than 100,000; patients who have uremic or pharmacologic (e.g., aspirin) platelet dysfunction may benefit from **desmopressin.** Reduction of systolic blood pressure to a target blood pressure of 160/90 is important to prevent rebleeding; If SBP is >200 mmHg or MAP is >150 mmHg, aggressive reduction of blood pressure with continuous IV infusion, with frequent blood pressure monitoring every 5 minutes is advised. If SBP is >180 mmHg or MAP is >130 mmHg and there is evidence of or suspicion of elevated ICP, then consider monitoring ICP and reducing blood pressure using intermittent or continuous IV medications to keep cerebral perfusion pressure >60 to 80 mmHg. Any clinical deterioration in association with reduction of BP should prompt reconsideration of ongoing BP management strategy. β-Blockers such as **labetalol** are preferred for blood pressure control, given their additional benefit of being antiarrhythmic; conversely, nitrates may paradoxically increase ICP by dilating the cerebral vasculature and are typically best avoided. IV calcium-channel blockers such as **nicardipine** may be useful if further reduction in blood pressure is needed. **Neurosurgical consultation** should be obtained early, **especially in cerebellar hemorrhage** of diameter 2 cm or greater, and an emphasis on surgical decompression and evacuation of hematoma should be considered (and not just placement of an extraventricular drain in cerebellar hemorrhage as this may promote upward transtentorial herniation). Resection of lobar or basal ganglia ICH

can be life saving but has not been well studied in large clinical trials; the large randomized international trial only included patients in whom the treating neurosurgeon felt there was clinical equipoise (leading to the exclusion of a large number of patients at certain treating centers that favored early surgical hematoma evacuation). Surgical methods include open craniotomy and stereotactic drainage. Intraventricular tPA may also improve outcome in patients with intraventricular extension of the ICH. **Obstructive or communicating hydrocephalus** may develop and usually requires external ventricular drainage, although it may not need permanent ventricular shunting (Fig. 30.4). Corticosteroids do not appear to be of benefit in ICH. **Anticonvulsant therapy** is indicated in patients with clinical seizure but not for prophylaxis.

4. When **ICH** is suspected **in patients who received thrombolysis for acute stroke,** a head CT should be obtained immediately, along with neurosurgical and hematologic consultation, PT, aPTT, complete blood count (CBC), and D-dimer and fibrinogen concentrations. Treatment of verified symptomatic hematoma includes use of 2 U of **FFP** to replete

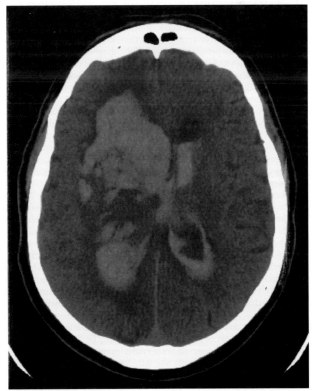

FIGURE 30.4 Axial image from an unenhanced CT of the brain showing a large right intracerebral hemorrhage with extension into the lateral ventricles and early obstructive hydrocephalus requiring ventriculostomy.

factors V and VII, 10 U of **cryoprecipitate** to replete fibrinogen, and 6 U of **platelets.** Patients treated with heparin should receive **protamine** by slow IV push, 1 mg per each 100 units of unfractionated heparin given in the preceding 4 hours. If an anticoagulant dose of low-molecular-weight heparin had been used, the maximum dose of protamine (50 mg) should be given as slow IV push. The foregoing laboratory values should be repeated every hour for the next 4 hours until bleeding is brought under control. If these measures fail to control bleeding, **aminocaproic acid,** 5 g IV over 1 hour, may be given.

C. **Cerebral Venous Thrombosis (CVT)** most commonly occurs in the sagittal, transverse, or straight sinus (often called venous sinus thrombosis), although the clot may extend into the vein of Galen or the internal jugular vein. Smaller, cortical venous thrombosis can also occur, as can cavernous sinus thrombosis. CVT may occur in the setting of infection, tumor, trauma, hypovolemia, coagulation disorders, systemic inflammatory diseases, oral contraceptive use, pregnancy, and the puerperium. Despite a thorough diagnostic evaluation, nearly 25% of cases will be deemed idiopathic.

1. The **clinical syndrome** includes signs of increased ICP such as headache, nausea, and vomiting, often more pronounced after prolonged recumbency. Focal neurologic signs or seizures may be seen in the setting of vasogenic edema or venous infarction. Without recanalization, altered sensorium can progress to coma. If the diagnosis is not considered, it is often overlooked until venous hemorrhage has occurred.

2. **Acute evaluation** relies on an imaging. CT with contrast may demonstrate filling defects in the superior sagittal sinus and torcula ("empty delta" sign) in up to 30% of patients, parenchymal abnormalities suggestive of deranged venous drainage in up to 60% of patients, small ventricles from increased ICP, or contrast enhancement of the falx and tentorium from venous hypertension. CT or MR venography provides enhanced sensitivity. Conventional cerebral angiography is diagnostic if MR is inconclusive. Lumbar puncture may demonstrate an elevated opening pressure, increased protein and red cells, and mild pleocytosis.

3. **Acute treatment** is effective if initiated early, but prognosis for recovery worsens significantly without treatment. Continuous IV unfractionated **heparin** titrated to aPTT of 60 to 80 should be given and maintained until the patient stabilizes or improves. Heparin should be given even in the presence of hemorrhage. In certain cases of extensive thrombosis or rapid deterioration in patient condition, transvenous thrombolysis with locally injected chemical thrombolytic or mechanical clot disruption should be considered at experienced centers. Measures to control ICP elevation should be instituted, prophylaxis for seizures can be considered, and factors that exacerbate clotting (e.g., dehydration) must be avoided.

D. **Subarachnoid hemorrhage** (SAH) may be traumatic or nontraumatic. Nontraumatic SAH is caused most commonly by the **rupture of a cerebral aneurysm.** The majority of aneurysms arise from the carotid artery circulation, most commonly the ACA and less frequently the posterior communicating artery or the MCA. Posterior circulation aneurysms commonly arise from the basilar tip or may also result from intradural vertebral dissections with pseudoaneurysm formation and rupture. Aneurysms may exist on a congenital basis, arise in the setting of atherosclerosis, or more rarely occur due to infection (mycotic) or emboli.

Rupture of cerebral aneurysms releases blood into the subarachnoid space and causes up to 30% mortality in the first 24 hours. The primary brain injury may be anything from minimal to lethal, and abrupt loss of consciousness at onset is characteristic. Rebleeding of untreated aneurysms occurs in up to 30% of patients in the first 28 days, with up to a 70% mortality if rebleeding occurs. Hypotension, aspiration pneumonia, neurogenic pulmonary edema, seizures, obstructive hydrocephalus, or ischemia due to vasospasm may produce secondary brain injury. Serial examination and brain imaging can identify symptoms suggestive of most of these complications, but separate techniques are necessary to distinguish vasospasm.

1. **Clinical syndromes.** The **"worst headache of my life" (WHOL)** complaint should raise suspicion of SAH. Nausea, vomiting, altered sensorium, and focal cranial nerve defects (especially third-nerve palsy) are associated with SAH. A warning headache ("sentinel headache") may occur due to a structural change in the aneurysm wall or minor self-limited bleeding. Clinical grading predicts outcome with the Hunt and Hess Classification used most frequently in the United States (Table 30.3) and risk of vasospasm (Table 30.4).

TABLE 30.3 Classification of Patients with Intracranial Aneurysms According to Surgical Risk (Hunt and Hess Classification System)

Grade	Characteristics
I	Asymptomatic or minimal headache and slight nuchal rigidity
II	Moderate to severe headache, nuchal rigidity, no neurologic deficit other than cranial nerve palsy
III	Drowsiness, confusion, mild focal deficit
IV	Stupor, moderate to severe hemiparesis, possibly early decerebrate rigidity, vegetative disturbances
V	Deep coma, decerebrate rigidity, moribund

In the original classification, one grade was added if major concurrent health problems were present such as lung, heart, liver, or kidney comorbities. In current practice, many centers do not add a grade for medical comorbidities.

TABLE 30.4 Classification of Subarachnoid Hemorrhage According to Risk of Vasospasm[a]

Group	Characteristics of Subarachnoid Hemorrhage on Computed Tomography Scan
1	Focal or diffuse thin SAH, no IVH
2	Focal or diffuse thin SA, with IVH
3	Thick SAH present, no IVH
4	Thick SAH present, with IVH

[a] Modified Fisher Group Classification System
Adapted from Frontera JA, Claassen J, Schmidt JM, et al. Prediction of symptomatic vasospasm after subarachnoid hemorrhage: the modified Fisher scale. *Neurosurgery* 2006;59(1):21–27.

2. **Acute evaluation. CT scan** is the best initial test for SAH, and modern-day (3rd-generation or better) CT will detect SAH in approximately >97% of cases if scanned within 6 hours of symptom onset. Lumbar puncture should be performed in cases where SAH is suspected and CT is negative, especially if presenting >6 hours after onset of headache. Xanthochromia is a helpful sign of old blood products in the CSF, but it takes at least 4 hours to develop. Detection of the breakdown of blood products in the CSF is best performed with spectrophotometry if available. Angiography should be performed urgently if SAH is confirmed. A small proportion of SAH cases will have normal angiography. Follow-up imaging is needed in most cases, and attention should be given to base-of-skull arteriovenous fistulas and aneurysms compressed by hematoma. MR or CTA may also reveal aneurysms and may help with surgical planning. With improved surgical and anesthetic techniques, early aneurysm localization with angiography, early definitive aneurysm repair, and modern critical care management have greatly improved outcome.

3. **Subsequent evaluation.** Conventional cerebral angiography remains the gold standard for documenting vasospasm; however, it is invasive and carries some risk. **Vasospasm** may develop at any time, but is most frequent between days 4 and 14 post rupture. Many centers perform **serial transcranial Doppler ultrasound** to detect presymptomatic narrowing of cerebral vessels at the base of the brain as reflected in elevated flow velocities, especially when normalized to the extracranial parent vessel flow velocity (i.e., Lindegaard ratio). Risk of clinically significant vasospasm can be predicted by classifying the presence of focal collections of blood on the CT scan in the area around the circle of Willis arteries (modified Fisher groups 1–4; see **Table 30.4**). There is a growing interest in continuous EEG monitoring in patients with aneurysmal subarachnoid hemorrhage, both to detect subclinical or subtle seizures and in the detection of vasospasm. As a patient develops vasospasm, a shift toward more power in the slower frequencies occurs (i.e., less alpha [8–12 Hz], more delta [0–4 Hz]; or a decrease in the alpha/delta ratio).

4. **Acute treatment** consists of definitive obliteration of the culprit aneurysm (clipping or endovascular therapy) and prevention of delayed ischemic deficits. Systolic arterial blood pressure should be strictly controlled with short-acting IV agents such as labetalol or titratable infusions such as nicardipine (at least <160 mmHg is reasonable according to the AHA/ASA 2012 guidelines, many centers aim for a lower SBP goal) until the aneurysm is secured. There is a dearth of evidence for specific BP goals and the risk of acutely lowering SBP further should be based on institutional clinical care pathways and balancing the risk of stroke, hypertension-related bleeding, and maintaining cerebral perfusion pressure. Surgery, endovascular therapy, or both are performed urgently; intervention choice is based on aneurysm location, anatomy, patient comorbidities, surgical and endovascular risk, and operator experience. A calcium-channel antagonist, **nimodipine,** 60 mg orally every 4 hours given for 21 days, improves neurologic outcomes after aneurysmal SAH and is considered the standard of care. If vasospasm after aneurysmal subarachnoid hemorrhage occurs, therapy is focused on maximizing cerebral blood flow and oxygen delivery to minimize the clinical sequelae of vasospasm. This is generally accomplished by creating a hyperdynamic state with induced hypertension, maintaining euvolemia, and optimal oxygen-carrying capacity. Release of natriuretic

factors causes **cerebral salt wasting** and subsequent volume loss, with resultant serum hypo-osmolarity and urine hyperosmolarity. The **treatment for cerebral salt wasting is volume repletion** with IV saline, either normal saline (0.9%) or **hypertonic saline** solutions. Volume restriction, which would normally be appropriate for syndrome of inappropriate antidiuretic hormone secretion (SIADH), should be avoided because it leads rapidly to hypovolemia, hypotension, and decreased blood flow distal to areas of vasospasm. Oral NaCl tablets and mineralocorticoid administration (**fludrocortisone,** 0.1 mg orally twice a day) may also be useful. **Albumin** (250 mL of 5% albumin) is often used in addition to normal saline (or other isotonic fluids) to maintain euvolemia. The exact transfusion threshold with patients with aneurysmal subarachnoid and cerebral vasospasm is not known; the intention is to support an optimal balance of oxygen-carrying capacity and blood viscosity in areas with compromised cerebral perfusion yet minimizing the risks and potential harms of the transfusion of packed red blood cells. Induced hypertension with an α-adrenergic agonist such as **phenylephrine** is safe and effective at reversing ischemic symptoms due to decreased cerebral blood flow in patients with vasospasm. The hyper-catecholaminergic state following SAH can trigger the development of a stunned myocardium (e.g., Takotsubo cardiomyopathy) and acute heart failure; this condition, although usually fully reversible, can result in several days of marked global cardiac hypokinesis. When combined with the need for induced hypertension, this requires in some patients invasive hemodynamic monitoring and inotropic support with agents such as **norepinephrine** or **dobutamine.** In refractory vasospasm or in patients who cannot tolerate induced hypertension, intra-arterial vasodilators such as **verapamil** or **nicardipine** or the use of **balloon angioplasty** may alleviate cerebral ischemia. In spite of an increased risk for complications, they have become a mainstay of therapy because of their ability to reduce major ischemic events. Newer multimodal intracerebral monitors (including brain tissue oxygenation, regional cerebral blood flow monitors, and cerebral microdialysis catheters) may provide early warning signs of vasospasm and help to guide appropriate therapy. Evidence for prophylactic anticonvulsant therapy is limited and may be associated with potential adverse effects, but it may be helpful in immediate period after aneurysmal subarachnoid hemorrhage, especially when a seizure with the associated increase in systemic blood pressure and intracranial pressure could be catastrophic (i.e., prior to the aneurysm being secured and/or in the setting of elevated intracranial pressures). No benefit from corticosteroids has been demonstrated in patients with SAH.

II. **SEIZURES** occur in more than 10% of patients during their ICU stay. Repeated tonic-clonic seizures are easily recognized and must be treated early; uncontrolled generalized motor seizures that persist for >60 minutes are associated with neuronal injury and mortality. Conversely, nonconvulsive seizures can easily go unrecognized; up to 8% of comatose patients *with no outward signs of seizures* have been found to have ongoing nonconvulsive seizures. While single seizures should prompt a search for etiology and correction of inciting conditions and/or seizure prophylaxis, **status epilepticus** (continuous seizures lasting longer than 5 minutes, or more than one seizure without restoration of appropriate mental status) is a medical emergency. Table 30.5 summarizes common causes of seizures in the ICU.

	Common Etiologies of Seizures in the Intensive Care Unit

Neurologic Pathology
- Neurovascular: ischemic or hemorrhagic stroke, vascular malformation
- Tumor: primary or metastatic
- Infection: abscess, meningitis, encephalitis
- Inflammatory disease: vasculitis, acute disseminated encephalomyelitis (ADEM)
- Trauma
- Primary epilepsy
- Inherited central nervous system metabolic disturbance

Complications of Critical Illness
- Hypoxia
- Drug toxicity
- Drug withdrawal: anticonvulsants, barbiturates, benzodiazepines, alcohol
- Fever (febrile seizure)
- Infection
- Metabolic abnormalities: hyponatremia, hypocalcemia, hypophosphatemia, hypoglycemia, renal or hepatic dysfunction
- Surgical manipulation: craniotomy

Adapted from *J Neurosurg Anesthesiol* 2001;13:163–175.

A. **Clinical Syndrome.** Seizures may be categorized into multiple subtypes. The most relevant in the ICU are generalized tonic-clonic, complex partial, and an unremitting form of either (status epilepticus). In **generalized tonic-clonic seizures,** patients present with stiffening (tonic phase), followed by limb jerking (clonic phase) and impaired consciousness, often with hyperdynamic vital signs. Seizures with subtle motor manifestations can go unrecognized in critically ill patients, though careful observation of a patient may reveal subtle rhythmic limb or facial movements indicative of seizure activity. **Complex partial seizures** produce a decrease in responsiveness without a complete loss of consciousness. They may be accompanied by automatisms (e.g., chewing, blinking, swallowing), but not rhythmic limb jerking.

B. **Differential Diagnosis.** Conditions mimicking seizures include benign entities (myoclonus, fasciculations, tremor, spasticity) and potentially dangerous entities (brainstem ischemia, metabolic encephalopathy, rigors). Sudden onset of bilateral arm and leg posturing coupled with impaired eye movements can be seen in acute basilar artery occlusion. Neurologic consultation and electroencephalogram (EEG) should be requested if the diagnosis is in question.

C. **Acute Evaluation of Seizures** consists of confirming the diagnosis and identifying potential causes. In many cases, EEG is not required for diagnosis, due to obvious motor signs. All patients should undergo laboratory screening tests including CBC, electrolytes, blood urea nitrogen (BUN), creatinine, glucose, Ca, Mg, PO_4, liver function tests (including NH_3), blood and urine toxicology screen, and when indicated, anticonvulsant medications levels, pregnancy test, and arterial blood gases. Once seizures are controlled, brain imaging (CT or MRI) and lumbar puncture may be needed to establish the underlying etiology. Physical exam should assess for signs of occult head trauma, substance abuse or withdrawal, fever, meningismus, and diabetes. Long-acting muscle relaxants or paralytics in the absence of EEG monitoring have **no role** in the initial management of uncontrolled seizures, except in patients who cannot otherwise be adequately ventilated.

D. **EEG** is used both for diagnosis (determining whether unusual movements or poor mental status are due to seizures) and monitoring (for patients having frequent, subtle, or subclinical seizures). EEG patterns commonly seen in critically ill patients and the medical conditions associated with these patterns are shown in Figure 30.5. Of note, many EEG patterns seen in critically ill patients fall on an "ictal–interictal continuum," and there is often no clear dividing line between seizures (ictal) or less injurious (interictal) phenomena (*J Clin Neurophysiol* 2005;22:79–91). A benzodiazepine trial may be helpful in these cases (see Table 30.6).

E. **Long-Term EEG Monitoring** should be considered in critically ill patients with unexplained alterations in level of consciousness or fluctuating neurological exam with unclear etiology, to rule out ongoing subclinical seizures. How long to monitor depends on the risk of developing subsequent seizures, which can be stratified on the basis of whether epileptiform abnormalities are present in the first 30 minutes of EEG recording. In critically ill patients *with* epileptiform abnormalities, the probability of seizures within 72 hours falls below 10% and 5% if the patient remains seizure-free for 7 hours and 16 hours of monitoring, respectively. In patients *without* epileptiform abnormalities, the probability of seizures within 72 hours falls below 10% and 5% if the patient remains seizure-free for 15 minutes and 2 hours, respectively (*Clin Neurophysiol* 2015;126(3):463–471).

F. **Acute Treatment of Seizures** consists in safely aborting seizures as early as possible with the appropriate degree of intervention. Most patients require no intervention and will spontaneously recover after one seizure. Other patients may require a benzodiazepine or intravenous anticonvulsant medication to terminate seizures. Loading doses, maintenance doses, and therapeutic serum levels for **intravenous anticonvulsants** can be found in Figure 30.6. In patients presenting with generalized convulsive status epilepticus, management with a predefined protocol is the best way to ensure prompt and adequate treatment. Diagnosis of convulsive and nonconvulsive status epilepticus is outlined in Table 30.6. A suggested protocol for treatment of generalized convulsive status epilepticus is shown in Figure 30.6.

III. ENCEPHALOPATHY

A. **Toxic-Metabolic** injury to the CNS is a frequent and reversible cause of impaired cognition in the ICU, but always remains a diagnosis of exclusion. Frequent causes include medication effects; perturbations in electrolyte, water, glucose, or urea homeostasis; acute renal or hepatic failure; sleep disturbances; and psychiatric disturbances. Treatment is supportive, with removal of the offending agent when possible. Hyperammonemia with or without signs of liver abnormality can cause profound encephalopathy and increased ICP and may respond to oral **lactulose** and reduction of nitrogen (protein) intake. Wernicke's encephalopathy, secondary to thiamine deficiency (usually in alcoholics, occasionally in persons on severe diet regimens or other rapid reductions in nutrition), presents with ataxia, eye movement paralysis, nystagmus, apathy, or confusion. Treatment consists of **thiamine** 100 mg IV, which should be continued daily for at least 5 days.

B. **Hypertensive Encephalopathy** is due to sustained, severe hypertension or relative hypertension with impaired autoregulation. Early, reversible

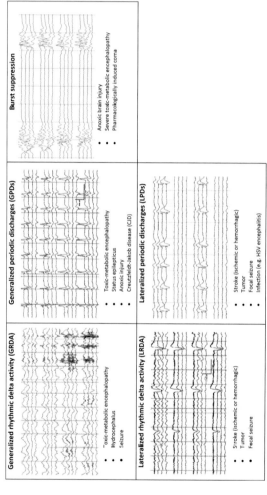

Generalized rhythmic delta activity (GRDA)

- Toxic-metabolic encephalopathy
- Hydrocephalus
- Seizure

Generalized periodic discharges (GPDs)

- Toxic-metabolic encephalopathy
- Status epilepticus
- Anoxic injury
- Creutzfeldt-Jakob disease (CJD)

Burst suppression

- Anoxic brain injury
- Severe toxic-metabolic encephalopathy
- Pharmacologically induced coma

Lateralized rhythmic delta activity (LRDA)

- Stroke (ischemic or hemorrhagic)
- Tumor
- Focal seizure

Lateralized periodic discharges (LPDs)

- Stroke (ischemic or hemorrhagic)
- Tumor
- Focal seizure
- Infection (e.g. HSV encephalitis)

FIGURE 30.5 EEG patterns and their associated conditions in the ICU.

TABLE 30.6 Diagnosis of Convulsive and Nonconvulsive Status Epilepticus

1) Generalized convulsive status epilepticus

Continuous convulsive seizure activity lasting >5 min

OR, ≥2 convulsive seizures without full return to baseline between seizures

2) Nonconvulsive status epilepticus (NCSE)

> **2a)** NCSE by strict electrographic criteria[a]
>
> An EEG pattern lasting ≥10 seconds and satisfying either of the following qualifies as an electrographic seizure[b]:
>
>> 1) Repetitive generalized or focal spikes, sharp-waves, spike-&-wave, or sharp-&-slow wave complexes at **≥3 Hz**.
>> 2) Sequential rhythmic, periodic, or quasiperiodic waves at **≥1 Hz** and unequivocal *evolution* in frequency (gradually increases/decreases by ≥1 Hz), morphology, or location (gradual spread into or out of a region involving two or more electrodes). Evolution in amplitude alone or in sharpness without other change in morphology is not enough to satisfy evolution in morphology.
>
> **2b)** NCSE by electroclinical or electroradiologic criteria
>
> Rhythmic/periodic EEG activity without evolution and with at least one of the following qualifies as NCSE:
>
>> 1) Benzodiazepine trial (see below) demonstrating electrographic or clinical improvement
>> 2) Clear correlation between rhythmic/periodic EEG activity and clinical symptoms
>> 3) CT-PET or MRI neuroimaging showing a pattern of hypermetabolism or diffusion restriction not clinically explained by another inflammatory or ischemic processes.

Benzodiazepine Trial[c]

Indication: rhythmic or periodic epileptiform discharges on EEG with concurrent neurological impairment

Monitoring required: EEG, pulse ox, blood pressure, EKG, respiratory rate with dedicated nurse

Give sequential small doses of rapidly acting, short-duration benzodiazepine (e.g., midazolam at 1 mg/dose) or a nonsedating IV anticonvulsant (e.g., levetiracetam, valproic acid, fosphenytoin, lacosamide). Between doses, repeat clinical and EEG assessment. Trial is stopped for any of the following:

> 1) Persistent resolution of the EEG pattern (and examination repeated)
> 2) Definite clinical improvement
> 3) Respiratory depression, hypotension, or other adverse effect
> 4) Maximum allowed dose is reached (e.g., 0.2 mg/kg midazolam)

Interpretation: POSITIVE test (i.e., seizure) if the ictal EEG pattern resolves and there is improvement in the patient's clinical state and/or appearance of previously absent normal EEG patterns (e.g., return of posterior dominant rhythm). EQUIVOCAL test if the ictal EEG pattern improves but the patient does not.

---

[a]Adapted from J Clin Neurophysiol 2005;22:79–91.
[b]Intracranial EEG may increase sensitivity of detecting electrographic seizures
(*Ann Neurol* 2014;75(5):771–778).
[c]Adapted from *Clin Neurophys* 2007;118:1660–1670.

ANTI-CONVULSANT THERAPY

CONCURRENT MANAGEMENT

STATUS EPILEPTICUS

1st line (seizures ongoing for 5–10 mins)

Lorazepam 4mg IV (push over 2 mins),
If seizures not controlled within 5 mins, repeat 4 mg IV × 1

If no IV access:
Diazepam 20 mg rectally (using IV solution)
or, **Midazolam** 10 mg intranasal/buccal/IM
(using IV solution).

1) Airway, Breathing, Circulation
2) Vital signs (cont. monitoring): HR, BP, O2, EKG
3) Finger stick blood glucose
   If glucose low or unknown: give thiamine 100mg IV,
   then D50 (50 mL IV)
4) Obtain IV access (≥2 IVs)
5) If febrile, treat w/ anti-pyretics, cooling, consider antibiotics
6) Labs: CBC, BMP, Ca, Mg, Phos, LFTs, troponin, ABG,
   tox screen (blood & urine), blood cultures (especially
   if febrile), AED levels (in patients w/ prior history of
   epilepsy), HCG (females)

If seizures persist

2nd line (10–30 mins)

Choose from the following (may be used in combination):
1) **Valproic acid** 40 mg/kg IV (max rate 6 mg/kg/min)
2) **Levetiracetam** 20 mg/kg IV (max rate 100 mg/min)
3) **Phenobarbital** 20 mg/kg IV (max rate 50–75 mg/min)
4) **Fosphenytoin** 20 mg PE/kg IV (max rate 150 mg/min PE/min)
   or, **Phenytoin** 20 mg/kg IV (max rate 25–50 mg/min)
   If no effect, can give additional dose:
   Fosphenytoin 10 mg PE/kg IV or Phenytoin 10 mg/kg IV
5) **Lacosamide** 400 mg IV over 5 min (need EKG pre/post)

Check anti-convulsant levels post-load and re-bolus if needed
(see box below for therapeutic levels):
   Phenytoin, valproic acid, phenobarbital - send level
   1 hr after load
   Fosphenytoin - send level 2 hrs after load

If seizures persist - - - - → INTUBATE.
Start continuous EEG monitoring

REFRACTORY STATUS EPILEPTICUS

3rd line (30–60 mins)

Choose from the following (may be used in combination):
1) **Midazolam** (good choice if BP unstable)
   Load 0.2 mg/kg IV.
   Repeat q5mins until seizures stop (max load 2 mg/kg)
   Maintenance infusion 0.1–2 mg/kg/hr
2) **Propofol**
   Load 2 mg/kg IV.
   Repeat q5mins until seizures stop (max load 10 mg/kg)
   Maintenance infusion 1–10 mg/kg/hr
   (<5 if treating for >48 hrs)

Titrate infusion to stop seizures or induce burst suppression (currently
no evidence to guide best depth / duration of suppression).

Use IV fluids and pressors to support BP (anesthetic doses required to tx
refractory SE are much higher than doses used for routine sedation).

Once seizure-free for >24–48 hrs, start slow taper of 3rd line meds over
24 hrs, while maintaining high therapeutic levels of AEDs to avoid
recurrent seizures. Continue EEG monitoring until seizure-free off 3rd line
meds for >24 hrs, to monitor for recurrence of non-convulsive seizures or
NCSE.

Continue maintenance anti-convulsants. Adjust doses for
therapeutic level:

MAINTENANCE DOSES	THERAPEUTIC LEVELS
1) **Valproic acid** 30–60 mg/kg/day (BID)	70–120 µg/mL
2) **Levetiracetam** 2–4 g/day (BID)	25–60 mg/L
3) **Phenobarbital** 1–4mg/kg/day (BID)	20–50 mg/L
4) **Fosphenytoin** 5–7 PE/kg/day (TID)	15–25 µg/mL* (total),
	1.5–2.5 µg/mL (free)
or, **Phenytoin** 5–7 mg/kg/day (TID)	"
5) **Lacosamide** 400–600 mg/day (BID)	Unknown

* Total dilantin level should be corrected for patient's renal function and albumin:
http://www.mdcalc.com/phenytoin-dilantin-correction-for-albumin-or-renal-failure/
If there is signifcant renal dysfunction or hypoalbuminemia, check a free dilantin
level.

Continue workup to determine underlying cause of SE
1) Neuroimaging - brain MRI (preferred) or head CT
2) Lumbar puncture – eval for infection, inflammatory,
   autoimmune causes

SUPER-REFRACTORY STATUS EPILEPTICUS

4th line (>72 hrs)

Choose from the following (may be used in combination):
1) Repeat burst suppression for 24–48 hrs
2) Add other AEDs (also consider carbamazepine, topiramate)
3) IV magnesium (bolus 4 g, then infuse 2–6 g/hr)
4) Ketamine
   Load w/ 1.5 mg/kg IV.
   Repeat q5mins until seizures stop (max load 4.5 mg/kg)
   Maintenance infusion at 1.2–7.5 mg/kg/hr
5) Pentobarbital (titrate to burst suppression)
   Load 5 mg/kg IV.(max rate 50 mg/min)
   Repeat q5mins until szs stop (max load 15 mg/kg)
   Maintenance infusion 1–10 mg/kg/hr
6) IV pyridoxine (200 mg/day)
7) Immune modulation
   Steroids (methylprednisolone 1g IV qd × 3–5 days)
   and/or IVIG (0.4 g/kg/day × 5 days)
   and/or plasma exchange (every other day × 5–7 days)
7) Ketogenic diet
8) Therapeutic hypothermia
9) Electroconvulsive therapy (ECT)
10) Neurosurgical treatment (eg, resection of focal lesion)
11) TMS

No strong evidence to guide best treatment here.

Treat underlying cause of status epilepticus.

FIGURE 30.6 Treatment protocol for generalized convulsive status epilepticus.

symptoms are likely due to blood–brain barrier disruption and vasogenic edema. With sustained hypertension, cerebral hemorrhage and irreversible injury may occur. Because acute elevations in blood pressure are commonly seen in many types of brain injury in which antihypertensive therapy could be deleterious (e.g., ischemic stroke, traumatic brain injury), accurate diagnosis is essential. Clinical manifestations range from headache and visual scotoma to confusion, seizures, and coma. The likelihood of recovery depends on the extent of injury prior to treatment. **Head CT** is insensitive and may reveal bilateral posterior predominant subcortical hypodensity. **MRI** reveals T2 and apparent diffusion coefficient hyperintensity with a posterior predilection, which may also involve diffuse subcortical white matter, cortical gray matter, and the cerebellum; gradient-echo sequences often reveal microscopic petechial hemorrhages. Management of hypertensive crisis is outlined in **Chapter 10**. Most patients with hypertensive encephalopathy have underlying chronic hypertension. This shifts upward the range of pressures at which cerebrovascular autoregulation occurs.

C. Infectious/Inflammatory

1. The most treatable **viral encephalitis** (and second most common after HIV) is acute **herpes simplex** infection. Patients present with headache, fever, seizure, or cognitive impairments. Early in the course, CSF shows a lymphocytosis (5–500 cells/mm^3) with normal glucose and mild increase in protein. Later, hemorrhagic necrosis is seen, with bloody CSF. The EEG often shows lateralized periodic discharges and MRI reveals temporal and inferior frontal lobe involvement. CSF polymerase chain reaction (PCR) is extremely sensitive, although false negatives can occur, especially in the first 72 hours, or in the setting of very high CSF leukocytosis. Therapy with **acyclovir** (10 mg/kg every 8 hours based on ideal body weight) reduces mortality and morbidity and should be instituted in any suspected case. Other forms of viral encephalitis, including those due to human herpes viruses 6 and 7, Epstein–Barr virus, cytomegalovirus, and varicella zoster virus, may respond to specific antiviral treatments. Encephalitis due to arboviruses (arthropod-borne viruses) such as eastern equine, California, and St. Louis encephalitis, do not respond to acyclovir but can present in a similar manner. West Nile encephalitis commonly presents with paraparesis in addition to headache, fever, and encephalopathy. Vasogenic edema, seizures, and increased ICP may occur in all of these disorders, and patients require close monitoring in an ICU setting.

2. **Bacterial meningitis** must be diagnosed and treated rapidly, although in the early hours it may be clinically indistinguishable from viral meningoencephalitis. Acute onset of headache, meningeal signs (neck stiffness, photophobia), fever, and altered sensorium should suggest the diagnosis of acute bacterial meningitis. Etiology, diagnosis, and treatment of meningitis are outlined in Chapter 28.

3. **Acute disseminated encephalomyelitis (ADEM) and acute hemorrhagic leukoencephalitis (AHL).** Often preceded by a routine viral illness or mycoplasma pneumonia, these infections present with cerebral demyelination (ADEM) or hemorrhage (AHL) and **malignant cerebral edema**. Initial presentations have variable localizing signs, but encephalopathy, stupor, and coma ensue rapidly. Early brain MR can reveal characteristic demyelination, edema, and/or widespread petechial hemorrhage, with markedly increased CSF protein. High-dose IV **methylprednisolone** and supportive care should be provided. ADEM has a better prognosis than AHL.

4. **Other infectious agents and inflammatory conditions.** Granulomatous diseases such as sarcoidosis as well as fungal, mycobacterial, and protein infectious (prion) agents can also affect the CNS and lead to encephalopathy. Characteristic imaging or CSF analysis may be helpful, but tissue biopsy is often required to diagnose these uncommon etiologies.

Selected Readings

Chong DJ, Hirsch LJ. Which EEG patterns warrant treatment in the critically ill? Reviewing the evidence for treatment of periodic epileptiform discharges and related patterns. *J Clin Neurophysiol* 2005;22(2):79–91.

Connolly ES Jr, Rabinstein AA, Carhuapoma JR, et al. Guidelines for the management of aneurysmal subarachnoid hemorrhage. *Stroke* 2012;43:1711–1737.

Jauch EC, Saver JL, Adams HP Jr, et al. Guidelines for the early management of patients with acute ischemic stroke. *Stroke* 2013;44:870–947.

Jirsch J, Hirsch LJ. Nonconvulsive seizures: developing a rational approach to the diagnosis and management in the critically ill population. *Clin Neurophysiol* 2007;118(8):1660–1670.

Kernan WN, Ovbiagele B, Black HR, et al. Guidelines for the prevention of stroke in patients with stroke and transient ischemic attack. *Stroke* 2014;45:2160–2236.

Morgenstern LB, Hemphill JC, Anderson C, et al. Guidelines for the management of spontaneous intracerebral hemorrhage: a guideline for healthcare professionals from the American Heart Association/American Stroke Association. *Stroke* 2010;41:2108–2129.

Varelas PN, Mirski MA. Seizures in the adult intensive care unit. *J Neurosurg Anesthesiol* 2001;13(2):163–175.

Westover MB, Shafi MM, Bianchi MT, et al. The probability of seizures during EEG monitoring in critically ill adults. *Clin Neurophysiol* 2015;126(3):463–471.

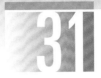

Acute Weakness

Sanjay Menon and Karen Waak

There are a myriad of causes that can lead to acute weakness in a patient in the intensive care unit. These include diseases affecting the central nervous system (CNS), the peripheral nervous system (PNS), the neuromuscular junction (NMJ), and the muscles (myopathic disorders). Other etiologic causes include effects of drugs/medication and injuries. Careful consideration hereof is crucial to reach a diagnosis with the aid of a full laboratory assessment along with specific testing such as lumbar puncture, electrophysiological studies (EMG/ENG), chest computed tomography (CT), and the like as warranted.

I. CNS CAUSES

A. Stroke
Patients being treated in a (nonneurological) intensive care unit can present with an acute muscle weakness caused by an ischemic or hemorrhagic stroke. Signs of lateralization and other focal neurological deficits ought to be recognized. Imaging of the brain with CT and/or magnetic resonance imaging (MRI) should be performed as soon as possible to assess the situation (hemorrhage, acute ischemic stroke), and to consider specific treatment (e.g., external ventricular drain, intravenous tPA, mechanical recanalization) when warranted.

B. Infection
Infections (meningitis or meningoencephalitis) and abscesses of the CNS are further causes that could lead to an acute muscle weakness in an intensive care unit (ICU) patient, which could typically go along with high fever, confusion, and focal defects like seizures. Careful evaluation of the serum lab work, cerebrospinal fluid (CSF) studies, and brain imaging is required to reach a diagnosis. Treatment will be goal directed (antibiotics, antiviral meds, surgical treatment for abscesses).

C. Central Pontine Myelinolysis
A progressive tetraparesis along with a decreased level of consciousness and brainstem dysfunctions (dysphagia, complexe III nerve palsy, weakness of respiratory muscles) should prompt the clinician to think of too rapid over- or undercorrection of serum sodium levels leading to central pontine myelinolysis. This osmotic demyelating disease occurs mainly in the pons and is supposed to happen because of dehydration of brain cells in the setting of a too rapid shift of water from the tissue; the exact mechanism is unclear. Extrapontine myelinolysis would include locations such as the cerebellum, basal ganglia, corpus callosum, and internal capsule. MRI would confirm the diagnosis. There is no specific treatment.

II. PNS CAUSES
A variety of conditions impacting the peripheral nervous system can lead to weakness, with the impact ranging from mild and isolated, to broad and severe. Patients with fractures should be screened for any associated nerve impairment. Compression injuries to peripheral nerves may result from

suboptimal patient positioning during surgery or periods of prolonged bed-rest. Many acquired polyneuropathies such as those resulting from vascular disease, diabetes, or alcohol use occur over time and thus do not typically present as an acute loss of strength. However, it is important to consider such conditions in the weak ICU patient who cannot provide a functional history. Infections, toxins, endocrine disorders, and vitamin B12 deficiency can also lead to polyneuropathy.

A. **Guillain-Barré Syndrome.** Guillain-Barré syndrome (GBS) describes a syndrome of acute, immune-mediated, inflammatory polyneuropathies that consist of several different forms. GBS is typically preceded by an infection or illness and is characterized by widespread, patchy areas of peripheral nerve demyelination that translates into weakness and paralysis. Acute inflammatory demyelinating polyneuropathy (AIDP) is interchangeably used with GBS. Variant forms of GBS including Miller Fisher syndrome (MFS), acute motor axonal neuropathy, and acute sensorimotor axonal neuropathy are less frequently seen in the US. Clinical presentation includes migrating, symmetrical paralysis, typically starting in the legs with absent or diminished deep tendon reflexes. Patients with MFS present with ophthalmoplegia, ataxia, and areflexia. Paresthesias and neuropathic pain are common. Symptoms usually progress over a 2-to-3-week period before reaching a nadir, followed by subsequent improvement. Degree of weakness can vary from mild to severe with complete paralysis. Approximately 25% to 30% of patients will have sufficient involvement of the respiratory muscles to require mechanical ventilation. Autonomic dysfunction including dysrhythmias, hypotension, and hypertension is common and may be fatal; thus, close monitoring is warranted.

  1. Diagnosis is based on clinical exam and confirmed with analysis of CSF and electrophysiology studies. Treatment in the acute phase includes supportive care with particular attention to the respiratory and cardio-vascular systems. Response to intravenous vasoactive drugs is often ex-aggerated and thus should be used with caution. Rehabilitation in the acute phase includes a focus on preventing secondary complications and initiating gentle active exercises, titrating to patient response. More intense rehabilitation is often indicated after the acute phase to restore function. Specific therapies to treat GBS include plasma ex-change and IV immunoglobulin (IVIG); treatment with either plasma exchange or IVIG is associated with improved recovery and expedited time to independent ambulation. Remyelination and functional re-covery occur over a period of weeks to months. Approximately 80% of patients return to independent ambulation by 6 months; 5% to 10% of patients have delayed and/or incomplete recovery. Relapses occur in approximately 7% of patients and are generally treated with the initial regimen. Deterioration after initial improvement and stabilization, or prolongation of symptoms beyond 8 weeks may indicate the presence of chronic inflammatory demyelinating polyneuropathy (CIDP).

B. **Critical Illness Polyneuropathy**

Critical illness polyneuropathy (CIP) is a sensorimotor neuropathy char-acterized by distal axonal degeneration. CIP frequently coexists with criti-cal illness myopathy (see later in chapter). Clinically, these two conditions can be difficult to distinguish, and it is not always necessary to do so. The alternative term "ICU-acquired weakness" (ICU-AW) is used extensively in the literature to describe more broadly weakness detected on clinical exam that develops as a *function of* critical illness, including both CIP and CIM. ICU-AW is common in critical illness, affecting 25% to 85% of patients, with increasing incidence in those with sepsis and multiorgan failure. The specific etiology of CIP is multifactorial, with inflammation, impaired perfusion, and altered permeability all potentially contributing. Typically CIP becomes apparent as the patient regains arousal and is noted to have profound weakness with inability to wean from the ventilator. It is characterized by flaccid, usually symmetrical weakness and diminished sensation with diminished or absent reflexes. Lower extremities may be more affected than upper extremities, and distal muscle groups more than proximal. Facial muscles are often spared; therefore, it is important to include assessment of facial movements when determining command following. Muscle atrophy will be present.

1. Formal diagnosis of CIP requires electrophysiology testing. Nerve conduction studies (NCS) will show evidence of a sensorimotor *axonal* neuropathy including decreased amplitude of compound motor and sensory action potentials, with absence of conduction block. Needle electromyography (EMG) will demonstrate resting fibrillation potentials. Bedside manual muscle testing procedures in cooperative patients will often provide adequate support for the diagnosis of "ICUAW" once other causes are ruled out (see Table 31.1). Electrophysiology studies should be considered in cases where a patient cannot be accurately examined at the bedside, and/or where weakness does not show improvement with time.

2. Strategies to prevent or minimize the development of ICU-acquired weakness should be incorporated into clinical practice as feasible. While robust, cause-effect evidence is limited, associations have been found among several critical care variables and ICU-AW and CIP. In particular, immobility contributes directly to muscle atrophy, and thus it is key to integrate exercise and mobilization into patient care as early as clinically appropriate. Early mobility pathways or algorithms can be helpful in facilitating safe, targeted, incremental activity in critically ill patients (see Fig. 31.1). Regular screening for participation in spontaneous awakening trials is encouraged in order to minimize oversedation, which in turn perpetuates immobilization. Similarly, when clinically acceptable, it is important to enable spontaneous breathing to facilitate diaphragm activation in order to minimize diaphragmatic atrophy.

   a. Prevention efforts may also include aggressive management of sepsis to minimize systemic inflammation and oxidative stress, as these conditions appear linked to ICU-AW and CIP. Consider early nutrition when appropriate to help mediate muscle catabolism. There is some evidence to show that intensive insulin therapy reduces the incidence of CIP; however, because other potential risks exist with this practice, it cannot be broadly recommended. The association between use of neuromuscular blocking agents (NMBA) and development of ICU-AW is not clear-cut. While NMBA have an apparent role in the management of select conditions (e.g., severe ARDS), it is probably wise to avoid prolonged use when possible.

3. Once present, treatment of ICU-AW and CIP ought to include the aforementioned considerations, as well as good supportive care and rehabilitation. Prognosis for recovery with CIP is variable and can be prolonged. CIP is associated with increased length of stay, time on the ventilator, mortality, and reduced functional outcomes. While most patients gradually recover over weeks to months, evidence suggests that a sizable portion of patients are not fully recovered at 1 year, particularly those with severe involvement.

	Right	Left
Abduction of the shoulder		
Flexion of the elbow		
Extension of the wrist		
Flexion of the hip		
Extension of the knee		
Dorsal flexion of the foot		

Sum Score (max 60): Test the six muscle groups listed above, bilaterally in sufficiently alert and attentive patients. Grade each muscle on score of 0–5. All grades can be combined for a "sum-score" out of 60. Sum-scores ≤48 may be associated with ICU-acquired weakness.

MRC strength grading scale: 0, no muscular contraction; 1, trace or flicker of contraction; 2, active movement with gravity eliminated; 3, active movement against gravity; 4, active movement against gravity and some resistance; 5, active movement against gravity and full resistance.

III. NEUROMUSCULAR JUNCTION DISORDERS

There are different etiologies for neuromuscular junction disorders (NMJD) discussed in the literature whereby myasthenia gravis (MG), belonging to the autoimmune category, is the most common form. Other causes are congenital or toxic (e.g., botulism).

A. Myasthenia Gravis

MG is a disease that interferes with the transmission of acetylcholine at the neuromuscular junction, leading to proximal muscle weakness and fatigue. In the majority of cases, it is caused through the binding of circulating autoantibodies to postsynaptic nicotinic ACh receptors. This in turn prevents acetylcholine, the neurotransmitter that is responsible for muscle contraction at the motor end plate, from connecting to its receptor. There is a generalized, an ocular, and a paraneoplastic variant of MG. The above-mentioned autoantibodies can be found in about 80% of those with the generalized form of MG. In about 10% of the MG patients, a thymoma can be detected, which goes along with anti-titin-antibodies.

1. The lead symptom of MG is general fatigue associated with a progressive proximal muscle weakness, especially upon activity and improving with rest. There is a typical progression during the course of the day, with a peak weakness during the evening hours. Facial, oropharyngeal, ocular, and neck muscles are as susceptible as skeletal muscles. Ocular involvement with diplopia and ptosis is frequently the initial sign. Further symptoms include dysarthria and dysphagia with severe cases affecting the respiratory muscles as well. *Myasthenic* crisis is a life-threatening condition with respiratory failure and aspiration that develops usually over days, rarely acutely. It is caused by infections, errors in intake of medication, and insufficient immunosuppression. Intensive care support and plasma exchange or IVIG are vital in these cases. Despite these measures, the mortality can be still as high as 5%.

2. A *cholinergic* crisis can present clinically in a similar fashion to the myasthenic crisis with flaccid paralysis; however, the underlying pathophysiology, and thus the therapy, is very different. Treatment with excess doses of cholinesterase inhibitors can lead to a cholinergic crisis by nonresponsiveness of ACh-receptors to abundant acetylcholine. Applying edrophonium (an ACh-esterase inhibitor) can distinguish both

	No activity	Phase 1: In bed; PROM/ Upright in bed	Phase 2: Sitting (Edge of bed or chair)	Phase 3: Standing	Phase 4: Ambulation
Criteria for Phase 1	a) Stable spine b) No excessive predicted mortality within the next 24 hrs c) ICP <20 cmH$_2$O				
Criteria for Phase 2		a) Follows 1-step commands b) Volitional movement present c) No SCI, no open lumbar drains, no open EVD's; no femoral-vein access for CVVH			
Criteria for Phase 3			a) ≥3/5 bilateral quadriceps strength b) Sits, no support c) No WB restrictions d) Grip strength >5 kg		
Criteria for Phase 4				a) Stands × 3 repetitions with minimal assist b) Steps-in-place with minimal assist	
Cardiovascular	Attempt to maintain blood pressure and heart rate in target range **_DURING_** mobilization: consider administration of vasopressors, volume, vasodilators, pain medication, etc as indicated. If not successful in stabilizing hemodynamics, then do not progress phases.				

FIGURE 31.1 Example of an early mobility pathway, the SICU Optimal Mobility Scale (SOMS).

forms of crises by worsening the cholinergic crisis and by improving the symptoms of a myasthenic crisis. There is no specific treatment for cholinergic crisis other than discontinuing the responsible agents and applying supportive measures like intubation and mechanical ventilation. Atropine, a blocking agent at the muscarinergic ACh receptor, has only limited impact on the muscle weakness component, which is triggered through nicotinergic acetylcholine receptors. Several medications can exacerbate symptoms of MG (Table 31.2).

3. A thorough history and a physical examination, especially with focus on the muscle groups, are essential. If MG is suspected with symptoms that can be objectified (important!) a pharmacological testing with neostigmine, edrophonium, or pyridostigmine with atropine at the bedside should be carried out to look for improvement of muscle strength, which occurs rapidly after the administration of the above-mentioned drugs. Careful documentation of the affected muscles is mandatory. A nonpharmacologic but unspecific test is the "ice-on-eyes" test that leads to an improvement of symptoms by decreasing the activity of ACh esterase due to low temperature. Additional neurophysiological testing with 3-Hz repetitive nerve stimulation (accessory or facial nerve) with evidence of a decrement of >10% further underscores the diagnosis. Laboratory testing should include anti-ACh-receptor antibodies (high yield in generalized and paraneoplastic MG forms), anti-MuSK (muscle-specific-kinase) antibodies (in 40%–70% positive in ACh receptor antibody "seronegative" MG) and anti-Titin antibodies (frequently associated with thymoma), beside general labs to assess complex comorbidities (e.g., diabetes, autoimmune thyroid disease) and for guidance of immune therapy. The autoantibody status is merely used for classification and has essentially no impact on management. Further studies should include imaging (chest CT or MRI) to rule out a thymoma.

4. Patients with suspected MG in the ICU should be stabilized first from the respiratory and, if necessary, cardiovascular standpoints. This might implicate intubation and mechanical ventilation. Symptomatic

T A B L E 31.2	Medications that Can Exacerbate Symptoms of Myasthenia Gravis
Substance Group	**Examples**
Analgesics	Morphine derivatives
Antibiotics	Aminoglycosides, macrolides, quinolones, sulfonamides, tetracyclines, polymyxines, penicillin in high doses
Antiarrhythmics	Procainamide, ajmaline, chinidine
Anticonvulsants	Benzodiazepines, gabapentin, carbamazepine, phenytoin
β-Blockers	Propranolol, pindolol, timolol
Calcium antagonists	Verapamil, nifedipine, diltiazem
Diuretics	Loop diuretics (furosemide), acetazolamide, hydrochlorothiazide
Statins	Different statins reported
Psychotropic agents	Chlorpromazine, promazine
Muscle-relaxing agents	Curare derivatives, suxamethonium

Note: These are merely examples of drugs that can cause a worsening of MG symptoms, and this list cannot be considered as complete!

treatment is achieved with acetylcholine esterase inhibitors such as pyridostigmine or neostigmine. Frequently intravenous administration is required in severe MG exacerbations but attention should be paid to their rather high side-effect profile (e.g., bronchial secretions). Glucocorticoids have a good efficacy on muscle weakness in MG with frequent initial deterioration of symptoms. The average onset of action, however, is 4 to 8 weeks in 70% to 80% of the cases. Thus, they are combined with other immunosuppressants, for example, azathioprine or cyclosporine A; an escalation therapy would include more potent immunomodulators like mycophenolate, cyclophosphamide, or methotrexate. Challenging courses might require off-label applications of agents like tacrolimus or monoclonal antibodies like rituximab or alemtuzumab. In refractory cases or in a myasthenic crisis, IVIG therapy or plasma exchange should be considered. Thymectomy should be considered after clinical stabilization in all patients with evidence of a thymoma and also in patients aged 15 to 50 years with generalized MG, without detected thymomas.

B. Lambert-Eaton Myasthenic Syndrome

A more uncommon disorder of the neuromuscular junction transmission is Lambert-Eaton myasthenic syndrome (LEMS) that presents with muscle weakness and is also an autoimmune disorder. The pathophysiology is based on antibodies directed against presynaptic voltage-gated calcium channels (VGCC), and there is a strong association with malignancy, especially with small cell lung cancer (SCLC). Treatment is focused on the underlying cause (removal of the tumor). Immune-directed therapy with steroids and plasma exchange are applied as well.

C. Botulism

Acute onset of symmetric descending weakness associated with bilateral cranial neuropathies (diplopia, nystagmus, ptosis, dysphagia, facial weakness) should raise red flags to consider botulism. Urinary retention and constipation can occur as well. Botulism is a rare potentially life-threatening disease caused through the toxin of the ubiquitously appearing gram-positive, spore-forming, obligate anaerobic bacterium *Clostridium botulinum*. There are different forms, namely, foodborne, infant, wound, adult enteric, and inhalational botulism. Foodborne botulism, for instance, is caused by consumption of these pathogens in home-canned foods like vegetables or fruits. When botulism is suspected, the clinician ought to contact the State Health Department instantly to obtain antitoxin as the treatment of choice. Equine serum heptavalent botulism antitoxin is used for adults. Wound botulism requires antibiotics (penicillin G or metronidazole) after the administration of antitoxin.

IV. MYOPATHIC CAUSES

A. Critical Illness Myopathy

Critical illness myopathy (CIM) is another acute neuromuscular disorder acquired during critical illness, impacting muscle. The incidence of isolated CIM is unknown as there is significant overlap with CIP, and distinguishing between the two is frequently not possible. Similar to CIP, CIM is thought to arise from a complex interaction of inflammatory processes, reduced microperfusion, and metabolic changes as well as muscle protein breakdown. The clinical presentation of CIM is quite similar to CIP, although proximal weakness may be more pronounced than distal and facial muscles may also be affected. In patients with pure CIM, reflexes are often normal and sensation intact. Patients may grimace in response to painful stimulation in the extremities, without producing a motor response in the limb.

1. Formal diagnosis of CIM requires EMG/NCS confirmation; these tests typically show increased duration of compound motor action potentials, normal sensory action potentials, and decreased muscle excitability with direct stimulation. Muscle biopsy (when performed) will show loss of myosin, fiber atrophy, and varying degrees of necrosis. Treatment for CIM is largely supportive. There is evidence suggesting increased risk for CIM in patients receiving IV glucocorticoids; thus, treatment includes minimizing glucocorticoids when possible. This entity can occur in conjunction or independent from a steroid-induced myopathy. There is literature to support physical therapy for strengthening in patients with CIM, although no dose–response relationship has been established. Additional preventative and treatment measures seem similar to those described for CIP. Prognosis for recovery varies but appears to be better than in CIP. Recovery frequently takes months; however, many patients with isolated CIM will be largely recovered within 6 months to 1 year.

B. Statin-Induced Myopathy

Muscle toxicity under statin therapy is rather uncommon (2%–11% for myalgias, 0.5% for myositis, and <0.1% for rhabdomyolysis); however, the possibility of muscle weakness caused through this generally widespread medication group should be considered. Statin-induced myopathy usually presents as proximal, symmetric muscle weakness with tenderness, potentially causing functional impairments. Typically, the onset of these symptoms after the initiation of statin therapy is weeks to months (although possible at any time of the treatment); however, it should be taken into consideration in a patient whose home medication includes statins. Fibrates have a direct muscle toxicity themselves and should be avoided in combination with statins. The temporal correlation with statin application, a rise in creatine kinase, and the improvement of symptoms after withdrawing statins are the cornerstones of the diagnosis. Discontinuation of the culprit is the treatment of choice and diuresis in cases of extreme elevations of CK levels to avoid renal failure. In patients where the continuation of statin treatment is required, a switch to less myotoxic statin (e.g., pravastatin) is recommended.

C. Rhabdomyolysis

Acute weakness caused by rhabdomyolysis is rather rare and occurs in the setting of myalgia, myoglobinuria, and elevated creatine kinase. Common causes of rhabdomyolysis are severe muscle injury with ensuing muscle necrosis. Complications that go along with this clinical entity are acute kidney injury, compartment syndrome, and disseminated intravascular coagulation. Treatment includes prompt correction of the above-mentioned manifestations and complications and identification of the trigger with appropriate management of the same (e.g., discontinuation of drugs causing rhabdomyolysis).

V. OTHER CAUSES

Transverse myelitis (TM) is an acute to subacute inflammatory insult to the spinal cord, frequently impacting one or two levels of the cord. TM may be idiopathic in nature or associated with other conditions. In many patients, TM is preceded by infection. Clinical presentation is consistent with an insult to the spinal cord below the level of the lesion (e.g., weakness and sensory changes). Pain and paresthesias are frequent complaints. MRI typically shows signal abnormality at the segment(s) of the lesion. CSF is abnormal in half of the patients, including elevated protein and lymphocytosis. Treatment for TM includes high-dose steroids with plasma exchange in therapy-refractory cases, as well as treatment of any other associated diseases. Most patients show signs of improvement by 3 months, although recovery is frequently incomplete. Patients with an acute aortic dissection or those undergoing surgery to repair the thoracoabdominal aorta are at risk for spinal cord infarct in the setting of decreased perfusion to the cord, notably to the anterior spinal artery (ASA). This can lead to acute weakness, for example, in form of flaccid paralysis and areflexia, which can later turn into hyperreflexia and urinary and bowel retention.

Selected Readings

Desart K, Scali ST, Feezor RJ, et al. Fate of patients with spinal cord ischemia complicating thoracic endovascular aortic repair. *J Vasc Surg* 2013;58:635–642.

Dowell VR Jr. Botulism and tetanus: selected epidemiologic and microbiologic aspects. *Rev Infect Dis* 1984;6(suppl 1):S202.

Drachman DB. Myasthenia gravis. *N Engl J Med* 1994;330:1797.

Elmqvist D, Lambert EH. Detailed analysis of neuromuscular transmission in a patient with the myasthenic syndrome sometimes associated with bronchogenic carcinoma. *Mayo Clin Proc* 1968;43:689–713.

Gupta A, Gupta Y. Glucocorticoid-induced myopathy: pathophysiology, diagnosis, and treatment. *Indian J Endocrinol Metab* 2013 Sep-Oct;17(5):913–916.

Kress JP, Hall JB. ICU-acquired weakness and recovery from critical illness. *N Engl J Med* 2014;370:1626–1635.

Latronica N, Bolton CF. Critical illness polyneuropathy and myopathy: a major cause of muscle weakness and paralysis. *Lancet Neurol* 2011;10:931–941.

Pati S, Goodfellow JA, Iyadurai S, et al. Approach to critical illness polyneuropathy and myopathy. *Postgrad Med J* 2008;84:354–360.

Sathasivam S, Lecky B. Statin induced myopathy. *BMJ* 2008;337:a2286.

Schweickert WD, Hall JI. ICU-acquired weakness. *Chest* 2007;131:1541–1549.

West TW. Transverse myelitis—a review of the presentation, diagnosis and initial management. *Discov Med* 2013;16(88):167–177.

Yuki N, Hartung H-P. Guillan-Barre syndrome. *N Engl J Med* 2012;336:2294–2304.

Drug Overdose, Poisoning, and Adverse Drug Reactions

Kevin Blackney and Jarone Lee

I. INTRODUCTION

A. Overdose, poisonings, and adverse drug reactions are common diagnoses treated by intensivists. According to the Centers for Disease Control (CDC), there was a 102% increase in fatalities from overdoses from 1999 to 2010 in the United States. Many of these poisonings rapidly deteriorate requiring intensive care unit (ICU) admission.

B. The initial approach to a patient with an overdose, poisoning, or adverse drug reaction varies. The American Association of Poison Control Centers is available 24 hours a day to assist—1-800-222-1222. There are also local poison control centers (PCC) that can be called as well. In addition to a thorough history and physical (including tests such as a basic metabolic panel, complete blood count, bedside blood glucose, liver panel, substance specific blood levels, urine toxicological screens, and an electrocardiogram), it is imperative to know the following:

  1. What substance, or substances, was used?
  2. What time and amount of the substance was taken?
  3. What was the route of intake (e.g., ingestion, inhalation, injection, etc.)?
  4. What treatment has already been rendered at home by the emergency medical services (EMS) and the emergency department (ED)?

C. While the answers to these questions are being sought, supportive care and stabilization should be initiated. Once the substance and its effects have been identified, additional treatment such as administration of an antidote, enhancing elimination, or decreasing absorption should begin. Activated charcoal in doses of 25 to 100 g for adults (1–2 g/kg) is effective if given within the first hour of ingestion, except when hydrocarbons, metals, and alcohols are ingested. Traditional treatment methods designed to minimize absorption through the GI tract, such as inducing emesis with syrup of ipecac or whole bowel irrigation, are no longer recommended except in specific situations. Similarly, gastric lavage is now out of favor, but can be considered when a known lethal dose of a substance, that does not have an antidote or bind activated charcoal, was ingested within an hour of presentation.

II. DRUG OVERDOSE

A. Drug overdoses can present in a variety of settings, from intentional (e.g., suicide), to unintentional (e.g., child ingesting pills), iatrogenic (e.g., unintentional overdose of acetaminophen from multiple products), and work related (chemical plant exposures).

B. Acetaminophen (APAP) is the leading cause of acute liver failure (ALF) in the United States and was associated with 401 overdose deaths as recently as 2009. As of 2008, because of timely administration of N-acetylcystiene (NAC), the nontransplanted survival rate has increased to 66%.

  1. In overdose of APAP, less than 10% of the total dose is needed to develop liver injury. Damage occurs when CYP2E1 metabolizes APAP to the

active metabolite, N-acetyl-p-benzoquinone-imine (NAPQI). NAPQI is normally neutralized by glutathione; however, toxicity ensues when NAPQI concentration exceeds that of glutathione. Excess NAPQI binds hepatocyte mitochondrial proteins, which inhibits cellular respiration. This leads to necrosis and apoptosis, ultimately causing ALF.

2. Patients may present without obvious illness, but then rapidly deteriorate to fulminant liver failure within 24 to 96 hours of ingestion, including profound encephalopathy, coagulopathy, hepatorenal syndrome, and metabolic acidosis. Cerebral edema typically develops within 2 weeks, leading to uncal herniation and death. The King's College Criteria can be used to help predict the need for liver transplantation among patients with ALF from both APAP overdoses, as well as non-APAP ALF as shown in Table 32.1. Please note that there is a modified King's College Criteria that incorporates lactate to increase the sensitivity (not shown).

3. To determine the severity risk, serum APAP levels are plotted on the Rumack-Matthew nomogram (see Fig 32.1). Ideally, the Tylenol level should be taken and plotted at exactly 4 hours postingestion.

   a. NAC should be administered in any of the following circumstances: (1) confirmed lethal toxicity by the Rumack-Matthew nomogram; (2) a confirmed lethal dose of APAP is ingested (>150 mg/kg); (3) the patient is at risk for hepatic injury; or (4) the ingestion time and amount is unknown. Error should be on overtreating with NAC as it is very efficacious with few side effects. Ideally, NAC should be started within 8 hours of ingestion as NAC has a close to 100% success rate in eliminating the need for liver transplantation among APAP overdoses if given within 8 hours. For example, the obtunded overdose patient that had access to Tylenol, but without anyone to corroborate history, should be started on NAC as soon as possible. Though there is an intravenous (IV) form available, NAC is usually administered enterally often via a nasogastric tube. Dosing can be found in Table 32.2.

C. **Salicylates** are widely available for overdose as it is one of the most popular over-the-counter analgesics and also used routinely in both primary and secondary prevention of cardiovascular disease.

   1. Absorption is variable, depending on the amount ingested and if the formulation was enteric coated. Salicylates are absorbed in an ionized form through the stomach and upper intestine and then undergo hydrolysis in the liver, intestinal wall, and erythrocytes before being

 King's College Criteria for Need for Liver Transplantation

Tylenol-Associated Acute Liver Failure	Other Causes of Acute Liver Failure
pH <7.3	INR >6.5
or all of the following:	or three of the following:
INR >6.5	Age <10 or >40 y
Creatinine >3.4 mg/dL	Non-A or non-B hepatitis or drug reaction
Grade III–IV	>7 d of jaundice before encephalopathy
encephalopathy	INR >3.5
	Serum bilirubin >17.5 mg/dL

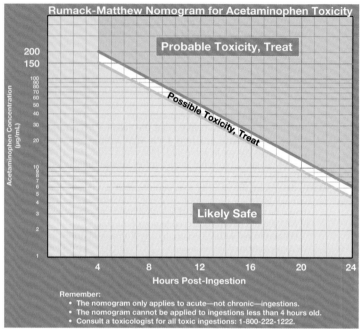

FIGURE 32.1 The Rumack-Matthew nomogram is designed to help determine the risk of hepatotoxicity based on hours since ingestion (*x*-axis) versus the serum acetaminophen level in mcg/mL (*y*-axis). Any acetaminophen level greater than the "150-line" at any time since ingestion should be treated with NAC. (Courtesy Graham Walker, MD, Emergency Physician, Kaiser San Francisco, Assistant Clinical Professor, UCSF and MDCalc.com)

TABLE 32.2	Dosing Regimen for N-acetylcystiene	
Route	**Loading Dose**	**Additional Doses**
Oral	140 mg/kg	70 mg/kg q4h × 17 doses
Intravenous	150 mg/kg over 15 min	50 mg/kg in 4 h, then 100 mg/kg over 16 h

excreted by the kidneys. The half-life is 2 to 4 hours, but is prolonged to up to 20 hours or longer in high doses or enteric-coated formulation. Levels >30 mg/dL are toxic while >75 mg/dL are lethal causing cerebral edema and cardiac and renal failure.

2. Salicylate toxicity presents with respiratory alkalosis due to CNS excitation, accompanied by tinnitus. Later, metabolic acidosis develops due to uncoupling of oxidative phosphorylation and inhibition of the tricarboxylic acid cycle in the liver. Stupor, coma, and gastrointestinal (GI) bleeding may also be seen.

3. Treatment is primarily supportive. Removal of salicylates is the most important aspect, either through aggressive gastric decontamination and/or early hemodialysis (HD). Indications for HD include severe metabolic acidosis, end-organ damage including seizures, pulmonary edema, acute renal failure, and a serum salicylate level >100 mg/dL. Alkalinization of both the serum and urine has also been shown to improve outcomes. Alkalinizing the serum decreases central nervous system penetration, while alkalinization of the urine improves renal excretion.

D. **Cardiovascular drug** overdoses, including β-blockers (BB), calcium-channel blockers (CCB), and cardiac glycosides (e.g., digoxin), generated over 50,000 calls to PCC nationally in 2012 and was the second most frequent cause of single-substance-exposure death. With an aging population and the associated increases in prescriptions for cardiovascular drugs, overdoses of these medications are expected to increase in the United States.

1. **BB** are used for a variety of medical conditions. They work by blocking β-adrenergic receptors, thus decreasing cAMP and decreasing catecholamine effects. This class of medications varies on its specificity for adrenergic receptors. Drugs blocking β1 receptors reduce the inotropic and chronotropic effects on the heart, while drugs blocking β2 receptors reduce bronchodilatation and gluconeogenesis. Drugs such as labetalol and carvedilol also block α1 receptors, which are involved in vasoconstriction.

a. Overdose can result in severe decreases in blood pressure and heart rate as well as hypoglycemia, atrioventricular (AV) block, bronchospasm, and seizures. In overdose, β-selectivity is often lost. If no symptoms are present 6 hours after ingestion, then the patient is cleared; however, sotalol requires a 12-hour period of observation.

b. Initial treatment in overdose includes charcoal, IV fluids, and supporting the heart rate with use of atropine or electrical pacing. Additionally, glucagon, in doses of 50 to 150 mcg/kg bolus followed by a continuous infusion of 2 to 5 mg/h, should be started. Glucagon works by activating adenylate cyclase through direct G-protein stimulation in cardiac tissue. Though less successful, other modalities include direct β agonist such as isoproterenol or amiodarone. Lastly, high-dose insulin therapy has been effective in case reports and is currently under evaluation in animal studies.

2. **CCB** are commonly used for hypertension, angina, supraventricular arrhythmias, and migraines. CCBs act at voltage-gated calcium channels in myocardial cells, smooth muscle cells, and β-islet cells in the pancreas during phase 2 of the action potential, thus reducing calcium entry. Dihydropyridines (e.g., amlodipine and nicardipine), act peripherally and reduce afterload, while nondihydropyridines (e.g., verapamil and diltiazem) act within the heart, reducing inotropy and chronotropy. In the pancreas, they decrease insulin secretion.

a. Overdose presents with hypotension, sinus bradycardia, AV block, and hyperglycemia. Hyperglycemia and decreased insulin secretion causes the body to convert to fatty acid oxidation, ultimately leading to metabolic acidosis.

b. Like with BB overdose, initial treatment aims at elimination through charcoal therapy, IV fluids, and cardiovascular support. Previous treatment modalities have included calcium, glucagon, epinephrine, and amiodarone. High-dose insulin therapy is also showing promise due to improved carbohydrate metabolism, which leads to improved cardiac function. Initial insulin dosing is 0.5 to 1 unit/kg/h. Insulin should be administered with a dextrose-containing fluid, an epinephrine infusion starting at 1 μg/min, and calcium supplementation.

3. **Digoxin** is still used for the treatment of atrial fibrillation and congestive heart failure. While overall use is declining, there is still an incidence rate of 48 digoxin-related admissions per 100,000 prescriptions. Digoxin is a sodium–potassium ATPase that increases intracellular sodium, leading to increased calcium and improved inotropy. Toxicity can occur with normal serum digoxin levels in the setting of hypokalemia, hypomagnesemia, or hypothyroidism. Conversely, serum digoxin levels can increase while on a stable dose if drugs such as amiodarone, verapamil, or erythromycin are coadministered.

   a. Toxicity leads to increased automaticity and dysrhythmias, including frequent premature ventricular contractions (PVCs), atrial fibrillation with slow ventricular response, or complete AV block. The classic "Salvadore Dali mustache" finding on ECG (ST depression) may be seen, but is not indicative of overdose. Other symptoms include gastric distress, anorexia, and visual halos.

   b. Digoxin is not effectively removed with HD. Treatment includes (1) withdrawal of the drug; (2) treatment of nonperfusing dysrhythmias (e.g., atropine or pacing for bradycardia, esmolol for supraventricular tachycardia, lidocaine 1–1.5 mg/kg IVP then 1–4 mg/min or phenytoin 15–20 mg/kg for ventricular arrhythmias); (3) correction of electrolytes such as hypokalemia or hypomagnesium in chronic toxicity; and (4) administering digoxin-specific immunoglobulin G (Dig IgG). Dig IgG works by binding digitalis before it interacts with sodium–potassium ATPase. Dosing varies slightly on the basis of the two commercially available forms of Dig IgG and depends on whether the serum concentration of digitalis is known. Traditionally, it was recommended to avoid giving calcium due to concern for worsening the dysrhythmia and "stone heart"; however, in retrospective studies this has been shown to be false.

E. **Antipsychotics and Antidepressants** are some of the most prescribed medications in the United States and constitute a large volume of PCC encounters.

   1. Antipsychotics include traditional (a.k.a. "typical") medications, such as haloperidol and chlorpromazine, and newer classes (a.k.a. "atypical") antipsychotics such as quetiapine and risperidone, which have less antidopaminergic effects. All antipsychotics can produce adverse reactions such as neuroleptic malignant syndrome (see Adverse Drug Reactions below), extrapyramidal side-effects (parkinsonism and dystonia), and tardive dyskinesia (irreversible, purposeless movements of the face and neck), though atypical antipsychotics produce these less frequently. In overdose, patients develop stupor and hypotension with reflex tachycardia, prolongation of the QT interval on electrocardiogram (ECG).

   2. Among antidepressants, overdose with tricyclic antidepressants (TCA) are the most toxic due to their antagonism of sodium channels affecting the heart and central nervous system. In the heart, sodium-channel blocking prolongs conduction time and reduces inotropy. Treatment includes sodium bicarbonate and support care with vasopressors. Consider lidocaine as an antiarrhythmic.

F. **Lithium** is the cheapest and most effective pharmacologic intervention for long-term treatment of bipolar disorder, but has a very narrow therapeutic window with several adverse side effects, and it is a teratogen (e.g., Ebstein anomaly).

1. In the kidney, lithium causes progressive decreases in glomerular filtration rate (GFR) over time with a reduction in renal concentrating ability. In the thyroid, it produces decreased iodine uptake and inhibition of iodotyrosine coupling with decreased thyroxine secretion. In the parathyroid gland, it causes a reduction in the calcium-sensing receptor leading to primary hyperparathyroidism.

2. Toxicity, serum concentrations of 1.5 mEq/L or greater, from lithium can be acute (e.g., a suicide attempt), subacute (e.g., in the setting of an illness such as diarrhea, heart or renal failure), or chronic (e.g., secondary to changes in metabolism or from drug interactions such as with nonsteroidals or ACE inhibitors). Patients with toxicity from lithium may present with decreased renal function and/or nephrogenic diabetes insipidus (DI) acutely. Chronic toxicity may also show these symptoms in addition to hypothyroidism or hypercalcemia. Case reports of lithium-induced hyperthermia exist as well.

3. In acute overdose, gastric lavage should be instituted immediately, and fluid replacement with 0.45% NS should be given for dehydration associated with nephrogenic DI. Thiazide diuretics help control polyuria. HD may also be required.

III. POISONINGS

A. **Carbon Monoxide (CO)** is one of the leading causes of poison-related deaths and accounts for over 50,000 ED visits annually in the United States. CO is an inhaled and odorless poison, a byproduct of combustion such as in house fires or the burning of organic material without proper ventilation. Individuals that smoke cigarettes typically have serum levels of 3% to 5%, which rise 2.5% for every pack per day of cigarettes smoked.

1. CO avidly binds heme (200× stronger than oxygen), thus displacing oxygen and causing hypoxia. CO also causes direct cellular damage through both immunologic and inflammatory processes.

2. The symptoms of CO poisoning do not correlate well with absolute serum levels. Patients often present with dizziness, headaches, fatigue, confusion, chest pain, or shortness of breath. A traditional presentation of "cherry red skin" is rare and should not be relied upon for diagnosis. Oxyhemoglobin and carboxyhemoglobin (COHgb) absorb light at the same wavelength, and therefore pulse oximetry will be normal despite severe hypoxemia. A CO serum level of 3% to 4% in nonsmokers and >10% in smokers should raise suspicion for exposure. Diagnosis requires a high index of suspicion.

3. Treatment involves removing the patient from the source of CO and instituting oxygen therapy. Increasing the FIO_2 drastically speeds the removal of CO from heme; at 21% FIO_2, the half-life of COHgb is 320-minutes, versus 70-minutes in patients with 100% FIO_2 via facemask. Further accelerations in reducing CO levels are seen with 100% FIO_2 via endotracheal tube and with hyperbaric oxygen (HBO). HBO does not improve short-term survival, but has shown to be associated with less long-term neurologic sequelae. Regardless, treatment should continue until CO levels are normal and the patient is symptom free for a minimum of 6 hours.

B. **Cyanide** exposures can come in many forms. Hydrogen cyanide is a common by-product from burning of synthetic material such as polyurethane found in paints and many plastics. Additionally, it is generated from prolonged use of sodium nitroprusside infusions and exposures in the precious metal industry and may be used in chemical weapons.

1. The effects of cyanide are due to its binding of the ferric ion in mitochondrial cytochrome oxidase. This inhibits the electron transport chain (ETC) and stops oxidative phosphorylation. Lactic acidosis rapidly ensues because of decreased ATP production. The brain, heart, and liver, all rich in cytochrome oxidase, are most affected. In extremely low concentrations, the human body is able to metabolize cyanide through two mechanisms, combining with hydroxycobalamin to form cyanocobalamin or by conversion to thiocyanate by the rhodanese enzyme.

2. Signs and symptoms include tachypnea, confusion, agitation, dizziness, headaches, and nausea/vomiting. Late findings include more severe cardiac (hypotension and bradycardic heart failure with preservation of inotropy) and neurologic (including seizures and extrapyramidal) manifestations. In general, levels of 0.5 to 1 mg/L are considered mild, 1 to 2 mg/L moderate, 2 to 3 mg/L severe, and >3 mg/L lethal; but do not delay treatment as serum levels can take time.

3. Treatment consists of administering 100% oxygen, though HBO has not proven helpful. There are two antidote kits approved for use by the US Food and Drug Administration (FDA). The hydroxycobalamin kit "Cyanokit," approved in 2006, is now preferred since it chelates cyanide to form cyanocobalamin (Vitamin B_{12}), which is easily excreted by the kidneys and has the beneficial side effects of scavenging nitric oxide, which raises the blood pressure. The *traditional* cyanide kits, consisting of amyl nitrite/sodium nitrite/sodium thiosulfate, are out of favor because they generate up to 30% serum methemoglobin levels with hypotension, hemolysis, and nephrotoxicity. Dosing is shown in Table 32.3.

IV. ADVERSE DRUG REACTIONS

A. **Hyperthermia-Related Drug Reactions** are a broad category that often results in patients being admitted to the ICU. These are hyperpyrexic states and not the result of hypothalamic dysregulation as seen in infections, and therefore APAP is not indicated.

1. **Malignant hyperthermia (MH)** is caused by an autosomal dominant defect of ryanodine receptors in the sarcoplasmic reticulum. When exposed to triggering agents, either volatile anesthetics or succinylcholine, these mutated receptors lead to a hypermetabolic state from

TABLE 32.3	Dosing Regimens for Cyanide Poisoning
Kit	**Dosing**
Traditional kit	Inhale amyl nitrite perles for 30 s each min, replacing perles q3min.
	If no response, infuse 10 mL sodium nitrite, 3% solution over 5 min.
	Infuse 50 mL sodium thiosulfate, 25% solution over 10 to 20 min and repeat at half doses 30 min later if no response.
Cyanokit	5 g IV over 15 min, repeat X1 over 15 to 120 min

excessive calcium release. This results in increased oxygen use and CO_2 production, lactic acidosis, hyperthermia, and disseminated intravascular coagulation (DIC). Early presentation includes spasm of masseter muscles, tachypnea, and rigidity, while diagnostic testing will commonly show elevated end-tidal CO_2, hyperkalemia, and evidence of rhabdomyolysis. Hyperthermia is a late finding. Death is typically from cardiac dysrhythmias and multiorgan failure. Immediate administration of dantrolene (initial dose of 2.5 mg/kg IV every 15-minutes until a total dose of 10 mg/kg IV has been administered followed by 1 mg/kg IV every 4 hours for 2 additional days) has reduced the mortality rate from 80% to 5%. Additional supportive therapy to address hyperkalemia, bleeding and prevent kidney damage is also indicated. Further information and 24-hour support is provided by the Malignant Hyperthermia Association of the United States (www.mhaus.org).

2. **Neuroleptic malignant syndrome (NMS)** occurs in 0.5% to 3% of patients taking antidopaminergic drugs (antipsychotics and dopamine antagonists such as metoclopramide and hydroxyzine). This syndrome can also present after abrupt discontinuation of dopamine agonists, such as patients with Parkinson's disease taking amantadine, levodopa, or bromocriptine. The mechanism for NMS is believed to be related to alterations in central neurotransmission (e.g., hypothalamic temperature regulation), as well as peripheral calcium transport in skeletal muscles. This is typically a diagnosis of exclusion; patients present initially with muscle rigidity and altered mental status, later developing hyperthermia and autonomic instability. Treatment includes supportive care, cooling, and benzodiazepines for agitation and decreasing sympathetic outflow. Modulation of the dopamine pathway is also necessary (e.g., removal of antidopamine agents or reinstituting the dopamine agonist if due to rapid withdrawal). In either situation, initiating dopamine agonists should be considered (bromocriptine 2.5 mg PO TID, amantadine 100 to 200 mg PO BID or levodopa/carbidopa 25/250 PO QID). Dantrolene may also be effective, but should not be used alone.

3. **Serotonin syndrome (SS)** results when serotonin levels are elevated in 5-HT2A receptors centrally. Drugs and substances known to cause SS include serotonin agonists including triptans, dextromethorphan, and tramadol; serotonin reuptake inhibitors including antidepressants, meperidine, and methadone; monoamine oxidase inhibitors (MAOI); supplements such as St John's wort and ginseng; and street drugs such as ecstasy and cocaine. Patients present with neuromuscular and autonomic instability including muscular rigidity, hyperreflexia, myoclonus, hyperthermia, diaphoresis, mydriasis, agitation, and confusion. Treatment includes removal of offending agent(s), supportive therapy, and cooling. While supportive care is the mainstay of treatment, cyproheptadine (4–12 mg PO q2-hours up to a total dose of 32 mg, repeat 4 mg q6-hours for a total of 48 hours if effective), chlorpromazine, and dantrolene can be considered in refractory cases.

4. **Anticholinergic crisis** results from patients taking excessive amounts of drugs with anticholinergic properties (e.g., antihistamines, TCAs, parkinsonian drugs, neuroleptics, atropine, scopolamine, and antispasmodics). Hyperthermia is caused by central temperature control dysregulation and peripheral muscarinic blockade. Further symptoms include agitation, confusion, dry mouth, blurred vision, tachycardia,

flushing, and urinary retention. Treatment is primarily supportive with cooling and benzodiazepines. Physostigmine, a tertiary acetylcholinesterase inhibitor that crosses the blood–brain barrier and helps increase acetylcholine levels centrally and peripherally, can be considered for diagnostic situations and refractory cases. Normal doses are 1 to 2 mg IV q10 to 15 minutes for a total dose of 4 mg. Physostigmine is relatively short acting, and its effects may diminish over time.

5. **Drug fevers** are not uncommon in the ICU. They have a typical onset of 7 to 10 days after exposure. Many antimicrobials, antineoplastics, nonsteroidals, and immunosuppressives are known instigators, and symptoms reverse soon after the drug is discontinued.

B. **Propofol-Related Infusion Syndrome (PRIS)** was first defined in 1998 in the pediatric population as refractory bradycardia with any of the following: severe metabolic acidosis, rhabdomyolysis, lipemic plasma, and fatty liver. At that time, this syndrome had an 83% mortality rate among 18 reported cases. The specific mechanism of how PRIS develops is not clear, though it is believed to behave similar to mitochondrial myopathies with defects in the mitochondrial respiratory chain. Anion-gap metabolic acidosis develops, which suppresses cardiac function further than what propofol does under normal situations. Brugada-like ECG changes may be seen. Treatment includes stopping propofol, supportive care, and HD. Inotropes show little benefit, though pacing and extracorporeal membrane oxygenation has been used in case reports. Ultimately, prevention is the best measure by limiting prolonged propofol use and utilizing high carbohydrate, low-fat nutrition. A prospective study published in 2009 found that only 18% of patients that developed PRIS had infusion rates >5 mg/kg/h for greater than 24 hours.

C. **Anaphylaxis and Anaphylactoid Reactions** are indistinguishable in presentation, differing only in that anaphylactoid reactions are not IgE mediated. The incidence of anaphylaxis has been increasing nationally; one recent study showed a fourfold increase in hospitalizations in New York from 1999 to 2006. Overall, foods represent the most frequent cause of anaphylaxis, followed by drugs and insect envenomations. About 20% of anaphylactic reactions have no known trigger.

1. The most common presenting symptom is urticaria and angioedema (88%), followed by dyspnea and wheezing (50%), while hypotension (33%) is less commonly seen.

2. Immediate administration of epinephrine (0.3 mg IM or 0.1 mg IV repeated every 5–15 minutes) is the most effective and efficient intervention. Consider early intubation. Cardiac and respiratory arrest can occur within 5-minutes of onset, and nearly 50% of deaths occur in the first hour. Many cases require repeated dosing of epinephrine and ultimately a continuous infusion. Secondary drugs such as diphenhydramine and steroids are effective but take up to an hour for clinical effect. Obtain a serum tryptase if possible within 2 hours of symptom onset.

V. SUBSTANCES OF ABUSE AND ADDICTION

A. **Alcohols** are one of the most abused and addictive substances in the United States. Methanol, ethylene glycol, and isopropyl alcohol are more toxic and can require ICU care in acute ingestions.

1. **Ethanol** contributes to 20% of ICU admissions and is involved in 50% to 60% of trauma patients. Approximately 10% of Americans are considered excessive alcohol drinkers, while 3% state they have had

withdrawal symptoms. The LC50 in normal individuals is usually between blood alcohol concentration (BAC) of 0.3% and 0.4%.

  a. Ethanol is metabolized in the liver via zero-order kinetics, first by
  alcohol dehydrogenase and then by acetaldehyde dehydrogenase,
  yielding acetate. There is also a P-450 metabolism that increases
  activity in chronic use. In acute intoxication, the effects of ethanol
  are exerted on GABA$_A$ receptors and by limiting glutamate activation of NMDA receptors. In chronic use, there is a down-regulation
  of GABA$_A$ responses and up-regulation of NMDA subtype glutamate
  receptors. Additionally in chronic use, liver dysfunction and cirrhosis develop, leading to impaired hepatic function and portal hypertension. *Wernicke* (ophthalmoplegia/dementia/ataxia)-*Korsakoff*
  (amnesia + aphasia/agnosia/apraxia) syndrome can develop long
  term due to lack of thiamine.

  b. Acute intoxication presents with CNS depression and dehydration,
  and at higher BAC, cardiopulmonary dysfunction or collapse can
  occur. Withdrawal symptoms occur after abrupt discontinuation
  in chronic users and can include tremors, irritability, and anxiety.
  Seizures and delirium tremens usually present 72 to 96 hours after
  a chronic abuser's last drink. Alcoholic ketoacidosis develops secondary to decreased intake of proteins and carbohydrates during
  alcohol binges along with other metabolic changes that favor the
  conversion to free fatty acids and ketogenesis.

  c. Acute intoxication is generally treated with supportive care. Withdrawal from chronic alcohol abuse is lethal. Monitoring tools such
  as the Clinical Institute Withdrawal Assessment (CIWA) in awake
  patients, or the Sedation Agitation Scale (SAS) in sedated or intubated patients, have been developed to recognize and treat withdrawal. Benzodiazepines are the mainstay of treatment due to their
  effect on GABA$_A$ receptors. Clonidine, which limits sympathetic outflow, and haloperidol for psychosis are also useful adjuncts. Propofol, dexmedetomidine, and barbiturates may also be used.

2. Methanol and ethylene glycol are both common solvents found in household and industrial materials. They can be ingested intentionally for
  their sedating and euphoric properties, unintentionally such as children drinking antifreeze, or as a poison such as in suicides or for nefar-
  ious purposes. Methanol is the by-product of home distilleries such as
  in "moonshine."

  a. Both methanol and ethylene glycol are readily absorbed through the
  GI tract; there is no minimal toxic level known for either. Both are
  metabolized first by alcohol dehydrogenase; methanol metabolism
  yields aldehyde, while ethylene glycol produces glycoaldehyde. Both
  by-products undergo further metabolism by aldehyde dehydrogenase. Methanol metabolism generates formate, which behaves similar to cyanide; neurons in the retina, optic nerve, and basal ganglia
  are very sensitive. Ethylene glycol metabolism generates glycolic,
  glyoxilic, and oxalic acids, which stop cellular respiration and nucleic acid synthesis. Oxalic acid also forms calcium oxalate that pre-
  cipitates in the kidneys causing direct damage.

  b. Both alcohols produce sedation or stupor akin to early ethanol intoxication along with GI distress. Later, methanol can lead to total
  or bright-visual-field blindness described as "snow-field blindness,"
  while ethylene glycol produces acute kidney injury within 24 to 72
  hours from ingestion. Diagnosis is based on a known ingestion of

either substance since specific serum levels of methanol or ethylene glycol are difficult to obtain. An elevated osmolar gap is evident early after ingestion for both alcohols; however, over time, this normalizes while the anion gap increases from metabolite buildup. Diagnostically, calcium oxalate in urine from ethylene glycol poisoning glows under ultraviolet light.

   c. Treatment for methanol and ethylene glycol varies on the basis of the time from ingestion. Both lead to profound acidosis, with some case reports showing utility in use of sodium bicarbonate. Ethanol and fomepizole act as competitive inhibitors of alcohol dehydrogenase, which significantly limits the breakdown of both ethylene glycol and methanol to their toxic metabolites. Fomepizole, while more costly, has the benefit of no additive sedation and acts much longer than ethanol (see dosing in Table 32.4). Ethanol and fomepizole can be life preserving, but these drugs serve as temporizing measures until the patient can receive HD.

3. **Isopropyl alcohol** is a common household product and key component in antiseptic hand washes. Unlike ethylene glycol and methanol, isopropyl alcohol is the toxic mediator. Isopropyl alcohol is broken down in the liver to acetone. Serum levels >150 mg/dL lead to seizure and hypotension while levels exceeding 200 mg/dL are lethal. Symptoms range from mild GI upset to seizures and coma. Unlike methanol/ethylene glycol poisoning, isopropyl alcohol causes an osmolar gap *without* a metabolic acidosis. Treatment is generally supportive.

B. Opioid overdose, combined with other sedatives such as benzodiazepines, comprise the number one reason for calls to PCCs as well as the top cause of drug-related death. These include prescription opioids and street drugs such as heroin.

1. Opioids are metabolized in the liver by CYP2D6 and 3A4, with some, such as morphine, meperidine, and codeine, having active metabolites. Opioid overdose presents with somnolence and sedation. These patients develop respiratory depression and decreased central response to increasing $Paco_2$. Because of their effects on the Edinger-Westphal nucleus, a myotic pupil is often a classic finding that does not dissipate with chronic use. Always maintain a high index of suspicion for other coingestants, such as benzodiazepines, sleep aides, or alcohol. Treatment of opioid overdose is with naloxone 40 µg per dose to reverse

TABLE 32.4	Dosing Regimen Ethanol and Fomepizole
Medication	**Dose**
Ethanol: goal BAC of 100–150 mg/dL	Use 10% ethanol in sterile water w/ dextrose: load 7.6 mL/kg over 1 h. Maintenance of 0.83 mL/kg/h for nondrinkers and 1.96 mL/kg/h for chronic ethanol users
Fomepizole	Load 15 mg/kg over 30 min. Maintenance of 10 mg/kg over 30 min every 12 h for 4 doses[a]

[a]Dosing adjustments based on serum level/pH and if HD has been initiated.

respiratory depression. Close monitoring is needed as the half-life of naloxone (1–1.5 h) may be shorter than some opioid preparations in which case a naloxone drip may be necessary. Watch for noncardiogenic pulmonary edema when treating chronic opioid users.

   2. Opioid withdrawal symptoms may also present in the ICU. Withdrawal symptoms are the result of a reflex increase in sympathetic outflow resulting in tachycardia, hypertension, diaphoresis, and abdominal pain. Effective treatment includes reinstituting low-dose opioids, clonidine, benzodiazepines, and ketamine.

C. Benzodiazepines are used frequently for sedation in both inpatient and outpatient settings. While this class of drugs has a relatively high safety profile, when combined with other substances that have sedative properties (e.g., opioids, antidepressants, alcohol), their toxicity is additive.

   1. Benzodiazepines provide sedative-hypnosis, anterograde amnesia, muscle relaxation, and anxiolysis through their actions on GABA receptors. They differ within the class on the basis of their potency and length of action, with chlordiazepoxide being the longest acting of the benzodiazepines in practice. All of these medications are metabolized by the CYP450 system and renally excreted. Symptoms of benzodiazepine overdose are nondescript, but include neurologic and respiratory depression. Stopping, or titrating down the drug, with supportive measures are the primary components of treatment. Flumazenil, at a dose of 0.5 to 5 mg IV, can be considered but has been found to induce seizures. Because its half-life is 1 to 2 hours, observe closely if long-acting benzodiazepines were ingested.

   2. Withdrawal from benzodiazepines occurs after chronic use. Symptoms include anxiety, irritability, sleep disturbances, hallucinations, vomiting, diarrhea, tachycardia, tachypnea, sweating, and fever. Treatment is supportive care and a slow taper of benzodiazepines, similar to alcohol withdrawal.

D. Indirect sympathomimetics (bath salts, amphetamines, cocaine) increase catecholamine concentrations by blocking their reuptake presynaptically and blocking their breakdown by oxidases within the synapse. Each of these drugs are stimulants and lead to a large sympathetic outflow. Because of this, it is important to avoid β-blockade, which can lead to hypertensive emergency due to unopposed catecholamine stimulation of α-receptors. However, newer population studies have shown that giving β-blockade is most likely safe.

E. Designer drugs with street names like ecstasy, spice, and molly are a fast-growing class of drugs of abuse made popular because of their psychoactive effects with limited means of detection. They are often well known to law enforcement and PCCs, both of which should be able to provide assistance in management. Treatment in acute intoxication is generally supportive.

VI. NERVE AGENT TOXICITY

A. From the use of phosgene in World War I, to attacks by Iraq on the Kurds and Iran in the 1980s, and most recently with their use in Syria, chemical weapons have been deployed with devastating results. Of the many classes of chemical weapons, organophosphates (OP) nerve agents are the most toxic. There are two main classes, the G-agents and V-agents. The "G" from G-agents comes from Germany and Dr. Gerhard Schrader who developed these agents in the 1930s. The G-agents include GA (tabun), GB (sarin), and GD (soman). V-agents were developed in England and include agents such as VX. Organophosphates are also used as pesticides.

1. The toxic effects of OPs are due to their ability to irreversibly bind and inhibit acetylcholinesterase (AChE), thus drastically increasing acetylcholine (ACh) within nerve synapses at skeletal muscle motor endplates and within the autonomic nervous system. In the central nervous system, OPs cause a release of glutamate and stimulation of α-amino-3-hydroxy-5-methyl-4-isoxazolepropionic acid (AMPA) and N-methyl-D-aspartic acid (NMDA) receptors that result in seizures. Additionally, with prolonged and uninterrupted exposure to OPs, "ageing" occurs whereby the phosphorous moiety on the OP becomes less electrophilic and more resistant to displacement by oxime antidotes.

2. Symptoms occur within minutes of exposure and typically develop in the following order: miosis, hypersecretion and fasciculation, convulsions, coma, and death by cardiac and respiratory arrest. Diagnosis is usually clinical, but may be aided by confirmatory air sampling at the site of exposure—the most commonly used lab tests are cholinesterase activity testing.

3. The first goal of treatment is to ensure the patient is properly decontaminated with all clothing removed, a gentle water rinse, bathing with hypoallergenic soap, followed by two more rinses in clean water. This helps stop the topical absorption of the chemical and prevents exposure to other bystanders. For treatment, start with atropine 1 to 3 mg IV bolus along with pralidoxime 2 g IV over 20 to 30 minutes, followed by a pralidoxime infusion of 0.5 to 1 g/h. Every 5 minutes, reassess the patient, and if symptoms have not resolved, double the dose of atropine until therapeutic effect is reached. Once stable, start an atropine infusion at a rate of 10% to 20% of the total dose that was needed to reach stability and give every hour. Titrate atropine off slowly until symptoms remain controlled and continue the pralidoxime infusion for 12 to 24 hours after atropine is complete. Lastly, use benzodiazepines as needed for agitation and seizures.

Selected Readings

Anseeuw K, Delvau N, Burillo-Putze G, et al. Cyanide poisoning by fire smoke inhalation: a European expert consensus. *Eur J Emerg Med* 2013;20(1):2–9.
Awisi DK, Lebrun G, Fagnan M, et al. Alcohol, nicotine and iatrogenic withdrawals in the ICU. *Crit Care Med* 2013;41(9):S57–S68.
Blei AT. Selection for acute liver failure: have we got it right? *Liver Transpl* 2005;11(11):S30–S34.
Brooks DE, Levine M, O'Connor AD, et al. Toxicology in the ICU. Part 2. Specific toxins. *Chest* 2011;140(4):1072–1085.
Ciccarone D. Stimulant abuse: pharmacology, cocaine, methamphetamine, treatment, attempts at pharmacotherapy. *Prime Care Clin Office Pract* 2011;38(1):41–58.
Eddleston M, Buckley NA, Eyer P, et al. Management of acute organophosphate pesticide poisoning. *Lancet* 2008;37(9612):597–607.
Guzman JA. Carbon monoxide poisoning. *Crit Care Med* 2012;(28):537–548.
Hodgman MJ, Garrard AR. A review of acetaminophen poisoning. *Crit Care Clin* 2012;28:499–516.
Kanji S, MacLean RD. Cardiac glycoside toxicity. More than 200 years and counting. *Crit Care Clin* 28(2012):527–535.
Kanter MZ. Comparison of oral and IV acetylcysteine in the treatment of acetaminophen poisoning. *Am J Health-Syst Pharm* 2006;63:1821–1827.
Kruse JA. Methanol and ethylene glycol intoxication. *Crit Care Clin* 2012;28:661–711.
Levine M, Brooks DE, Truitt CA, et al. Toxicology in the ICU. Part 1. General overview and approach to treatment. *Chest* 2011;140(3):795–806.
Marraffa JM, Coehn V, Howland MA. Antidotes for toxicological emergencies: a practical review. *Am J Health-Syst Pharm* 2012;69:199–212.

McKnight RF, Adida M, Budge K, et al. Lithium toxicity profile: a systematic review and meta-analysis. *Lancet* 2012;379:721–728.

Nowak RM, Macias CG. Anaphylaxis on the other front line: perspectives from the emergency department. *Am J Med* 2014;127:S34–S44.

Paden MS, Franjic L, Halcomb SE. Hyperthermia caused by drug interactions and adverse reactions. *Emerg Med Clin N Am* 2013;(31):1035–1044.

Pearlman BL, Gambhir R. Salicylate intoxication: a clinical review. *Postgraduate Med* 2009;121(4):162–168

Reilly TH, Kirk MA. Atypical antipsychotics and newer antidepressants. *Emerg Med Clin N Am* 2007;25:477–497.

Shepherd G. Treatment of poisoning caused by β-adrenergic and calcium-channel blockers. *Am J Health-Syst Pharm* 2006;63(19):1828–1835.

Wong JM. Propofol infusion syndrome. *Am J Ther* 2010;17(5):487–491.

Adult Resuscitation

Peter L. Bekker and Richard M. Pino

I. **OVERVIEW.** The intensivist needs to be well versed in advanced cardio-pulmonary resuscitation (CPR) not only to administer care in the ICU but also to assist throughout the hospital. The algorithms and protocols presented here are based on the American Heart Association 2010 Guidelines for cardiopulmonary resuscitation. Formal training with routine recertification is essential to maintenance of skills. In addition to competence in resuscitation, the responsibilities of the intensivist include personnel and resource management that involves clear and deliberate communication and delegation of responsibilities in a crisis.

II. **CARDIAC ARREST**
   A. **Initial response** to a cardiac arrest can be quite rapid in the hospital setting. In the ICU, because of continuous ECG monitoring, the frequent use of arterial blood pressure determinations, the optimal nurse-to-patient ratios, abnormalities in the circulation, and dysrhythmias are identified immediately.
   B. **Etiologies.** Cardiac arrest in adults may be due to a number of causes, ranging from intrinsic cardiopulmonary problems to metabolic and anatomic abnormalities.
      1. Myocardial infarction
      2. Pericardial tamponade
      3. Pulmonary embolus
      4. Tension pneumothorax
      5. Hypoxemia
      6. Acid–base derangements
      7. Hypovolemia
      8. Hypothermia
      9. Electrolyte abnormalities, including potassium, calcium, and magnesium
      10. Adverse drug events
   C. **Pathophysiology.** A cascade of events begins with the systemic hypo-perfusion caused by cardiac arrest. Initially, hypoxemia leads to anaerobic metabolism and acidosis. This leads to systemic vasodilation, pulmonary vasoconstriction, and insensitivity to catecholamines. With resuscitation after a period of hypoxia, the different organs are susceptible to reperfusion injury.

III. **ADULT RESUSCITATION**
   A. **Basic Life Support (BLS) Primary Survey and Advanced Cardiac Life Support (ACLS) Secondary Survey.** ACLS relies on **proper BLS assessment and care**, including high-quality **CPR** and defibrillation, as appropriate. ACLS achieves definitive treatment by adding drug therapy and advanced airway management. Immediately starting CPR and defibrillating without delay increases the chance of return of spontaneous circulation (ROSC) and survival to discharge for ventricular fibrillation (VF) sudden cardiac

arrest (SCA), while interventions such as advanced airway management and pharmacologic therapy have not been shown to improve survival to discharge.

1. **Circulation.** Evaluation of appropriate circulation should take place immediately and involve palpation of the **carotid pulse for at least 5, but not more than 10, seconds.** If no definite pulse is palpated or the patient has a critically low blood pressure for the clinical situation, then chest compressions are begun at a rate of 100 compressions/min, alternating with ventilation in a 30:2 ratio. In the event of advanced airway placement, compressions continue at 100/min without stopping for ventilation at 8 to 10 breaths/min. **Compressions** should be performed with the rescuer's hands on the sternum at the level of the nipple, depressing the chest at least 2 inches and allowing the chest to completely recoil after each compression. Adequacy of compressions may be assessed by palpating a pulse or observing the pressure using invasive arterial pressure monitoring. Furthermore, the patient should be placed onto a hard surface to facilitate the quality of compressions. The evaluation for ROSC should be done after every five cycles, or 2 minutes. After successful return to a perfusing rhythm, chest compressions must continue for an additional 2 minutes.

2. **Airway.** The ICU patient may already have a secured airway. Otherwise, the airway patency needs to be initially assessed with a head tilt–chin lift maneuver, jaw thrust, or artificial airway. The patient should be evaluated for spontaneous ventilation, using the algorithm—**look** for rise and fall of the chest, **listen** for exhalation, and **feel** for airflow. During the first minutes of VF SCA, rescue breaths are probably not as important as chest compressions.

3. **Breathing.** In the absence of adequate ventilation, the rescuer will initiate **two breaths** via bag-valve mask ventilation with 100% oxygen. At this point, breaths should be evaluated and maintained at a rate of **8 to 10 breaths/min**, or alternating with compressions in a **30:2 ratio**. If appropriate rise and fall of the chest is not achieved, then the airway should be repositioned and examined for a foreign body. Additionally, **a definitive airway may be placed as long as it does not interfere** with other resuscitative efforts, and it should be done by the most experienced person. Proper placement of the endotracheal tube (ETT) is confirmed with end-tidal CO_2 measurement using a colorimetric CO_2 indicator or continuous waveform capnography and auscultation of the chest. In addition to confirming tracheal tube placement in the airway, continuous capnography can be used as a guide for further CPR. An $ETCO_2$ <10 mmHg indicates the CPR technique requires improvement (better chest excursions, higher rate of compressions). The persistence of $ETCO_2$ <10 mmHg suggests that ROSC is unlikely while an abrupt increase to 35 to 40 mmHg demonstrates that ROSC has likely been achieved. Excessive ventilation is unnecessary and is harmful because it increases intrathoracic pressure, decreases venous return to the heart, and diminishes cardiac output and survival.

   If intravenous access cannot be obtained immediately, epinephrine, atropine, naloxone, vasopressin, and lidocaine can be administered via the ETT. The dose is typically 2 to 2.5 times the intravenous dose, diluted in 5 to 10 mL of water or saline.

4. **Defibrillation**, with CPR, forms the basis of successful adult resuscitation for VF SCA, with the attention focused on minimal interruption of other interventions. As time progresses, the likelihood of ROSC decreases.

The successful utilization of **automated external defibrillators (AEDs)** has resulted in the training of additional responders, such as police, fire personnel, security guards, airline attendants, and so on. AEDs are available in many public areas and include adhesive electrode pads for both delivery of shock and sensing of the rhythm. In light of evidence supporting minimizing interruption of chest compressions, the current recommendation is for a single shock between cycles of CPR and the palpation for a pulse after an additional 2 minutes of chest compressions. This is to minimize any delays in coronary perfusion, despite ROSC.

a. **Biphasic waveform defibrillators** utilize a positive current in one direction then reversed in the opposite direction. Unless there is documentation of previous successful defibrillations, 200 J is recommended for the first shock. As mentioned above, CPR should continue through the charging, and it is the responsibility of the operator to make sure that all personnel are "cleared," or not in contact with the patient, during defibrillation.

b. **Monophasic waveform defibrillators** supply a shock in a single direction and have been replaced by biphasic defibrillators in most institutions.

5. **Diagnosis and cardioversion of dysrhythmias.** Although the most common nonperfusing waveforms are VF and ventricular tachycardia (VT), instability may be also due to bradycardia and supraventricular tachycardia (SVT). A useful diagnostic and therapeutic tool is **adenosine** that has the ability to reveal underlying atrial rhythms (Fig. 33.1) and possibly

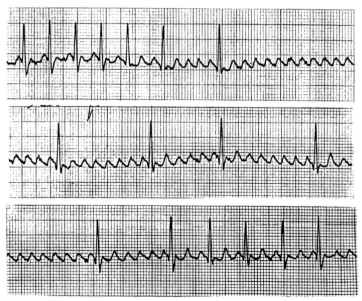

FIGURE 33.1 Diagnosis of a rhythm with adenosine. The initial ventricular response of 180 beats/min disappears after atrioventricular conduction is inhibited by adenosine, revealing an underlying rhythm of atrial flutter (300 beats/min, **top**), followed by a 6 to 8:1 block (**middle**), then a 2 to 3:1 block of atrial flutter with a ventricular rate of 120 beats/min.

convert an SVT to sinus rhythm. This diagnosis is complex, differentiating a wide-complex SVT from VT, and thus should not be used in the event of VT. A more sensitive method for diagnosing the atrial activity is the **atrial electrogram.** If the patient is not dependent on atrial pacing and has intraoperatively placed atrial pacing wires, these can be connected to a precordial lead and monitored temporarily. Additionally, a **transesophageal pacer** can be utilized to obtain the atrial electrogram (Fig. 33.2). If this is not immediately available, then a transvenous pacing wire can be passed through a No. 4 endotracheal tube inserted in the esophagus for the same purpose. In contrast to defibrillation during

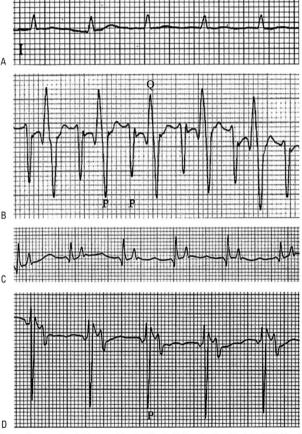

FIGURE 33.2 Suspected atrial flutter with a 2:1 block. **A:** Standard lead I of the ECG: The flutter waves are not distinct. **B:** Atrial electrogram obtained through an esophageal lead, showing an atrial rate of 300 beats/min with P waves (P) and Q waves (Q) easily seen. The polarity of the P wave is inverted because of the positioning of the esophageal probe. **C:** After treatment with amiodarone and cardioversion, normal sinus rhythm is seen on the standard ECG and the atrial electrogram **(D).**

which time electrical charges are administered on command when there are no discernible QRS complexes, with cardioversion, the shocks are synchronized to the R-wave. This prevents the electrical charge creating a lethal dsyrrhymia by falling on the T-wave. For synchronized cardioversion of a paroxysmal SVT (PSVT), the operator should choose a lower initial dose, such as 50 J (Fig. 33.3). With more resistant rhythms, such as **atrial fibrillation (AF) and atrial flutter,** an initial dose of 100 J may be indicated. For hemodynamically stable VT, an initial cardioversion at 100 J is warranted. In all dysrhythmias, the responder must be cognizant of the precipitating causes of the abnormality.

6. **Pacing** involves pharmacologic and electronic choices for symptomatic bradycardia. Initial pharmacologic treatments for bradycardia, such as with atropine, are often effective, but lack precision in heart rate control and are not universally efficacious. Atropine should not be used in Mobitz type II second-degree block or complete heart block in which case pacing should be attempted. Transcutaneous pacing is often the most feasible method of control with sedation required for patient comfort.

7. **Intravenous access** is important for effective medication administration, although **it should not interfere with prompt initiation of CPR** and delivery of shocks. Central circulation access is ideal for resuscitation medications, as circulation time is greatly accelerated over peripheral access. It should be noted that the drawback of central access is that it may not be feasible during active resuscitation or compressions. Upper extremity veins are well suited for peripheral access, while intraosseous cannulation is also safe and effective in the absence of peripheral access. Many patients will have additional central access, including hemodialysis ports, portacaths, and peripherally inserted central catheters (PICC).

8. **Medications** are used to treat hypotension, myocardial ischemia, and dysrhythmias. For treatment of dysrhythmias, current guidelines recommend attempts at CPR and defibrillation, if necessary, before medical therapy. A few critical drugs may be given via the endotracheal tube (naloxone, atropine, vasopressin, epinephrine, and lidocaine) if IV access is not present. The dose is typically 2 to 2.5 times that of the IV dose diluted in 5 to 10 mL of saline or sterile water. **Adenosine** is an endogenous purine nucleotide with an extremely short half-life of 5 seconds. It is useful for its ability to slow

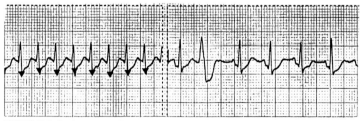

FIGURE 33.3 Synchronous cardioversion of a supraventricular tachycardia. Arrowheads (**left**) indicate synchrony of the defibrillator with the patient's rate (300 beats/min) prior to cardioversion (**right**) to a rate of 140 beats/min that was followed with pharmacologic therapy.

atrioventricular (AV) nodal conduction to convert SVT to a sinus rhythm. Because it exerts its primary effect on the AV node, it is not useful for ventricular dysrhythmias or atrial fibrillation/flutter (Fig. 33.1). In fact, the more common transient vasodilatation may manifest as hypotension if given inappropriately during VT. Other adverse effects may include angina, bronchospasm, and dysrhythmias. For peripheral intravenous administration, an initial dose of 6 mg should be given rapidly with a fluid flush. If this is nondiagnostic or ineffective, the dose can be increased to 12 mg for successive doses, although other, longer-duration agents may be required for recurrent PSVT. With central venous administration, the dose is reduced by half; the initial dose should be 3 mg, followed by 6 mg as needed.

a. **Amiodarone** is a versatile antiarrhythmic agent with effects on sodium, potassium, and calcium channels, as well as α- and β-adrenergic blocking properties. Indications include unstable VT, defibrillation with VF, rate control of VT, conversion of AF to sinus rhythm, ventricular rate control with atrial arrhythmias unresponsive to digitalis and due to accessory pathways, and as adjunctive treatment to cardioversion for SVT and atrial tachycardia. Typical acute side effects include hypotension, bradycardia, and QT-interval prolongation. **Dosing for unstable VT and VF** is **300 mg** in 20 to 30 mL saline or D_5W, given rapidly. For more stable dysrhythmias, such as AF with rapid ventricular response, the initial dose is 150 mg over 10 minutes, followed by an infusion of 1 mg/min for 6 hours, and 0.5 mg/min, with a maximum daily dose of 2 g.

b. **Atropine** is an anticholinergic agent that reverses hemodynamically significant bradycardia or AV block. However, atropine is not suitable for treatment of Mobitz type II heart block or complete heart block, in which case pacing should be initiated. Dosing for symptomatic bradycardia is 0.5 mg, repeated every 3 to 5 minutes to a maximum dose of 0.04 mg/kg. It is no longer indicated for asystole.

c. β-**Blocking agents.** The utility of β-blockers in ACLS is limited to rate control in patients with preserved ventricular function and narrow complex tachycardias from a reentry SVT or automatic focus that is not controlled with vagal maneuvers or adenosine. These agents can be used for heart rate control in AF and atrial flutter. Typical side effects include hypotension, bradycardia, possible exacerbation of reactive airway disease, and AV conduction delays. Contraindications include second- or third-degree heart blocks, hypotension, acute or severe congestive heart failure, and preexcitation syndrome such as Wolf-Parkinson-White (WPW). **Esmolol** is a very short-acting β_1-blocker, with a half-life of approximately 5 minutes. It is administered as a 0.5 mg/kg IV bolus (over 1 minute), with a 4-minute infusion of 0.05 mg/kg/min. A repeat dose of 0.5 mg/kg IV can be given, with an infusion of 0.1 mg/kg/min, up to 0.3 mg/kg/min. **Metoprolol** is another selective β_1-blocker, and it is given as a 5-mg IV bolus at 5-minute intervals. **Propranolol** is a nonselective β-blocker (β_1 and β_2), given as an IV bolus of 1 to 2 mg at 2-minute intervals and has a slightly longer duration of action than does metoprolol.

d. **Calcium chloride** is used specifically for treatment of symptomatic hypocalcemia, symptomatic hyperkalemia, magnesium intoxication, or reversal of calcium-channel blocker toxicity. When given as calcium chloride, doses of 200 to 1,000 mg IV, over 5 minutes, are given as needed.

e. **Dopamine** is a δ-, α-, and β-adrenergic receptor agonist. Although not frequently used in ACLS, dopamine can be used to increase heart rate in the event of bradycardia refractory to atropine treatment and to increase vascular tone to raise the blood pressure and end-organ perfusion. Most common side effects include tachyarrhythmias. The initial dose should be started low (150 µg/min, or 2–3 µg/kg/min) and titrated to desired result or limited by adverse effects.

f. **Epinephrine** continues to be the primary pharmacologic agent in cardiac arrest due to its α-adrenergic effects in increasing coronary and cerebral perfusion. The limitation of efficacy lies in β-adrenergic activation by increasing myocardial oxygen demands, ischemia, and myocardial toxicity. Even though it is a mainstay of treatment, this is no good evidence that demonstrates an improvement in survival to discharge after cardiac arrest. High-dose epinephrine was supported by early ROSC and survival reports, but several randomized trials have failed to show any benefit with escalating doses in cardiac arrest. Theoretically, a higher dose may be justified in β-blocker or calcium-channel blocker overdose. Dosing for intravenous administration is 1 mg (10 mL of a 1:10,000 solution) every 3 to 5 minutes during cardiac arrest. Epinephrine can be given via the endotracheal route at 2 to 2.5 mg per dose, until IV/IO access is established.

g. **Ibutilide** is an antiarrhythmic agent that is utilized to convert or control AF and flutter by prolonging the action potential and refractory period of cardiac tissue. In patients with normal cardiac function, it is used to convert AF or atrial flutter of duration less than 48 hours and for rate control in AF or atrial flutter in patients unresponsive to β-blockers or calcium-channel blockers. Additionally, it is useful for cardioversion of AF or AD in patients with preexcitation syndrome (WPW). The most common side effects of ibutilide are ventricular arrhythmias, requiring continuous monitoring for 6 hours after dosing. Additionally, it carries minor incidence of hypotension and bradycardia. It is contraindicated with prolonged QTc >440 ms. Dosing is based on weight; for patients more than 60 kg, the intravenous dose of 1 mg is administered over 10 minutes, with an additional 1 mg IV dose given similarly in 10 minutes, if necessary. For patients less than 60 kg, the initial dose should be 0.01 mg/kg, administered as above.

h. **Lidocaine** is a local anesthetic that has been relegated as an alternative to amiodarone as an adjunct to defibrillation and prevention of VF after myocardial infarction. This change in status over the years is due to randomized controlled trials showing inferior rates of ROSC and higher rates of asystole. Dosing is 1 to 1.5 mg/kg IV, with additional doses at 0.5 to 0.75 mg/kg IV push, at 5 to 10 minute intervals.

i. **Magnesium** is a cofactor in many enzyme reactions, and hypomagnesemia can worsen hypokalemia in addition to inducing VT. The utility of magnesium as therapy is based on two observational studies in treating *torsades de pointes*. Adverse effects include hypotension and bradycardia. Emergent administration is 1 to 2 g diluted in 10 mL D_5W over 5 to 20 minutes.

j. **Procainamide** is useful for conversion of AF and atrial flutter to sinus rhythm, controlling rapid ventricular response in SVT, and converting wide complex tachycardia. It has largely been replaced by amiodarone. Dosing is begun with an infusion of 20 to 30 mg/min for a total loading dose of 17 mg/kg or until arrhythmia is terminated, the patient has nausea, there is hypotension, or the QRS widens by 50%. A maintenance infusion should be maintained at 1 to 4 mg/min. Procainamide administration should be followed with serum levels of procainamide and *N*-acetylprocainamide, the active metabolite. It is rarely used today.

k. **Sodium bicarbonate** is not recommended for routine use in most cardiac arrests due to harmful effects, including paradoxical worsening of intracellular acidosis. The exceptions include treatment of hyperkalemia, tricyclic antidepressant, and phenobarbital overdose. Bicarbonate may be considered in severe metabolic acidosis unresponsive to standard ACLS treatments. The initial bicarbonate dose is 1 mEq/Kg IV, with repeat doses of 0.5 mEq/kg administered at 10-minute intervals.

l. **Sotalol** is a class III antiarrhythmic agent with nonselective β-blocking properties. Similar to ibutilide, it is used in patients with preserved ventricular function and monomorphic VT, AF with rapid ventricular response, atrial flutter, and preexcitation syndrome such as WPW. Most common side effects include bradycardia, arrhythmias, including *torsades de pointes*, and hypotension. IV dosing is 1 to 1.5 mg/kg administered at a rate of 10 mg/min. The required slow rate of infusion is a limiting factor in emergent situations.

m. **Vasopressin** is a noradrenergic vasoconstrictor and antidiuretic hormone analogue. It is useful as an alternative to epinephrine during treatment of VF and requires less frequent dosing due to a longer half-life. Although retrospective data indicate a possible survival benefit in patients with asystole, randomized controlled trials fail to display any advantage over epinephrine in regard to ROSC, early survival, or survival to discharge. Dosing is 40 units intravenously, replacing the first or second dose of epinephrine.

n. **Verapamil and diltiazem** are calcium-channel blockers that slow AV nodal conduction and increase refractoriness, with depressant effects on myocardial contractility. They are used for reentry SVT unresponsive to adenosine or vagal maneuvers and rate control in AF and atrial flutter. Because of their vasodilator and negative inotropic effects, side effects include hypotension, worsening of congestive heart failure, bradycardia, and exacerbation of accessory pathways in WPW syndrome. Verapamil dosing is initially 2.5 to 5 mg IV over 2 minutes, with repeat doses 5 to 10 mg given every 15 to 30 minutes up to 20 mg. Diltiazem dosing is 0.25 mg/kg (20 mg), followed by a repeat dose of 0.35 mg/kg (25 mg). Diltiazem can also be infused at a rate of 5 to 15 mg/h, titrated to heart rate. In the event of significant hypotension due to calcium-channel blocker use, calcium chloride 500 to 1,000 mg is recommended.

9. **Specific ACLS algorithms**
   a. Pulseless arrest (Fig. 33.4)
   b. Tachycardia with pulse (Fig. 33.5)
   c. Bradycardia (Fig. 33.6)

10. **Direct cardiac compression with open chest** is an option for patients with penetrating chest trauma, pericardial tamponade, chest wall deformity, or any recent chest surgery. This allows for direct assessment and compression of the myocardium and direct defibrillation with internal paddles starting at 5 to 10 J.

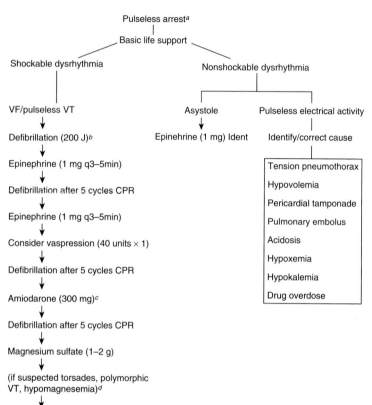

FIGURE 33.4 Algorithm for pulseless arrest. VF, ventricular fibrillation; VT, ventricular tachycardia. [a]When rhythm is unclear and could be VF, treat as shockable rhythm. [b]Biphasic. One cycle of CPR should follow any successful defibrillation. [c]Amiodarone bolus should be administered in 20 to 30 mL saline or D_5W. This is followed by an infusion of 1 mg/min for 6 hours and then 0.5 mg/min thereafter. An additional dose of 150 mg IV can be readministered for recurrence of VF or pulseless VT. [d]Consider earlier in the algorithm in addition to the other interventions if these are suspected.

11. **Termination of CPR** is warranted after a prolonged, competent trial of CPR and ACLS. The likelihood of survival to discharge becomes exceedingly small in the absence of ROSC after a prolonged BLS and ACLS attempt of 15 to 20 minutes. Although there is a paucity of significant data, intermittent ROSC may delay the termination of resuscitative efforts. The circumstances and decision to terminate efforts should be documented.

12. **Unique situations in resuscitation**

    a. **Do not resuscitate (DNR)** orders are advance directives that express the patient's wishes in the event resuscitation is an option. These orders

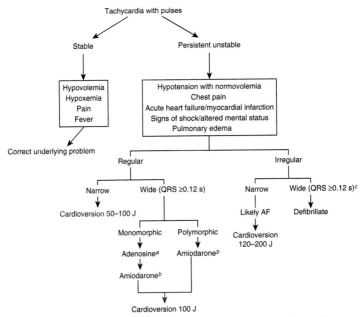

FIGURE 33.5 Protocol for tachycardia with pulse. AF, atrial fibrillation. [a]Adenosine: rapid peripheral IV push 6 mg, and 12 mg if second dose is needed; central access: initial dose 3 mg, second dose 6 mg. [b]Amiodarone bolus should be administered in 20 to 30 mL saline or D_5W. This is followed by an infusion of 1 mg/min for 6 hours and then 0.5 mg/min thereafter. [c]When rhythm is unclear and could be VF, treat as shockable rhythm (Fig. 33.4).

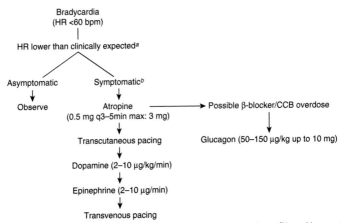

FIGURE 33.6 Protocol for bradycardia. HR, heart rate; bpm, beats per minute. [a]Normal heart rate goal may be <60 bpm for patients receiving therapeutic nodal agents (e.g., β-blocker). [b]Symptoms may include altered mental status, hypotension, pulmonary edema, congestive heart failure, myocardial infarction. [c]Calcium-channel blocker.

are not automatically modified or suspended in the perioperative period, but instead each situation needs to be carefully addressed. This includes the patient's desire for perioperative resuscitation, limits of perioperative resuscitation, and reinstatement of the original DNR orders. The intensivist may be asked to respond to arrests and incubate outside the intensive care unit. In those situations, the patient's code status should be determined, as the responder is ethically and legally bound to follow the patient's directives.

Selected Readings

American Heart Association. 2010 American Heart Association Guidelines for cardiopulmonary resuscitation and emergency cardiovascular care science. *Circulation* 2010;122(suppl):S722–S729.

Bella BS, Alvarado JP, Myklebust H, et al. Quality of cardiopulmonary resuscitation during in-hospital cardiac arrest. *JAMA* 2005;293:305–310.

Eisenberg MS, Mengert TJ. Cardiac resuscitation. *N Engl J Med* 2001;344:1304–1313.

Martens PR, Russell JK, Wolcke B, et al. Optimal response to cardiac arrest study: defibrillation waveform effects. *Resuscitation* 2001;49:233–243.

Niemann JT, Stratton SJ, Cruz B, Lewis RJ. Endotracheal drug administration during out-of-hospital resuscitation: where are the survivors? *Resuscitation* 2002;53:153–157.

Wik L, Hansen TB, Fylling F, et al. Delaying defibrillation to give basic cardiopulmonary resuscitation to patients with out-of-hospital ventricular fibrillation: a randomized trial. *JAMA* 2003;289:1389–1395.

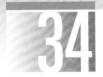

Burn Critical Care

Benjamin Levi, Victor W. Wong, and Robert Sheridan

I. INTRODUCTION

A. Scope of the Problem in the United States

1. Burns are a major source of morbidity: approximately two million burns occur per year. Burns result in more than 60,000 hospitalizations and nearly 6,000 deaths per year. Total health care expenditures approach 4 billion dollars per year. Recent reports demonstrate a 50% decline in burn-related deaths and hospital admissions over the last 20 years.

2. Large-burn patients should be cared for as other critical care patients—providers should make sure to assess all organ systems. Though formulas for fluid resuscitation are well known, it is important to assess the resuscitative progress similar to the resuscitative efforts of other critically ill patients. While, critical illness in burned patients is most often caused by sepsis, burn wound sepsis is no longer seen as frequently due to aggressive early debridement. In fact, pneumonia is now most common cause of sepsis in burn patients.

B. The first steps of the overall critical care management plan are the initial assessment and resuscitation, followed by early wound excision and biologic closure either with autograft (if available) or allograft within 96 hours. Subsequently definitive wound closure is achieved and rehabilitation can begin. Throughout the execution of this plan, the physiologic effects of burn injury must also be kept in mind. They are as follows:

1. Early hypodynamic "ebb" phase: Early hours after injury with hypodynamic state requiring aggressive critical support.

2. Hyperdynamic "flow" phase: After first few hours, patient will develop increased cardiac output, increased muscle catabolism, and decreased peripheral vascular resistance.

3. Massive capillary leak thought to result from burn wound inflammatory mediators.

4. Postresuscitative phase: Volume requirements often decline after the first 24 hours and capillary leak decreases. Patient then has a hyperdynamic phase with fever and increased protein catabolism. Inflammatory mediators such as TNF-α, IFN-γ, IL-6, and IL-10 are released.

II. COMPONENTS OF PRIMARY AND SECONDARY SURVEY IN BURN PATIENTS

During their initial evaluation, burn patients should have a primary and secondary survey according to advanced trauma life-support guidelines. The components of this are the following:

A. **Airway.** Objective measurements include respiratory rate, respiratory effort, breath sounds, skin assessment, and intraoral and intranasal examination for soot and mucosal inflammation. It is important to establish definitive airway before transport, especially if large fluid requirements are estimated (>30% TBSA). Even without airway injury, patients develop progressive mucosal edema from massive inflammation and fluid requirements. For airway burns, it is crucial to evaluate for burns of the face, eyes, neck, and nasopharynx, including soot in these regions. Get a detailed history of where the patient sustained their burn as inhalation injuries rarely occur in nonenclosed spaces. Assess if patient was exposed to chemicals or carbon monoxide. If carboxyhemoglobin levels are >20%, consider hyperbaric oxygen (only if patient is stable enough) or 100% FIO_2. When intubating, make sure an airway assessment is performed initially. If patient has difficult anatomy, it is important to have fiberoptic setup, bougie, and surgical consultation in case a surgical airway is needed. The patient's hemodynamics should be assessed prior to intubation. Typical induction medications can include propofol (make sure patient is not hypotensive) or etomidate (may get delayed adrenal insufficiency) and rocuronium as the paralytic (avoid succinylcholine). All of these induction agents cause hypotension, so providers should be ready with a vasopressor such as IV neosynephrine. Newer studies demonstrate ketamine might represent alternative with less hypotensive effects.

B. **Breathing.** Once patient is intubated, it is crucial to assess location of the tube through auscultation, visualization of moisture in the endotracheal tube, bilateral chest rise, and CO_2 detection. Take care when securing the endotracheal tube around the head to prevent a potential tourniquet effect as the patient becomes edematous during resuscitation.

C. **Circulation.** It is important to have large-bore IV access with 16 or 18G peripheral IVs. It is better to place access in nonburned areas though this is not always possible. If the patient is going to require invasive monitoring, a central line should be placed under sterile conditions. If a PiCCO device (Pulsion Medical Systems AG, Munich, Germany) is used to monitor the patient, it is best to have central line in the internal jugular vein and the arterial line in the groin. This technology uses thermodilution to determine cardiac performance. Studies have demonstrated feasibility of this technology compared to pulmonary artery catheter. Blood pressure cuffs can be difficult to obtain an accurate read, making arterial lines useful.

D. **Disability/Neurologic Assessment.** Using the "AVPU" mnemonic, evaluate if patient is **A**lert, responsive to **V**erbal stimuli, responsive to **P**ainful stimuli only, or **U**nresponsive, which might help assess if patient is hypoxic, hypercarbic, or altered. Obtain a baseline Glasgow Coma Score, and make sure there are no other injuries.

E. **Exposure and Environmental Control.** It is important to remove all clothing, especially if a chemical injury is sustained, and it is necessary to decontaminate (copious water irrigation until pH = 7) the patient prior to transport. Make sure to remove any jewelry that can create a tourniquet effect once swelling sets in.

III. BURN-SPECIFIC SECONDARY SURVEY

A. **History:** mechanism and timing of injury; was there chemical exposure and, if so, what are the side effects of this chemical; was the patient inside or outside; was there any risk of inhalation injury; neurologic status; extrication time; fluids and mediations given on scene and during transport; tetanus status; code status; and decision makers

B. **Face:** detailed orbital and periorbital exam. Electrical injury increases risk of glaucoma. Massive fluid resuscitation can cause intraocular compartment syndrome. Ophthalmology consult should be obtained if there is concern for corneal injury, and they should perform a fluorescein dye test. If conjunctival swelling, patient may not be able to close their eyelids. If this is the case, consider temporary tarsorrhaphy. Large-volume irrigation of globes with neutral pH solution is required, especially if chemical injury. Examine the nose for singed vibrissae. Perform an intraoral exam to look for swelling and carbonaceous sputum.

C. **Neurologic:** Abnormal neurological exam may indicate carbon monoxide exposure.

D. **Chest:** Assess chest compliance and if eschar is limiting chest excursion and decreasing compliance.

E. **Genitourinary System:** Early Foley catheter placement allows for close monitoring of urine output and therefore kidney perfusion. Deeply burned foreskin may affect penile perfusion.

F. **Extremities:** Important to examine all extremities (proximal and distal) for compartment syndrome. Unlike crush injury or electrical injury (caused by immobile fascia), flame and scald burns cause compartment syndrome by creating immobile skin layer. Most sensitive exam finding for compartment syndrome is pain with passive movement; however, this may not be possible in intubated patient. Important to assess distal two-point discrimination (normal <6 mm) and arterial pulses. By time there is a change in neurologic or vascular exam of the extremity, it is usually too late. If electrical injury, it is important to monitor serum creatine kinase (CK), and, in addition to escharotomy, patient will require fasciotomy to release deeper compartments.

G. **GI:** Patient may require abdominal escharotomy for large-volume resuscitation to avoid abdominal compartment syndrome. If patient develops abdominal compartment syndrome, it should be addressed by making sure adequate escharotomy is done, laying patient supine, making sure the patient has a nasogastric tube, treating pain, and starting a paralytic (not succinylcholine) if needed. If these measures fail, the patient will need a laparotomy, which has extremely high mortality in burn patients.

H. **Initial Wound Evaluation:** crucial to assess location and depth of all burns using a burn diagram. Rule of 9s estimate that surface area for each upper extremity is 9%, lower extremity 18%, anterior chest/abdomen 18%, back 18%, and head 9% (Fig. 34.1). Alternatively, you can use the patient's palm, which represents 1% to estimate burn area. In children, the head is 18% and the lower extremities are each 14%. Burn wound often has three zones of injury (Fig. 34.2). Zone of coagulation has full-thickness burn through the epidermis and dermis. The zone of stasis can go on to heal or progress to become zone of coagulation. Zone of hyperemia is superficial and will go on to heal.

I. **Burn Depth**
   1. Superficial partial thickness: Burn down to papillary dermis
   2. Deep partial thickness: Burn down to reticular dermis

J. **Laboratories and Radiographs**
   1. Carboxyhemoglobin if concern for inhalation injury (normal up to 3% in nonsmokers, up to 15% is normal in smokers)
   2. Chest x-ray to assess placement of endotracheal tube
   3. CBC, chemistries, LFTs, coags, T&S, ABG

IV. TOOLS TO HELP IN HEMODYNAMIC MONITORING

The provider should also consider the different tools to help in hemodynamic monitoring, including the following:

A. Central venous pressure trend can be used to assess progress of resuscitation, though the absolute numbers have limited value.

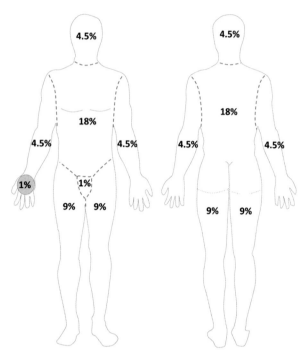

FIGURE 34.1 Schematic of "Rule of 9s" to estimate burn surface area in adults. Anterior (left panel) and posterior (right panel) views of body. Area of palm approximates 1% total body surface area.

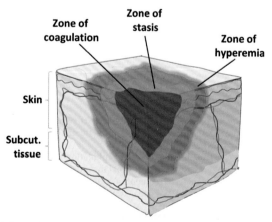

FIGURE 34.2 Zones of burn injury. The central zone of coagulation describes coagulation necrosis and irreversible full thickness burn injury. The zone of stasis describes an intermediate level of injury severity and depth that may be reversible. The zone of hyperemia describes increased vasodilation surrounding the burn area which should heal once the acute inflammatory phase subsides.

B. Arterial lines can be helpful given difficulty using cuff pressures in very edematous extremities.

    1. The arterial line with central venous catheter can also be used to assess cardiac output when using the PiCCO system. This allows the provider to trend values, which may be more valuable than absolute numbers.

C. Pulmonary Artery Catheters. As in other areas of critical care, the PA catheter allows for goal-directed therapy. Studies have failed to show improvements in outcomes using PA catheters. They may be more useful in older patients with histories of cardiac disease.

V. MECHANICAL VENTILATION
Similarly mechanical ventilation can be employed with the following considerations:

A. Early endotracheal intubation is important in patients with inhalation injury or who have burns covering a lot of body surface areas. Airway protection is needed in patients requiring large-volume resuscitation. Other common indications for intubation include hypoxia and hypercarbia as well as inhalation injury.

B. Follow ARDSnet protocol recommendations. Low-volume protective lung ventilation: 4 to 6 mL/kg; plateau airway pressures should not exceed 30 cmH$_2$O. Assess best PEEP trial to set PEEP, but a PEEP of at least 5 cmH$_2$O should be used to avoid derecruitment. Consider esophageal manometry to aid in pleural pressure measurements if patient is obese. Recruitment maneuvers may be needed. Permissive hypercapnea is preferred over large tidal volumes. Limited studies have shown a potential role for high-frequency percussive ventilation in burn patients. Keep HOB 45° to decrease swelling and to prevent aspiration and ventilator-associated pneumonia in all ventilated patients. Daily mouth care with chlorhexidine should be used for ventilated patients.

VI. CONSIDERATIONS SURROUNDING RESUSCITATIVE STRATEGIES
Similarly, the following considerations surrounding resuscitative strategies should be employed and are temporally bound:

A. First 24 hours. Expect massive fluid shifts in both burned and nonburned tissues. Release of proinflammatory mediators such as TNF-α, histamine, and leukotrienes lead to increased microvascular permeability, edema, and shock. In general, resuscitation should be considered only in patients who have more than 30% total body surface area (TBSA) burns. It is important to get at least two large bore peripheral IVs. Starting point for fluids includes lactated ringers at 2 to 4 mL/kg × %TBSA burn with the first half given in the first 8 hours from injury (not arrival) and the second half given in the subsequent 16 hours. Children weighing less than 20 kg do not have large liver glycogen stores and should receive 0.45% saline with 5% dextrose at 3 to 4 mL/kg/h in addition to resuscitative fluid.

B. During resuscitation, it is imperative to follow the clinical response by monitoring: urine output, lactate, base deficit, mixed venous O$_2$ (and central venous O$_2$ if a PA line is in), central venous pressure, and cardiac output if using PiCCO or pulmonary artery catheter. It has been recommended to maintain urine output of about 0.5 mL/kg/h in adults and 0.5 to 1.0 mL/kg/h in kids; however, urine output can lag behind resuscitation and care must be taken not to overresuscitate. Studies do not necessarily demonstrate improved outcomes with either of these devices. PA catheters may lead to overresuscitation in healthy patients but are helpful in patients with cardiac diseases and those at risk of cardiac shock and congestive heart failure. It is important to assess for the presence of compartment syndrome of the extremities. This is done by clinical exam and by pulse examination. Monitoring for abdominal compartment syndrome is done by transducing bladder pressures and noting if there is increased difficulty ventilating and oxygenating, due to decreased venous return. Ocular compartment syndrome can be assessed using a tonometer.

C. Second 24 hours. All patients should receive crystalloid to maintain urine output and to maintain parameters of perfusion. Monitoring for adequacy of perfusion is done by measuring lactate, pulse volume variation, and cardiac outputs. Nutritional support should be started, usually by employing enteral nutrition within 24 to 48 hours. After 24 to 36 hours, intravenous fluids can be decreased by one-third, as long as the patient continues to produce adequate urine. Intravenous fluids can again be decreased by one-third for hours 36 to 48 (assuming urine output does not drop off). Colloids can be given after initial crystalloid resuscitation (5% albumin at 0.3–0.5 mL/kg/%TBSA over 24 hours) if blood pressures are not adequate.

D. After 48 hours, intravenous fluid should be administered to maintain urine output at 0.5 to 1 mL/kg body weight/h. Insensible losses and hyperthermia are associated with a hyperdynamic state. Daily weights can be helpful to determine insensible fluid loss or fluid retention.

E. Overresuscitation. If during the first 24 hours, resuscitation exceeds 6 mL/kg/%TBSA burn/24 h, the physician should reassess the clinical picture. An exuberant administration of intravenous fluid can lead to abdominal or extremity compartment syndrome, decreased chest wall compliance, and elevated peak airway pressures. Hourly neurovascular exams should be performed of all extremities at risk. Since patients are frequently intubated, physical exams can be limited. However, capillary refills can be assessed, as can pulse oximetry and compartment pressures with a Stryker needle or arterial line setup. If circumferential eschar is causing concern for compartment syndrome, extremity escharotomy should be made through the dermis down to the underlying adipose tissue but not through the muscular fascia (Fig. 34.3). Incisions should be made laterally and medially across affected extremities. Carpal tunnels may also need to be released (Fig. 34.4).

1. **Chest compartment syndromes.** The diagnosis is based on decreased chest wall compliance and increased peak airway pressures. Chest escharotomy should be performed along the anterior axillary line and connected at the infraclavicular and subcostal lines.

2. **Abdominal compartment syndrome.** The diagnosis is based on exam and bladder pressures >30 mmHg. Escharotomies laterally can also help prevent abdominal compartment syndrome. Once present, however, a bedside decompressive laparotomy may be needed, especially if high bladder pressures and high peak airway pressures remain after completion of the escharotomy.

3. **Orbital** compartment syndrome is relieved with lateral canthotomy.

VII. INHALATION INJURY AND CARBON MONOXIDE POISONING

A. Inhalation injury is divided into (1) upper airway (pharynx and trachea), (2) lower airway and parenchyma, and (3) toxicity due to toxic gases.

1. **Upper airway.** Swelling maximal at 12 to 24 hours. It can be diagnosed at the time of direct laryngoscopy. Upper airway has large absorptive capacity and prevents most burns to lower airway. Decision to intubate should be based on patient exam, pharyngeal swelling, carbonaceous

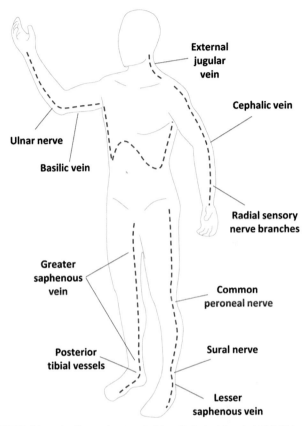

FIGURE 34.3 Schematic of burn escharotomy incisions. Dashed red lines depict full thickness incisions through burned skin down to subcutaneous fat. Labels point to key anatomic structures that should be preserved whenever possible when performing escharotomies.

sputum below the vocal cords, and mucosal swelling. Treatment of upper airway burns includes admission to hospital, humidified oxygen, general pulmonary toilet, and bronchodilators if indicated. Intubation is provided if indicated by experienced provider with access to fiberoptic technology and surgical intervention. If intubated, larger tube allows for better bronchoscopy and pulmonary toilet.

2. **Lower airway.** Caused by smoke combustion products and inhaled steam. It results in loss of ciliary clearance of damaged mucosa and debris leading to a high incidence of pneumonia (50%).

VIII. SIGNIFICANT MORBIDITY AND MORTALITY ASSOCIATED WITH THERMAL BURNS WITH INHALATIONAL INJURIES

A. Mortality for burn patients on ventilator for more than 1 week is similar to that of ARDS. Burn patients are unique in their development of ALI and

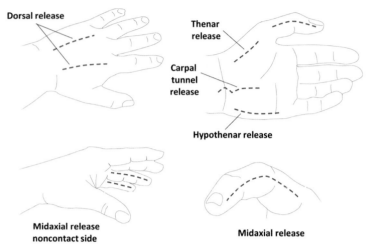

FIGURE 34.4 Schematic of burn escharotomy incisions for hand burns. Because these incisions are identical to those performed for hand compartment release, dissection should proceed bluntly through the muscular fascia if concern for hand compartment syndrome. Dorsal incisions should overlie the second and fourth metacarpals. Midaxial incisions should be on non-contact digit surfaces and avoid the volarly positioned neurovascular bundle.

ARDS, as they suffer smoke inhalation, causing respiratory insufficiency, hypoxia by increased capillary permeability, ciliary dysfunction, and interstitial edema. Damaged necrotic respiratory mucosa will slough, causing bronchial plugging and atelectasis. Usually hypoxemia and ARDS do not develop until 4 to 8 days postburn. Whether smoke inhalation is a separate condition from ALI/ARDS is still debated. Treatment is supportive.

B. Standard Diagnostics: bronchoscopy of upper and lower airway to look for soot tissue sloughing, mucosal necrosis, and carbonaceous material in the airway. Prophylactic antibiotics are not indicated. In all, 96% of patients will have positive bronchoscopy for inhalation injury if clinical triad of history of closed-space fire, increased serum carbon monoxide >10%, and the presence of carbonaceous sputum.

C. Treatment for Inhalational Injury. If inhalation injury is present, the patient should have airway assessment and be placed on supplemental oxygen. Aerosolized agents, including β-agonists, can improve pulmonary toilet in some patients. Do not continue these treatments if the patient does not respond. Necrotic endobronchial debris sloughing can make secretion clearance difficult. Therapeutic bronchoscopy may help clearance of debris, but data do not show improved outcomes with bronchoscopy performed to improve pulmonary toilet.

D. Pulmonary Infection. Occurs in 30% to 50% of patients. Patients with purulent sputum, fever, and impaired gas exchange should be treated for pneumonia. Chest radiographic findings and leukocytosis should make the provider suspicious that the patient has a chest infection. If the patient has pneumonia and been in the hospital for more than 48 hours, he or she should be treated for hospital-acquired pneumonia. Sputum should be sent for aerobic, anaerobic, and quantitative cultures. Empiric antibiotics including coverage of *Pseudomonas* should be started until cultures come back. Empiric treatment should cover MRSA, and thus vancomycin or linezolid are preferred. If vancomycin is used, it is important to check vancomycin levels to avoid renal toxicity.

E. Ventilator-Associated Pneumonia (VAP). *Staphylococcus aureus* and *Streptococcus* are common causes of early VAP. *Pseudomonas aeruginosa* is the most common cause of late VAP. The normal diagnosis of pneumonia (fever, purulent sputum, or leukocytosis) may not be helpful in burn patients, since almost all patients are febrile, tachypneic, and have elevated white blood cell counts. The best diagnostic test in this situation is probably a bronchoscopy-obtained bronchial alveolar lavage sample with quantification of the bacteria, $>10^3$ CFU. This level of bacteria is considered significant, as per ABA recommendations for VAP treatment. Antibiotic treatment duration for pan-sensitive organisms is 8 days. Duration of antibiotic treatment for multidrug-resistant organisms is 15 days. Providers should consider prophylactic antifungals (diflucan) if the patient has received prolonged broad-spectrum antibiotics.

F. Carbon Monoxide. Increased carbon monoxide is found commonly in fires from enclosed settings. Injury occurs from a combination of increased concentrations of carbon monoxide, the presence of both anoxia and hypotension. Carbon monoxide binds to heme-containing enzymes, such as hemoglobin, more avidly than oxygen. If carboxyhemoglobin is greater than 25%, patient should receive hyperbaric oxygen, if they are stable enough to tolerate movement to a chamber. Typical hyperbaric oxygen regimens include exposure to three atmospheres for 90 minutes with 10-minute breaks. Contraindications to HBO include unstable hemodynamics in patient with wheezing or auto-PEEP, high fevers, and a risk of seizures.

IX. METABOLIC RESPONSE AND NUTRITION

A. Metabolic rates in burn patients are significantly greater than other critically ill patients, leading to lean body mass wasting. Positive nitrogen balance is the key to prevent skeletal muscle breakdown.

B. General composition of the enteral feeding should include at least 60% calories from carbohydrates, but not exceeding 1,600 kcal/d, 12% to 15% lipids and essential fatty acids, and 20% to 25% protein. Failure to meet large energy and protein requirements can impair wound healing and alter organ function. Adequate nutrition is crucial and overfeeding must be avoided. Previously, a randomized, double-blind, prospective study demonstrated that aggressive high-calorie feeding with enteral and parenteral nutrition was associated with increased mortality. The daily caloric requirements should be calculated using the Curreri formula: [(25 kcal) (body wt kg)] + [(40) (%TBSA burn)] 1 to 2 g/kg/day of protein for synthetic needs of the patient. Burn patients should receive less percentage calorie requirements from fat than other ICU patients. Livers in burn patients have less VLDL, causing hepatic TG elevation. Increased fat consumption leads to increased complications including fatty liver, infection, hyperlipidemia, hypoxia, and mortality.

C. Micronutrients. There is decreased gastrointestinal absorption and increased urinary losses of micronutrients. Thus, burn patients can develop deficiencies in vitamin C, vitamin E, zinc, iron, and selenium. Burn patients have been shown to benefit from glutamine supplementation.

D. Acute response to thermal injury is biphasic, with the hypodynamic shock state at 24 to 72 hours and hyperdynamic catabolic state on the 5th postburn day. Patients have supraphysiologic cardiac outputs, elevated body temperatures, supranormal oxygen consumption, supranormal glucose consumption, altered glucose metabolism, and increased CO_2 production due to accelerated tissue catabolism. This hyperdynamic catabolic state is thought to be caused by an excessive release of catabolic hormones, including catecholamines, glucagon, and cortisol. A shift from an anabolic–catabolic homeostasis to this hypercatabolic state leads to an increased need for energy, leading to skeletal muscle loss, which is broken down to maintain a sufficient supply of glucose and amino acids. The increased resting metabolic rate is directly related to the severity of the burn injury. A persistent hypermetabolic state is unsustainable. To decrease this hypermetabolic state, the provider should attempt to decrease the catabolic response by treating sepsis, performing early excision and skin grafting, and maintaining the core body temperature between 38 and 38.5°F. A nonselective β-blocker, such as propranolol, can also be used, as it inhibits the effect of catecholamines and slows muscle catabolism. Herndon et al. demonstrated that the usage of propranolol for the treatment of acute burns in the pediatric population improved net muscle synthesis and increased lean body mass.

E. Other medications to consider include pharmacological agents that convert catabolism to anabolism: oxandrolone (a testosterone analog given 0.1 mg/kg q12h) improves muscle synthetic activity, increases expression of muscle anabolic genes and increases net muscle protein synthesis. These effects improve lean body mass composition and have reduced weight loss. This also improves donor site wound healing and decreases the duration of the hospital stay. The provider needs to check liver function tests weekly due to the risk of transaminitis when receiving anabolic steroids. The practice has been to continue oxandrolone for 6 months. Human growth hormone and insulin-like growth factors have also been investigated, but the results of their administration have been mixed.

F. Glucose Control. Increase in hepatic gluconeogenesis and impaired insulin-mediated glucose transport into skeletal and cardiac muscle and adipose tissue occur regularly in burn patients. Hypermetabolism leads to hyperglycemia and insulin resistance. Data do not support strict glucose control (<110 mg/dL), but moderate blood glucose control is recommended (should be kept <180 mg/dL).

X. ELECTROLYTE ABNORMALITIES AND ACUTE RENAL FAILURE

A. The immediate effect of burn injury on kidney function occurs when there is hypovolemia (see above) and because of the release of cytokines.

B. A diuretic phase is seen at 48 to 72 hours after "third space" fluid is reabsorbed.

C. Hyponatremia is often seen due to large-volume resuscitation with hypotonic IV fluids. This will self-correct. Open burn wounds or use of topical silver nitrate can also cause hyponatremia. Be aware that renal hypoperfusion exacerbates hyponatremia by decreasing glomerular filtration.

D. Hypernatremia is due to insensible and evaporative water losses.

E. Providers should monitor patients for hyperkalemia and hypokalemia.

F. Hypophosphatemia can result from dilution or when a refeeding syndrome occurs.

G. Hypocalcemia can result from the use of silver nitrate.

H. Acute Kidney Injury. Risk factors for acute kidney injury include sepsis, TBSA burns, organ failure, and antibiotic administration. Physiologically in burns, there is a decrease in renal perfusion, glomerular filtration rate, and renal plasma flow. The renal medulla is the most sensitive to hypoxia, and renal tubular cells are the most vulnerable.

1. **Presentation:** oliguria and decreased creatinine clearance
2. **Early renal failure:** often results from hypovolemia-induced ischemic injury. Early fluid resuscitation is important to prevent this. Overresuscitation can cause abdominal compartment syndrome, which will also compromise renal perfusion. Renal failure can also be caused from rhabdomyolysis, most commonly seen in burns due to electrical injury.
3. **Late renal failure:** occurs after the fifth postburn day. Can be caused by sepsis. And nephrotoxic antibiotics. Renal replacement therapy (CRRT) is thought to improve outcomes in patients with burns and AKI, but studies are still underway.
4. **Pharmacologic treatments:** Dopamine has **not** been shown to improve outcomes. However, the dopamine-1 receptor agonist, fenoldapam, at low doses has showed promise in studies by increasing urine output and decreasing serum creatinine. Lasix and mannitol will improve urine output, but have not been shown to improve outcomes in burn patients.
5. Initial care of ARF patients should focus on reversing the underlying cause, as well as correcting any fluid and electrolyte imbalances. Ensure adequate volume status, avoid nephrotoxins, and dose medications appropriately. A high aldosterone response often necessitates potassium supplementation.

XI. CHEMICAL BURNS

A. General Approach to Chemical Burn Treatment. Protect yourself with personal protective equipment—always consider that the chemicals are still present and must be neutralized or temporized. With few exceptions (see below), all chemical burns should be copiously irrigated with water. Water dilutes, but does not neutralize, the chemical and cools the burning area. Neutralization of chemical burns is generally contraindicated because neutralization may induce a hyperthermic reaction. Water irrigation is contraindicated or ineffective in several scenarios, including the following:
   1. Elemental sodium, potassium, and lithium: these both may precipitate an explosion.
   2. Dry lime, which should be brushed off and, not irrigated.
   3. Phenol, which is water insoluble and should be wiped from the skin with polyethylene glycol-soaked sponges.

B. Types of Chemical Burns
   1. **Alkali:** causes liquefaction necrosis and protein denaturation. Found in oven and drain cleaning products, fertilizers, and industrial cleaners. Alkali injuries extend deeper into tissues until the source is removed or diluted and are especially disruptive to the eye.
   2. **Acids:** damage tissue via coagulation necrosis and protein precipitation
   3. **Organic compounds (phenol and petroleum):** cause damage via cutaneous damage due to fat solvent action (cell membrane solvent action) and systematic absorption with toxic effects on the liver and kidneys. These can also cause significant erythema in the surrounding areas that may be mistaken for cellulitis.

C. Specific Types of Chemical Burns
   1. **Hydrofluoric acid (HF):** potent and corrosive acid used as a rust remover, in glass etching, and to clean semiconductors. Although a weak acid, the fluoride ion is toxic. It causes severe pain and local necrosis.

Treatment is copious water irrigation. Fluoride ion is neutralized with topical calcium gel (one amp calcium gluconate in 100 g lubricating jelly). If symptoms persist, intra-arterial calcium infusion (10 mL calcium gluconate diluted in 80 mL of saline, infused over 4 hours) and/or subeschar injection of dilute (10%) calcium gluconate solution are recommended. Fluoride ion binds free serum calcium; make sure to check the serum calcium and replace with IV calcium as needed.

2. **Phenol:** commonly used in disinfectants and chemical solvents. Phenoal is an acidic alcohol with poor water solubility and causes protein disruption and denaturation, resulting in coagulation necrosis. It is responsible for cardiac arrhythmia and liver toxicity: cardiac and liver function should be monitored. It is cleared by the kidneys. Phenol causes demyelination and has a local anesthetic effect, and thus pain is not a reliable indicator of injury. Recommended treatment is copious water irrigation and cleansing with 30% polyethylene glycol or ethyl alcohol. EKG monitoring is required.

3. **Tar:** used in the paving and roofing industry. It can be heated to 260°C (~500°F) prior to application and causes thermal injury; tar solidifies as it cools and will become enmeshed with hair and skin. It should be cooled with copious water irrigation to stop the burning process. Tar removers promote micelle formation to break the tar–skin bond. Sterile surfactant mixture (De-Solv-it or Shur-Clens) allows tar to be wiped away in real time. Applying wet dressings using polysorbate (Tween 80) or Neomycin cream for 6 hours prior to tar removal can also be effective.

4. **White phosphorus:** used to manufacture military explosives, fireworks, and methamphetamine. Obvious particles should be brushed off. Skin should be irrigated with a 1% to 3% copper sulfate solution. Copper sulfate stains the particles black for identification. Copper sulfate will also prevent ignition when particles are submerged in water. After copper sulfate irrigation, the exposed area should be placed in a water bath and the white phosphorous should be removed.

5. **Anhydrous ammonia:** alkali used in fertilizer. Skin exposure is treated with irrigation and local wound care. Exposure is associated with rapid airway edema, pulmonary edema, and pneumonia. Always consider early intubation for airway protection.

6. **Methamphetamine:** causes tachycardia (greater than expected with a similar size burn), hyperthermia, agitation, and paranoia

D. **Injury to Eyes:** Treat with prolonged irrigation with Morgan lenses. Eyelids may need to be forced open due to edema or spasm. Utilize a topical ophthalmic analgesic and consult an ophthalmologist.

XII. ELECTRICAL INJURY
A. Unlike other burns, TBSA is not necessarily associated with prognosis and TBSA does not quantify damage to deeper tissues.
B. Mechanism of injury
1. Thermal: can generate temperatures above 100°C
2. Electroporation: electrical force drives water into lipid membrane, causing cell rupture
3. Difficult to determine type and severity of damage between entrance and exit
4. Tissue resistance in decreasing order = bone, fat, tendon, skin, muscle, vessel, nerve
5. Bone heats to a high temperature and burns surrounding structures.

C. **Injury Severity.** Determined by voltage, current type, and resistance. High-voltage burns are considered to be those involving >1,000 volts. Alternating current causes tetanic muscle contraction and the "no let-go" phenomenon. This occurs due to simultaneous contraction of (stronger) forearm flexors and (weaker) forearm extensors.

D. Current flow through tissue can cause burns at entrance/exit wounds and burns to deep tissue. A current will preferentially travel along low-resistance pathways. Current will pass through soft tissue, contact high-resistance bone, and travel along bone until it exits to the ground. Vascular injury to nutrient arteries through damage to their intima and media leads to thrombosis.

E. **Cardiac Effects.** Arrhythmia. Recommend an EKG monitor for at least 24 hours, watching for coronary artery spasm, myocardial injury, and infarction.

F. **GI Effects.** Injury to solid organs, acute bowel perforation, and gallstones after myoglobinuria

G. Initial monitoring:
   1. Airway maintenance: C-collar until c-spine cleared
   2. Breathing and ventilation—100% oxygen
   3. Circulation and cardiac status: Cardiac monitor, two large-bore IVs, assess peripheral perfusion, EKG
   4. 24-hour monitoring indicated if any of these is present: ectopy or dysrhythmia, loss of consciousness, cardiac arrest, or abnormal rate or rhythm
   5. Disability, neurological deficit, and gross deformity: Assess level of consciousness, note any neurological deficit, and note any gross deformity.
   6. Exposure and environmental control: Stop the burning process, then remove clothes and avoid hypothermia.
   7. Perform renal function analysis and urine myoglobin.

H. **Fluid Resuscitation.** TBSA provides inadequate estimation of electrical burn severity. Unlike thermal injury, electrical injury often occurs deep to the skin and is not visible. Standard fluid resuscitation models (Parkland) may underestimate fluid resuscitation needs. If no urine pigmentation is present, the minimum acceptable urine output is 0.5 mL/kg/h. Pigmented urine can be caused from myoglobin (secondary to rhabdomyolysis) and/or free hemoglobin (from damaged RBCs). For myoglobinuria, the urine dipstick will be positive for blood and microscopy will not demonstrate RBCs. The goal for urine outputs when rhabdomyolysis and myoglobinuria has occurred is 2 mL/kg/h or about 75 to 100 cc/h. Insufficient volume resuscitation can predispose to myoglobin-induced acute tubular necrosis. In addition to adequate fluid resuscitation, myoglobin excretion can be enhanced using mannitol (12.5 g/h osmotic diuresis) and/or urine alkalinization with 50 mEq/L of bicarbonate. Follow urine myoglobin levels every 6 hours until a downward trend is seen.

I. **Compartment Syndrome** can occur after high-voltage injury to an extremity. Current travels along bone, which has high resistance. The bone serves as a conductor and "cooks" adjacent tissue from deep to superficial. In the upper extremity, FDP and FPL will be most severely affected (closest to bone). Overaggressive fluid resuscitation can worsen tissue edema, resulting in increased tissue pressures and exacerbating raised compartment pressures, typically occurs within 48 hours of injury. Clinical concern for raised compartment pressures mandates an evaluation of compartment pressures or a trip to the operating room. The 6 "P" signs/

symptoms include pain out of proportion, paresthesia, pallor, paralysis, pulselessness, and poikilothermia. Elevated compartment pressures can be used as an adjunct to clinical diagnosis or for cases where the patient is unable to participate in clinical exam. Absolute pressure ≥30 mmHg or elevated pressure within 20 mmHg of the diastolic blood pressure is also diagnostic of compartment syndrome. Forearm compartment syndrome is managed via surgical release of volar and extensor compartments and the mobile wad. In the hand, release carpal tunnel, Guyon's canal, and the nine compartments of the hand. Lower extremity compartment syndrome is managed with fasciotomies of the anterior, lateral, superficial posterior, and deep posterior compartments.

XIII. BURN WOUND MANAGEMENT
A. Topical Antimicrobials
1. **Silver sulfadiazine.** Broad-spectrum antimicrobial activity due to silver ion. Soothing sensation that does not cause significant metabolic or electrolyte complications. Does not penetrate eschar. Can cause neutropenia but this is often self-limited. Assess if patient has sulfa allergy.
2. **Sulfamylon (mafenide acetate).** Penetrates eschar and is useful on ears to prevent suppurative chondritis. Can be used as a cream or as a soak (2.5% or 5%). It does not stop fungi, which silver nitrate does. Can also cause metabolic acidosis due to its inhibition of carbonic anhydrase. Can be painful on partial-thickness burns.
3. **Silver nitrate.** Offers broad-spectrum antimicrobial coverage against gram-positive and gram-negative bacteria and fungal coverage. Delivered as an aqueous 0.5% solution every 4 hours to keep dressing moist and prevent precipitation of the silver nitrate. Side effects include staining skin (and anything it contacts) black, hyponatremia, and hypomagnesemia. Rare instances of methemoglobinemia necessitating methylene blue treatment.
4. **Mupirocin:** Effective against MRSA and can be used in addition to other topicals to expand coverage

XIV. COLD INJURY
A. Frostbite occurs in response to a slow rate of cooling with ice crystal formation in tissue when tissue temperature <28°F.
B. Concentrated solutes draw fluid out of cells and ice crystals subsequently cause cell membrane puncture.
C. Intravascular ice crystals cause direct vascular damage and indirect vascular sludging.
D. With rewarming, tissue thaws from the blood vessels outward.
E. Freeze-induced endothelial damage allows capillary leaking to occur. This allows extravasation of PMNs and mast cells, causing inflammation, edema, microvascular stasis, and occlusion.
F. Blisters will form at 6 to 24 hours when extravasated fluid collects beneath the detached epidermal sheet. If the dermal vascular plexus is disrupted, hemorrhagic blisters will be present.
G. Stages of Frostbite
1. **1st degree:** hyperemia, intact sensation, no blisters on rewarming, no tissue loss expected
2. **2nd degree:** blisters containing clear or milky fluid, local edema, no tissue loss expected
3. **3rd degree:** hemorrhagic blisters, edematous tissue, shooting or throbbing pain, and likely tissue loss

4. **4th degree:** mottled or cyanotic skin, hemorrhagic blisters, and frozen deeper structures. Mummification occurs over several weeks.

H. Treatment

Multiple freeze–thaw cycles causes multiplicative, not additive, damage to the affected tissues. Intact blisters should be left alone. Debride ruptured blisters and apply bacitracin ointment or silvadene. Beware of the "after-drop" phenomenon during rewarming, where central rewarming results in peripheral vasodilation. This returns cold blood from the extremities to central circulation and can result in systemic hypothermia. Rapid re-warming of affected area in 104° to 108°F water bath, not radiant heat. Additional strategies include ibuprofen 400 mg PO q12h; penicillin 600 mg q6 × 48 to 72 hours; elevation of limb with splinting to decrease movement; no smoking, caffeine, or chocolate; and tetanus prophylaxis. Three-phase bone scan may identify "at risk" tissue.

I. Acute Interventions after Warming

1. For stable patients with severe frostbite, rapid extrication to a center with interventional radiology capabilities within 12 hours is indicated. Arterial catheterization can identify and treat vasospasm and micro-vascular thrombosis with tPA or heparin. Catheter-directed tPA should be given for 24 hours and then the patient should be placed on a hep-arin gtt.
2. Reversal of local microvascular thrombosis may restore perfusion be-fore irreversible necrosis and ischemia occur.
3. Several studies have shown significant decrease in amputation rates and tissue loss with this aggressive protocol.
4. Early regional sympathectomy of an affected extremity is controversial.

XV. STEVENS JOHNSON SYNDROME (SJS) AND TOXIC EPIDERMAL NECROLYSIS SYNDROME (TENS)

A. Both SJS and TENS have widespread necrosis of the superficial portion of the epidermis.

B. SJS/TENS is commonly associated with sulfonamides, trimethoprim-sulfamethoxazole, oxicam NSAIDs, chlormezanone, and carbamazepine. A single offending drug is identified in less than 50% of cases. Antibiotic-associated SJS/TENS presents ~7 days after drug is first taken. Anticonvulsant-associated SJS/TENS can present up to 2 months after drug is first taken.

C. TENS can also be caused by staphylococcal infections in immuno-compromised patients.

D. SJS—total involvement less than 10% TBSA. Widespread erythematous or purpuric macules or flat atypical targets are present.

E. Overlap SJS-TENS—total cutaneous involvement of 10% to 30%. Widespread purpuric macules or flat atypical targets are present.

F. TENS with spots—total cutaneous involvement of greater than 30% TBSA. Widespread purpuric macules or flat atypical targets are present.

G. TENS without spots—total cutaneous involvement greater than 10% TBSA. Large epidermal sheets present. No purpuric macules or targets.

H. Initial symptoms can be a 2-to-3-day prodrome of nonspecific findings such as fevers, headaches, and chills. Symptoms of mucosal irritation like conjunctivitis, dysuria, and/or dysphagia may be present. These symptoms are followed by mucosal and cutaneous lesions.

I. Mucosal irritation typically occurs at two or more sites. Involved sites may include vaginal, urinary, respiratory, gastrointestinal, oral, and/or conjunctival.

J. Skin lesions are diffusely present. Lesions are typically erythematous macules with purple, possibly necrotic, centers. Nikolsky's sign is typically positive (rubbing the skin causes exfoliation of outermost layers and/or a new blister to form).

K. Differential diagnosis of acute, diffuse blistering includes staphylococcal-scalded skin syndrome, pemphigus vulgaris, pemphigus folaceus, paraneoplastic pemphigus, bullous pemphigoid, acute graft-versus-host disease, and linear IgA dermatosis.

L. Diagnosis of SJS/TENS is largely clinical and can be confirmed by both skin biopsy and histology.

M. Treatment. Discontinue all potentially offending drugs. Transfer to a burn ICU for fluid/electrolyte monitoring, dressing changes, and temperature regulation is recommended. Debride flaccid bullae. Administer initial wound care with dressing changes until extent of skin loss is known. All necrotic epidermis should be debrided to reduce bacterial growth, and area should be covered with biological or synthetic dressings. Recommend human allograft and porcine xenograft placement to the denuded areas to reduce pain, decrease fluid loss, and promote healing. Empiric systemic antibiotics have been associated with increased mortality and are not indicated. Topical antimicrobials such as silver sulfadiazine, silver nitrate, and polymyxin-bacitracin can help prevent infection; however, silver sulfadiazine should be avoided due to its sulfonamide component. Consider hemodialysis to remove potentially offending drugs with long half-lives. Corticosteroid and cyclosporine A therapy has not been supported by current data and is not recommended. Early ophthalmology consultation is recommended. More than 50% of SJS/TENS patients can develop symblepharon or entropion. Treatment can involve other consultant services (pulmonary, urology, gynecology, gastroenterology) as needed. Administration of steroids and IVIG is controversial. TENS is known to overexpress FAS, which promotes apoptosis of keratinocytes by binding to the FAS/CD95 receptor. IVIG blocks the CD95 receptor and has been efficacious in small series of TENS patients.

XVI. PRESSURE ULCERS

A. Definition. Necrosis and tissue breakdown from pressure.

B. Etiology. Tissue ischemia from external pressures exceeding the closing pressure of nutrient capillaries (32 mmHg) for a prolonged duration. Pressures exceeding 70 mmHg for 2 hours cause ischemia. Shear forces cause vessel stretch, leading to thrombosis. Friction causes epidermal injury (e.g., during transfers). Excess moisture causes skin maceration and increased pressure sore risk. Ischemia–reperfusion cycle plays a role. Decreased autonomic control lead to spasm, loss of bladder, and bowel control, and excessive sweating lead to increased moisture. Advanced age causes decreased skin tensile strength. Malnutrition depletes patient of protein and vitamins needed for wound healing. Sensory loss causes inability to experience discomfort or tissue ischemia.

C. Epidemiology/Natural History. Prevalence is 15% in general acute care setting. Incidence is 0.5% to 38% in general care settings. More than 60% of patients with pressure sores are >70 years of age. Additional risk factors include cerebrovascular disease, previous pressure sore, immobility (debilitated or paralyzed), malnutrition, end-stage renal disease, and diabetes mellitus. Chronic polymicrobial colonization is defined as count >1 × 10^5 per mm^3 tissue. *Staphylococcus aureus* and *Streptococcus* are the most common bacteria. Chronic wound has possibility of malignant degeneration (Marjolin's ulcer).

D. Prevention: Avoid moisture through bladder/bowel hygiene, avoiding soilage. Control of spasticity facilitates proper positioning, and baclofen or diazepam treatment can also help with spasticity. Proper pressure distribution using air fluidized, low air-loss, and alternating air cell mattresses. Pressure relief protocols recommend repositioning recumbent patients every 2 hours.

E. Diagnosis/Workup. Perform laboratory studies and imaging, complete blood cell count (CBC) with differential, glucose/hemoglobin A1c, albumin/prealbumin, erythrocyte sedimentation rate (ESR)/C-reactive, protein (CRP), and MRI.

1. Stages defined by National Pressure Ulcer Advisory Board (NPUAP) (Fig. 34.5):
    a. **Stage I:** nonblanchable erythema present for >1 hour after pressure relief. Skin intact
    b. **Stage II:** partial-thickness skin loss
    c. **Stage III:** full-thickness skin loss into subcutaneous tissue but not through fascia
    d. **Stage IV:** through fascia into muscle, bone, tendon, or joint
    e. **Note:** If eschar is present, wound cannot be staged until fully debrided.
2. Muscle is more susceptible to ischemia than is skin. Muscle necrosis may have occurred with skin erythema as the only sign.
3. **Nutritional status:** Serum albumin <3.5 mg/dL may be a risk factor for developing pressure sores.
4. **Osteomyelitis:** Presence of bone infection must be determined. Initial studies include ESR, CRB, CBC, with ESR >100 usually indicative of osteomyelitis. MRI can identify osteomyelitis and extent of disease. T2-weighted images will show enhancement in region of osteomyelitis. Bone biopsy remains the gold standard for diagnosis: Send one sample to pathology and one sample for quantitative microbiology.
5. Identify contractures and spasticity in paraplegic and quadriplegic patients.
6. Assess bowel/bladder routine and continence.
7. Assess motivation and support structure including adherence to pressure relief protocols, adherence to wound care routines, maintenance of adequate nutrition, and participation in risk factor modification (e.g., smoking cessation).

F. Treatment Overview. Excise and treat infection and avoid new pressure sores. Surgical closure is not attainable in all patients (e.g., poor surgical candidates, nonoptimal social circumstances). Debridement of nonviable tissues is recommended. Provide wound care with dressing if wound is not ready to be closed. Continue with antibiotics for 6 weeks if osteomyelitis is present. Primary surgical closure is not ideal as maximal pressure point is directly under incision. Local rotational or advancement flaps using skin and/or fascia offer more robust coverage. Recurrence of ulcers is the rule, not the exception.

G. Wound Dressings

1. **General:** Achieve warm, moist, and clean environment for wound healing; desiccated wound needs hydration, and wound with excess drainage needs an absorbent. A wound with necrosis needs debridement, and infected wounds need antimicrobial dressings. Wet-to-moist dressing is recommended for debrided, clean-looking wound with

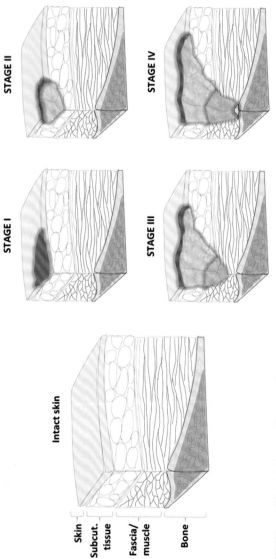

FIGURE 34.5 Schematic of stages of pressure ulcer formation. Stage I involves superficial injury with non-blanching erythematous changes but intact skin. Stage II describes partial thickness skin injury. Stage III ulcers have full thickness skin loss with exposed subcutaneous tissue. Stage IV ulcers extend through muscular fascia into muscle, tendon, or bone.

normal saline and mesh gauze. In clean wounds, this prevents desiccation for optimal fibroblast and keratinocyte development and epithelial migration.

2. **Debriding dressings:** Chemical topicals include enzymatic agents such as collagenase and papain, which liquefy devitalized tissue. If using these dressings, it should be asked why patient cannot have the tissue surgically debrided.

3. **Antiseptic dressings:** Oxychlorosene, Dakin's solution, and dilute bleach are applied in wet-to-moist fashion. These are used in heavily contaminated wounds to decrease bacterial counts. Acetic acid is thought to be effective in controlling *Pseudomonas*. Several of these agents have detrimental effects on wound healing (e.g., impair fibroblast proliferation). Switch to other dressings when the wound is clean.

4. **Negative pressure wound therapy:** no guidelines for the role in pressure sore management. Appropriate for stage III and IV wounds. Contraindicated with bleeding, osteomyelitis, necrotic tissue, malignancy, and fistulas. Easier for nursing/home health care given it only needs to be changed every 3 to 4 days.

H. **Soft Tissue Infections.** Cellulitis—skin warmth, spreading erythema, edema due to skin breakdown. Subcutaneous abscess, a fluctuant, tender, erythematous wound, if draining can have malodorous purulent discharge. Abscesses can lead to systemic infections with leukocytosis, fever, and sepsis. Obtain specimens after debridement for quantitative bacterial counts, culture, and sensitivity. *Staphylococcus, Streptococcus, E. coli,* and *Pseudomonas* are the most common culprits. Mixed aerobic/anaerobic infections are not uncommon. Treat promptly with drainage, irrigation, wide debridement, and antibiotics guided by culture.

I. **Osteomyelitis**

1. **Diagnosis.** Exposed/palpable bone on initial evaluation: osteomyelitis until proven otherwise. Bone biopsy is gold standard for diagnosis. Obtain bone biopsy during initial evaluation with a rongeur if patient is insensate, and send one sample to pathology and one sample to quantitative microbiology. Bone scans are not specific for diagnosing osteomyelitis but can rule out osteomyelitis if negative. MRI has 98% sensitivity and 88% specificity in diagnosis of osteomyelitis. T2 images will show enhancement of infected areas and can also be used to determine extent of disease and to plan out surgical resection.

2. **Operative treatment of pressure sores.** Wide debridement of devitalized and infected bone. Six-week IV antibiotic course tailored to causative organism. Bring patient back to the operating room for further debridement and flap closure. Resend quantitative cultures and pathology at that time. When resection is impossible (extension to acetabulum and pubic rami), flap closure is contraindicated. Management is chronic suppressive antibiotics and wound dressings indefinitely.

J. **Postoperative Care.** Pressure dispersion: for example, air-fluidized mattress, pressure-relief protocols, protection of flap from pressure, shear and friction, optimize nutrition, control spasticity/spasms, bladder and bowel regimen, surgical drains essential, antibiotic treatment if indicated by intraoperative cultures, and no pressure on the flap/wound bed for 6 weeks

XVII. CALCIPHYLAXIS

Rare condition of extraskeletal calcifications causing overlying tissue necrosis. Associated with disorders that alter calcium–phosphate balance

Part 2 Specific Considerations

(often patients with renal failure or recent renal transplantation). Patients develop painful cutaneous lesions of tissue necrosis with underlying calcification of the vessels. Distal lesions of the extremities have better survival (60%) compared with more proximal lesions of the trunk (30%). Diagnosis is based on history and biopsy. Treatment includes working with the renal team to change hemodialysis. Aggressive surgical excision followed by negative pressure wound therapy is recommended, followed by skin graft closure.

Selected Readings

Branski LK, Mecott GA, Herndon DN, et al. The use of exenatide in severely burned pediatric patients. *Crit Care* 2010;14(4):R153. doi: 10.1186/cc9222. Epub ahead of publication 2010.

Mosier MJ, Pham TN. American Burn Association practice guidelines for prevention, diagnosis and treatment of VAP in burn patients. *JBCR* 2009;30:910–928.

Herndon DN, Hart DW, Wolf SE, et al. Reversal of catabolism by beta-blockade after severe burns. *N Engl J Med* 2001;345(17):1223–1229.

Pruitt BA, Ciofi WG. Thermal injuries. In: Davis JH, Sheldon GF, eds. *Surgery: a problem solving approach.* 2nd ed. St. Louis: Mosby, 1995:643–720.

Sharer SR, Heimbach DM. Management of inhalation injury in patients with and without burns. In: Haponik EF, Munster AM, eds. *Respiratory injury—smoke inhalation and burns.* New York: McGraw-Hill, 1990:195–215.

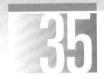

Transfusion Medicine

Christopher R. Tainter and Kenneth Shelton

I. **INDICATIONS FOR TRANSFUSION THERAPY.** Blood component transfusion is usually performed because of decreased production, increased utilization/destruction or loss, or dysfunction of a specific blood component (red cells, platelets, or coagulation factors).

A. **Anemia**

1. **Red cell mass.** The primary reason for red blood cell transfusion is to maintain an adequate oxygen-carrying capacity of the blood. Healthy individuals or individuals with chronic anemia can usually tolerate a hematocrtit (Hct) of 20% to 25%, assuming normal intravascular volume. The Hct assumes red blood cell normocytosis and appropriate hemoglobin (Hgb) content. A patient with hypochromic normocytic anemia may have an Hct within normal range but a decreased oxygen-carrying capacity. For this reason, **many institutions use Hgb (g/dL) in lieu of Hct (%)** as an indicator of red blood cell mass. Modern techniques assay total red cell Hgb and the red blood cell count to calculate the Hct instead of measuring the packed cell volume by centrifugation.

2. Anemia may be caused by **decreased production** (marrow suppression), **increased loss** (hemorrhage), or **destruction** (hemolysis). Acute blood loss generally does not change the relative concentration of red blood cells immediately (as other intravascular volume is lost at the same rate), but the infusion of intravenous fluid may contribute to a dilutional effect.

3. Anemia in critically ill adults is common. The exact Hgb level that should prompt red blood cell transfusion may be different for various scenarios, but even among a homogenous population remains controversial. Results from the two largest randomized controlled trials of critically ill patients suggest that a "restrictive" transfusion policy improves hospital survival when compared with a more liberal transfusion strategy (maintaining Hgb 7–9 g/dL vs. 10–12 g/dL in one study, Hct ≥24% vs. ≥30% in the other). Another large randomized trial of patients after hip fracture with a history of or risk factors for cardiovascular disease showed no reduction in death or functional outcome with a Hb target of >10 versus >8 g/dL.

4. Estimating the volume of blood to transfuse can be calculated as follows:

$$\text{Volume to transfuse} = (\text{Hct}_{\text{desired}} - \text{Hct}_{\text{present}}) \times \text{BV}/\text{Hct}_{\text{transfused bood}}$$

where BV is blood volume, which may be estimated at 70 mL/kg actual body weight in male adults and 65 mL/kg in female adults. Higher values may be used in infants (80 mL/kg) and neonates (85 mL/kg). The Hct of transfused blood is approximately 70 ± 5%.

B. **Thrombocytopenia.** Spontaneous bleeding is unusual with platelet counts more than 5,000 to 10,000 per µL, but in the immediate postoperative period, platelet counts of more than 20,000 to 50,000 are sometimes recommended. Thrombocytopenia may be due to decreased bone marrow production (e.g., chemotherapy, tumor infiltration, or alcoholism) or increased consumption (e.g., trauma, sepsis, drug effects like histamine-2 antagonists or ticarcillin, or immune-mediated reactions like idiopathic thrombocytopenic purpura or heparin-induced thrombocytopenia). A relative deficiency of platelets may also be caused by large volume intravenous infusions or red blood cell transfusions.

II. BLOOD TYPING AND CROSS-MATCHING
Donor blood and **recipient blood** are typed in the red cell surface **ABO** and **Rh systems** and screened for antibodies to other cell antigens. **Cross-matching** involves directly mixing the patient's plasma with the donor's red cells to establish that hemolysis does not occur from any undetected antibodies.

A. An individual's red cells have either A, B, both (type AB), or neither (type O) ABO-type surface antigens. If a person's red cells are lacking either A or B surface antigen, then antibodies will be produced against it. Consequently, a person with type B red blood cells will have anti-A antibodies in the serum, while a type O individual, that is, a person having neither A nor B surface antigens will have circulating anti-A and anti-B antibodies. Conversely, a person who has type AB red blood cells will not have antibodies to either A or B, thus can receive red blood cells from a person of any blood type (universal recipient). Type O blood has neither A nor B surface antigens, and a person with this blood type is a universal red cell donor.

B. **Rh Surface Antigens** are either present (Rh-positive) or absent (Rh-negative). Individuals who are Rh-negative will develop antibodies to the Rh factor when exposed to Rh-positive blood. This is not a problem with the initial exposure, but hemolysis will occur due to the circulating antibodies with subsequent exposures. This can be particularly problematic during pregnancy. The anti-Rh antibodies are immunoglobulin (IgG) and freely cross the placenta. In Rh-negative mothers who have developed Rh antibodies, these antibodies are transmitted to the fetus. If the fetus is Rh-positive, massive hemolysis will occur, termed hemolytic disease of the newborn. **Rh-immune globulin**, an Rh-blocking antibody, prevents the Rh-negative patient from developing anti-Rh antibodies. Rh-immune globulin is routinely administered to Rh-negative women when possible exposure to Rh surface antigens occurs (e.g., disruption of the placenta with an Rh-positive fetus). Rh-immune globulin should be considered for all Rh-negative individuals who receive Rh-positive blood, especially women of childbearing age. The recommendation is one dose (approximately 300 µg/vial) for every 15 mL of Rh-positive blood transfused.

III. BLOOD COMPONENT THERAPY
A. Whole Blood
1. Whole blood has been largely replaced by component therapy because of storage impediments and no demonstrable superiority of the former. The exceptions may be for children younger than 2 years undergoing complicated cardiovascular surgery, exchange transfusions, where whole blood may have an outcome benefit in reduced transfusions, and during warfare due to limited storage capacity and availability of healthy donors.
2. Whole blood must be ABO and Rh identical because transfusion includes antibodies from the donor.

TABLE 35.1   Transfusion Compatibility

Recipient	Donor					
	A	B	O	AB	Rh+	Rh−
1. Red Blood Cells						
A	X		X			
B		X	X			
O			X			
AB	X	X	X	X		
Rh+					X	X
Rh−						X
2. Fresh Frozen Plasma						
A	X			X		
B		X		X		
O	X	X	X	X		
AB				X		
Rh+					X	X
Rh−					X	X

Compatible transfusions are marked by X.

B. Red Blood Cells

1. Packed red blood cells (pRBCs) contain concentrated ABO-specific red blood cells from a single donor. One unit (typically containing 250–300 mL) can be expected to raise the Hb of a euvolemic adult by approximately 1 g/dL once equilibration has taken place.

2. pRBCs must be ABO compatible (Table 35.1). If an emergency blood transfusion is needed, type-specific (ABO) red cells can usually be obtained within minutes if the patient's blood type is known. If type-specific blood is unavailable, type O red cells may be transfused. Rh-positive blood may be transfused to Rh-negative individuals in some situations and may be accompanied by Rh-immune globulin. Type-specific blood should be substituted as soon as possible to conserve resources and minimize the amount of type O plasma (containing anti-A and anti-B antibodies) transfused.

C. Platelets

1. One unit of random donor platelets contains approximately 10^{11} platelets and 60 mL of plasma from a single donor. These are typically grouped into "pools" of 4 to 6 units (often called a "6-pack"), from random or single donors. Each unit of platelets is expected to increase the platelet count by 5,000 to 10,000 per µL. If thrombocytopenia is due to increased destruction (e.g., due to the presence of antiplatelet antibodies), platelet transfusions will be less efficacious. A posttransfusion platelet count drawn 10 minutes after completion of platelet transfusion confirms platelet refractoriness if the count fails to increase by 5,000/µL for each unit transfused (30,000 µL for a 6-unit pool).

2. **ABO-compatible platelets** are not required for transfusion, although they may provide a better response as measured by the posttransfusion platelet count. Single-donor platelets are obtained from one individual by platelet pheresis. Single-donor platelets may be used to reduce

exposure to multiple donors or in cases of poor response to random donor platelets where destruction is suspected. In cases where allo-immunization causes platelet refractoriness, HLA-matched platelets may be required for effective platelet transfusion. Rh-negative women of childbearing age should receive Rh-negative platelets if possible because some RBCs and plasma are transfused with platelets. If this is impossible, Rh-immune globulin may be considered.

D. Fresh Frozen Plasma (FFP) is the liquid portion of blood after the red blood cells and platelets have been removed. It contains primarily coagulation factors and immunoglobulins and is generally filtered to remove white blood cells. One unit is approximately 220 to 250 mL.

   1. Factors V and VIII are most labile and quickly become depleted in thawed FFP. A typical dose of 10 to 20 mL/kg will increase plasma coagulation factors by about 20%. Fibrinogen levels increase by 1 mg/mL of plasma transfused.

   2. Acute reversal of warfarin generally requires 5 to 8 mL/kg of FFP. It is important to note that the International Normalized Ratio **(INR) of FFP is approximately 1.6**, so infusion of FFP alone is unlikely to lower a patient's INR below this level.

   3. ABO-compatible FFP transfusion is required (Table 35.1), but Rh-negative patients may receive Rh-positive FFP.

   4. Six units of platelets (one pool) contain the equivalent of one unit of FFP.

E. Cryoprecipitate is formed by cold precipitation and centrifugation of FFP. Each unit is approximately 15 mL and is typically provided in pools of 6 to 10 units.

   1. Each unit of cryoprecipitate typically contains 80 units of factor VIII and approximately 200 to 300 mg of fibrinogen. It also contains factor XIII, von Willebrand factor, and fibronectin.

   2. Indications for cryoprecipitate include hypofibrinogenemia, von Willebrand disease, hemophilia A (when factor VIII is unavailable), and preparation of fibrin glue (although commercially available virally inactivated concentrates have a higher fibrinogen concentration and are preferred for this purpose). **One unit/7–10 kg raises the plasma fibrinogen concentration by approximately 50 mg/dL** in a patient without massive bleeding.

   3. ABO compatibility is not required for transfusion of cryoprecipitate, but it is preferred because of the presence of 10 to 20 mL of plasma per unit.

F. Factor Concentrates. Individual coagulation factors are available for patients with discrete factor deficiencies. These may be derived from pooled human plasma or synthesized by recombinant gene technology.

   1. Activated recombinant factor VII (rFVIIa) was originally developed to control bleeding in patients with hemophilia A or B who had developed circulating inhibitors to factors VIII and IX. Subsequently, rFVIIa has been used to treat hemorrhage related to trauma, disseminated intravascular coagulation (DIC), intracranial hemorrhage, and perioperative bleeding. rFVIIa is thought to facilitate local coagulation by complexing with a tissue factor after endothelial injury and subsequent stimulation of the coagulation cascade. It has a half-life of approximately 2 hours and is very expensive. Current evidence supports only a very **limited role for factor VIIa in massively bleeding patients**. It should be considered only in carefully selected patients with diffuse coagulopathy (as opposed to a surgically correctable source of hemorrhage) who fail to respond to conventional component therapy, and its administration should be governed by an institutional protocol.

G. Technical Considerations

1. **Compatible infusions.** Many transfusion guidelines recommend avoiding coinfusion of pRBC with solutions other than normal saline. Dextrose-containing solutions may contribute to hemolysis, although this has not been demonstrated (Keir, 2014). Infusion with lactated Ringer's (LR) carries a theoretical concern of inappropriately activating clotting, but this has not been demonstrated either (Lorenzo 1998). Sodium chloride, albumin, and FFP are all compatible with pRBC.

2. **Blood filters** (80 μm) should be used for all blood components except platelets to remove debris and microaggregates. **Leukocyte filters** may be used to remove white blood cells to prevent transmission of cytomegalovirus in the immunocompromised, to prevent alloimmunization to foreign leukocyte antigens, and to diminish the incidence of febrile reactions. **Platelets** should be transfused through a 170-μm blood filter.

IV. SYNTHETIC BLOOD SUBSTITUTES

Blood product availability is limited and stored products maintain their integrity for a limited time. They continue to carry risks for infection and other adverse events (see Section VII), and some cultures have an aversion to homologous blood transfusion (e.g., Jehovah's Witnesses). **Oxygen-carrying blood substitutes** are being developed, and used in other countries, with some success. Primarily, these materials are hemoglobin-based oxygen carriers (HBOC) and perfluorocarbon-based oxygen carriers (PFBOC). Unfortunately, none are able to completely replicate the complex functions and efficiency of human red blood cells, but they may serve as a useful adjunct, particularly in areas with limited resources.

There are several products in clinical trials in the United States and Europe, a few available for veterinary use, but none currently available for clinical use in humans in the United States.

V. PHARMACOLOGIC THERAPY

A. Erythropoietin is an endogenous hormone that stimulates proliferation and development of erythroid precursor cells. Exogenous administration has been used to correct anemia in patients with chronic renal failure and to increase red cell mass prior to preoperative autologous donation. Current evidence does not support the routine administration of erythropoietin for critically ill patients. It may be considered for the severely anemic patient who refuses blood transfusion. Iron and folate supplementation are also recommended for patients receiving erythropoietin. Initial recommended doses in renal failure patients range from 50 to 100 units/kg IV or SQ three times a week.

B. Granulocyte Colony-Stimulating Factor (GCSF) and Granulocyte-Macrophage Colony-Stimulating Factor (GMCSF) are myeloid growth factors useful for shortening the duration of neutropenia induced by chemotherapy. GCSF is specific for neutrophils, and GMCSF increases production of neutrophils, macrophages, and eosinophils. Administration of these drugs enhances both neutrophil count and function. As such, they are frequently used for the treatment of febrile neutropenia. Treatment results in an initial brief decrease in the neutrophil count (due to endothelial adherence), then a rapid (usually after 24 hours) sustained leukocytosis that is dose dependent. Recommended doses are GCSF 5 μg/kg/d or GMCSF 250 μg/m^2/d until absolute neutrophil count is more than 10,000 mm^3.

C. Other interventions to enhance hemostasis are discussed in **Chapter 25.**

VI. **BLOOD CONSERVATION AND SALVAGE TECHNIQUES.** Blood transfusion of critically ill patients is common, with approximately 40% of patients being transfused during an ICU stay. Those patients who are older and stay longer in the ICU are more likely to receive a transfusion. Increasing evidence supporting the deleterious effects of homologous blood transfusion in critically ill patients reinforces the importance of techniques to diminish or eliminate the need for blood transfusion.

A. **Phlebotomy Losses** from critically ill patients can be significant, ranging from 40 to 400 mL/d, with higher losses in surgical units versus medical units. Patients with more severe illness and a greater number of dysfunctional organs suffer higher phlebotomy losses due to a greater number of blood draws. Techniques demonstrated to reduce phlebotomy losses include (a) a **"closed" system** of blood sampling where the initial aspirated blood is reinjected into the patient instead of discarded, (b) use of **small-volume phlebotomy tubes**, and (c) **"point-of-care" testing** at the bedside, which frequently requires less blood than the clinical laboratory. Finally, the presence of both arterial and central venous catheters in critically ill patients is correlated with higher phlebotomy losses, suggesting another reason to repeatedly evaluate the need for such catheters with respect to hemodynamic monitoring or medication/nutritional support administration.

B. **Surgical Drain Salvage Devices** allow the reinfusion of shed blood. Most commonly used in patients with blood collected from chest tubes, these are useful for reducing homologous transfusions in the immediate postoperative period. Use of these devices requires skilled nursing for proper administration and sterile technique. They are contraindicated in conditions where the drained cavity is infected. A potential danger is hyperkalemia from reinfusion of hemolyzed cells, which may be life threatening.

VII. **COMPLICATIONS OF BLOOD TRANSFUSION THERAPY**
A. **Transfusion Reactions**
1. **Acute hemolytic transfusion reactions** are estimated to occur in 1 in 250,000 transfusions and are usually due to clerical errors. Symptoms include anxiety, agitation, chest pain, flank pain, headache, dyspnea, and chills. Nonspecific signs include fever, hypotension (or cardiovascular collapse), unexplained bleeding (or DIC), and hemoglobinuria (or renal failure). Fatal reactions are estimated at 1 in 1,250,000 units. Table 35.2 describes the steps to be taken if a transfusion reaction is suspected.
2. **Nonhemolytic transfusion reactions** are usually due to antibodies against donor white cells or plasma proteins. These patients may complain of anxiety, pruritus, or mild dyspnea. Signs include fever, flushing, hives, tachycardia, and mild hypotension. The transfusion should be stopped and a hemolytic transfusion reaction considered (see above).
   a. If the reaction is only urticaria, the transfusion should be slowed and antihistamines (**diphenhydramine**, 25–50 mg IV) or glucocorticoids (**hydrocortisone**, 50–100 mg IV) may be administered.
   b. In patients with known febrile or allergic transfusion reactions, leukocyte-poor red cells (leukocytes removed by filtration or centrifugation) may be given and the patient pretreated with antipyretics (**acetaminophen**, 650–975 mg) and an antihistamine.

	Treatment of Suspected Acute Hemolytic Transfusion Reaction

1. Stop transfusion
2. Send remaining donor blood and fresh patient sample to blood bank for re–cross-match
3. Send patient sample to laboratory for free hemoglobin, haptoglobin, Coombs' test, DIC screen
4. Treat hypotension with fluids and/or vasopressors as necessary
5. Consider use of corticosteroids
6. Consider measures to preserve renal function and maintain brisk urine output (intravenous fluid, furosemide, mannitol)
7. Monitor patient for DIC

DIC, disseminated intravascular coagulation.

     c. Anaphylactic reactions occur rarely and may be more common in patients with an IgA deficiency. These reactions are usually due to plasma protein reactions. Patients with a history of transfusion anaphylaxis should only be transfused with washed red cells (plasma free).

B. Metabolic Complications of Blood Transfusions

  1. Potassium (K^+) concentration changes are common with rapid blood transfusion, but seldom of clinical importance. With storage or hemolysis, red cells leak $K+$ into the extracellular storage fluid. This is rapidly improved after transfusion, due to replenishment of erythrocyte energy stores.

  2. Calcium (Ca^{2+}) is bound by citrate, which is used as an anticoagulant in stored blood products. Rapid transfusion may decrease the ionized calcium level. Citrate is even more concentrated in FFP, and thus an equal volume is more likely to cause citrate toxicity compared with packed pRBC. Usually, the decreased ionized calcium level is transient because the citrate is rapidly metabolized by the liver, but the effect is cumulative in large volume transfusions. Severe hypocalcemia, manifested as hypotension, QT-segment prolongation on the electrocardiogram, and narrowed pulse pressure may occur in patients who are hypothermic, who have impaired liver function, or who have decreased hepatic blood flow. Ionized calcium levels should be monitored during rapid transfusions and aggressively repleted if signs or symptoms of hypocalcemia are present.

  3. Acid–base status. Although banked blood is acidic due to citrate anticoagulant and accumulated red cell metabolites, the clinical effect to the patient is minimal. Acidosis in the face of severe blood loss is more likely due to hypoperfusion and will improve with volume resuscitation. Alkalosis (from metabolism of citrate to bicarbonate) is common following large-volume blood product transfusions.

C. Infectious Complications of blood transfusions have been markedly reduced due to improved testing of donated blood. Recent changes to U.S. blood bank screening for viral pathogens include addition of specific nucleic acid testing of small pooled donated samples to enhance detection of hepatitis C virus (HCV) and human immunodeficiency virus (HIV) before serologic antibody conversion has occurred. Pooled products (e.g., cryoprecipitate) have an increased risk of infection proportional to the number of donors.

1. **Hepatitis B.** The current risk of HBV transmission is estimated to be 1 in 220,000 units transfused. Although the majority of infections are asymptomatic (only 35% of infected individuals demonstrate acute disease), approximately 1% to 10% become chronically infected with potentially significant long-term morbidity.

2. **Hepatitis C.** The risk of transfusion-related HCV is approximately 1 in 1,935,000 units. Risks of HCV infection are more serious than those with HBV, however, because 85% of patients suffer chronic infection, 20% develop cirrhosis, and 1% to 5% of infections cause hepatocellular carcinoma.

3. **HIV.** Because of improved screening and testing, the risk of transfusion-associated HIV has been estimated to be approximately 1 in 2.1 million units transfused in the United States.

4. **Cytomegalovirus (CMV).** The prevalence of antibodies to CMV in the general population is approximately 70% by adulthood. The incidence of transfusion-associated CMV infection in previously uninfected patients is quite high. CMV infection in healthy individuals is usually asymptomatic, but immunosuppressed patients, such as those who have received bone marrow or stem cell transplantation, are at high risk for serious complications, including death. Thus, the American Association of Blood Banks recommends that either CMV-seronegative or leukoreduced blood be administered to transplant recipients who are CMV-negative and to patients undergoing chemotherapy with severe neutropenia as an expected consequence.

5. **West Nile virus** is a seasonal epidemic causing febrile and neurological illnesses including meningoencephalitis and acute flaccid paralysis. Transfusion transmission was first documented in 2002, and screening is done in endemic regions. The current risk in these areas is estimated at 1 in 1 million units transfused.

6. **Bacterial infections.** Exclusion of donors with evidence of infectious disease and the storage of blood at 4°C reduces the risk of transmitted bacterial infection. However, the necessity of room-temperature storage of platelets to maintain functional integrity creates favorable medium for bacterial growth. Infection rates for platelets are estimated at 1 in 1,000 to 2,000 units, with an estimated 15% to 25% of infected transfusions causing severe sepsis. Organisms likely to infect platelet concentrates include *Staphylococcus aureus*, coagulase-negative *Staphylococcus*, and diphtheroids. Red blood cells are much less likely to become contaminated with bacteria, but the most commonly cultured organism is *Yersinia enterocolitica*, and the mortality rate from transfusion-acquired sepsis is approximately 60%.

D. **Transfusion-Related Acute Lung Injury (TRALI)** is a syndrome of acute lung injury (see Chapter 19) after blood product transfusion. Symptoms may include severe hypoxemia, dyspnea, and pulmonary edema, often accompanied by fever and hypotension, and usually occur 4 to 6 hours after transfusion. The pathophysiology is incompletely understood, and it is likely underrecognized. Possible mechanisms of injury include (a) donor blood containing WBC antibodies to recipient WBC antigens, resulting in granulocyte or lymphocyte activation and subsequent pulmonary endothelial injury, and (b) donor blood containing biologically active lipids, which similarly activate granulocytes.

Incidence of TRALI has decreased over the past several years, partly due to increased recognition of risk factors (e.g., FFP from female donors). It is currently estimated at 1 per 12,000 units transfused. Any transfused product that contains plasma may cause TRALI. Mortality from TRALI is approximately 5%. Treatment is similar to other forms of acute lung injury and frequently requires mechanical ventilation. Most patients show dramatic clinical improvement within 48 hours and radiographic clearing of edema within a few days.

E. **Transfusion-Associated Circulatory Overload (TACO)** has been described as a syndrome associated with rapid transfusion of a large volume of blood products, which overwhelms the circulatory system. It may manifest with hypertension and signs of right and left heart failure (peripheral edema and pulmonary edema).

VIII. MASSIVE TRANSFUSIONS (see Appendix 35.1)

A. **Massive transfusion** is arbitrarily defined as the administration of at least 8 to 10 units of blood transfused within a 6-to-12-hour period.

1. Transfusion of 10 to 12 units of red blood cells can cause a 50% drop in the platelet count and produce a **dilutional thrombocytopenia** that can result in diffuse oozing and failure to form clot.

2. Adequate hemostasis may occur with plasma clotting factor concentrations as low as 30% of normal. There is approximately a 10% decrease in clotting factor concentration for each 500 mL of replaced blood loss. Small quantities of the stable clotting factors are also present in the plasma of each unit of red cells transfused. Bleeding from factor deficiency during a massive transfusion is usually due to diminished levels of fibrinogen and labile factors (V, VIII, and IX), which may be replaced with FFP or cryoprecipitate. Bleeding from hypofibrinogenemia is unusual unless the fibrinogen level is less than 75 mg/dL.

3. **Additional complications** of massive transfusion include **hypothermia** from the rapid infusion of blood, **citrate toxicity** (Section VII.B.2), and dysrhythmias secondary to **electrolyte abnormalities** (hypocalcemia and hypomagnesemia). Hypotension and acidosis may also be a result of ongoing bleeding and ischemic- or septic-mediated myocardial depression.

4. Once bleeding has begun from a **dilutional coagulopathy** and thrombocytopenia, it can be very **difficult to control**. Therefore, it is recommended that 1 unit of FFP be administered for every 1 to 2 units of pRBCs. Additionally, 6 units of platelets should be administered for every 10 units of pRBCs. Careful attention must be paid to the use of cell saver units of blood. Like banked blood, these are nearly devoid of clotting factors and must be included in the transfusion count.

5. In addition to transfusion of appropriate blood products, the strategy for massive transfusion includes **maintaining intravascular volume**, administering **calcium** as needed to offset the effects of citrate, and the consideration of **vasopressors with inotropic properties** as a temporizing measures to maintain adequate perfusion until resolution of the underlying pathology can be established. Antifibrinolytic agents (see **Chapter 24**) may be considered and employed if fibrinolysis is contributing to bleeding. Frequent laboratory measures of coagulation status may be needed because these parameters change rapidly in the setting of massive hemorrhage and transfusion. Finally, direct **communication with the blood bank** is fundamental to expedite component preparation.

6. Unfortunately, there are no good markers to determine when further transfusion is futile.

APPENDIX 35.1 ABRIDGED MASSIVE TRANSFUSION PROTOCOL OF THE MASSACHUSETTS GENERAL HOSPITAL TRAUMA SERVICE

1. The protocol can be initiated at any time during the trauma patient's hospitalization, including prior to arrival to MGH
2. Appropriate candidates include the following:
   a. Any patient with an initial blood loss of at least 40% of blood volume, or in whom it is judged that at least 10 units of blood replacement is immediately required
   b. Any patient with a continuing hemorrhage of at least 250 mL/h
   c. Any patient, when clinical judgment is made such that blood loss as identified in "A" and "B" is imminent
3. Once the decision is made to initiate this protocol, the appropriate physician needs to do the following:
   a. Notify the blood bank with the age and gender of the patient
   b. Ensure that a blood bank sample is obtained
4. The blood bank fellow is available to assist in decision making.
5. RBC selection
   a. At least 4 units of emergency-release, uncross-matched group O negative pRBCs will be released for all Rh-negative or Rh-unknown patients.
   b. All patients will receive Rh-negative cells as long as inventory is adequate. An effort will be made to provide Rh-negative cells to females age less than 50. The blood bank will decide to switch the patient to Rh-positive RBCs on the basis of the available inventory and the anticipated requirement.
   c. Group O RBCs will be used until the patient's blood group is known after which the patient will be switched to group-specific RBCs.
6. Blood components requests
   After the initial assessment, if >10 total units are expected to be needed, the clinical team should request the following:
   a. 10 pRBCs
   b. 10 FFPs
   c. 1 dose of platelets
7. It is essential that the clinical team communicates to the blood bank when the patient is being moved to a different ward.
8. Laboratory monitoring for ongoing blood support in cases requiring >10 units of RBCs:
   a. Transfusion support should be individualized for each patient.
   b. The following general guidelines apply:
      1. Check Hb, platelet count, INR, and fibrinogen after each blood volume lost/infused.
      2. Include the number of "cell saver" units in the tally of pRBCs.
      3. Target a ratio of 2 pRBCs to 1 FFP during the course of acute bleeding.
      4. Anticipate fibrinolysis and treat with antifibrinolytics if there is ongoing diffuse bleeding.
      5. Verify that the INR is <2 and fibrinogen >100. Values outside these ranges may indicate systemic fibrinogenolysis, DIC, or hemodilution.
      6. In the absence of platelet transfusion, anticipate a halving of the platelet count with each blood volume resuscitation. Transfuse platelets to maintain an anticipated platelet count >50,000 μL.
      7. A stat AST or ALT can be used to document shock liver (values >800), which is an independent indication for antifibrinolytic therapy.
   c. Monitor and treat abnormalities of ionized Ca^{2+}, K^+, pH, and temperature.
9. Not all massively injured patients can be saved. The decision to withdraw support for the massively injured patient should be made by consensus of the treating team.

Selected Readings

American Society of Anesthesiologists Task Force on Blood Component Therapy. Practice guidelines for perioperative blood transfusion and adjuvant therapies. *Anesthesiology* 2006;105:198–208.

Boffard KD, Riou B, Warren B, et al. Recombinant factor VIIa as adjunctive therapy for bleeding control in severely injured trauma patients: two parallel randomized, placebo-controlled, double-blind clinical trials. *J Trauma* 2005;59:8–18.

Carson JL, Grossman BJ, Kleinman S, et al; Clinical Transfusion Medicine Committee of the AABB. Red blood cell transfusion: a clinical practice guideline from the American Association of Blood Banks. *Ann Intern Med* 2012;157(1):49–58.

Carson JL, Terrin ML, Noveck H, et al; FOCUS Investigators. Liberal or restrictive transfusion in high-risk patients after hip surgery. *N Engl J Med* 2011;365(26):2453–2462.

Chang TM. From artificial red blood cells, oxygen carriers, and oxygen therapeutics to artificial cells, nanomedicine, and beyond. *Artif Cells Blood Substit Immobil Biotechnol* 2012;40(3):197–199.

Corwin HL, Gettinger A, Fabian TC, et al. Efficacy and safety of epoetin alfa in critically ill patients. *N Eng J Med* 2002;357:965–976.

Dutton RP, Hess JR, Scalea TM. Recombinant factor VIIa for control of hemorrhage: early experience in critically ill trauma patients. *J Clin Anesth* 2003;15:184–188.

Dutton RP, Shih D, Edelman BB, et al. Safety of uncrossmatched type-O red cells for resuscitation from hemorrhagic shock. *J Trauma* 2005;59(6):1445–1449.

Gunter OL, Au BK, Isbell JM, et al. Optimizing outcomes in damage control resuscitation: identifying blood product ratios associated with improved survival. *J Trauma* 2008;65:527–534.

Hajjar LA, Vincent JL, Galas FR, et al. Transfusion requirements after cardiac surgery: the TRACS randomized controlled trial. *JAMA* 2010;304(14):1559–1567.

Hébert PC, Wells G, Blajchman MA, et al. A multicenter, randomized, controlled clinical trial of transfusion requirements in critical care. *N Engl J Med* 1999;340:409–417.

Hess JR, Holcomb JB. Transfusion practice in military trauma. *Transfus Med* 2008;18(3):143–150.

Holcomb JB, Wade CE, Michalek JE, et al. Increased plasma and platelet to red blood cell ratios improves outcome in 466 massively transfused civilian trauma patients. *Ann Surg* 2008;248:447–458.

Holland LL, Brooks JP. Toward rational fresh frozen plasma transfusion: the effect of plasma transfusion on coagulation test results. *Am J Clin Pathol* 2006;126(1):133–139.

Keir AK, Hansen AL, Callum J, et al. Coinfusion of dextrose-containing fluids and red blood cells does not adversely affect in vitro red blood cell quality. *Transfusion* 2014;54(8):2068–2076.

Lake CL, Moore RA, eds. *Blood: hemostasis, transfusion, and alternatives in the perioperative period*. New York: Raven, 1995.

Lorenzo M, Davis JW, Negin S, et al. Can Ringer's lactate be used safely with blood transfusions? *Am J Surg* 1998;175(4):308–310.

O'Connell NM, Perry DJ, Hodgson AJ, et al. Recombinant FVIIa in the management of uncontrolled hemorrhage. *Transfusion* 2003;43:1711–1716.

Perel P, Roberts I, Ker K. Colloids versus crystalloids for fluid resuscitation in critically ill patients. *Cochrane Database Syst Rev* 2013;2:CD000567.

Simpson E, Lin Y, Stanworth S, et al. Recombinant factor VIIa for the prevention and treatment of bleeding in patients without haemophilia. *Cochrane Database Syst Rev* 2012;3:CD005011.

Spinella PC, Perkins JG, Grathwohl KW, et al. Effect of plasma and red blood cell transfusions on survival in patients with combat related traumatic injuries. *J Trauma* 2008;64:S69–S78.

Stainsby D, MacLennan S, Thomas D, et al. Guidelines on the management of massive blood loss. *Br J Hem* 2006;135:634.

The SAFE Study Investigators. A comparison of albumin and saline for fluid resuscitation in the intensive care unit. *N Engl J Med* 2004;350:2247–2256.

Toy P, Gajic O, Bacchetti P, et al; TRALI Study Group. Transfusion-related acute lung injury: incidence and risk factors. *Blood* 2012;119(7):1757–1767.

Zarychanski R, Turgeon AF, McIntyre L, et al. Erythropoietin-receptor agonists in critically ill patients: a meta-analysis of randomized controlled trials. *CMAJ* 2007;177(7):725–734.

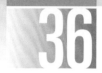

Obstetric Critical Care

Olof Viktorsdottir and Rebecca D. Minehart

 Fetal Heart Rate Monitoring

I. **INTRODUCTION.** The obstetric patient population is in general healthy, but preexisting comorbid conditions and several pregnancy-related disorders may be associated with significant morbidity and mortality. The incidence of ICU admission for pregnant and postpartum women ranges from 0.7 to 13.5 per 1,000 deliveries.

   A. When caring for the critically ill pregnant woman, it is important to consider how management affects the fetus.

   B. Any pregnant patient admitted to the ICU should prompt multidisciplinary care plan formation, including potential labor and delivery plan. Preterm labor and delivery are common in setting of critical illness.

II. **GENERAL CONSIDERATIONS RELEVANT TO THE OBSTETRIC, CRITICALLY ILL POPULATION**

   A. Physiologic Changes of Pregnancy

   1. Pregnant women undergo normal physiologic changes associated with pregnancy, labor, and delivery. See Table 36.1 for details. Maintenance of these physiological changes is critical for placental perfusion and fetal oxygenation. Thus, common treatments in the ICU such as high levels of PEEP, diuretics, and vasopressors must be weighed against the risk of decreased venous return, decreased cardiac output, and changes in maternal blood flow distribution—all of which may affect placental perfusion and fetal oxygenation.

   2. After 20 weeks' gestation (uterus palpable above the umbilicus), patients should be positioned with left uterine displacement or in the lateral position to minimize aortocaval compression.

   3. Physiologic changes of pregnancy can alter pharmacokinetics and pharmacodynamics.

   B. Viability of the Fetus and Fetal Heart Rate Monitoring (reference video)

   1. Most sources define the age of fetal viability as being about 24 weeks of gestation. After 24 weeks, fetal heart rate monitoring is recommended to evaluate fetal well-being. Normal fetal heart varies between 110 and 160 beats per minute. A heart rate that does not vary or is too low or too high may signal a potential problem with the fetus.

   C. Teratogenic Agents

   1. **Teratogens** are substances that act to irreversibly alter growth, structure, or function of the developing fetus.

   2. Timing of exposure as well as the drug-dosing regimen can influence teratogenicity. The classic period of susceptibility to teratogenic agent is between 2.5 and 8 weeks after conception, or during the period of organogenesis. Later effect is more prominent on growth and/or nervous system and gonadal tissue. The US FDA issued a drug classification system with five categories (A–D and X) implying a progressive fetal risk from Category A to X. Category X drugs are contraindicated in pregnancy.

Parameter	Change (Relative to Nonpregnant State)
Blood volume	+45%
Plasma volume	+55%
Red blood cell volume	+30%
Tidal volume	+45%
Cardiac output	+50%
Stroke volume	+25%
Heart rate	+25%
Systemic vascular resistance	−20%
Left ventricular end diastolic volume	↑
Ejection fraction	↑
Left ventricular stroke work index	No change
Central venous pressure	No change
Pulmonary capillary wedge pressure	No change
Maternal oxygen consumption	+20%
Inspiratory reserve volume	+5%
Expiratory reserve volume	−25%
Residual volume	−15%
Vital capacity	No change
Total lung capacity	−5%
Inspiratory capacity	+15%
Functional residual capacity	−20%
Minute ventilation	+45%
Alveolar ventilation	+45%

TABLE 36.1 Physiologic Changes of Pregnancy

3. Medications commonly encountered in the ICU setting and have known teratogenic properties include antiepileptics (phenytoin, carbamazepine, phenobarbital, valproic acid), lithium, statins, ACE inhibitors, warfarin, tetracyclines, and ribavirin.

4. Multiple Internet resources are available for further drug and teratogen information, including the websites of the American College of Obstetrician and Gynecologists (ACOG) and the Centers for Disease Control and Prevention (CDC).

5. Most drugs are safe for use during lactation. Typically only 1% to 2% of the maternal dose appears in breast milk. The Drugs and Lactation database (LactMed) of the National Library of Medicine's Toxicology Data Network is an up-to-date source of further information.

D. Vasopressor Use and Potential Effects on the Fetus

1. Little data exist regarding vasopressor use for maternal hypotension or shock due to critical illness. Traditionally, there have been concerns with vasopressor use during pregnancy regarding the potential adverse effects on uterine blood vessels and fetal blood flow.

2. When managing hypotension, it is reasonable to attempt other interventions initially, such as administering intravenous fluids and placing the patient in left lateral decubitus position to prevent compression of the inferior vena cava by the gravid uterus.

3. In the setting of persistent hypotension, restoring maternal perfusion pressure is of paramount importance, and it should override

any theoretical concerns of vasopressor-induced uterine vasculature constriction. Increasing the MAP will improve perfusion pressure to organs, including the gravid uterus. Norepinephrine, an endogenous catecholamine that crosses the placenta, is often used as first-line vasopressor. Second-line vasopressors such as epinephrine or vasopressin may be considered. No good data exist regarding the use of vasopressin in pregnant women. Therefore, caution is recommended if this agent is used since it may theoretically activate uterine V1a receptors, leading to uterine contractions.

E. Ventilation and Blood Gases (Table 36.2)

   1. Most aspects of mechanical ventilation are the same for pregnant and nonpregnant women. An exception is the target arterial carbon dioxide tension ($Paco_2$). Ventilator settings should be adjusted to maintain mild respiratory alkalosis with $Paco_2$ between 30 and 32 mmHg and arterial pH between 7.40 and 7.47. This replicates normal physiology during pregnancy due to respiratory stimulation by progesterone.

   2. Significant respiratory alkalosis with $Paco_2$ <30 mmHg should be avoided because it may decrease uterine blood flow. Maternal hypercapnia ($Paco_2$ >40 mmHg) may result in decreased removal of CO_2 from the fetus, causing fetal acidosis, in addition to increased fetal breathing movements, which may increase fetal oxygen use. Thus, it seems prudent to avoid maternal hypercapnia even though studies have not identified any adverse sequelae in fetuses that were exposed to $Paco_2$ levels as high as 60 mmHg during permissive hypercapnia. Maternal oxygen consumption increases in pregnancy by 20% to 30% at term, largely because of increased consumption by the fetus and placenta. To minimize fetal effects, the maternal Pao_2 should be maintained at more than 60 mmHg.

III. **PREECLAMPSIA** is part of a spectrum of hypertensive disorders specific to pregnancy. Although the precise etiology of preeclampsia remains unknown, it is a disease that occurs only in the presence of placental tissue. The maternal manifestations are consistent with a process of vasospasm, ischemia, and changes in the normal balance of humoral and autocoid mediators. Preeclampsia is diagnosed in 3% to 5% of all pregnancies in the United States and is most common in nulliparous women. A patient meets the criteria for a diagnosis of preeclampsia if she has persistently elevated blood pressure after 20 weeks' gestation in the setting of previously normal blood pressure, and proteinuria of greater than 300 mg in 24 hours or signs of end-organ dysfunction. The diagnosis of preeclampsia is divided into

TABLE 36.2 Blood Gas Measurements during Pregnancy

Parameter	Nonpregnant	Trimester		
		First	Second	Third
$Paco_2$ (mmHg)	40	30	30	30
Pao_2 (mmHg)	100	107	105	103
pH	7.40	7.44	7.44	7.44
$[HCO_3^-]$ (mEq/L)	24	21	20	20

mild and severe on the basis of the presence or absence of specific signs, symptoms, and abnormal laboratory values (Table 36.3).

A. Two additional diagnoses, **eclampsia and potentially HELLP syndrome,** are a part of this spectrum of disease.

   1. **Eclampsia** is defined as the occurrence of **seizures or coma** in a woman with preeclampsia that cannot be attributed to other causes. Eclamptic seizures may occur antepartum, intrapartum, or postpartum. Eclampsia is a cause of significant maternal and fetal morbidity and is present in approximately 50% of maternal deaths associated with preeclampsia. Eclamptic seizures are usually preceded by headache and visual disturbances. Seizures are generally abrupt and self-limited, but may be complicated by cardiopulmonary arrest or pulmonary aspiration of gastric contents.

   2. **HELLP syndrome** (**H**emolysis, **E**levated **L**iver enzymes, and **L**ow **P**latelets) involves a constellation of laboratory abnormalities and was previously regarded as a subset of severe preeclampsia; however, it is now

TABLE 36.3	Diagnostic Criteria for Mild and Severe Preeclampsia
Blood pressure	≥140 mmHg systolic or ≥90 mmHg diastolic on two occasions at least 4 hours apart after 20 weeks of gestation in a woman with a previously normal blood pressure
	≥160 mmHg systolic or ≥110 mmHg diastolic, hypertension can be confirmed within a short interval (minutes) to facilitate timely antihypertensive therapy
and	
Proteinuria	≥300 mg per 24-h urine collection (or this amount extrapolated from a timed collection)
	or
	Protein–creatinine ratio ≥0.3 (each measured by mg/dL)
	Dipstick reading of 1+ (used only if other quantitative methods are not available)
Or in the absence of proteinuria, new-onset hypertension with the new onset of any of the following:	
Thrombocytopenia	Platelet count <100,000/µL
Renal insufficiency	Serum creatinine concentrations >1.1 mg/dL or a doubling of the serum creatinine concentration in the absence of other renal disease
Impaired liver function	Elevated blood concentrations of liver transaminases to twice normal concentration
Pulmonary edema	
Cerebral or visual symptoms	

Adapted from American College of Obstetricians and Gynecologists. *Hypertension in pregnancy.* Washington, DC: American College of Obstetricians and Gynecologists, 2013.

recognized as potentially a distinct clinical entity. The diagnosis of HELLP syndrome is also associated with an increased risk of adverse outcomes including abruption, renal failure, hepatic subcapsular hematoma formation, liver rupture, and fetal and maternal death. Management is generally aimed at administering magnesium, supportive care with normalizing blood pressure in the face of severe hypertension, and delivery of the fetus with recognition of the increased risk of hemorrhage in this population. Platelet counts can fall precipitously, and platelet transfusions are indicated in any parturient with significant bleeding or with a platelet count of less than 20,000/mm³. Subcapsular hematoma, if it occurs, is an emergency and can result in shock and fulminant hepatic failure. Death is typically due to exsanguination and coagulopathy. Prompt surgical intervention and resuscitative measures have led to improvement in maternal survival.

B. Management
   1. **Delivery**. The only definitive treatment for preeclampsia, eclampsia, or HELLP syndrome is delivery of the fetus and placenta. The decision of when to deliver is made on the basis of the gestational age and the severity of the disease. Each patient and clinical situation should be individualized with a management strategy that seeks to balance and minimize both maternal and fetal morbidity.
   2. **Pharmacologic therapy**
       a. **Seizure prophylaxis**. Although the mechanism of action is unknown, **magnesium sulfate** is the medication of choice for prophylactic prevention and treatment of eclamptic seizures. Dosage of magnesium is 4 g intravenous (IV) bolus over 30 minutes followed by 2 g/h IV, but because it is renally cleared, this may need to be adjusted if severe renal dysfunction is present. The drug is administered during active labor, delivery, and for 24 to 48 hours postdelivery. Because of its relaxant effect on vascular and visceral smooth muscle, magnesium may decrease maternal blood pressure and predispose to postpartum atony and hemorrhage. It also inhibits acetylcholine release at the motor endplate, leading to potentiation of neuromuscular blocking agents.
       b. **Antihypertensive medications** such as **labetalol, hydralazine,** and **calcium-channel blockers** are frequently administered for control of blood pressure. The goal is not to normalize blood pressure, but to keep patients from progressing to a hypertensive crisis, encephalopathy, or stroke. When administering antihypertensive medications, it is important to remember that the placenta has no ability to autoregulate flow. Thus, a sudden drop in maternal blood pressure may decrease placental perfusion and result in significant compromise to the fetus.

IV. ACUTE FATTY LIVER OF PREGNANCY (AFLP) is a rare but potentially fatal complication of pregnancy, involving microvesicular fat deposition in the liver and characterized by liver dysfunction, DIC, severe and refractory hypoglycemia, encephalopathy, and renal insufficiency. Patients usually present in the third trimester, although the disease has been described as early as 23 weeks' gestation. More than half (50%–70%) of AFLP patients can have associated preeclampsia. Some authors consider AFLP and HELLP to be part of a spectrum of a single disease, but AFLP can be distinguished from HELLP on the basis of severe hepatic dysfunction, rather than merely elevated liver transaminases (as occurs in HELLP). The precise pathogenesis of AFLP remains unknown although believed to be due to defective mitochondrial β oxidation of fat either in the mother or the fetus, which is hepatotoxic. Mortality remains high for both mother and fetus.

- **A. Clinical Manifestations.** Patients frequently present with nonspecific symptoms such as malaise, nausea and emesis, jaundice, epigastric or right upper-quadrant pain, headache, and anorexia. Hypoglycemia may be present and severe and accounts for some of the mortality associated with AFLP.
- **B. Diagnosis and Laboratory Findings.** One distinct laboratory finding of acute fatty liver of pregnancy is **hyperbilirubinemia** with serum levels of 3 to 40 mg/dL reported. Patients also have profound elevation of alkaline phosphatase with mild to moderate transaminase elevations. Progression to hepatic failure can be rapid, and large elevations in hepatocellular enzymes may be missed. In addition to hepatic dysfunction, renal failure, coagulopathy, profound hypoglycemia, and metabolic acidosis are early complications.
  1. Hyponatremia from diabetes insipidus can be present in up to 10% of patients. Liver biopsy is rarely required and should be performed only when absolutely necessary because of the concomitant coagulopathy.
- **C. Management.** The liver dysfunction and failure associated with AFLP is reversible in most patients, and **supportive care** and **delivery** are the mainstays of treatment. AFLP is a medical emergency that requires immediate evaluation. The most important component of treatment is the delivery of the fetus. Careful attention to **fluid balance** is crucial due to the increased risk of pulmonary and cerebral edema secondary to low colloid osmotic pressure. There is almost always early onset of **acute renal dysfunction** (90%), which is usually reversible, but renal support is often required.
  1. **Serum glucose levels** should be checked every 1 to 2 hours and hypoglycemia aggressively treated; all patients should receive an infusion of at least 5% dextrose, and many will require higher concentrations with intermittent boluses to maintain normoglycemia. **Coagulation studies** should be followed at regular intervals and postpartum hemorrhage anticipated. Regardless of the mode of delivery, patients should have adequate IV access and cross-matched blood products available. If the patient requires a cesarean section, improving or correcting the coagulopathy prior to incision should be considered.
  2. There is often a worsening of liver function, renal function, and coagulopathy for 48 hours after delivery, but then improvement should be expected. Transplantation is generally not required for AFLP, but may be necessary in severe cases.

V. NEUROLOGIC DISEASE

- **A. Stroke.** Pregnant women are at higher risk than nonpregnant women with the incidence of stroke being 5 to 15 per 100,000 deliveries with cerebrovascular events accounting for 5% of maternal deaths. A significant proportion of strokes occur late in pregnancy, with the highest incidence in the peripartum period. **Ischemic events appear to** account for one-half to two-thirds of cerebrovascular events in pregnancy, whereas **hemorrhagic strokes** may be slightly less common.
  1. **Etiologies.** Ischemic cerebral infarctions may be divided into primarily arterial or venous etiologies. **Arterial etiologies** include vasculopathies, dissections, and embolic events; **venous infarctions** may result from hypercoagulable states, dehydration, or infections. **Hemorrhagic events**

are largely a result of aneurysms, vascular malformations, preeclampsia, or trauma. Treatment may be challenging, as up to 50% of venous infarctions manifest in areas of hemorrhage, making anticoagulation difficult.

2. **Clinical manifestations** are similar as in nonpregnant women. **Headache** is the most common presenting symptom. Other symptoms include focal neurologic deficits and seizures.

3. **Diagnosis.** In addition to physical examination, neurologic imaging is critical for establishing the diagnosis and etiology. Attempts should be made to minimize fetal exposure to radiation, but appropriate diagnostic imaging should not be avoided. The fetal radiation exposure from noncontrast CT scan is less than 1 rad.

4. **Management** in the pregnant patient is similar to the treatment of nonpregnant patients. Care is supportive, and thrombolytic therapy should be considered if indicated for ischemic stroke. Thrombolysis with recombinant tissue plasminogen activator (r-tPA) has been reported during pregnancy and appears to be safe for the fetus; there is minimal transplacental passage of r-tPA. However, retroplacental bleeding with pregnancy loss has been reported. The therapeutic window (i.e., time from onset of symptoms to administration of the agent) is 4.5 hours.

   a. For preservation of fetal well-being, oxygenation and intravascular volume should be maintained, and hypotension, hyperglycemia, and fever avoided. Delivery of the fetus may be complicated by the risk of aneurysm or arteriovenous malformation (AVM) rupture, thrombolytic therapy, or anticoagulation; both the route of delivery and anesthetic management should be tailored to each individual patient.

B. **Seizure Disorders.** Approximately 0.5% of all parturients have a chronic, preexisting seizure disorder. A third of women will experience an increase in their seizure frequency, 50% will experience no change, and the remainder will note a decrease in seizures. Because many antiseizure medications carry an elevated risk of teratogenicity to the fetus, patients and providers must weigh the risks and benefits of continuing these medications in pregnancy. Many patients begin monotherapy, and folate supplementation is a necessity. Uncontrolled generalized seizures pose serious risk to both mother and fetus. Serum levels of antiseizure medications may fall due to greater drug clearance and decreased protein binding in pregnancy. In addition, epileptic parturients appear to be at increased risk for preeclampsia, preterm labor, and placental abnormalities.

1. **Status epilepticus** (see **Chapters 10 and 30**). Although the frequency of seizure activity is increased in a significant portion of parturients, pregnancy itself does not increase the likelihood of status epilepticus.

   a. Should status epilepticus occur in a pregnant patient, **treatment goals** include (a) maintaining an adequate airway, (b) ensuring adequate oxygenation, (c) determining the cause of the seizure, and (d) stopping the seizure. The patient should be placed in full lateral position and supplemental oxygen administered, in addition to receiving advanced airway support if needed.

   b. **Pharmacologic therapy** should be initiated after 2 to 5 minutes of prolonged seizure activity and consists of the same medications used in the nonpregnant population; benzodiazepines should be considered.

    c. For **intractable seizure activity,** electroencephalographic monitoring, suppression of seizure activity with medications, tracheal intubation, and mechanical ventilation may be necessary. Fetal bradycardia may occur and necessitate prompt delivery.

  2. Eclampsia. The diagnosis of eclampsia should be entertained and ruled out in any pregnant woman who presents with a new-onset seizure disorder after 20 weeks' gestation. Management of eclamptic seizures includes magnesium sulfate and prompt delivery. See section above for further discussion.

VI. ACUTE RESPIRATORY DISTRESS SYNDROME (ARDS, see **Chapter 19)** is a rare but serious complication in pregnancy and, when present, may result in significant maternal and fetal mortality. No large studies are available, but data from the last several decades place maternal mortality rates in the range of 30% to 40% and fetal mortality over 20%.

  A. Risk Factors Specific to Pregnancy include gastric aspiration, medications used for tocolysis, preeclampsia, amniotic fluid or trophoblastic embolism, and abruption.

  B. Management. As in the nonpregnant population, the mainstay of treatment is supportive care. However, the following should be considered when managing a pregnant patient with ARDS.

    1. Ventilation. Goals of ventilation should strive to maintain physiologic alterations of pregnancy (see section II.E).

    2. Maintenance of maternal cardiac output is critical for placental perfusion and fetal oxygenation. Thus, standard treatments in ARDS therapy such as high levels of PEEP, diuretics, and vasopressors must be weighed against the risk of decreased venous return, decreased cardiac output, and changes in maternal blood flow distribution—all of which may decrease placental perfusion and fetal oxygenation. Additionally, after 20 weeks' gestation (uterus palpable above the umbilicus), patients should be positioned with left uterine displacement or in the lateral position to minimize aortocaval compression.

  C. Obstetric Considerations. Fetal assessment should be performed at regular intervals to evaluate fetal well-being. Lastly, some authors suggest that delivery of the preterm fetus after 28 weeks' gestation in patients with ARDS may improve maternal outcome.

VII. CARDIOVASCULAR DISORDERS

  A. Valvular Heart Disease (see Chapter 16)

    1. Chronic **regurgitant lesions** are well tolerated with the normal physiologic changes of pregnancy. A decrease in systemic vascular resistance, reduced left ventricular afterload, and a modest increase in heart rate all lead to a reduction in regurgitation. However, in the immediate postpartum period, the sudden increase in venous return and vascular resistance may lead to decompensation, and patients should be carefully monitored for the first 24 to 48 hours. **Endocarditis prophylaxis** is not recommended in this patient population.

      a. Aortic regurgitation (AR) with preserved LV function is well tolerated in pregnancy. In symptomatic, severe AR, the treatment is **salt restriction, diuretics,** and **digoxin.** Vasodilators such as **hydralazine** and **nitrates** may be used as substitutes to ACE inhibitors, which are contraindicated in pregnancy.

      b. Mitral regurgitation (MR) during pregnancy is usually due to rheumatic valvular disease or the myxomatous degeneration of mitral valve prolapse. Patients with MR in pregnancy will rarely become symptomatic, but if decompensation occurs, medical management with **vasodilators** and **diuretics** may be helpful.

c. As in the nonpregnant population, **acute regurgitant lesions** are poorly tolerated and constitute a medical and surgical emergency.

2. In contrast to regurgitant lesions, **stenotic lesions** are not well tolerated in pregnancy. Increased intravascular volume, increased heart rate, and the decreased systemic vascular resistance of pregnancy adversely affect these patients. Known predictors of poor maternal–fetal outcome include prior cardiac event or arrhythmia, impaired left ventricular function, pulmonary hypertension, severe stenotic lesions, and impaired New York Heart Association functional class at the initiation of prenatal care. The autotransfusion and increased venous return associated with delivery and the immediate postpartum period (where cardiac output is highest) may lead to further decompensation, and patients should be closely monitored for the first 24 to 48 hours postpartum. **Endocarditis prophylaxis** is not recommended in patients with stenotic lesions. Considerations for invasive blood pressure monitoring using arterial lines, continuous EKG to evaluate for arrhythmias, as well as central venous access (via a central venous line or a peripherally inserted central catheter) for CVP monitoring and potential vasopressor administration should be part of the multidisciplinary planning discussion regarding these patients.

a. **Aortic stenosis (AS)** in pregnant women is usually congenital. Women with mild to moderate disease will tolerate pregnancy provided they are followed closely and managed appropriately. In contrast, women with severe AS are at risk of deterioration with development of heart failure and preterm delivery.

   1. **Medical management** consists of **diuretics** and **maintenance of sinus rhythm**.
   2. If possible, patients with severe disease should undergo preconceptual valve replacement or valvuloplasty. In the setting of an established pregnancy, valvuloplasty is the procedure of choice to minimize the risk of fetal loss.
   3. For delivery, hemodynamic monitoring, early epidural placement, and an assisted second stage are recommended (which may require a dense sacral block if forceps delivery is attempted).

b. **Mitral stenosis (MS)** is the most common acquired valvular lesion in pregnancy. The increased stroke volume and heart rate in the setting of a significantly narrowed valve lead to increased left atrial pressure, arrhythmias, and worsened symptoms.

   1. Patients contemplating pregnancy with severe stenosis should be offered valvuloplasty or replacement; in patients who are already pregnant, valvuloplasty is preferred.
   2. Optimal **medical management** of the pregnant patient involves administration of $\beta1$-**blockers** for reducing heart rate and left atrial pressure. **Diuretics** and **salt restriction** may also be necessary. **Anticoagulation** should be considered in patients with severe MS and an enlarged left atrium, even in the absence of atrial fibrillation.
   3. Hemodynamic monitoring, early epidural anesthesia, and an assisted second stage are recommended for delivery. Patients with MS are particularly vulnerable to failure following delivery, and diuretics may be necessary to prevent failure.

    c. Isolated **pulmonic stenosis (PS)**, even when severe, is well tolerated in pregnancy. In symptomatic patients, balloon valvuloplasty is a treatment option.

3. **Prosthetic cardiac valves** are associated with additional risks during pregnancy. Despite the replacement of a malfunctioning valve, some degree of myocardial, valvular, or pulmonary dysfunction usually persists.

    a. Anticoagulation. Thromboembolic events are of particular concern in pregnancy, and all obstetric patients with mechanical valves or bioprosthetic valves in atrial fibrillation should receive anticoagulation. Women with bioprosthetic valves and no risk factors do not require anticoagulation. Anticoagulation in pregnancy is usually accomplished with **unfractionated heparin** or **low-molecular-weight heparin (LMWH)** because warfarin carries with it a risk of embryopathy, with exposure between gestational weeks 6 to 9, and a high risk of warfarin fetopathy (CNS abnormalities, ocular abnormalities, fetal loss, and stillbirth), with fetal exposure occurring later in pregnancy. **Endocarditis prophylaxis** is recommended in this patient population.

B. Congenital Heart Disease. Pregnant women with a history of repaired congenital disease are becoming increasingly common as more survive to childbearing age, and congenital heart lesions are now the most common cause of cardiac disease in the pregnant population. Many will be **asymptomatic** with relatively normal pressures and flow patterns, and such patients will not require special treatment during pregnancy. However, others will **present with a partially repaired or completely uncorrected lesion**, making management considerably more complex. Known predictors of poor maternal–fetal outcome include the following markers: elevated pulmonary artery pressure, depressed right or left ventricular function, cyanosis, and impaired New York Heart Association functional class. **Endocarditis prophylaxis** should be given to patients with unrepaired cyanotic heart disease, repaired disease with residual defects adjacent to prosthetic material, or a repair involving placement of prosthetic material within the previous 6 months. Essentially, all patients with congenital heart disease should be assessed by a cardiologist, ultimately understanding the anatomy of these patients (since corrections of the lesions may differ). Everyone is a unique case.

    Please refer to more detailed texts (e.g., Chestnut's, Schneider) for specific disorders.

C. Myocardial Infarction is uncommon in pregnancy, with an estimated incidence of 3 to 10 per 100,000 deliveries and a case fatality rate of 5% to 20%. Possible etiologies include atherosclerotic disease, and coronary arterial dissection, vasospasm, or thrombus. Risk factors for MI in pregnancy include advanced maternal age, hypertension, diabetes, thrombophilia, smoking, cocaine abuse, transfusion, and postpartum hemorrhage.

1. The balance between **myocardial oxygen supply and demand** is affected by the physiologic changes of pregnancy, leading to an increase in myocardial mass, heart rate, contractility, and wall tension. Additionally, labor and delivery are associated with a significant increase in cardiac output, myocardial oxygen consumption, and elevated levels of circulating catecholamines. While pregnancy itself is not thought to be a risk factor for MI, the changes of pregnancy may place high-risk individuals at even greater risk; compared with nonpregnant individuals of the same age, the incidence of MI may be three- to fourfold higher in pregnancy.

2. **Diagnosis.** As in nonpregnant individuals, the diagnosis of MI is made by history, examination, and appropriate diagnostic tests. **Troponins** remain sensitive and specific in the pregnant population (although are elevated at baseline in preeclamptic patients). However, in pregnancy, minor electrocardiographic (ECG) changes such as T-wave inversions and ST-segment depressions are common, diminishing specificity of ECG interpretation for ischemia. **Cardiac catheterization** should be considered despite the small risk of ionizing radiation to the fetus; with shielding and limited fluoroscopy, the total radiation dose may be limited to approximately 1 rad, well below the 5-rad teratogenic threshold. Lastly, an echocardiogram may be useful for evaluating ventricular function.

3. **Management** of an acute MI in pregnancy is guided by the same principles as in the nonpregnant population, with several important considerations.

   a. **Medical management.** β1-**Blockers** and **nitrates** may be used safely in pregnancy, although hypotension should be avoided. **Low-dose aspirin** has been shown to be safe even with chronic use. Conversely, ACE inhibitors and statins are contraindicated in pregnancy, and both should be avoided.

   b. **Anticoagulation** may be safely achieved with **unfractionated heparin** or **LMWH.** There is very limited information about the safety and efficacy of **thrombolytic therapy** in pregnancy; although successful use has been reported, there is an increased risk of puerperal hemorrhage and placental abruption.

   c. **Revascularization.** Both **PCI** and **CABG** have been successfully used to treat pregnancy-associated acute MI. Pregnancy is not a contraindication to cardiopulmonary bypass and good maternal and fetal outcomes are possible, although fetal loss is estimated to be between 20% and 40%.

   d. **Obstetrical management.** The fetus should be carefully monitored and, if viable, a plan for delivery established in the event of sudden maternal or fetal decompensation.

D. **Peripartum Cardiomyopathy (PPCM)** is a rare dilated cardiomyopathy, which has an estimated incidence of 1 in 4,000 to 15,000 live births. The etiology remains unclear, although risk factors include multiple gestation, advanced maternal age, obesity, and preeclampsia.

   1. **Clinical presentation and diagnosis.** Patients present with symptoms of heart failure such as dyspnea, fatigue, and edema that may be difficult to distinguish from normal changes in pregnancy. The diagnosis requires echocardiographic evidence of cardiomyopathy and three criteria: (1) onset within a 6-month period, from the last month of pregnancy to 5 months postpartum; (2) no prior history of cardiomyopathy or preexisting heart failure; and (3) exclusion of all other identifiable causes of cardiomyopathy.

   2. **Medical management** is supportive and similar to the treatment of other forms of heart failure. Patients may benefit from **inotropic support, diuretics,** and **ventricular afterload reduction.** Patients with PPCM are at high risk of thromboembolism, and **anticoagulation** should be considered. Pregnant patients should not receive ACE inhibitors, and nitroprusside should be used cautiously because of the risk of fetal cyanide toxicity with prolonged use. Finally, mechanical support with a **ventricular assist device** or **intra-aortic balloon pump** should be considered as a bridge to transplant in patients who fail to respond to medical management.

3. **Obstetrical management.** Delivery should be strongly considered in pregnant patients diagnosed with PPCM, particularly if the fetus is at risk, the patient is not responding to medical management, or if the patient also has preeclampsia.

4. **Prognosis and recurrence.** Fifty percent of patients diagnosed with PPCM will have a significant improvement in cardiac function. The remainder will have progression of their disease requiring heart transplant or resulting in an early death. The overall estimated mortality of patients who acquire PPCM ranges from 15% to 50%. There is no clear consensus on the recurrence of PPCM in subsequent pregnancies, but the data would suggest patients with residual left ventricular impairment at the time of conception have an increased risk of recurrence and mortality.

E. **Pulmonary Hypertension (pHTN)** in pregnancy is associated with considerable risks of maternal mortality and morbidity. Mortality rates of 16% to 38% have been described despite modern treatment modalities. Right ventricular failure can rapidly ensue when pregnancy-induced increases of blood volume and cardiac output are superimposed on preexisting pulmonary hypertension. pHTN is currently classified into five groups by etiology. Women with pHTN are usually advised against pregnancy.

1. **Pulmonary arterial hypertension (PAH) (group 1)** includes idiopathic pulmonary arterial hypertension and pulmonary hypertension due to congenital heart disease. PAH is defined as mean pulmonary arterial pressure (PAP) ≥25 mmHg at rest assessed by right heart catheterization and normal pulmonary artery occlusion pressure (PAOP) or <15 mmHg. The pathophysiology involves pulmonary vasoconstriction, which leads to right ventricular (RV) overload, vascular wall remodeling, and RV hypertrophy and later dilation leading to right ventricular failure and death.

   a. **Medical management** should be individualized in each case, and a multidisciplinary team approach adopted. **Oxygen,** either continuous or for several hours each day, reduces PAP and improves cardiac output. **Anticoagulation** with unfractionated heparin or LMWH is often recommended to prevent pulmonary emboli, which may be fatal. **Specific pulmonary vasodilator therapy** includes **inhaled nitric oxide;** inhaled, subcutaneous, or IV **prostacyclin;** and **sildenafil.** Use of **bosentan** is contraindicated in pregnancy due to teratogenicity.

   b. Throughout pregnancy and delivery, the hemodynamic goals should be (1) to avoid pain, hypoxemia, acidosis, and hypercarbia; (2) to maintain intravascular volume and preload, but with careful monitoring to avoid volume overload and RV failure in the peripartum period; (3) to maintain systolic blood pressure greater than PAP to ensure adequate coronary perfusion of the RV; (4) to augment cardiac output as needed; and (5) to avoid tachydysrhythmias.

2. **Secondary pulmonary hypertension** can develop from long-standing mitral valve disease or untreated left-to-right shunts. The mortality rate in pregnancy of these patients is 25% to 50% and may be due to embolism, dysrhythmia, right ventricular failure, or myocardial infarction. Treatment should focus on the underlying disease.

VIII. **VENOUS THROMBOEMBOLISM (VTE)** remains one of the leading causes of maternal mortality in the United States. Several normal physiologic changes of pregnancy increase the risk of VTE, including venous stasis in the lower extremities from mechanical compression of the uterus, increased production of coagulation factors, and increased platelet activation.

Antepartum bed rest, cesarean delivery, and postpartum tubal ligation further increase the risk.

A. The incidence of pulmonary thromboembolism (PE) in pregnancy is estimated to be 0.5%. Up to one-quarter of pregnant patients with untreated deep vein thrombosis will experience a pulmonary embolus, and of those who do, the mortality rate is 12% to 15%.

B. Risk Factors. In addition to the factors listed above, obesity, increased age and parity, and acquired or congenital hypercoagulable states are associated with an increased risk of VTE.

C. Diagnosis. Pregnant patients present with the same signs and symptoms as the nonpregnant population. However, confirming the diagnosis may be more complex. **Doppler ultrasonography** of the lower extremities may be used without safety concern in pregnancy. Although the imaging studies commonly used to diagnose PE (**spiral computerized tomography, perfusion scan,** and **pulmonary angiography**) do expose the fetus to radiation, the exposure is considerably less than 5 rad.

IX. HEMORRHAGE. Blood volume increases 30% to 40% during pregnancy, which helps to compensate for the blood loss that may occur at the time of delivery. Even with significant bleeding, most parturients will recover quickly and completely; however, a small number require ICU care for treatment of hemorrhage. Despite improvements in resuscitation strategies, hemorrhage, both antepartum and postpartum, remains a significant source of maternal morbidity and is the second most common cause of maternal mortality.

A. Antepartum Vaginal Bleeding occurs in approximately 6% of pregnancies and is frequently a marker for abnormal placentation. The patient at greatest risk is the fetus, and premature delivery may be required. **Etiologies** include the following:

1. Placenta previa, which is diagnosed when the placenta comes up to or covers the internal cervical os. **Risk factors** for previa include a uterine scar from a previous surgery or procedure, increasing multiparity, and advanced maternal age. The classic presentation is painless vaginal bleeding. Ultrasound confirms the diagnosis.

2. Placental abruption, which is defined as a premature separation of the placenta from the uterus. Bleeding occurs because of the exposed vessels, and fetal distress may ensue from a loss of placental surface for oxygen and nutrient exchange. Etiology remains unclear, but **risk factors** are hypertension, advanced maternal age, increasing multiparity, trauma, prior history of abruption, tobacco and cocaine use, and preterm premature rupture of membranes. The classic presentation is vaginal bleeding, uterine tenderness, and painful, frequent contractions. The diagnosis is largely clinical, although ultrasound and laboratory tests such as a Kleihauer-Betke, a blood test which measures the amount of fetal hemoglobin transferred into maternal circulation, may be helpful.

3. Uterine rupture is an uncommon complication of pregnancy with potential for significant maternal and fetal morbidity. The major **risk factor** is a previous uterine scar; in patients with a previous lower uterine segment incision, the incidence is less than 1%. However, in patients with a history of a classical uterine incision, the incidence is higher; in these patients rupture is associated with greater morbidity because of the vascularity of the anterior uterine wall and the possible disruption of the placental bed.

4. **Management.** In all cases of antepartum bleeding, the first steps are maternal stabilization and assurance of fetal well-being. Adequate IV access should be obtained and preliminary laboratory tests sent. Placental abruption and previa may be expectantly managed, depending upon the degree of bleeding and gestational age. For significant bleeding, prompt delivery and aggressive volume resuscitation is critical. Previa and abruption place patients at increased risk for atony and development of coagulopathy, which should be anticipated and aggressively treated. Uterine rupture requires immediate delivery of the fetus. The uterus may be repaired, but hysterectomy is sometimes required.

B. **Postpartum Hemorrhage.** The average blood loss for a vaginal delivery and cesarean delivery is <500 cc and <1,000 mL, respectively. Postpartum hemorrhage may be defined as blood loss in excess of the above, or clinically as a 10% decrease in hematocrit from admission to the postpartum period. **Etiologies** include the following:

1. **Uterine atony,** which is the most common cause of primary postpartum hemorrhage and a frequent indication for peripartum hysterectomy. The incidence of unanticipated uterine atony (e.g., no known maternal risk factors) appears to be rising. **Risk factors** include prolonged labor, multiple gestation, high parity, chorioamnionitis, augmented labor, precipitous labor, tocolytic agents, and use of volatile anesthetics. Once the diagnosis is made, initial treatment should include bimanual massage, placement of large-bore IV access, and **oxytocin** infusion. Further pharmacologic therapy may include administration of uterotonic medications such as oxytocin, **methergine 0.2 mg IM, misoprostol 800 to 1,000 μg PR,** and **15-methyl prostaglandin F2a 250 μg IM.** Surgical intervention may be required, including a peripartum hysterectomy.

2. **Placenta accreta,** which is defined as a placenta adherent to the uterine wall. There are two additional types of placenta accreta: **placenta increta,** defined as invasion into the myometrium, and **placenta percreta,** defined as invasion through the uterine serosa. **Risk factors** for placenta accreta include a previous uterine incision or instrumentation, advanced maternal age, multiparity, assisted reproductive techniques, and a low-lying placenta or placenta previa. The incidence of accreta rises significantly when placenta previa is present in a patient with one or more previous uterine incisions. Management includes having a high index of suspicion in patients with risk factors and preparing appropriately for a large-volume resuscitation. Although in some cases the uterus may be preserved, peripartum hysterectomy is frequently necessary.

3. **Uterine inversion,** which is the turning inside out of all or part of the uterus. A rare event, it may cause significant hemorrhage due to ischemia of the fundus, leading to atony. In addition to basic resuscitation and management of potential hemodynamic collapse, the first-line treatment is the manual replacement of the uterus, which is facilitated by discontinuation of uterotonic agents and administration of uterine relaxants (e.g., nitroglycerin IV or sublingual, terbutaline, magnesium). This is followed by aggressive medical management (readministration of uterotonic medications) to improve uterine tone and limit further blood loss.

4. **Retained placenta,** which is a frequent cause of postpartum hemorrhage. Management involves removal of the placenta manually or with curettage, and volume resuscitation as required.

X. **SEPSIS (see Chapter 29)** is a significant cause of maternal mortality and morbidity and seems to be on the rise. In a recent large study, sepsis was found to complicate 1:3,300 deliveries, severe sepsis 1:11,000, and sepsis-related death 1:105,000. In the developing countries, maternal mortality secondary to sepsis is as high as 10%. Seven percent of OB ICU admissions in the United Sates are due to sepsis. Diagnosis can be challenging. Pregnancy is associated with an increase in heart rate, a decrease in blood pressure, and an increase in cardiac output. These changes may mask some early signs of sepsis and may further compromise organ perfusion in the septic patient.

   A. **Causes.** Obstetrical sepsis primarily arises from chorioamnionitis, endometritis, urologic infections, septic abortions, wound infections, and pneumonia. Most obstetric infections are polymicrobial. Common pathogens implicated with maternal sepsis are *E. coli*, staphylococcus, streptococcus, and gram-negative and anaerobic organisms.

   B. **Risk Factors for Maternal Sepsis** include advanced maternal age, African American race, Medicaid insurance, cerclage placement, PPROM, retained products of conception, and medical comorbidities such as congestive heart failure and chronic liver or renal disease.

   C. **Management.** Early diagnosis with prompt and aggressive treatment is critical for minimizing morbidity and mortality. Although no studies have specifically addressed the management of sepsis in obstetric patients, most evidence-based recommendations for improving survival in sepsis may be applied to pregnancy. Pregnant patients who develop sepsis are at high risk for preterm delivery and fetal loss. In the setting of sepsis, fetal compromise is usually the result of maternal decompensation and, thus, initial efforts toward maternal resuscitation should be priority. Regular and frequent cardiotocographic monitoring should be performed for assessment of fetal well-being and for surveillance for preterm labor as well as serving as a measure of end-organ function. When choosing antibiotics, attempts should be made to maximize the effectiveness for the mother and minimize fetal harm, although this may not always be possible. Finally, the physiologic changes of pregnancy may change the pharmacokinetics of antibiotics and require adjustments in dosing and monitoring.

XI. **ENDOCRINE DISORDERS** (see Chapter 27)

   A. **Diabetic Ketoacidosis (DKA)** is infrequent in pregnancy, with an estimated incidence between 1% and 3% in pregnancies complicated by preexisting or gestational diabetes. In recent years, maternal mortality associated with DKA has improved, but fetal loss remains high, with estimates ranging from 10% to 25% in affected pregnancies.

      1. **Clinical presentation** and **laboratory abnormalities** may be identical to those in the nonpregnant population; however, studies have shown that pregnant women are more likely to present with much lower glucose values, including normoglycemia, than their nonpregnant counterparts, making this a diagnostically challenging situation. More rapid development in the pregnant patient may also lead to a delayed diagnosis and treatment, necessitating a raised awareness of this condition. In addition, evidence of fetal compromise is frequently present.

      2. **Risk factors** for DKA in pregnancy include emesis of any cause, use of f3-sympathomimetics, infection, previously undiagnosed diabetes, and poor patient compliance with using insulin.

      3. Several **physiologic changes of pregnancy** predispose patients to developing DKA. Pregnancy is a state of relative insulin resistance and

increased lipolysis, with a tendency toward ketone body formation. Additionally, increases in minute ventilation cause a mild respiratory alkalosis that is compensated by increased renal excretion of bicarbonate; this compensated respiratory alkalosis leaves patients less capable of buffering serum ketone acids. Accelerated starvation, dehydration, reduced caloric intake, and stress are additional risk factors unique to the pregnant state.

4. **Fetal concerns.** Maternal acidosis decreases uterine blood flow and causes a leftward shift in the maternal oxyhemoglobin dissociation curve, both of which compromise fetal oxygenation. Ketoacids dissociate and cross the placenta, contributing to a metabolic acidosis in the fetus. Lastly, glucose readily crosses the placenta, causing fetal hyperglycemia, osmotic diuresis, and hypovolemia.

5. **Medical management** is unchanged from the nonpregnant population. Aggressive fluid resuscitation, glucose control with insulin, search for and treatment of the underlying etiology, and control of electrolyte abnormalities are the mainstays of treatment.

6. **Obstetric management.** Fetal status may be measured indirectly by fetal heart rate tracings or biophysical profile. Maternal resuscitation is imperative to improving the fetal outcome, and delivery for fetal indications should be reserved for fetal compromise, which continues after appropriate maternal resuscitation. Nonreassuring fetal heart tracings may revert to normal after correction of the maternal acidemic and hypovolemic state.

B. **Ovarian Hyperstimulation Syndrome (OHSS)** is a rare, iatrogenic complication of ovulation induction, which may occur in response to almost every agent used to stimulate the ovaries. It usually occurs in the luteal phase or within the first week postconception. The seminal event in the genesis of OHSS is ovarian enlargement, with an acute fluid shift out of the intravascular space, resulting in ascites and intravascular hypovolemia.

1. The reported **prevalence** of the most severe form is 0.5% to 5% with an estimated mortality of 1 per 450,000 to 1 per 50,000 patients.

2. **Clinical presentation.** Signs and symptoms result from increased vascular permeability and arterial dilation, which leads to extravasation of intravascular fluid into the extravascular spaces. Patients may present with ascites, oliguria, renal failure, hydrothorax, or ARDS. Laboratory abnormalities include electrolyte imbalances (hyponatremia and hyperkalemia), elevated creatinine, hemoconcentration, leukocytosis, and thrombocytosis.

3. **Management.** Treatment of OHSS is supportive. Patients should be carefully monitored, administered isotonic fluids to restore intravascular volume, and treated for electrolyte disturbances. Increased intra-abdominal pressure from ascites may result in poor pulmonary function and impaired renal perfusion and may have significant deleterious effects on maternal circulation. **Ultrasound-guided paracentesis** has been shown to improve creatinine clearance, urine output, dyspnea, and osmolarity, but care must be taken to avoid inadvertent puncture of ovarian cysts with subsequent intraperitoneal hemorrhage. These patients are also at risk of developing thrombosis in either the arterial (25%) or venous (75%) circulations, and prophylactic **anticoagulation** should be initiated.

4. **Resolution.** After a period of several days, patients begin to mobilize the extravascular fluid and a natural diuresis occurs. Complete resolution typically takes 2 weeks from the onset of symptoms.

XII. AMNIOTIC FLUID EMBOLISM (AFE) is a rare but possibly catastrophic complication of pregnancy. Because AFE remains a diagnosis of exclusion, the true incidence is unknown but is estimated to be between 3 and 5 per 100,000 live births. However, the mortality rate among affected parturients is as high as 85%, and the disease accounts for up to 12% of all maternal deaths overall. Among survivors, significant and permanent neurologic sequelae are common. Approximately 50% of patients who have an AFE are at risk for cardiac arrest, according to one recent epidemiologic study.

A. Clinical Presentation. Classically, patients present during labor or delivery, or in the immediate postpartum period (up to 4 hours after delivery in some case reports), with acute hypoxia and hypotension that rapidly deteriorates to cardiovascular collapse, coagulopathy, and death. In the initial phase, systemic and pulmonary hypertension are present along with profound hypoxemia and are then followed by left ventricular dysfunction and coagulopathy.

B. Pathophysiology. The etiology is likely multifactorial and is poorly understood. AFE is a uniquely human event and thus is difficult to study in animal models. While some believe the inciting event is a breach in the barrier between the maternal and fetal compartments leading to the presence of fetal cells, amniotic fluid, and inflammatory mediators in the maternal circulation, others believe in more of a humoral response to an unknown instigator, since many asymptomatic pregnant women may be found to have fetal cells present in their blood and never manifest AFE. Ultimately, recent thought is that "amniotic fluid embolus" is a misnomer, yet the name persists despite an unclear pathophysiologic basis for the syndrome that occurs.

C. Manifestations affect multiple organ systems, and presentation may vary depending upon the predominant physiologic change.

1. Cardiovascular. Hypotension is a hallmark feature, present in 100% of patients with severe disease. A biphasic model of shock has been proposed to explain the findings seen in patients with AFE. The initial transient response is pulmonary hypertension, likely from the release of vasoactive substances, causing hypoxia and right heart failure. Patients who survive the initial insult develop a second phase of left heart failure and pulmonary edema.

2. Pulmonary. Hypoxia is an early manifestation, arising from acute pulmonary hypertension with subsequent ventilation–perfusion mismatch. Later, pulmonary edema develops in association with left ventricular dysfunction. A substantial portion of patients will also manifest non-cardiogenic pulmonary edema after left ventricular function improves.

3. Coagulation. Disruption of the normal clotting cascade occurs in up to two-thirds of patients. It remains unclear whether the coagulopathy is the result of a consumptive process or from massive fibrinolysis. However, patients may experience significant bleeding, massive hemorrhage, and DIC.

D. Management involves aggressive resuscitation; supportive care is aimed at minimizing additional hypoxia and subsequent end-organ damage. Goals of therapy include maintenance of oxygenation, circulatory support, and correction of the coagulopathy. (1) Most patients will require tracheal intubation, mechanical ventilation, and supplemental oxygen. (2) Hemodynamic instability should be corrected with fluid resuscitation and pressor support as needed. (3) **Lines and monitors** should include central and peripheral large-bore IV access, continuous pulse oximetry, invasive blood pressure monitoring and possibly a pulmonary artery catheter, and/

or transesophageal echocardiography to assess ventricular function. (4) **Laboratory studies** should be sent at regular intervals, and coagulopathy aggressively treated. (5) If the event occurs before delivery, the fetus should be delivered as quickly as possible to minimize fetal hypoxia and to aid maternal resuscitation. (6) Rescue therapies such as cardiopulmonary bypass, extracorporeal membrane oxygenation, and intra-aortic balloon counterpulsation have been described in the literature as successful options for the treatment of refractory AFE. In addition, an area of future study appears to be the role of inflammatory cytokines in the pathophysiology of this disease, which may be targeted for treatment strategies to improve survival.

XIII. **TRAUMA (see Chapter 9)** is the leading cause of nonobstetric mortality and morbidity in pregnancy accounting for 45% to 50% of all maternal deaths in the United States and complicates up to 1 in every 12 pregnancies. Common causes include motor vehicle accidents, domestic violence, and falls. As for the general population, hemorrhagic shock and head trauma are leading causes of death. Risk factors for maternal trauma include young age, low socioeconomic status, minority race, and use of illicit drugs or alcohol. It is important to remember that any female patient of reproductive age who is a victim of trauma could be pregnant at the time of injury.

   A. **Management.** Standard guidelines for care of trauma patients apply to pregnant patients, with several important modifications.

   1. Patients at 20 weeks' gestation or more who are placed on a backboard should be placed in left uterine displacement, to minimize aortocaval compression.

   2. Efforts should be made to transfuse only O-negative blood in the event that transfusion is required before a type and cross can be performed.

   3. It is crucial to preserve maternal cardiac output, blood pressure, and oxygen delivery to optimize maternal recovery and protect fetal well-being.

   4. Early evaluation for pregnancy complications and assessment of fetal well-being should be performed. Fetal evaluation should include a thorough **ultrasound evaluation** of the fetus and placenta and continuous **fetal heart-rate monitoring** for the first 2 to 6 hours or longer.

   B. **Complications** will vary based upon the mechanism and severity of injury. Uterine rupture or placental abruption are common complications of major trauma.

   1. **Placental abruption** may be present in up to 60% of women with severe maternal trauma and usually occurs from 16 weeks' gestation onward. It can cause occult hemorrhage and coagulopathy and should be considered as a source of bleeding in an unstable pregnant trauma victim. Early, frequent contractions are a sensitive indicator of abruption. The period of monitoring and observation should be increased in women with contractions, abdominal tenderness, or significant maternal injury.

   2. **Preterm labor** is a common complication of trauma (up to 25%), even with minor trauma.

   3. **Amniotic fluid embolism** is an uncommon complication of trauma but should be considered if resuscitation is refractory.

   C. **Testing.** Additional testing specific to pregnancy may include a **Kleihauer-Betke test,** which can indicate the severity of uterine-placental trauma by measuring fetal blood in the maternal circulation. All patients should have a type and screen, and Rh-negative patients with a positive Kleihauer-Betke should be given **Rh-immune globulin.**

1. **Blunt trauma is more common than penetrating trauma or burns.** Because of increased vascularity and shifting of abdominal contents by the gravid uterus, splenic and retroperitoneal injury is more common in pregnant women, while bowel injury is less frequent.

2. **Penetrating trauma.** Because of anatomical changes, pregnant women have a fourfold decrease in death from penetrating trauma, as opposed to nonpregnant women. However, the same anatomic changes lead to an increased risk of bowel injury when penetrating trauma occurs in the upper abdomen.

D. **Fetal Outcome** is dependent upon maternal outcome and the mechanism of injury. The risk for direct fetal trauma increases with gestational age. Prior to 13 weeks´ gestation the maternal pelvis shields the uterus and fetus. Maternal death is the most common cause of fetal death, and severe maternal injuries result in fetal death in 20% to 40% of cases. In significant penetrating abdominal trauma, fetal injuries are common with fetal mortality ranging from 40% to 70%, due to direct fetal injury or premature delivery.

XIV. **LOCAL ANESTHETIC SYSTEMIC TOXICITY (LAST).** Systemic absorption or inadvertent intravascular injection of local anesthetics may result in toxicity that is typically manifested by central nervous system (CNS) symptoms and cardiovascular compromise. Toxicity of local anesthetics is correlated to potency and their rank in order of increasing toxicity is as follows: 2-chloroprocaine, mepivacaine, lidocaine, etidocaine, tetracaine, and bupivacaine.

A. **CNS Symptoms** reported by patients correlate with increased plasma concentrations of local anesthetics. At lower levels, **periorbital numbness** and **metallic taste** are reported. As the serum concentration increases, **loss of consciousness, seizures,** and **respiratory arrest** may occur.

B. **Cardiovascular Manifestations** occur at much higher serum concentrations than do CNS symptoms. They may progress from **increased blood pressure to bradycardia, ventricular dysfunction, ventricular tachycardia, and fibrillation.** As in nonpregnant patients, the more potent amide local anesthetics such as bupivacaine have a smaller margin of safety and may cause refractory arrhythmias. Despite this, bupivacaine remains the most common local anesthetic in obstetric anesthesia.

C. Pregnancy increases the risk of adverse outcomes from local anesthetic toxicity by several mechanisms: decreased concentrations of plasma proteins result in a higher free serum concentration, and vascular engorgement may increase the risk of epidural catheter placement into an epidural vein. Additionally, resuscitation is more difficult because of unclear symptomatology, rapid development of hypoxemia, and the technical difficulty of performing effective chest compressions in pregnant patients.

D. **Management** is largely supportive. Seizures should be terminated with **benzodiazepines** or **barbiturates.** Additionally, resuscitation with **intralipid** therapy should be considered standard practice. All patients should be given supplemental oxygenation, and tracheal intubation should be considered early, as acidemia may worsen the outcome. Monitoring should include the fetal heart rate. Blood pressure should be supported with fluids, vasoactive medications, and, if needed, ACLS. If LAST is suspected, epinephrine dose should be reduced to 1 mcg/kg (a significantly smaller dose than usual) and vasopressin should be avoided on the basis of small but compelling animal studies. See section XIII for additional critical modifications to ACLS in the obstetric patient.

XV. CARDIOPULMONARY RESUSCITATION (CPR). Cardiac arrest complicates roughly 1 in 12,000 pregnancies, with a higher incidence in women with underlying cardiopulmonary disease; the most common precipitating cause is hemorrhage in a recent study. In general, CPR algorithms are unchanged for pregnant women, since maternal resuscitation is the best therapy for the fetus. However, there are a few critical modifications that must be performed such as higher hand position for chest compressions, manual left uterine displacement, and consideration of perimortem cesarean delivery if gestational age is ≥24 weeks. **Vasoactive medications** and **defibrillation** should be administered as in the nonpregnant population. There are some important differences:

  A. Airway. The pregnant patient should be intubated soon after initiation of CPR to protect the airway from aspiration and facilitate oxygenation and ventilation. A difficult airway should be anticipated.

  B. Circulation. Cardiac output is significantly affected by patient positioning after approximately 20 weeks' gestation. Uterine compression of the IVC and aorta can considerably compromise preload and cardiac output. A critical component of resuscitation in the obstetric population involves manual left uterine displacement, or, if this cannot be performed, left uterine displacement accomplished with a wedge or pillow under the patient's right hip.

  C. Delivery. If cardiac arrest occurs before 24 weeks' gestation (age of fetal viability), the rescuer's efforts should be directed exclusively toward the mother. If arrest occurs after 24 weeks, the fetus should be delivered within 5 minutes if CPR has not been successful in achieving return of spontaneous circulation, to optimize both maternal and fetal outcomes. Prompt delivery of the fetus minimizes the risk of hypoxic insult to the mother and improves maternal cardiac output by relieving aortocaval compression, decreasing metabolic demands, and allowing for more effective chest compressions. Delivery may be considered even in a nonviable pregnancy to improve resuscitation of the mother.

  D. Venous Access should be secured in the upper extremities. If no venous access is obtainable after attempts, intraosseous line placement in the humeral heads should be considered.

  E. Both **cardiopulmonary bypass** and **open cardiac massage** have been advocated if closed-chest resuscitative efforts are unsuccessful.

Selected Readings

American College of Obstetricians and Gynecologists. ACOG Committee Opinion No. 299. *Guidelines for diagnostic imaging during pregnancy.* Washington, DC: ACOG, September 2004.

Bandi VD, Munnur U, Matthay MA. Acute lung injury and acute respiratory distress syndrome in pregnancy. *Crit Care Clin* 2004;20:577–607.

Bauer ME, Bateman BT, Bauer ST, et al. Maternal sepsis mortality and morbidity during hospitalization for delivery: temporal trends and independent associations for severe sepsis. *Anesth Analg* 2013;117(4):944–950.

Budev MM, Arroliga AC, Falcone T. Ovarian hyperstimulation syndrome. *Crit Care Med* 2005;33:S301–S306.

Carroll MA, Yeomans ER. Diabetic ketoacidosis in pregnancy. *Crit Care Med* 2005;33:S347–S353.

Dennis AT. Heart failure in pregnant women: is it peripartum cardiomyopathy? *Anesth Analg* 2015;120(3):638–643.

Duhl AJ, Paidas MJ, Ural SH, et al. Antithrombotic therapy and pregnancy: consensus report and recommendations for prevention and treatment of venous thromboembolism and adverse pregnancy outcomes. *Am J Obstet Gynecol* 2007;197:457e1–457e21.

Elkayam U, Bitar F. Valvular heart disease and pregnancy. I. Native valves. *J Am Coll Cardiol* 2005;46:223–230.

Fernandez-Perez ER, Salman S, Pendem S, et al. Sepsis during pregnancy. *Crit Care Med* 2005;33:S286–S293.

Grear KE, Bushnell CD. Stroke and pregnancy: clinical presentation, evaluation, treatment, and epidemiology. *Clin Obstet Gynecol* 2013;56(2):350–359.

Vidovich MI. Cardiovascular disease. In: Chestnut DH, Wong CA, Tsen LC, et al, eds. *Obstetric anesthesia: principles and practice.* 5th ed. Philadelphia: Saunders, 2014: 960–996.

James AH, Jamison MG, Biswas MS, et al. Acute myocardial infarction in pregnancy: a United States population-based study. *Circulation* 2006;113:1564–1571.

Lansberg MG, O'Donnell MJ, Khatri P, et al; American College of Chest Physicians. Antithrombotic and thrombolytic therapy for ischemic stroke: antithrombotic therapy and prevention of thrombosis, 9th ed: American College of Chest Physicians Evidence-Based Clinical Practice Guidelines. *Chest* 2012;141:e601S–e636S.

Mendez-Figueroa H, Dahlke JD, Vrees RA, et al. Trauma in pregnancy: an updated systematic review. *Am J Obstet Gynecol* 2013;209(1):1–10.

Mhyre JM, Tsen LC, Einav S, et al. Cardiac arrest during hospitalization for delivery in the United States, 1998–2011. *Anesthesiology* 2014;120(4):810–818.

O'Shea A, Eappen S. Amniotic fluid embolism. *Int Anesthesiol Clin* 2007;45:17–28.

Rajasri AG, Srestha R, Mitchell J. Acute fatty liver of pregnancy (AFLP)––an overview. *J Obstet Gynaecol* 2007;27(3):237–240.

Stout KK, Otto CM. Pregnancy in women with valvular heart disease. *Heart* 2007;93:552.

Turan TT, Stern BJ. Stroke in pregnancy. *Neurol Clin* 2004;22:831–840.

Viktorsdottir O. Pulmonary hypertension in pregnancy and anesthetic implications. *Curr Anesthesiol Rep* 2015;5(1):82–90.

Wanderer JP, Leffert LR, Mhyre JM, et al. Epidemiology of obstetric-related ICU admissions in Maryland: 1999–2008. *Crit Care Med* 2013;41(8):1844–1852.

Wilson W, Taubert KA, Gewitz M, et al. Prevention of infective endocarditis: guidelines from the American Heart Association. *Circulation* 2007;116:1736–1754.

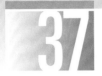

ICU Handoffs and Transitions

Jeffrey Bruckel, Fiona D. Roberts, and Daniel Yagoda

ACKNOWLEDGMENTS

The authors of the current chapter gratefully acknowledge the contributions of David Shahian, MD, Vice President, and Laura Rossi, RN, Staff Specialist, Center for Quality and Safety, Massachusetts General Hospital.

I. **HANDOFFS DEFINED**—A handoff is defined by the Joint Commission as "the process of transferring primary authority and responsibility for providing clinical care to a patient from one departing caregiver to one oncoming caregiver."

  A. In the ICU setting, caregivers include, but are not limited to, attending, fellow and resident physicians; nurse practitioners; physician assistants; nurses; respiratory therapists; physical therapists; occupational therapists; and pharmacists.

II. **ESSENTIAL ROLE OF COMMUNICATION IN ADVERSE EVENTS**—Handoff quality is heavily dependent on good communication, and it is widely accepted that poor communication plays a substantial role in adverse events. Below are two examples that highlight these relationships.

  A. **Joint Commission Sentinel Event Alerts**—The Joint Commission collects voluntarily submitted sentinel event reports from hospitals nationwide. Data collection began in 1996, and resulted in publication of Sentinel Event Alerts since 1998.

   1. Communication is among the top three root causes of sentinel events resulting in patient harm or death each year.

   2. In 2013, communication was the second most commonly reported root cause, playing a role in 563 out of 887 total reported cases.

   3. From 2004 to 2013, communication was the most commonly reported root cause in cases of delayed treatment, playing a role in 728 out of 903 total reported cases.

  B. **Closed Malpractice Claims**—Analysis of closed malpractice claims has identified communication as a significant factor in adverse patient events leading to litigation.

   1. **Obstetric anesthesia**—Of all adverse events, 31% are related to communication problems. Obstetric newborn death/brain damage cases

involving anesthesia had an increased proportion involving poor communication.

2. **Surgical cases**—Systems factors contributed to error in 82% of malpractice cases, with communication breakdown comprising 24% of system factors.

3. **Cases involving trainees**—Teamwork breakdowns contributed to 70% of malpractice cases, with handoff problems being a leading cause of teamwork breakdown.

III. **COMMUNICATION AND TEAMWORK STRATEGIES IN OTHER INDUSTRIES**—Many high-risk industries have realized the importance of standardized communication and have devised strategies for structuring communication between team members. Notable examples include the aviation industry and the military.

A. **Airline Industry**

1. **Sterile cockpit rule**

a. In the early 1980s, the FAA identified that crew distractions by non–flight-related activities contributed significantly to a large number of air accidents and incidents.

b. A review of the aviation safety reporting system database demonstrated incidents related to issues such as extraneous conversation (including with the control tower), distractions from the flight attendants, nonpertinent radio calls and PA announcements, and sight-seeing. Some of these incidents resulted in fatalities.

c. These incidents led directly to the implementation of the Sterile Cockpit Rule in 1981. This rule states that during "critical phases of the flight" (ground operations, takeoff, landing, and all flight operations below 10,000 feet), crew are prohibited from performing duties other than those required for safe operation of the aircraft.

2. **Crew resource management**

a. Root cause analysis of plane crashes in the 1970s revealed that failures of communication and teamwork resulted in significant risk. These investigations resulted in a recommendation for teamwork training programs for flight crews, the first of which was held by NASA in 1979.

b. The improvement program is designed to enhance team situational awareness and communication by using standardized techniques called inquiry and advocacy and fosters a questioning attitude among team members. This involves standardized communication, outlined below, to escalate concerns or questions:

1. Get the person's attention.
2. State your concern.
3. State the problem as you see it.
4. State a solution.
5. Obtain agreement.

IV. **COMMUNICATION STRATEGIES ADAPTED FOR HEALTH CARE: TeamSTEPPS**
This evidence-based program for improving teamwork in hospitals was developed and distributed by the Agency for Healthcare Research and Quality (AHRQ) and the Department of Defense (DoD). With the goal of enhancing team situational awareness, TeamSTEPPS involves a readiness assessment, implementation, and sustainment phases. The program was field-tested and then fully implemented at many hospitals throughout the country, with plans

to disseminate to all hospitals nationwide. There are four core competencies that are crucial for ensuring effective team performance:

A. Team Leadership
B. Situation Monitoring
C. Mutual Support
D. Communication

TeamSTEPPS promotes an environment of open communication and candor, where everyone on the team feels comfortable "speaking up."

V. TYPES OF HANDOFFS IN THE ICU—There are several different types of handoffs. Below are several of the major categories in which an effective and efficient transfer of patient responsibility is necessary.

A. Shift-to-shift Handoff—This is a direct transfer of responsibility for the patient from one clinician to another for a defined period of time. With changes in resident work hours, health care delivery models have required more handoffs as day teams sign out to their night teams to ensure continued clinical coverage. The departing clinician must deliver an efficient and informative overview of the patient's current clinical condition over the past shift (8–12 hours) and provide an update on any anticipated events over the next 8 to 12 hours.

B. Permanent Unit-to-unit Handoff—This is a permanent (or semipermanent) change in location of a patient from a sending clinical unit to a receiving clinical unit. Examples include emergency room or operating room to ICU and ICU to floor.

C. Temporary Unit-to-unit Handoff—As implied, this is a temporary transfer of clinical responsibility of a patient for some length of time, typically for a procedure or diagnostic test. For example, locations for temporary transfer may include interventional radiology, imaging, or operating room with plans to return to the ICU.

D. External Transfer—patient being admitted to or discharged from the hospital. This is a handoff between the referring facility and the accepting facility. It should cover all of the same information as an internal transition of care, plus additional information that may be less readily available to the receiving provider outside the organization (such as copies of reports for procedures, tests, etc.).

E. Escalating an Acute Situation—If there is a rapid and significant change in a patient's clinical condition, it is paramount that that information be efficiently and effectively communicated up the chain of command.

F. Ongoing, Living Record of Patient History of Hospital Course—Included as part of written sign-out only, the background and history of the patient's hospital course should be updated at least daily and can reside in the electronic record.

VI. WRITTEN AND VERBAL HANDOFFS—In both the written and verbal handoffs, it is important that the giver of the handoff dedicate time to prepare a comprehensive, well-organized synopsis of the patients being transferred to the receiving clinician.

A. Verbal Handoff—should include an efficient synopsis of the patient's clinical condition given by the sending clinician to a receiving clinician. There are several different styles by which verbal handoffs are given, but generally they should include the following information, as exemplified by several recently published handover studies, including I-PASS (see below):

1. Patient's current clinical condition, in brief—This should be communicated so that all clinicians are speaking the same "language" and have the same perception of the terminology (e.g., "LOL" has several meanings).

2. A brief summary of patient's treatment, condition, and history. The length and amount of detail will depend on the clinical complexity of the patient.

3. A sign out of tasks that require attention (e.g., ordering medications, checking test results, actions to be taken, etc.)

4. Anticipatory planning for potential events and who needs to be notified (e.g., suggested actions for clinical deterioration—if "X" happens, do "Y.")

5. An opportunity for the receiver of the handoff to ask questions and convey their understanding or concerns

B. **Written Handoff:** This is typically a paper or electronic document to accompany the verbal handoff.

1. Usually follows a more detailed format than a verbal handoff

2. Many electronic medical record (EMR) solutions include a handoff tool that is integrated into the system. This is designed to improve communication, allowing each role group access to view each other's handoff notes (i.e., physician can see a nurse's sign out on the same patient and vice versa).

VII. **COMMONLY USED HANDOFF TOOLS**—There are a variety of tools available for handoffs. Two common approaches are detailed below:

A. **SBAR**

1. Components and mnemonic

a. **S = Situation:** a concise statement of the problem

b. **B = Background:** pertinent and brief information related to the situation

c. **A = Assessment:** analysis and considerations of options—what you found/think

d. **R = Recommendation:** action requested/recommended—what you want

2. This tool was developed by the Navy—it is not health care specific

3. Intended for unexpected or escalation situations, but has been adapted successfully for other scenarios, as well

4. Provides clinicians with a predictable and structured framework for communication that is standardized across settings

B. **I-PASS**

1. Components and mnemonic (Fig. 37.1)

a. **I = Illness Severity:** Standard language of stable, "watcher," or unstable

b. **P = Patient Summary:** summary statements of events leading up to admission, the hospital course, ongoing assessment, and the plan of care

c. **A = Action List:** a "to-do" list with timeline and assigned ownership

d. **S = Situational Awareness/Contingency Planning:** high-level context of patient care and plans for potential complications or events (i.e.. if "X" happens, do "Y.")

e. **S = Synthesis by receiver:** receiver recaps handoff, restating key items and asking questions; encourages active listening and participation of receiver

2. Two multisite studies published the following:

a. Ten site study with ~50% reduction in medical errors

b. Twenty-three site study in children showing ~30% reduction in medical errors

3. Adaptable for all clinical disciplines, though originally created for physicians

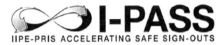

I Illness Severity • Stable, "watcher," unstable

P Patient Summary
- Summary statement
- Events leading up to admission
- Hospital course
- Ongoing assessment
- Plan

A Action List
- To do list
- Timeline and ownership

S Situation Awareness & Contingency Planning
- Know what's going on
- Plan for what might happen

S Synthesis by Receiver
- Receiver summarizes what was heard
- Asks questions
- Restates key action/to do items

FIGURE 37.1 I-PASS framework (From Starmer A, Spector N, Srivastava R, et al. I-PASS, a mnemonic to standardize verbal handoffs. *Pediatrics* 2012;129:201–204, with permission).

VIII. IMPLEMENTING HANDOFF TOOLS IN THE ICU

A. Identify and recruit a multidisciplinary team consisting of all stakeholders involved in the handoff process. (E.g., Neurosurgeon, anesthesiologist, OR nurse, intensivist, ICU bedside nurse, and ICU resource nurse all play a role in OR-to-neuro ICU handoffs.)

B. Set up regular meetings with your team to discuss project status and opportunities for improvement (e.g., weekly or biweekly preferred initially).

C. Agree on a set of shared values or guiding principles that describes the team's shared vision for an ideal handoff. (E.g., Handoffs should be (1) documented electronically, (2) include face-to-face communication, (3) include all team members involved in the care of the patient, (4) conducted efficiently, and (5) include all pertinent information related to the patient's care.)

D. Use process maps to develop a shared understanding of the current state, that is, the existing handoff process. Mapping software like Vizio may be helpful, or use sticky notes on a wall to depict the process if doing this exercise with your team (preferred).

E. Compare current process with values set forth by the team to determine if there is alignment. Observe and audit key steps in the process to assess reliability of current process and accuracy of the process map. (E.g., What percentage of the time that a patient is transferred (1) does the team actually meet to give handoff; (2) is an anesthesia and surgical report given; (3) does the receiving team ask questions and recap the plan?)

F. For any gaps, perform a root cause analysis to assess why certain steps in the process are not occurring. Use a fishbone diagram to help visualize the issues, as needed.

G. Brainstorm solutions to address root causes. (E.g., (1) Implement a handoff tool, like I-PASS to standardize handoff content; (2) develop a communication process to alert senders and receivers of impending handoff time and location; (3) build an electronic template to capture handoff documentation; (4) create an education campaign to inform clinicians about the expectations for proper handoff.)

H. Prioritize solutions on the basis of ease of implementation and level of impact; use a prioritization matrix to visualize this exercise with the team.

I. Test solutions by implementing and measuring progress (e.g., PDSA cycles). Use "run" or "control" charts to help visualize progress over time.

J. Perform additional improvement cycles, repeating steps above, as needed.

IX. SUSTAINING IMPROVEMENTS—It is essential to sustain focus on handoffs even after an initial implementation, especially in high-turnover environments (such as teaching hospitals).

A. Incorporate handoff education materials into onboarding documents and orientation curriculum.

B. Establish regular auditing and reporting frequency on key measures in the handoff process; establish regular review frequency with ICU leadership.

C. Review handoff and communication-related safety reports, and share lessons learned with unit staff.

D. Conduct periodic safety culture surveys to assess staff perceptions on handoffs and communication, and discuss results with staff to understand how handoffs can be further improved.

E. Incorporate redundancies into handoff process to ensure any missed steps do not hinder patient care.

Selected Readings

Bigham MT, Logsdon TR, Manicone PE, et al. Decreasing handoff-related care failures in children's hospitals. *Pediatrics* 2014;134(2):e572–e579.

Clancy CM, Tornberg DN. TeamSTEPPS: assuring optimal teamwork in clinical settings. *Am J Med Qual* 2007;22(3):214–217.

Cooper GE, White MD, Lauber JK. *Resource management on the flightdeck: proceedings of a NASA/Industry Workshop.* NASA CP-2120. Moffett Field: NASA-Ames Research Center, 1980.

Crewmember Duties. Code of Federal Aviation Regulations. Title 14. §121.542 (1981) and §135.100 (1981).

Davies JM, Posner KL, Lee LA, et al. Liability associated with obstetric anesthesia: a closed claims analysis. *Anesthesiology* 2009;110(1):131–139.

Flight Safety Foundation. Cockpit chatter leads to crash. Accident/incident briefs. Flight Safety Digest. August 1992. http://flightsafety.org/fsd/fsd_aug92.pdf. Accessed July 25, 2014.

Institute for Healthcare Improvement. Toolkit on SBAR. http://www.ihi.org/resources/Pages/Tools/SBARToolkit.aspx

International Association of Fire Chiefs. Crew resource management: a positive change for the fire service. 2003. Accessed July 25, 2014.

National Transportation Safety Board. United Airlines, Inc. McDonnell-Douglas DC-8-61, N8082U Portland, Oregon: December 28, 1978. http://libraryonline.erau.edu/online-full-text/ntsb/aircraft-accident-reports/AAR79-07.pdf. Accessed July 25, 2014.

Rogers SO Jr, Gawande AA, Kwaan M, et al. Analysis of surgical errors in closed malpractice claims at 4 liability insurers. *Surgery* 2006;140(1):25–33.

Singh H, Thomas EJ, Petersen LA, et al. Medical errors involving trainees: a study of closed malpractice claims from 5 insurers. *Arch Intern Med* 2007;167(19):2030–2036.

Starmer AJ, O'Toole JK, Rosenbluth G, et al. Development, implementation, and dissemination of the I-PASS handoff curriculum: a multisite educational intervention to improve patient handoffs. *Acad Med* 2014;89(6):876–884. doi:10.1097/ACM.0000000000000264.

Starmer AJ, Spector ND, Srivastava R, et al; I-PASS Study Group. I-PASS, a mnemonic to standardize verbal handoffs. *Pediatrics* 2012;129:201–204.

Sumwalt RL. The sterile cockpit. *ASRS Directline* 1993;4. http://asrs.arc.nasa.gov/publications/directline/dl4_sterile.htm. Accessed July 25, 2014.

The Joint Commission. The Joint Commission history. http://www.jointcommission.org/assets/1/6/Joint_Commission_History.pdf. Accessed July 2014.

The Joint Commission Office of Quality Monitoring. Sentinel event data: root causes by event type 2004–2014. http://www.jointcommission.org/assets/1/18/Root_Causes_by_Event_Type_2004-2014.pdf

Timmel J, Kent PS, Holzmueller CG, et al. Impact of the comprehensive unit-based safety program (CUSP) on safety culture in a surgical inpatient unit. *Jt Comm J Qual Patient Saf* 2010;36(6):252–260.

White AA, Pichert JW, Bledsoe SH, et al. Cause and effect analysis of closed claims in obstetrics and gynecology. *Obstet Gynecol* 2005;105(5, pt 1):1031–1038.

Wiener EL, Kanki BG, Helmreich RL. *Cockpit resource management.* San Diego: Harcourt Brace, 1993.

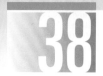

Long-Term Outcomes of ICU Patients

Laurie O. Mark and Ronald Hirschberg

LONG-TERM OUTCOMES OF ICU PATIENTS

The intensive care unit (ICU) serves to provide acute care to patients with severe and life-threatening illnesses or injuries that require immediate care, as well as close and constant monitoring. Once the patient has recovered from the inciting insult, they are discharged to the floor, often lost to follow-up. The ICU treats various complicated conditions, but not much information is provided to clinicians in the ICU about the long-term outcomes of our patients. Over the past 50 years in trauma and ICU care, there has been a paradigm shift in outcome assessment from that of pure mortality–survival (i.e. death or life), to specific morbidity for the survivors. Progress continues in this area as we attempt to show functional gains and abilities in the continuum of care, from ICU to community. This chapter serves to discuss the long-term outcomes of ICU patients who survive trauma, acute respiratory distress syndrome (ARDS), sepsis, and traumatic brain injury (TBI)—some of the most common conditions encountered in this setting.

I. TRAUMA
   A. Trauma can range from blunt trauma (e.g., motor vehicle accidents, falls), to penetrating trauma (e.g., gunshot, stab wounds).
   1. The established studies do not differentiate between blunt and penetrating trauma, but "major trauma in the ICU" is associated with the following:
   a. Requiring urgent surgery
   b. Admission to an intensive care unit for >24 hours
   c. Requiring mechanical ventilation
   d. An injury severity score >15
   e. Death occurring after injury.
   B. The available data suggest that the trauma population is greatly affected in all aspects of life postdischarge from the ICU, and in all measured dimensions the scores are lower than the general population. These effects are most pronounced within the first year, but scores remain consistently low even after several years.
   1. One reason for such a drastic change is that trauma patients are usually previously healthy individuals (compared with, for example, septic patients), so the changes in quality of life seem drastic.
   2. As a general rule many of our trauma patients are of a younger age, with vocational and social expectations at prime time in their lives, and taking this into consideration with respect to return to work, pain issues, emotional and social health, and so forth is essential.
   C. Trauma ICU survivors consistently have a lower health-related quality of life (QOL) in the years after ICU discharge. Although QOL is certainly subjective, the most common measurement tool for QOL is the Short Form 36 Health Survey (SF-36) questionnaire, which evaluates individual health status, enables comparison across diseases or injuries, and determines how QOL is affected by treatment.

1. The eight sections included (each with a score 0–100; the lower the score, the greater the disability) are vitality, physical functioning, bodily pain, general health perception, physical role functioning, emotional role functioning, social role functioning, and mental health.

2. In short-term follow-up (3–12 months after ICU discharge), an increase in physical function, bodily pain, and social functioning scores was observed in one study but the scores plateaued by 12 months and of note were still consistently lower than the general population.

3. After 2 years of follow-up, a large decrease in HRQOL was also evident, predominantly in the physical dimensions section, which was attributed to musculoskeletal effects and secondary pain. Extending the follow-up period even further to 7 years demonstrated the same results.

4. Demographics (age, area of the country, personal wealth), trauma characteristics (MVA vs. violence related), the injury severity score, preexisting disease (especially psychological disorders and abuse problems), and pain issues were all shown to be predictors of poor HRQOL among trauma survivors.

5. Patients who obtained higher levels of education, had greater family and social support, and better material and housing conditions were perhaps predisposed to optimism and might "see the positive side of things after a severe illness".

D. ICU survivors of trauma had a lower incidence of returning to work and a higher incidence of early retirement compared with the nontrauma, non-ICU general population.

   1. Only 52% of survivors returned to work (of the approximately 80% who survived after the ICU) and 20% pursued an early retirement.

   2. The odds of returning to work increased within the first year after ICU discharge but plateaued after 12 months. Again, pain and physical disability were the main reasons for a lower return-to-work rate.

   3. Interestingly, spouses and close family members of trauma survivors had a low rate of return to work. This may speak to the "outcome" of primary care givers themselves in the home and care giver burden.

E. Importantly, a common theme found between studies was an increased incidence of chronic pain after trauma. Pain scores were reported to be the highest during the 6-to-12-month period after ICU discharge, with mild improvement after 12 months. The only reliable predictor identified for the development of chronic pain was the prevalence of pain prior to trauma.

F. Physical and emotional recovery from a significant trauma can take multiple years. The vast majority of studies only looked at the first year after injury. The trend of HRQOL, return to work, and chronic pain within the first decade after injury might be more informative. However, such long-term follow-up is difficult to perform once the patient has been discharged.

II. ACUTE RESPIRATORY DISTRESS SYNDROME

ARDS is an inflammatory process in the lungs that significantly reduces gas exchange and can be triggered by infection, sepsis, or trauma. Recovery from ARDS can be more extensive than recovery from sepsis or trauma in that patients must overcome the initial insult and then recover from the massive insult to their lungs, which includes mechanical ventilation in and of itself, excessive fluid requirements, and relative hypoxemia. As a result, patients can have significant impairment after discharge that can last for months to years.

A. Survivors of ARDS have poorer HRQOL compared with the general population. The main features affected are mobility, energy, social relationships, domestic tasks, and professional tasks. Mobility is greatly impaired in patients with long ICU and hospital courses, and especially in those who have had long intubation or sedation times. Although modern ICU treatment supports early mobilization, there is indeed significant relative immobilization, which quickly can lead to deconditioning of the muscle, bone and joints, soft tissue, skin, and cardiovascular systems in particular. Overcoming ICU-acquired weakness after ARDS requires weeks to months of rehabilitation and depending on functional level of the patient post-ICU will require admission to a rehabilitation hospital or discharge home with planned outpatient therapies.

B. Fatigue or "lack of energy" are common long-term complaints experienced post-ARDS treatment that likely has multifactorial contributions (e.g., direct sarcopenia, decreased sleep secondary to other impairments, low cardiopulmonary endurance, depression). Social and family relationships can be affected because patients are in the acute care hospital and potentially rehabilitation hospital undergoing treatment and are discharged to recuperate at home following weeks to months of relative isolation, and relationships can be strained. In addition, patients may feel they are a burden to their family, or caretakers may feel resentful for having to give up their time, job, and money to care for the patient.

C. The incidence of depressive symptoms in the ARDS population is increased. Recovery is long and grueling, which can be a significant stressor or trigger for depression. Some patients lack the necessary social support to get through their recovery, which compounds the problem further.

D. ARDS causes significant damage to the lungs and adversely affects pulmonary physiology. Survivors typically can regain baseline or normal pulmonary function after 12 months, and strict follow-up with imaging and pulmonary function tests after discharge are needed. Follow-up studies and appointments are expensive and the time and commitment required to make the appointments is significant, which may contribute to the lack of return to work.

E. Long-term neuropsychological impairment is *not* uncommon in survivors of ARDS. In addition to the psychological effects of hospitalization itself and "ICU delirium," physiological repercussions from ARDS treatment have been documented. Hypoxemia and hypotension can be detrimental and have been associated with impaired executive function on follow-up examinations.

   1. Poor fluid management can prolong a disease course, such as liberalizing fluid administration leading to pulmonary edema and worsening of ARDS, which in turn contributes to a prolonged intubation and hospitalization.

   2. In ICU patients with hypoxemia and/or hypotension, the brain receives less oxygen than is needed and the effect on brain functioning can be apparent even in the long term.

   3. Observational studies have demonstrated cognitive impairments at 1 year from ARDS from 30% to 55% prevalence. The cognitive changes (executive functioning, memory, attention, processing speed, etc.) can impact further recovery of physical functioning because of the need for optimal mentation for the rehabilitation process.

F. Outcome studies for ARDS have several limitations, especially lack of emphasis on differences regarding age, patient comorbidities, demographics, and inciting event. Significant differences have been noted between survival and recovery between the young and previously healthy and the elderly with preexisting cardiac and pulmonary disease and should be considered for future outcome studies.

III. SEPSIS

Sepsis is one of the leading causes of death in the ICU. Over 1,665,000 cases of sepsis occur in the United States each year, and even with optimal treatment, mortality due to severe sepsis or septic shock is approximately 40% and can exceed 50% in the sickest patients. Sepsis affects all organ systems, and recovery can be long and difficult. Much like trauma, patients who survive sepsis in the ICU demonstrate an impaired QOL, with continued reduction in scores as compared with the general population. Most of the studies available use mortality at 28 days as the clinical end point, but it is important to note that patients with varying comorbidities and degrees of sepsis die or decompensate in months and years after this; only 61% of all comers will survive to 5 years.

A. Morbidity. From a morbidity standpoint, the most common long-term adverse effects of sepsis are neurologic or cognitive impairment, psychological symptoms, and impaired physical or emotional QOL.

   1. Survivors demonstrate deficits in attention, verbal fluency, executive function, and verbal memories, even in the absence of psychiatric disturbances. Many display significant exhaustion and fatigue, which can manifest as irritability, lack of concentration, and lack of stamina to perform tasks they were previously able to perform.

   2. Some evidence suggests that patients who experience ICU delirium are at higher risk of cognitive dysfunction, and neuropsychological test scores are frequently low in these survivors.

B. Emotional disturbances were also commonly noted in survivors of sepsis in the ICU.

   1. Patients can feel traumatized because their body is "failing" or when interventions are being performed. For example, they may feel a threat of suffocation when a central line is being placed, have a feeling of impending death when they are being induced for intubation, or feel frustrated when they cannot communicate with an endotracheal tube in place.

   2. Memories of actual events from the ICU can have more of an effect on a patient in the long run than episodes of delusion or hallucinations they may have experienced during this time. These factual memories can lead to acute stress disorders or even posttraumatic stress disorder.

   3. Mood disruptions have been observed in survivors of sepsis, and premorbid anxiety and depression might play a part in this development, but further studies are needed to confirm this hypothesis.

C. The QOL dimensions most affected after sepsis are social functioning (ability to engage in old relationships, hobbies, or recreational activities), and physical functioning in activities of daily living (ADLs). Much like trauma, the return-to-work rate of sepsis survivors is fairly low because of physical and mental/cognitive limitations. One study reported a negative impact on employment of 33% by 6 months and 28% by 1 year.

D. As with ARDS patients, considerable muscle wasting and weakness after surviving a sepsis syndrome in the ICU is common and places strain on the patient and family, and, given the extended recovery process, on the health care system as a whole, as patients require several months of rehabilitation to regain function. It is important to note that the affected functional dimensions are interrelated.

   1. Physical limitations are directly the result of impairments at the physiological level, as well as the result of cognitive, psychological, and/

or social stressors or limitations that affect the ability to rehabilitate optimally.

   2. Conversely, emotional and social functioning typically are directly impacted upon by the physically functional level of the individual.

   3. Lastly and of key importance is the introduction of the emotional stress when patients become dependent on their spouses or primary caretakers, which can affect overall outcome poorly on both the patient and the family.

E. Of interest, the longest follow-up period of any study of septic ICU patients was 1 year.

   1. Patients who show improvement or decline in multiple areas of their life in many years after discharge have not been studied. The data also fail to stratify patients on the basis of premorbid conditions and age.

     a. An elderly patient with end-stage renal disease on hemodialysis 3 days a week who became sick in the ICU is different from a 30-year-old patient who developed an infection and multiorgan dysfunction after a routine gynecologic surgery.

     b. As discussed, we have come far in some respects regarding outcomes post-ICU; however, further work is needed with respect to not only premorbidity and age, but also pre-ICU functional status.

IV. TRAUMATIC BRAIN INJURY

Traumatic brain injury (TBI) affects approximately 1.4 million people in the United States every year and is classified as mild, moderate, or severe. Outcomes after TBI can range from full functional recovery to death. The Glasgow Coma Scale is the most commonly used scale to determine severity and is used along with adjunctive tests, such as CT scans. The severity is also determined by the nature, speed, and location of the injury and complicating factors, such as hypoxemia, hypotension, intracranial hemorrhage, or increased intracranial pressure. Many survivors will experience long-term disabilities, from the purely cognitive, to physical and psychosocial, and all of the above.

A. Understanding outcomes in TBI includes knowledge of some of the neurological and medical-expected morbidities.

   1. Seizures are common sequelae of most types of TBI. Within the first 24 hours of injury, 25% of patients with brain contusions or hematomas and 50% of patients with penetrating TBI will develop seizures. Injury severity is correlated with the chance of developing seizures, but no evidence suggests that these patients will develop epilepsy.

   2. Development of neurodegenerative disorders (such as dementia of the Alzheimer's type and Parkinson disease) is associated with mild to moderate TBI.

   3. The risk of disease development is correlated with chronic damage to the brain, as is seen in professional boxers and more recently observed in the professional football player.

   4. Other known sequelae of TBI include aphasia, dysarthria, dysphagia, incontinence, muscle pain and spasticity, deep-vein thrombosis, heterotopic ossification, and posttraumatic stress disorder.

B. The vast majority of studies on outcome after TBI have focused short-term outcomes, approximately 6 to 12 months after injury. Initial literature discusses mortality in these time intervals, and more recently there are more data on severe TBI outcome. More recently, efforts have been made to examine outcomes several years after injury.

1. There is a twofold increased risk of mortality for patients with TBI compared with the general population; studies have demonstrated evidence for risk factors that contribute to premature death in these patients post-TBI.
   a. Head-injury-associated deaths range from 15 to 30 per 100,000 population (the majority being young adults) and are associated with motor vehicle accidents and falls.
   b. Documented history of prior problems with alcohol or substance abuse, personal problems, and social/behavioral issues were found to contribute to the mortality rate.
   c. People with disabilities post-TBI have a higher risk of death after TBI than able-bodied individuals, and functional limitations upon discharge from rehab were also noted to correlate with increased mortality.
2. Overall, differentiating between death as a direct or indirect result of TBI is difficult. For example, patients with significant disability following TBI have prolonged hospitalizations and are prone to developing complications that include pneumonia, ICU-acquired weakness, and cognitive impairments. Interestingly, the cognitive impairments could contribute to accidents that would have otherwise not have occurred had the patient been in their preinjury state of health.

C. The most frequent complications seen after TBI are cognitive, such as memory loss, loss of reasoning ability and concentration, and various behavioral issues (depression, anxiety, personality changes, and lack of social situational awareness).
   1. The severity of a patient's cognitive disability after TBI depends on the severity of the injury as well as preinjury characteristics (such as educational level, emotional variability, physical condition, and personality disorders, in addition to substance use). Preinjury intelligence, volume of brain tissue lost, and brain region injured also affect the severity of cognitive dysfunction.
   2. In penetrating brain injury, the cognitive effects of normal aging are exacerbated.
   3. TBI decreases the chance of returning to work and to the same position held preinjury.
      a. Long-term disability was predicted by older age, preinjury unemployment, substance abuse, and more severe disability upon discharge from a rehabilitation center.
      b. Long-term unproductivity was predicted by preinjury unemployment, longer posttraumatic amnesia, substance abuse, and more disability upon admission to a rehabilitation center.
   4. TBI adversely affects recreational activities, social and familial relationships, functional status, and independence.
   5. Severity of injury is correlated with social outcome, but the evidence is insufficient to specify which type of injury will produce a specific adverse outcome.

D. Factors known to influence long-term survival include basic functional skills (such as mobility and the ability to feed oneself), the type and severity of injury, and specific neuro-functional impairments (cognitive changes, risk-taking behavior, and mood disorders).
   1. The Community Integration Questionnaire (CIQ) is frequently used to assess long-term home and social integration and productivity after TBI.
      a. Three months postinjury, a decline in CIQ score compared with preinjury condition in regard to home and social integration and productivity

    b. Maximal improvement was achieved within the first year, but slight improvement continued up to 3 years after the injury.

    c. The major determinants of community integration were preinjury community integration, age, and destination after hospital discharge.

    d. Lower CIQ scores were found among males, older patients, those living with others preinjury, longer hospitalizations, abnormal CT scans, those who were more dependent on others, those with motor and cognitive impairment, and those who were discharged to an inpatient rehabilitation center or nursing home.

E. It should be noted that the Glasgow Coma Scale as a single variable may have limited value as a predictor of functional outcome.

    1. GCS assessment is not useful in day-to-day ICU assessment and neurological change and has not been shown to predict longer term outcome.

    2. The highly vetted Coma Recovery Scale–Revised (CRS-R) was established first in 1991 with the goal of tracking levels of consciousness over weeks to months following severe TBI. The scale incorporates detailed assessments of auditory, visual, motor, verbal, communication, and level of arousal as patients emerge from vegetative state (VS) through the levels of minimally conscious state (MCS).

    3. The standard in functional outcome assessment (as opposed to specific levels of consciousness) for moderate to severe TBI is the Disability Rating Scale (DRS) established by Wright. This scale incorporates visual, motoric, and verbal aspects of impairment akin to the GCS, in addition to level of functional limitation (ADLs, etc.) as well as disability (employability, social integration). Both highly reliable and valid, the DRS demonstrates functional changes of TBI survivors over months to years.

Selected Readings

Adhikari NK, Tansey CM, McAndrews MP, et al. Self-reported depressive symptoms and memory complaints in survivors five years after ARDS. *Chest* 2011;140(6):1484–1493.

Bazarian JJ, Cernak I, Noble-Haeusslein L, et al. Long-term neurologic outcomes after traumatic brain injury. *J Head Trauma Rehabil* 2009;24:439–451.

Carlson CG, Huang DT. The Adult Respiratory Distress Syndrome Cognitive Outcomes Study: long-term neuropsychological function in survivors of acute lung injury. *Crit Care* 2013;17(3):317.

Gabbe BJ, Simpson PM, Sutherland AM, et al. Evaluating time points for measuring recovery after major trauma in adults. *Ann Surg* 2013;257(1):166–172.

Griffiths J, Hatch RA, Bishop J, et al. An exploration of social and economic outcome and associated health-related quality of life after critical illness in general intensive care unit survivors: a 12-month follow-up study. *Crit Care* 2013;17(3):R100.

Kalmar K, Giacino JT. The JFK Coma Recovery Scale—Revised. *Neuropsychol Rehabil* 2005;15(3–4):454–460.

Korosec Jagodic H, Jagodic K, Podbregar M. Long-term outcome and quality of life of patients treated in surgical intensive care: a comparison between sepsis and trauma. *Crit Care* 2006;10(5):R134.

Kowalczyk M, Nestorowicz A, Fijałkowska A, et al. Emotional sequelae among survivors of critical illness. *Eur J Anaesthesiol* 2013;30(3):111–118.

Lazosky A, Young GB, Zirul S, et al. Quality of life after septic illness. *J Crit Care* 2010; 25(3):406–412.

Misak C. Cognitive dysfunction after critical illness: measurement, rehabilitation, and disclosure. *Crit Care* 2009;13:312.

Neviere R. Sepsis and the systemic inflammatory response syndrome: definitions, epidemiology, and prognosis. *Up To Date* May 2014. http://www.uptodate.com/contents/sepsis-and-the-systemic-inflammatory-response-syndrome-definitions-epidemiology-and-prognosis.

Orwelius L, Bergkvist M, Nordlund A, et al. Physical effects of trauma and the psychological consequences of preexisting diseases account for a significant portion of the health-related quality of life patterns of former trauma patients. *J Trauma Acute Care Surg* 2012;72(2):504–512.

Overgaard M, Hoyer CB, Christensen EF. Long-term survival and health-related quality of life 6 to 9 years after trauma. *J Trauma* 2011;71(2):435–441.

Ribbers GM. Brain injury: long term outcome after traumatic brain injury. In: Stone JH, Blouin M, eds. *International encyclopedia of rehabilitation.* http://cirrie.buffalo.edu/encyclopedia/en/article/338/

Safaz I, Alaca R, Yasar E, et al. Medical complications, physical function and communication skills in patients with traumatic brain injury: a single centre 5-year experience. *Brain Inj* 2008;22(10):733–739.

Toien K, Bredal I, Skogstad L, et al. Health related quality of life in trauma patients. Data from a one-year follow up study compared with the general population. *Scand J Trauma Resusc Emerg Med* 2011;19–22. doi:10.1186/1757-7241-19-22.

Ulvik K, Kvale R, Wentzel-Larsen T, et al. Quality of life 2–7 years after major trauma. *Acta Anaesthesiol Scand* 2008;52(2):195–201.

Ware JE. SF-36 Health Survey Update. In: Maruish M, ed. *The use of psychological testing for treatment planning and outcomes assessment.* 3rd ed. Mahwah: Lawrence Erlbaum Associates, 2004:693–718.

Willemse-van Son AH, Ribbers GM, Hop WC, et al. Community integration following moderate to severe traumatic brain injury: a longitudinal investigation. *J Rehabil Med* 2009;41:521–527.

Willemse-van Son AH, Ribbers GM, Verhagen AP, et al. Prognostic factors of long-term functioning and productivity after traumatic brain injury: a systematic review of prospective cohort studies. *Clin Rehabil* 2007;21:1024–1037.

Zafonte RD, Hammond FM, Mann NR, et al. Relationship between Glasgow Coma Scale and functional outcome. *Am J Phys Med Rehabil* 1996;75(5):364–369.v

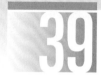

The Economics of Critical Care: Measuring and Improving Value in the ICU

Andrea T. Tull and J. Perren Cobb

I. COSTS AND BURDEN OF CRITICAL CARE

A. Caring for the critically ill or injured is a complex and resource-intensive endeavor. There are roughly 6,000 intensive care units in the United States, representing 10% of the total hospital beds but a disproportionate share of hospital operating costs—roughly one-third. Today's ICUs are highly specialized units dedicated to care for very specific populations of patients at risk for or experiencing overt, critical organ dysfunction. Many hospitals, typically in larger centers, further subdivide patients into burn or neurosurgery subspecialty ICU's. This increased specialization, coupled with growing demand for intensive care services, presents challenges to hospitals seeking to control costs. Applying a family- and patient-oriented, value-based framework to intensive care helps practitioners focus on optimizing outcomes while simultaneously reducing costs.

B. Detailed analysis indicates that critical care represents 13.4% of hospital charges, 4.1% of US health care expenditures, and 0.66% of gross domestic product. This is due in part to high overhead costs—on average, an ICU bed costs $3,500 to $4,000 per day—together with the expense of high-intensity nurse and therapist staffing. Moreover, critical care expenditures in the United States are projected to increase as a proportion of total health care costs as the population ages, the prevalence of chronic disease increases, and technological advances help people live longer following serious illness and injury. In 2000, for example, roughly 12% of the US population was age 65 years or older; by 2050, persons age 65 years and older are projected to comprise 21% of the US population. More people are expected to live to advanced ages, with the percentage of US adults age 85 and older projected to increase from less than 1% in 2000 to 5% in 2050. This growth in the elderly population will fuel demand for intensive care services, further straining resources. In addition, health care economists suggest technological advances combined with greater access to health insurance increased demand for critical care services in recent years, a trend that is likely to continue. New technology includes a broader array of pharmaceuticals, devices, and new medical procedures (most of which tend to be expensive), as well as a deeper understanding of the clinical process of care. These advances in aggregate have substantially improved outcomes for patients, but drive up demand for critical care services and costs, accordingly. Thus, for most hospitals with shrinking margins in a difficult policy environment, critical care represents a potential high-impact opportunity for focusing on efficiencies and improving care.

C. Evidence suggests that the supply of intensivists, critical care nurses, respiratory therapists, and other clinical staff required to effectively manage critically ill patients is not keeping pace with the demand for critical care services, putting increasing pressure on critical care providers. Some estimate a 35% shortage of intensivists by 2020, with even greater shortages in specialty areas such as surgical and pediatric critical care, or those with dual-board certification in emergency medicine and critical care, or palliative medicine and critical care. Yet, ICU clinicians and administrators have several potential levers to improve the quality and efficiency of ICU care and therefore reduce costs, such as preventing hospital-acquired infections, reducing length of stay, and ensuring proper staffing of the ICU with intensivists.

D. All of these factors combine to create a challenging matrix for providing high-value, patient- and family-centered care to critically ill patients. Measuring the value of the care provided in our ICUs is an essential first step in addressing these challenges and can help identify opportunities to create efficiencies and improve clinical outcomes.

II. THE VALUE OF CRITICAL CARE EXPENDITURES

A. A new paradigm, "the value proposition," has gained traction as the US health care system tries to balance the tension found in delivering the highest quality care at the lowest possible cost. Value in health care is defined as the outcomes experienced by the patient (typically a quality metric) divided by the cost of delivering those outcomes/metrics. Value can therefore be maximized by either improving outcomes and/or reducing costs. Measuring hospital costs is challenging because health care costs are much less transparent than that in other industries. The prices charged by providers and the amounts reimbursed by insurers often do not reflect the actual cost of the care provided. In addition, high-margin treatments and procedures are used to subsidize other areas where reimbursements do not cover the costs. Determining costs for patients in the ICU is particularly challenging because of the interdisciplinary nature of the care provided and the heterogeneity of the ICU patient population. The value measurement framework includes equal emphasis on achieving goals for both quality outcomes and costs. The value of medical care can be improved either by reducing costs or improving quality. Ideally, both scenarios would be met to maximize value. There are many opportunities to apply this lens to critical care and drive improvement on both fronts.

B. Quality Care: Traditionally, measures of quality for critical care were focused solely on the ICU portion of the patient's hospital stay, using metrics (like length of stay) that are easy to measure but less important to patients and families (functional status, long-term survival, and quality of life). The new value framework provides a structure for measuring the impact and value of critical care services over the long term, using patient- and family-centered outcomes. One popular approach groups health outcomes into three tiers: health status achieved or retained, process of recovery, and sustainability of health (Table 39.1).

This approach provides a framework for measuring value for critically ill patients that includes a continued focus on survival but also calls attention to duration of recovery and ultimate health obtained.

1. Measures of outcomes that drive up overall cost: hospital-acquired infection rates, pressure ulcer rates, falls and injury rates, readmissions to the ICU, and readmissions to the hospital postdischarge (within specified time periods, typically 30 days)

2. Measures of overall quality that are value-producing: adherence to protocols for managing specific diseases such as sepsis, early mobilization, monitoring for delirium, etc.

Tier	Domain	Measure
1. Health Status Achieved or Maintained	Survival	• In-hospital mortality • Postdischarge mortality (30 d, 6 mo, 1 y)
	Degree of Health or Recovery	• Discharge location (LTACH, SNF, Home) • Ability to live independently • Ability to return to work • Related readmissions • For end-of-life patients, ability to access palliative care and hospice services in accordance with patient/family goals
2. Process of Recovery	Time to Recovery	• Critical care unit length of stay • Overall hospital length of stay • Time to return of full functionality (reanimation)
	Disutility of Care	• Hospital-acquired infections (e.g., CLABSI, CAUTI, MRSA, *C. difficile*, SSI) • Incidence of pressure ulcers • Delirium
3. Sustainability of Health	Sustainability of health recovery and nature of recurrences	• Quality of life years • Return to full functionality (reanimation)
	Long-term consequences of therapy	• Long-term cognitive deficits • Depression/anxiety/other mental health diagnoses

Adapted from Porter ME, Teisberg EO. *Redefining health care.* Cambridge, MA: Harvard Business School Press, 2006.

C. Costs: There are many different approaches to measuring health care costs, each with advantages and disadvantages. Many analyses of costs are completed retrospectively using **administrative (billing) data.** This approach is often used because data are readily available and in a structured format that lends itself to analysis. However, hospital billing data are complex, with many assumptions built in regarding direct, indirect, variable, and fixed costs. Direct costs are directly related to patient care (labor and supplies); indirect costs refer to shared resources that are allocated to individual patients on the basis of a set of assumptions (e.g., salaries of administrators). Fixed costs are those that do not change with the volume of patients; these tend to represent the operational costs of the ICU, such as clinician salaries, or the purchase of specialized equipment. Variable costs will change with the volume of patients, such as the cost of mechanical ventilation or the cost of lab tests. Conventional wisdom is that roughly 80% of costs in the ICU are fixed costs, although new thinking on costing methodology for the health care industry is challenging that notion. Alternatively, costs can be measured prospectively using a framework of **Time-Driven Activity-Based Costing (TDABC)**, which involves tracking the amount of time it takes each clinician to conduct patient care tasks and then calculating the costs of the labor and supplies on the basis of the actual amount of time spent on each task. This approach is much more accurate in terms of determining the actual costs for a specific procedure or patient with a particular clinical condition because it views every resource as variable and fungible. However, TDABC is a more labor-intensive method that involves process mapping and time studies, which may not be practical in all situations.

1. The approach to measuring costs will depend on the question of interest and the amount of time and resources available for the analysis. Administrative data are best suited to address basic questions of utilization (e.g., number of central line days, number of CT scans) and the associated labor and supply costs. This approach is a simple way to determine whether key metrics around resource utilization are trending in the desired direction and is therefore often used in ongoing monitoring. Yet it is often challenging to disentangle the total costs of a particular patient's ICU stay using administrative data. Physician billing data are often located in a separate data system. Nursing costs are typically included in "room and board" charges, with no ability to track the actual costs of the time providers spend with patients.

2. TDABC, on the other hand, provides a more robust and reliable analysis of the actual labor and supply costs for patients with particular medical conditions or procedures. This approach is most helpful in answering questions about capacity, or measuring the cost savings of a particular intervention, such as a quality improvement project. TDABC is also very useful in determining the potential cost savings from substitutions; for example, substituting a nurse practitioner for an MD for a particular patient care task. However, TDABC requires process maps, time studies, and observational data collection, all of which are time-consuming and add cost to the analysis.

3. By understanding the tradeoffs between these two costing strategies—administrative data *versus* TDABC—ICU leaders can choose the approach that best suits the question. If using administrative data, we recommend focusing efforts on measuring direct costs that clinicians can readily affect, both from a cost and quality approach. Some examples include measures of utilization such as ventilator days, catheter days, utilization of high-cost drugs, ICU length of stay, and total average length of stay. When using TDABC, it is important to scope the project so it is achievable and easily replicated in other environments.

III. INFLUENCE OF POLICY ENVIRONMENT

A. Health care reform is redefining the way we think about and measure quality and costs in the ICU. Under a traditional fee-for-service model, ICU care was viewed as a distinct and separate part of the patient's hospital stay. As reimbursement policy evolves from fee-for-service to bundled payments for episodes of care and population health management, the care provided in the ICU must be measured in a broader context. In addition, pay-for-performance programs are increasingly focused on outcomes and costs rather than clinical process of care, consistent with the shift to patient- and family-centered care. This shift in financial incentives puts additional pressure on ICUs to improve the quality and efficiency of care provided. Although this policy environment is challenging, critical care units that effectively improve performance on key metrics will cultivate a competitive advantage while also providing high-value care to the sickest patients.

In the following pay-for-performance programs, ICU care will have either a direct or indirect effect on hospital performance:

1. **Value-based purchasing (VBP):** VBP is a CMS annual pay-for-performance program incenting optimized process of clinical care, pat ent experience, outcomes, and efficiency. Under this program, for example, hospitals have an opportunity to gain or lose up to 1.75% of their base DRG payments in fiscal year 2016 (increasing to 2% in FY17). Although process of care measures were initially 70% of the VBP program, by fiscal year 2016 these measures will represent only 10% of the dollars at risk. Outcome and efficiency measures, in contrast, will comprise 65% of the dollars at risk in VBP by fiscal year 2016. Outcome measures in the VBP program include many ICU-related phenotypes, such as mortality from heart failure, AMI and pneumonia, hospital-acquired infections (CLABSI and CAUTI), the AHRQ composite patient safety indicator (PSI-90), and surgical-site infections. The efficiency score is based on Medicare Spend Per Beneficiary, a risk-adjusted measure of total expenditures for 3 days prior to and 30 days after an inpatient hospital stay.

2. **Hospital-acquired condition reduction program (HAC):** The CMS annual HAC reduction program is a payment penalty assessed on hospitals with poor performance (7th to 10th decile) on hospital-acquired infection rates; the penalty is currently 1% of base DRG payments. In the first year of the program, metrics included AHRQ PSI-90 (a composite score of several Patient Safety Indicators), CLABSI, and CAUTI (ICU rates only). In future years, the program will include surgical-site infection rates for hysterectomy and colon surgery, MRSA bacteremia, and *C. difficile* rates. Hospitals that work to reduce the rate of these potentially preventable, hospital-acquired conditions in the ICUs will have a competitive advantage in this performance program.

3. **Readmissions penalty program:** The CMS Readmissions Reduction Program represents another effort to incent efficiency and improve the value of care by reducing readmissions within 30 days of discharge for selected conditions and procedures. Up to 3% of the hospital's base DRG payments are at risk in this program. Conditions and procedures currently included in the program include AMI, heart failure, pneumonia, COPD, and hip and knee arthroplasty (additional conditions and procedures will be added in the future). It is not uncommon for patients with these diagnoses and procedures to spend some portion of their inpatient stay in the ICU. Thus, care provided in the ICU has the potential to influence the trajectory of recovery and therefore the likelihood of readmission within 30 days.

4. **Medicaid and commercial P4P programs:** State Medicaid programs and commercial insurers often model their incentive programs on Medicare programs, with similar focus on improving efficiency, reducing hospital-acquired conditions, and improving value. Hence, pressure will likely increase on those who provide critical care to demonstrate evidence of sufficient value and return on the invested resources.

B. **Interventions that Affect Value: The 5 Do's and 5 Don'ts of Critical Care**

1. A new term, post–intensive care unit syndrome or PICS, was coined recently to refer to phenotypes associated with survival after severe, debilitating, critical illness. PICS describes new or worsening problems for patients and/or their families during recovery from critical illness, including physical, cognitive, and/or mental health deterioration. Two recent, complementary, national campaigns illustrate how

TABLE 39.2	Five "Don'ts" of Critical Care: the Choosing Wisely Campaign

1. Don't order diagnostic tests at regular intervals (such as every day), but rather in response to specific clinical questions.
2. Don't transfuse red blood cells in hemodynamically stable, nonbleeding ICU patients with a hemoglobin concentration greater than 7 g/dL.
3. Don't use parenteral nutrition in adequately nourished critically ill patients within the first 7 d of an ICU stay.
4. Don't deeply sedate mechanically ventilated patients without a specific indication and without daily attempts to lighten sedation.
5. Don't continue life support for patients at high risk for death or severely impaired functional recovery without offering patients and their families the alternative of care focused entirely on comfort.

Adapted from Angus DC, Deutschman CS, Hall JB, et al. Choosing wisely(R) in critical care: maximizing value in the intensive care unit. *Crit Care Med* 2014;42(11):2437–2438.

performance improvement interventions can be used to improve the value of care provided in ICUs and to potentially avoid the ravages of PICS. For example, both the American Association of Critical Care Nursing and the Society of Critical Care Medicine promote the ABCDE Bundle, which couples five best-practice protocols into a coherent approach to care redesign: coordination of spontaneous awakening and spontaneous breathing trials, delirium assessment and management, and early mobilization. Use of this bundle in a study of medical and surgical patients was associated with less time on the ventilator, less delirium, and less immobility in the ICU. The cost-saving implications are therefore significant (and should be compelling to hospital administrators responsible for performance improvement). Similarly, the American Board of Internal Medicine, partnering with the Critical Care Societies Collaborative, identified by consensus five ICU care areas in which to "choose wisely": the ICU Choosing Wisely Campaign (Table 39.2). These items are intended to educate and to prompt discussions between ICU clinicians, patients, and their families to evaluate critically use of therapies that may not be helpful (and may even be harmful) under certain conditions. Lack of benefit and/or avoiding harm both increase quality and decrease costs, supporting the value proposition.

Selected Readings

Angus DC, Deutschman CS, Hall JB, et al. Choosing wisely(R) in critical care: maximizing value in the intensive care unit. *Crit Care Med* 2014;42(11):2437–2438.

Balas MC, Vasilevskis EE, Olsen KM, et al. Effectiveness and safety of the awakening and breathing coordination, delirium monitoring/management, and early exercise/mobility bundle. *Crit Care Med* 2014;42(5):1024–1036.

Bloomfield EL. The impact of economics on changing medical technology with reference to critical care medicine in the United States. *Anesth Analg* 2003;96(2):418–425.

Centers for Medicare and Medicaid Services. Hospital-acquired condition (HAC) reduction program. http://www.cms.gov/Medicare/Medicare-Fee-for-Service-Payment/AcuteIn-patientPPS/HAC-Reduction-Program.html. Accessed March 9, 2014.

Centers for Medicare and Medicaid Services. Hospital value-based purchasing. https://www.cms.gov/Medicare/Quality-Initiatives-Patient-Assessment-Instruments/hospi-tal-value-based-purchasing/index.html?redirect=/hospital-value-based-purchasing/. Accessed March 9, 2014.

Centers for Medicare and Medicaid Services. Readmissions reduction program. http://www.cms.gov/Medicare/Medicare-Fee-for-Service-Payment/AcuteInpatientPPS/Re-admissions-Reduction-Program.html. Accessed March 9, 2014.

Duke EM; US Department of Health & Human Services, Health Resources & Services Administration. The critical care workforce: a study of the supply and demand of critical care physicians. 2006. http://bhpr.hrsa.gov/healthworkforce/reports/studycritical-carephys.pdf. Accessed September 10, 2014.

Kaplan RS. Improving value with TDABC. *Healthc Financ Manage* 2014;68:76–83.

Napolitano LM, Fulda GJ, Davis KA, et al. Challenging issues in surgical critical care, trauma, and acute care surgery: a report from the Critical Care Committee of the American Association for the Surgery of Trauma. *Trauma* 2010;69:1619–1633.

Needham DM, Davidson J, Cohen H, et al. Improving long-term outcomes after discharge from intensive care unit: report from a stakeholders' conference. *Crit Care Med* 2012;40(2):502–509.

Pandharipande P, Banerjee A, McGrane S, et al. Liberation and animation for ventilated ICU patients: the ABCDE bundle for the back-end of critical care. *Crit Care* 2010;14(3):157.

Population Division, U.S. Census Bureau. Table 12. Projections of the Population by Age and Sex for the United States: 2010 to 2050 (NP2008-T12). August 14, 2008. http://www.census.gov/population/projections/

Porter ME. What is value in healthcare? *N Engl J Med* 2010;363:2477–2481.

Porter ME, Teisberg EO. *Redefining health care.* Cambridge: Harvard Business School Press, 2006.

Shorr AF. An update on cost-effectiveness analysis in critical care. *Curr Opin Crit Care* 2002;8(4):337–343.

Society for Critical Care Medicine. Critical care statistics. http://www.sccm.org/Communications/Pages/CriticalCareStats.aspx. Accessed August 1, 2014.

The American Association for the Surgery of Trauma. Critical care illness. http://www.aast.org/generalinformation/criticalcareillness.aspx. Accessed August 1, 2014.

Wunsch H, Gershengorn H, Scales DC. Economics of ICU organization and management. *Crit Care Clin* 2012;28:25–37.

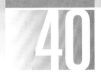

Telemedicine and Remote Electronic Monitoring Systems in ICU

Sanjeev V. Chhangani

I. INTRODUCTION

A. "Telemedicine," as defined by the American Telemedicine Association, is the use of medical information exchanged from one site to another via electronic communications to improve a patient's clinical health status. Many forms of technology have been used to support telemedicine. Telemedicine and telehealth are often used interchangeably. Telehealth, in broad term, encompasses population health care management using telemedicine technology. Telemedicine is not a separate medical specialty, but is meant to supplement traditional models of health care as a delivery tool or system. Consultation is a cornerstone of modern hospital care, particularly in the intensive care unit (ICU). The focus of telemedicine in the ICU ("Tele-ICU") is to supplement traditional ICU care by delivering collaborative, multiprofessional care using telemedicine technology. Goran defined tele-ICU as the provision of team-based critical care via a computer in combination with audio-visual or telecommunication systems.

B. Currently only 10% of hospitals in the United States use tele-ICU technology to provide intensive care. Given the aging of the U.S. population and a continued shortage of available intensivists nationally, tele-ICU has been utilized to bridge the gap between supply and demand for intensive care expertise. Tele-ICU can also expand access to intensivist expertise in rural and critical access hospitals alike. This chapter addresses a number of applications of telemedicine and electronic monitoring systems in the ICU, describing potential benefits as well as barriers of implementation.

II. TELE-ICU MODELS AND ORGANIZATION OF SERVICE

Grundy et al. published the first report of a clinical trial of tele-ICU in 1982. This was a teleconsultative model providing intermittent consultative advice to an inner-city hospital via two-way video and telephones. The report concluded that patients were more likely to survive when intensivists' suggestions were implemented. The around-the-clock model whereby a remote intensivist provides telemedicine care to adult ICU patients was first reported in 2000 by Rosenfeld et al. Since then, three basic delivery models of tele-ICU have been popularized. Each of them can be used to deliver tele-ICU care recommendations successfully.

A. Centralized (Hub-and-Spoke) Model

The centralized model, also known as the hub-and-spoke model, is the most commonly utilized model for Tele-ICU (Fig. 40.1). In this model, tele-ICU intensivists and support personnel are located in a central location in an urban hospital (the hub) and provide tele-ICU interventions to several types of outlying units or rural/community hospitals (the spokes). The intensivists and support personnel work in shifts providing 24 × 7 (i.e., around the clock) monitoring and recommended interventions for these ICU patients. Recent reports suggestions that compliance with

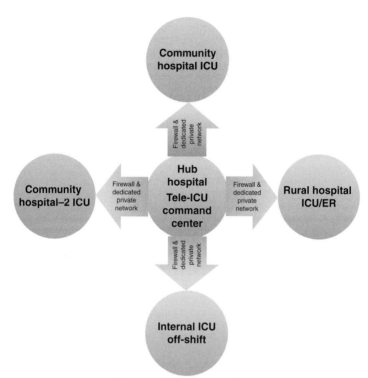

FIGURE 40.1 Centralized Tele-ICU model.

evidence-based ICU protocols is improved with this centralized tele-ICU care model. This model is typical with the commonly used term "electronic ICU" or "eICU care." This model typically has higher setup and operational costs (in thousands of dollars per bed).

B. Decentralized Model

The decentralized model allows intensivists in different locations to access the tele-ICU via desktop or laptop without relying on a central hub from which to practice (Fig. 40.2). This is associated with significantly reduced startup cost for both the consulting and receiving organization.

C. Hybrid Model

This model combines features of both the centralized and decentralized models. The consulting intensivists are not located in one central location, but may be in multiple facilities, and the model has the ability to provide tele-ICU care to multiple facilities. Similar to the decentralized model, startup and operational costs for the hub are typically lower with this model.

III. ORGANIZATION OF TELE-ICU SERVICE

Successful organization of tele-ICU service requires clinical, business/administrative, and legal collaboration between two or more health care facilities with the common goal of improving access to high-quality critical care. The collaborative domains include personnel, technology, and patient populations.

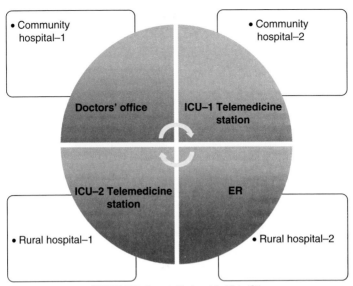

FIGURE 40.2 Decentralized model of Tele-ICU.

A. Personnel

Critical care clinicians and business administrators at both the consulting and receiving facility must collaborate for the service to work. Optimally, physician and business administration champions must be identified from each facility to facilitate discussions during the formative and implementation stages and to monitor progress of the tele-ICU service. All critical care physician consultants from the consulting organization must be fully licensed to practice their specialty in the state or province where the receiving facility is located. In addition, the critical care consultants must be credentialed by the receiving hospital's medical staff office. Typical care providers at the receiving facility include hospitalists, advanced care practitioners, critical care nurses, respiratory therapist, and/or emergency room physicians. Health care providers participating in tele-ICU services should have the necessary orientation and education to ensure they possess necessary competencies in clinical care, communication, documentation, and safety protocols, consistent with the clinical environment encountered.

B. Technology

All components of tele-ICU technology must comply with federal and state regulations to protect personal privacy, confidentiality, and health care–related patient information. Consent for tele-ICU consultation should be included in the patient registration process at the consulting and receiving facility. Electronic and video connections between the two facilities should have multiple levels of security, and a firewall built for transmission of encrypted information. Providers at both institutions should have full access to the electronic heath record. The ideal hardware solution should be located on a mobile cart at the receiving facility. The institutional IT infrastructure on both ends must be committed to providing technical support for hardware and software.

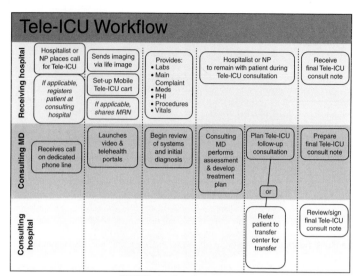

FIGURE 40.3 Tele-ICU workflow.

C. Patient Population
Tele-ICU services may be provided to all types of patients at the receiving hospital, regardless of status. The patient may be located in the ICU, on the general care unit, or the emergency room. Triage decisions—to transfer the patient to another hospital or not—are made during the tele-ICU consult. Figure 40.3 is a schematic representation of the organizational flow required to set up tele-ICU services.

IV. TELE-ICU OUTCOMES AND QUALITY METRICS
There are many reports in the literature documenting significant positive impact on outcomes of critically ill patients using intensivist-supported tele-ICU service. Two recent meta-analyses concluded lower ICU mortality after implementation of tele-ICU service, although the topic remains somewhat controversial as benefit of tele-ICU-based care is dependent on both the patient phenotype and care environment. Besides the reported benefit to mortality, tele-ICU has been shown to improve adherence to best practices, decreased medication errors, and foster early intervention and consultation by providing additional provider resources for critical care access. Additional potential benefits of implementing tele-ICU include decreased length of stay in ICU, cost savings from decreases in transportation costs, and improved patient and family satisfaction with care provided "close to home" (avoiding unnecessary transfers). In addition to standard ICU value measures, quality metrics for tele-ICU service should also include the number of consults performed and transfer data, patient and family acceptance of tele-ICU services, consultant provider response time, quality of audio and video transmissions, and reasons for patient transfers and their attendant costs.

V. BARRIERS AND CHALLENGES TO TELE-ICU

Several barriers to adoption of tele-ICU technology have been identified. The startup costs, both in terms of financial and human capitol, may be substantial. This is particularly true if a large number of ICU beds in different locations require tele-ICU coverage. In addition, lack of provider experience with communication technology or unwillingness to change practice patterns and processes of care are major barriers to adoption of tele-ICU technology. A range of options are available, from built-in, fixed systems for each bed added to existing hospital IT infrastructure (more expensive) to stand-alone, mobile carts using out-of-the-box computer video software and wireless communications (less expensive). Finally, many third-party payers (insurance agencies) provide little to no reimbursement for tele-ICU services, although the evidence for improved value is motivating change.

VI. SUMMARY

Tele-ICU services can accomplishes the "triple aims" of reducing costs, improving access to and quality of care, and improving patient and family experiences, especially in rural areas. Despite the challenges described, tele-ICU is here to stay and is expected to expand as health care shifts from volume-based care to value-based care for population management. In addition to tele-ICU, telemedicine has been successfully applied in radiology, emergency medicine, psychiatry, pain medicine, neurology, and dermatology. Many wearable sensors and alert systems report and store patient data providing insight to changes in their health status. At-home monitoring technology helps avert hospital (re-)admissions by allowing clinicians to keep close watch on patients with chronic health conditions such as diabetes mellitus, renal, lung, and cardiac diseases after they are discharged from home. Lessons learned in these environments will drive in-patient telemedicine innovations and close gaps in patient information, improving continuity of care across the spectrum, from prehospital to rehabilitation.

Selected Readings

American Telemedicine Association. http://www.atmeda.org. Accessed May 22, 2015.

Breslow MJ, Rosenfeld BA, Doerfler M, et al. Effect of a multiple-site intensive care unit telemedicine program on clinical and economic outcomes: an alternative paradigm for intensivist staffing. *Crit Care Med* 2004;32:31–38.

Duke E. The critical care workforce: a study of the supply and demand for critical care physicians. Rockville: Health Resources and Services Administration, 2006. http://bhpr.hrsa.gov/healthworkforce/reports/studycriticalcarephys.pdf. Accessed May 23, 2015.

Goran S. A new view: tele-intensive care unit competencies. *Crit Care Nurse* 2011;31(5)17–29.

Grundt BL, Jones PK, Lovitt A. Telemedicine in critical care: problems in design, implementation, and assessment. *Crit Care Med* 1982;10:471–475.

Kohl B, Gutsche J, Kim P, et al. Effect of telemedicine on mortality and length of stay in a university ICU. *Crit Care Med* 2007;35(12):A22.

O'Reilly KB. Tele-ICU technology improves patient outcomes, study finds. American Medical News, May 30, 2011. http://amednews.com/article/20110530/profession/305309936/7/. Accessed May 23, 2015.

Reynolds HN, Rogove H, Bander J, et al. Working lexicon for the tele-intensive care unit: we need to define for the tele-intensive care unit to grow and understand it. *Telemed J E Health* 2011;17:773–783.

Rogove H. How to develop tele-ICU model? *Crit Care Nurse Q* 2012;35:357–363.

Rosenfeld BA, Dorman T, Breslow MJ, et al. ICU telemedicine: alternative paradigm for providing continuous intensivist care. *Crit Care Med* 2000;28:1–7.

Rosenfeld BA, Dorman T, Breslow MJ, et al. Intensive care unit telemedicine: alternate paradigm for providing continuous intensivist care. *Crit Care Med* 2000;28:3925–3931.

Shaffer JP, Breslow MJ, Johnson JW, et al. Remote ICU management improves outcomes in patients with cardio-pulmonary arrest. *Crit Care Med* 2005;33(12):A5.

Wilcox ME, Adhikari NK. The effect of telemedicine in critically ill patients: systematic review and meta-analysis. *Crit Care* 2012;16(4):R127.

Yeo W, Grass-Ahrens SL, Wright T. A new era in the ICU: the case for telemedicine. *Crit Care Nurse Q* 2012;35:316–321.

Young LB, Chan PS, Lu X, et al. Impact of telemedicine intensive care unit coverage on patient outcomes: a systematic review and meta-analysis. *Arch Intern Med* 2011;171(6): 498–506.

Zawada ET, Herr P, Larson D, et al. Impact of an intensive care unit telemedicine program on a rural health care system. *Postgrad Med* 2009;121:160–170.

Quality Improvement and Standardization of Practice

Jessica Hahn and Brian M. Cummings

I. QUALITY IMPROVEMENT (QI)

A. **Background:** The current health care environment places increasing emphasis on improving the quality of medical care. Almost half of patients do not receive recommended care while hospitalized, for a variety of reasons. The complexities of care present in the critical care environment make it particularly prone to medical error, and the patient population is particularly susceptible to experiencing morbidities related to their hospitalization. With better clinical studies, process improvement, and focus on quality and safety, ICU mortality rates [in the U.S.?] have decreased 35% between 1988 and 2012, despite an increase in age and severity of illness in the ICU population. Ensuring that all patients receive the best evidence-based treatment, proactively preventing morbidity and eliminating the occurrence of medical errors is the goal of all quality programs. Delivering safe, high-quality care remains a moral imperative: Do No Harm.

B. **Definition of Quality Care:** The Institute of Medicine (IOM) has benchmarked quality care using six metrics: care that is safe, timely, effective, efficient, equitable, and patient centered.

C. **Financial Implications:** Reimbursement for care is increasingly linked to performance, as measured by quality metrics and the prevention of patient harm. For example, Medicare no longer reimburses hospitals for certain preventable, hospital-acquired infections. Financial incentives are now a tool to enforce desired behavior and decrease unwanted practice variance.

D. **Components.** There are three standard quality of care components: structure, process, and outcome.

   1. **Structure.** The structure of intensive care units varies between individual units, hospitals, and regions. Elements of the structure of an intensive care unit include the training and experience of care providers, staffing organization, and the diagnostic and treatment technology available. Changing unit structure is challenging and requires coordination with hospital and health care system infrastructure. There are insufficient data to recommend which of many existing models is best.

   2. **Process.** Process refers to both the actual care provided to patients (and how well this care complies with best practices) as well as certain nonclinical issues that may have an indirect effect on patient care. Examples of processes of care including number of patients utilizing a central line as well as use of a checklist for line placement. Hundreds of process studies are published annually to guide consensus on ICU best practice.

   3. **Outcome.** Outcome refers to the results realized and has been the traditional metric to judge performance of critical care clinicians and researchers. The usual benchmark is 28-day, risk-adjusted mortality. Length of stay, hospital-acquired infections, and quality-adjusted life years (QALY) serve as other outcome measure in clinical trials. However, advances in patient- and family-centered ICU care increasingly

argue for use of patient-related outcome measures (PROMs), such as early, full functional recovery and return to work.

   4. **Focus on Process in QI.** While we should continue to address outcome measures, quality improvement that focuses on process has certain advantages. In addressing the process, we can concentrate on different aspects of care, there is less need for risk adjustment as with outcome measures, sample sizes are smaller, and less time is needed to acquire results. Additionally, it can provide direct feedback to providers. Regardless, the quality measures we use should be meaningful, scientifically sound, generalizable, and interpretable.

E. **Leadership and Culture**: For any quality effort to take hold, there must be an enthusiastic and motivated core of people dedicated to the hard work of sustained improvement. In the ICU, this requires a multidisciplinary team that has insight into many different facets of care. A leader in quality improvement needs to be amenable to change, able to foster a culture of safety, and willing to resist the argument "because we've always done it that way." An environment that fosters the "ground" team at the point of care is critical to understand issues and implement improvement process. Improving the safety culture may be needed before any improvement project is undertaken; there are various measures to assess the safety climate of a unit.

F. **Model for Approaching Quality Improvement.** The Institute for Healthcare Improvement (IHI) recommends a model for improvement developed by the Associates in Process Improvement (see Fig. 41.1).

   1. **Formulate the right questions.** As seen in the Figure, three fundamental questions are used to focus the quality improvement effort, moving from a general concept to a specific target.

   2. **Target measure and goal.** The target measure must be carefully defined and should use discrete, measurable components. The ability to quantify the target measure should be easily extracted from existing databases both to establish a baseline and to continue to monitor over time. A specific improvement goal should be explicitly stated.

   3. **Plan-Do-Study Act (PDSA cycle).** The PDSA cycle involves creating a course for change as well as methods for evaluating the impact of these changes. It is often initially instituted in a limited or test population. The first step is developing an approach to institute an improvement (Plan). The most effective process change strategies are tailored to the environment and the improvement they are hoping to create. They rely on audit and feedback of recent performance and are augmented by a variety of educational modalities including interactive teaching methods, brief informal discussion, and more structured lectures and dissemination of written information. After an intervention is initiated (Do), the results on the target measure should be evaluated (Study), as well as feedback as to what worked and what did not. This information should be incorporated into the improvement effort (Act) and the intervention modified appropriately, restarting the plan–do–study–act cycle. Once an intervention has been optimized, it should be expanded and more universally applied.

   4. **Impact of quality improvement:** The potential impact of a quality improvement effort can be measured in terms of five dimensions. As individual providers, hospitals, and health care systems institute quality improvement programs, they should address most, if not all, dimensions.

      a. **Reach**: How much of the target population participated?

      b. **Efficacy**: What is the success rate if implemented as intended?

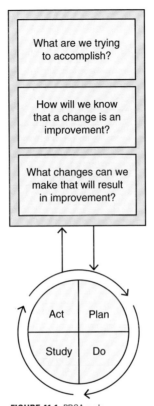

FIGURE 41.1 PDSA cycle.

     c. Adoption: What proportion of target institutions and practitioners adopt the intervention?

     d. Implementation: To what extent is it implemented as intended?

     e. Maintenance: How is the intervention sustained over time?

II. STANDARDIZATION

    A. Checklists. As the number of quality improvement initiatives increase, with both individual items and bundles, ensuring that each patient receives all appropriate interventions is increasingly a challenge. The use of a checklist, often incorporated as part of daily rounds, brings attention to these interventions and helps coordinate care. Checklists have been shown to increase implementation of best practices and are strongly associated with improved outcomes. Checklists may also be used to ensure that all best practice elements in a particular process are completed, like central line insertion. Figure 41.2 shows the central line insertion checklist at our hospital. Importantly, the existence of a checklist *per se* is not sufficient to insure quality care; in most studies, compliance rates reported in ICUs are low (30%–70%), indicating opportunities for improvement.

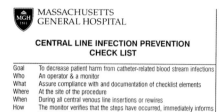

FIGURE 41.2 MGH Central Line Infection Prevention Checklist

B. Care Bundles: Care bundles are aggregated, evidence-based interventional practices that are designed to improve outcomes by delivering structured, measureable processes of care. They consist typically of three to six separate elements supported by evidence from clinical trials. These elements are more successful when implemented together than when used individually and should be delivered to every patient every time. Bundles should decrease unwanted practice variance while still allowing for individualized care when indicated.

1. **Compliance.** Measurement of compliance with bundles is integral to their success, and completion of a bundle is an all-or-nothing event. Bundles should be dynamic and evolve over time as new evidence changes best practice. The greatest effect on outcomes occurs when >90% bundle compliance is reached.

2. **Patient care.** Bundles have been shown to have success in reducing ventilator-associated pneumonia (VAP), reducing central line–associated blood stream infections (CLABSI), and improving the management of sepsis and septic shock. A new example is the ABCDE bundle, which links Awakening and Breathing Coordination of daily sedation and ventilator removal trials, Delirium monitoring and management, and Early exercise and mobility. ABCDE has been reported to minimizing sedative exposure, reducing duration of mechanical ventilation, and help manage ICU-acquired delirium and weakness (see Fig. 41.3). Patients cared for following implementation of this bundle spent 3 more days breathing without assistance, experienced less delirium, and were more likely to be mobilized in their ICU stay. There were no significant differences in self-extubation and reintubation rates.

3. Multiple examples of checklists and care bundles are provided under the section on quality metrics.

III. QUALITY METRICS, MORBIDITY, AND SAFETY IN THE ICU

   A. **Background.** The ICU is an high-stakes environment. Critical illness itself, the treatments we provide, and the methods of monitoring we use can each be associated with significant morbidity and mortality. Here we discuss some of the key elements to prevent ICU-related harm.

   B. **Central Line–Associated Bloodstream Infection (CLABSI).** ICU patients often require central venous access to allow for stability of access, the ability to deliver certain medications or nutrition (e.g., vasopressors, TPN), and central monitoring. However, these benefits are balanced by risks, including CLABSI and thrombus formation. The high attributable costs of CLABSI have led federal agencies to base a significant fraction of annual reimbursement on better outcomes (that is, low CLABSI rates compared with peer institutions).

   1. **Costs.** Estimates vary from $6,000 to $45,000 per CLABSI due to attributed costs of care related to central line infections, with annual health care costs exceeding $1 billion.

   2. **Prevention.** The most direct way to reduce the occurrence of CLABSI is to restrict line use and to remove the line as soon as is prudent.

   3. **Infectious sources.** Line contamination can occur at time of placement, either extraluminally or intraluminally. Therefore, strict sterile technique should be employed, using full-barrier precautions. Bacteria that enter extraluminally from the skin surface are often responsible for infections that occur with short-term use (3–7 days). Infection from intraluminal spread is increasingly being recognized as a continued cause of CLABSI, especially with longer term use (>7 days).

   4. **Central venous catheter (CVC) bundle of care.** Below are process of care recommendations for reduction of CLABSI. They are frequently included in bundles and checklists for insertion. Daily review of indications for catheter use is indicated.

      a. All associated equipment should be maintained in a central line cart.

      b. Educate health care personnel on insertion, care, and maintenance of CVCs, with periodic assessment of this knowledge.

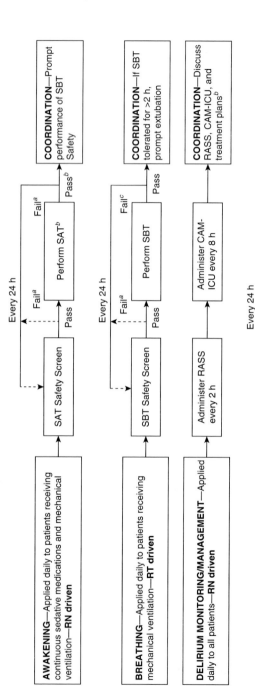

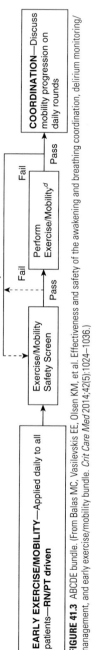

FIGURE 41.3 ABCDE bundle. (From Balas MC, Vasilevskis EE, Olsen KM, et al. Effectiveness and safety of the awakening and breathing coordination, delirium monitoring/management, and early exercise/mobility bundle. *Crit Care Med* 2014;42(5):1024–1036.)

[a]Continuous sedative medications maintained at previous rate if SAT safety screen failure. Mechanical ventilation continued, and continuous sedative medications restarted at half the previous dose only if needed due to SBT safety screen failure. [b]Continuous sedative infusions stopped, and sedative boluses held. Bolus doses of opioid medications allowed for pain. Continuous opioid infusions maintained only if needed for active pain. [c]Continuous sedative medications restarted at half the previous dose and then titrated to sedation target if SAT failed. Interdisciplinary team determines possible causes of SAT/SBT failure during rounds. Mechanical ventilation restarted at previous settings and continuous sedative medications restarted at half the previous dose only if needed if SBT failed. [d]SAT pass if the patient is able to open his/her eyes to verbal stimulation without failure criteria (regardless of trial length) or does not display any of the failure criteria after 4 hr of shutting off sedation.

    c. Perform hand hygiene prior to insertion and any manipulation of CVC.

    d. Wear cap, mask, gown, and sterile gloves for insertion.

    e. Use maximal sterile barrier precaution with drapes during CVC insertion.

    f. Avoid the femoral vein as an access site in adult patients if able.

    g. Use >0.5% chlorhexidine-based antiseptic skin preparation in patients >2 months old.

    h. Use ultrasound guidance to place catheters to reduce cannulation attempts and mechanical complications.

    i. Use a chlorhexidine-impregnated sponge dressing if CLABSI rates remain high despite implementation of other guidelines.

    j. Consider use of antimicrobial-impregnated catheters in high-risk populations or if CLABSI rates remain high despite instituting other guidelines.

    k. Disinfect catheter hubs, needleless connectors, and injection ports before accessing catheters.

    l. Change administrations sets used for blood, blood products, or fat emulsions every 24 hours. Change other continuous-use administration sets no more frequently than every 96 hours but at least every 7 days.

    m. Change dressings sterilely when soiled or loose, and at least every 7 days even if clean, dry, and intact.

    n. Remove catheter as soon as clinically able.

    o. Do not rewire lines if infection is the reason for a line change.

C. Catheter-Associated Urinary Tract Infection (CAUTI). Indwelling urinary catheters are frequently used in the ICU for monitoring and skin protection. However, like intravenous catheters, urinary catheters carry significant risk of infections, including UTI and urosepsis.

    1. Costs. The cost associated with CAUTI is significantly less than other health care–associated infections, approximately $750 per patient, which translates to $300 million annually in the United States. However, urinary catheters and the associated asymptomatic bacteriuria represent a significant reservoir for drug-resistant organisms. Like CLABSI, CAUTI rates are now monitored nationally and factor into pay for performance by federal agencies.

    2. Causes. Absence of sterile technique during insertion, retrograde flow of urine from urinary collection devices, and duration of catheter use all increase the risk for CAUTI and asymptomatic bacteriuria.

    3. Prevention and care bundle. Below are recommendations for avoiding CAUTI.

        a. Only use indwelling urinary catheters for appropriate indications.

            1. Acute urinary retention or bladder outlet obstruction

            2. Need for accurate measurement of urine output in critically ill, hemodynamically unstable patients

            3. Perioperative use for selected surgical procedures and/or epidural use

            4. To assist healing in sacral or perineal wounds in incontinent patients

            5. Patients requiring prolonged immobilization

            6. To improve comfort in end-of-life care

        b. Remove indwelling catheters as soon as clinically able (i.e., when initial indication is no longer present).

        c. Intermittent catheterization is preferable to indwelling catheters in patients with bladder-emptying dysfunction.

d. Perform hand hygiene immediately before and after inserting or manipulating indwelling urinary catheters.

e. Insert using aseptic technique and sterile equipment-sterile drapes, gloves, sponges, sterile antiseptic solution for periurethral cleaning, and single-use lubricant packets.

f. Properly secure catheters after insertion to prevent movement and urethral traction.

g. Maintain a closed drainage system and replace catheter and system if breaks occur.

h. Maintain unobstructed flow, avoiding kinks and keeping collecting bag below the level of the bladder at all times to avoid retrograde flow.

i. Bladder irrigation is not recommended, including routine irrigation with antimicrobials. If required due to obstruction, use closed continuous irrigation.

j. Use antimicrobial-impregnated catheters if CAUTI rates remain high despite implementing other guidelines. They may be helpful in at risk populations.

D. Ventilator-Associated Pneumonia (VAP) and Ventilator-Associated Events (VAE). All definitions of VAP combine three features of pulmonary infection in a mechanically ventilated patient: radiographic evidence, clinical signs, and laboratory and microbiologic results. Some of these data are subjective (e.g., new infiltrates on CXR) leading to variability in interpretation and weak interobserver concordance. Hence, the CDC recently released a new series of metrics on the basis of objective criteria. Events are now determined by changes in ventilator settings made by bedside clinicians to optimize patient status: VAE. Event triggers include infectious and noninfectious complications of mechanical ventilation, such as barotrauma, pulmonary embolus, ARDS, and pulmonary edema. There are three definition tiers within the VAE algorithm. The CDC offers examples and has a calculator on their website to help appropriately classify these events.

1. Ventilator-Associated Condition (VAC). The patient experiences worsening oxygenation following a period of stability or improvement on the ventilator (>2 calendar days of stable or decreasing daily minimum FIO_2 or PEEP values). Worsening oxygenation is defined as increase in daily minimum FIO_2 of >0.20 or daily minimum PEEP >3 cmH$_2$O.

2. Infection-Related Ventilator-Associated Complication (IVAC). After calendar day 3 of mechanical ventilation and within 2 calendar days before or after the onset of worsening oxygenation as in VAC, the patient has both (1) temperature >38°C or <36°C or WBC >12,000 or <4,000 cells/mm^3 AND (2) a new antimicrobial agent is started and continued for >4 calendar days.

3. Possible and Probable VAP. Both involve meeting the criteria for IVAC with additional requirements.

a. Possible VAP includes criteria for purulent respiratory secretions OR positive culture of sputum, endotracheal aspirate, bronchoalveolar lavage, lung tissue, or protected specimen brushing (culture of normal respiratory flora and certain other microorganisms excluded).

b. Probable VAP includes purulent respiratory secretions AND a positive culture (cannot be from sputum and there are minimum quantitative requirements with the same microorganism exclusions). Probable VAP is also diagnosed if criteria for IVAC are met and there is a positive pleural fluid culture, positive lung histopathology, positive diagnostic test for *Legionella*, or positive diagnostic test for

influenza virus, respiratory syncytial virus, adenovirus, parainfluenza virus, rhinovirus, human metapneumovirus, and coronavirus.
4. **Costs.** Ventilator-associated lung infection is associated with significant morbidity, including prolonged periods of mechanical ventilation, extended hospitalization, excess use of antimicrobial medications, and increased mortality. Health care costs are $14,000 to $29,000 per occurrence and about $1 billion annually.
5. **Risk factors.** Pneumonia risk factors include prolonged intubation, enteral feeding, witnessed aspiration, paralytic agents, underlying illness, and extremes of age. Pneumonia arises secondary to bacterial invasion of the formerly sterile lower respiratory tract from aspiration of secretions, colonization of the aerodigestive tract, or use of contaminated medications or equipment.
6. **Prevention and bundles of care.** Directed toward these sources of infection and risk factors, similar to preventing CLABSI and CAUTI
   a. Maintain hand hygiene.
   b. Minimize duration of ventilation.
      1. Use noninvasive ventilation to prevent intubation or to allow quicker extubation if indicated.
      2. Use daily assessment of readiness to wean.
   c. Prevent aspiration.
      1. Maintain in semirecumbent position (35°–45°).
      2. Avoid gastric overdistention.
      3. Avoid unplanned extubation and reintubation.
      4. Use cuffed endotracheal tube (with cuff maintained at 20 cmH$_2$O or less) with in-line or subglottic suctioning.
   d. Reduce colonization of aerodigestive tract.
      1. Orotracheal intubation is preferable to nasotracheal intubation.
      2. Avoid H$_2$-blocking agents or PPI in patients not at high risk for developing stress ulcers or stress gastritis.
      3. Perform regular oral care with an antiseptic solution; a chlorhexidine mouthwash or gel is the most studied.
   e. Minimize contamination of equipment.
      1. Use sterile water to rinse reusable ventilator equipment.
      2. Remove condensate from respiratory circuit, keeping circuit closed while removing condensate and avoiding retrograde flow of condensate.
      3. Change circuit only when visibly soiled or malfunctioning.
      4. Store and disinfect respiratory therapy equipment properly.

E. Deep Venous Thrombosis (DVT) and Thromboembolism
1. **Background.** Pulmonary embolus remains a significant proximal cause of morbidity and mortality among critically ill patients. Preventing the formation and mobilization of deep venous thrombi that can lead to pulmonary embolus is an important goal of critical care.
2. **Risk factors.** The risk of DVT and PE probably vary among the heterogeneous populations of ICUs but exists for all patients. Some proportion (2%–10%) of patients admitted to adult medical-surgical ICUs already have DVTs. An additional 10% to 30% of patients develop DVTs within the first 7 days of ICU admission.
3. **Medication thromboprophylaxis.** Unfractionated heparin thromboprophylaxis reduces acquired DVT rate by 50%. Low-molecular-weight heparin (LMWH) may have greater risk reduction of pulmonary embolus and DVT in some populations. The comparative bleeding risk is still being examined.

4. **Mechanical thromboprophylaxis.** Graduated compression stockings and pneumatic compression devices have not been as well studied in the ICU population, especially in comparison with heparin prophylaxis. Existing studies show mixed results with either no effect or up to 30% reduction in DVT risk. Mechanical devices should be utilized if there is a contraindication to medication-based prophylaxis, but should not be used as a substitute for heparin.

5. **Screening.** Periodic screening with venous ultrasound may be conducted for patients that have contraindications to anticoagulation and in high-risk populations (e.g., in patients with pelvic fractures and illness resulting in prolonged immobilization).

6. **High risk for thrombosis with heparin contraindications.** Inferior vena cava filters do not prevent DVT but may be considered to prevent pulmonary embolism.

F. **Stress Ulcer Prophylaxis**

1. **Background.** Gastrointestinal bleeding in critically ill patients has been documented since the 1800s. This is thought to be secondary to compromised mucosal perfusion and/or reperfusion injury that interfere with the normal protective mechanisms of the gastric mucosa. Endoscopic studies show that up to 75% to 100% of critically ill patients have gross gastric lesions in the first 1 to 3 days of illness. Determining the incidence and prevalence of clinically significant bleeding is a little more difficult to quantify; however, it is likely to be in the range of 1.5% to 4% of critically ill patients. The relative risk of mortality is approximately two to four times compared with those without clinically significant bleeding, controlling for other factors.

2. **Risk factors.** Includes respiratory failure, acute hepatic failure, coagulopathy, hypotension, chronic renal failure, prolonged duration of NG tube, history of alcohol abuse, sepsis, *Helicobactor pylori*, IgA >1.

3. **Prevention.** To reduce morbidity and mortality, a variety of acid suppressors and mucosal protectants have been utilized. These include histamine 2 receptor antagonists (H2RA), proton pump inhibitors (PPIs), misoprostal, sucrafalate, and antacids. PPIs allow greater acid suppression compared with H2RA and may provide better reduction in gastric bleeding. Additionally, there may be rapid development of tolerance to H2RA. However, the risks of acid suppression include increased rates of hospital-acquired infections, including VAP and *Clostridium difficile* infection. Small studies have suggested decreased gastrointestinal bleeding with acid suppression, but there are no high-quality data to reliably identify optimal therapy with minimal risk. Early enteral nutrition may help minimize gastric ulceration and reduce the risk of bleeding. More information on which patients should receive stress ulcer prophylaxis, which agents should be used, and how enteral feedings change these recommendations will hopefully be provided with future studies.

IV. **INFECTION CONTROL AND THE ICU**

A. **Background:** As noted above, hospital-acquired infection (HAI) is a potentially preventable, serious complication in ICU patients. These are associated with statistically significant worsening of important ICU quality measures, including morbidity, mortality, length of stay, and costs of care. An important element of delivering quality care is prevention of these infections and further transmission.

B. **Transmission.** Transmission of infection requires three elements: a source or reservoir of infectious agents, a susceptible host with a portal of entry the infectious agent can access, and a mode of transmission for the agent. Patients admitted to the ICU are at particular risk for the acquisition of new infections while in the hospital. Critical illness itself increases susceptibility to new infections due to "immune paralysis" secondary to lymphocyte depletion and down-regulation of adaptive immunity. Additionally, many ICU patients have underlying risk factors for infection, such as extremes of age, diabetes, malignancy, and drug-induced immunosuppression. Medications delivered in the ICU such as antibiotics, gastric acid suppressants, and corticosteroids alter the patient's normal microbial flora and responses to microbes. Lastly, many devices used to monitor or treat patients breach the natural barriers to infection, including skin and mucosal surfaces, creating ports of entry for infectious agents. The source of the infectious agent transmission is usually other people (health care workers, other patients, visitors, etc.). Health care providers are regularly exposed to multiple sources of infection; hence, strict hygiene is paramount, as described below. Physical elements of the hospital environment may also participate in the transmission of infections and are minimized by contemporary methods of room cleaning and disinfection.

C. Standard Precautions
   1. **Background**. Standard infectious precautions should be used with all patient interactions. They are based on the principle that all blood, body fluids, secretions, excretions (except sweat), nonintact skin, and mucous membranes may contain transmissible infectious agents.
   2. **Standard precautions include the following:**
      a. **Hand hygiene:** Use of alcohol-based products or washing with soap or water after any contact with body fluids, after removing gloves, and between all patient contacts (that is, before entering and upon exiting each patient's room).
      b. **Personal protective equipment (PPE)**
         1. **Nonsterile gloves:** When touching body fluids, any mucous membrane, or nonintact skin
         2. **Nonsterile gown:** Wear a single-use impermeable gown during procedures and during any patient interaction in which clothing or exposed skin may contact patient body fluids, mucous membranes, or nonintact skin.
         3. **Mask, eye protection (goggles), or face shield:** Wear during procedures and patient care activities that may generate a splash or spray of blood, body fluid, secretion, or excretion.
   3. **Environmental surfaces and devices:** Soiled patient care equipment is handled with gloves or other PPE until appropriately discarded or cleaned, followed by hand hygiene. Environmental surfaces are routinely cleaned and disinfected. Laundry and textiles are handled to prevent transmission of infection.
   4. **Sharps injury prevention**
      a. **Background:** Injuries from needles and other sharps have been associated with the transmission of HBV, HCV, and HIV to health care providers. Direct costs associated with sharp injuries range from $71 to $5,000 per incident. Six devices cause nearly 80% of injuries: disposable syringes, suture needles, winged steel needles, scalpel blades, IV catheter stylets, and phlebotomy needles. In one study, 56% of sharp injuries occur with hollow bore needles, which are associated with the highest likelihood of HIV transmission to health care workers. Safe handling of these devices is an essential

element of standard precautions. Hospital sharp injury prevention programs typically include a well-defined process for reporting sharps injuries as well as providing evaluation and potential infection prophylaxis for health care workers following a sharp injury. Education and intervention should be targeted to areas with prior incidents as well as those at high risk (e.g., emergency and operating rooms).

b. Injury prevention strategies
   1. Use needleless systems and devices when able.
   2. Use needles and sharps engineered with safety devices.
   3. During procedures,
       a. the user of the sharp should be in control of its location and ensure that others are aware a sharp is in use
       b. use instruments, not fingers, to grasp needles, retract tissues, and load/unload needles and scalpels
       c. do not directly pass sharps to another person; instead pass through a preidentified neutral zone
   4. Avoid recapping needles and if necessary do so using a one-handed technique.
   5. Avoid leaving sharps with sharp end exposed.
c. Ensure all sharps are appropriately disposed of immediately in designated and marked disposal containers.

D. Transmission-Based Precautions: These precautions are utilized when a specific infectious etiology is known or suspected. They are based on how that microorganism may be transmitted. They are used, singly or in combination, in addition to standard precautions.

1. Contact transmission and precautions:
   a. Contact transmission can be separated into two types:
       1. Direct contract transmission occurs when microorganisms are transferred from one infected person to another, without an intermediate object or person. It includes passage of infectious agents through blood or body fluid that contacts mucous membranes or nonintact skin or transfer from skin to skin.
       2. Indirect contact transmission involves transfer of an infectious agent using another person or object as an intermediary. It includes transfer by nondisinfected hands of health care professionals, common patient care devices or toys, or improperly sterilized surgical equipment.
   b. Contact precautions are utilized with a variety of conditions that are usually spread via direct contact transmission. These include infectious agents such as MRSA, RSV, parainfluenza, lice, rotavirus, vancomycin-resistant enterococcus and *Clostridium difficile*. They are also utilized with wound drainage or other excessive amounts of body fluid.
   c. Health care professionals should wear gown and gloves with all interactions with patients on contact precautions to prevent exposure from patients or their environment.
   d. Patients should be placed in single rooms or cohorted with other patients infected with the same microorganism.

2. Droplet transmission and precautions. Microorganisms that are transferred by droplet transmission travel in droplets directly from the infected person's respiratory tract to another person's susceptible mucosal surfaces over short distances (approx. 3 ft). They may also be transferred by contact transmission.

    a. Infectious agents transmitted by droplet include *Bordatella pertussis*, influenza virus, adenovirus, rhinovirus, *Mycoplasma pneumonia*, group A strep, and *Neisseria meningitidis*.

    b. Health care professionals should wear a mask, usually in addition to contact precaution gear, when interacting with patients on droplet precautions.

    c. Patients should be placed in private rooms and wear masks when outside the room.

  3. **Airborne transmission and precautions**: Airborne transmission occurs by airborne droplet nuclei and small particles that remain infective over time and distance. They may traverse large distances and infect people who have not been in the same room with the patient.

    a. Infectious agents transmitted by the airborne route include *Mycobacterium tuberculosis*, *Varicella zoster*, and rubeola.

    b. Health care professionals should wear an N95 mask or respirator during all interactions with the patient.

    c. The patient should be placed in a private isolation room with special ventilator capacity ("negative pressure room") that allows 12 air exchanges per hour. The patient should wear a mask whenever out of the isolation room.

E. **Infection Control Surveillance Programs**

  1. It is essential for ICUs to have real-time tracking of hospital-acquired infections to prevent further morbidity and mortality. A close working relationship with the hospital's infection control staff is very helpful.

  2. Weekly or monthly reports should be displayed for staff to promote accountability and a culture of safety. Practices adopted from industry such as prominent displays of "weeks from last infection," for example, are effective and increasingly popular.

Selected Readings

Alhazzani W, Lim W, Jaeschke RZ, et al. Heparin thromboprophylaxis in medical-surgical critically ill patients: a systematic review and meta-analysis of randomized trials. *Crit Care Med* 2013;41:2088–2098.

Attia J, Ray JG, Cook DJ, et al. Deep vein thrombosis and its prevention in critically ill adults. *Arch Intern Med* 2001;161:1268–1279.

Balas MC, Vasilevskis EE, Olsen KM, et al. Effectiveness and safety of the awakening and breathing coordination, delirium monitoring/management, and early exercise/mobility bundle. *Crit Care Med* 2014;42(5):1024–1036.

Byrnes MC, Schuerer DJE, Schallom ME, et al. Implementation of a mandatory checklist of protocols and objectives improves compliance with a wide range of evidence-based intensive care unit practices. *Crit Care Med* 2009;37(10):2775–2781.

Centers for Disease Control and Prevention. Ventilator-associated event protocol. http://www.cdc.gov/nhsn/acute-care-hospital/vae/. Accessed June 17, 2015.

Centers for Disease Control and Prevention. Workbook for designing, implementing, and evaluating a sharp injury prevention program. http://www.cdc.gov/sharpssafety/pdf/sharpsworkbook_2008.pdf. Accessed June 17, 2015.

Chenoweth C, Saint S. Preventing catheter-associated urinary tract infections in the intensive care unit. *Crit Care Clin* 2013;29:19–32.

Coffin SE, Klompas M, Classen D, et al. Strategies to prevent ventilator-associated pneumonia in acute care hospitals. *Infect Control Hosp Epidemiol* 2008;29(S1):S31–S40.

Cook DJ, Crowther M. Thromboprophylaxis in the intensive care unit: focus on medical-surgical patients. *Crit Care Med* 2010;38(suppl):S76–S82.

Cook D, Crowther M, Meade M, et al. Deep venous thrombosis in medical-surgical critically ill patients: prevalence, incidence, and risk factors. *Crit Care Med* 2005;33(7):1565–1571.

Curtis JR, Cook DJ, Wall RJ, et al. Intensive care unit quality improvement: a "how-to" guide for the interdisciplinary team. *Crit Care Med* 2006;34:211–218.

Gould CV, Umscheid CA, Agarwal RK, et al. Guideline for prevention of catheter-associated urinary tract infections 2009. *Infect Control Hosp Epidemiol* 2010;31(4):319–326.

Langley GL, Moen R, Nolan KM, et al. *The improvement guide: a practical approach to enhancing organizational performance.* 2nd ed. San Francisco: Jossey-Bass, 2009.

Marik PE, Vasu T, Hirani A, et al. Stress ulcer prophylaxis in the new millennium: a systematic review and meta-analysis. *Crit Care Med* 2010;38:2222–2228.

Marwick C, Davay P. Care bundles: the holy grail of infectious risk management in hospital? *Curr Opin Infect Dis* 2009;22:364–369.

Miller SE, Maragakis LL. Central line-associated bloodstream infection prevention. *Curr Opin Infect Dis* 2012;25:412–422.

Mietto C, Pinciroli R, Patel N, et al. Ventilator associated pneumonia. Evolving definitions and preventive strategies. *Respir Care* 2013;58(6):990–1003.

Morandi A, Brummel NE, Ely EW. Sedation, delirium and mechanical ventilation: the 'ABCDE' approach. *Curr Opin Crit Care* 2011;17:43–49.

O'Grady NP, Alexander M, Burns LA, et al. Guidelines for the prevention of intravascular catheter-related infections. *Am J Infect Control* 2011;39(4, suppl 1):S1–34.

Rossi PJ, Edmiston CE. Patient safety in the critical care environment. *Surg Clin N Am* 2012;92:1369–1386.

Sagana R, Hyzy RC. Achieving zero central line-associated bloodstream infection rates in your intensive care unit. *Crit Care Clin* 2013;29:1–9.

Siegel JD, Rhinehart E, Jackson M, et al. 2007 guideline for isolation precautions: preventing transmission of infectious agents in health care settings. *Am J Infect Control* 2007;35(10, suppl 2):S65–S164.

Tambyah PA, Oon J. Catheter-associated urinary tract infection. *Curr Opin Infect Dis* 2012;25:365–370.

Tauseef A, Harty R. Stress-induced ulcer bleeding in critically ill patients. *Gastroenterol Clin N Am* 2009;38:245–265.

Zimlichman MD, Henderson D, Tamir O, et al. Health care-associated infections: a meta-analysis of costs and financial impact on the US health care system. *JAMA Intern Med* 2013;173(22):2039–2046.

Zimmerman JE, Kramer AA, Knaus WA. Changes in hospital mortality for United States intensive care unit admissions from 1988 to 2012. *Crit Care* 2013;17:R81.

Ethical and Legal Issues in ICU Practice

Alexandra F. M. Cist, Rebecca I. Kalman, and Sharon Brackett

I. INTRODUCTION

In caring for critically ill patients, it is inevitable that ethical issues will arise. Patients often have complex medical conditions, multiple providers, and uncertain prognosis or treatment plans. This can lead to **conflict and moral distress** among patients, family, health care providers, and support staff. We describe a **proactive approach** to ethical issues in the ICU. Adoption and adaptation of these measures may help minimize conflict and moral distress. Key **ethical concepts** and **practical guidelines** are provided in order to optimize care in a variety of circumstances in which ethical tensions may arise because of conflicts over values or decision-making authority. It is hoped that you will build trust and connect with your patients and their families through empathy, seeking to understand them, confronting (rather than avoiding) problems, managing expectations well, and providing optimal clinical care.

II. PROACTIVE APPROACH

A. A proactive approach to ethical issues in the ICU can minimize conflict and moral distress. Conflict is common in the ICU and is considered to be dangerous or harmful. Yet, 70% of conflicts are perceived to be preventable. Conflicts arise within teams and between staff and families. Disagreements regarding value-laden clinical decisions may be exacerbated by interpersonal tension, poor communication, mistrust, and difficult end-of-life care. The costs of unreconciled conflict are high and include misguided treatment, moral distress, staff burnout, and high job turnover. Such poor outcomes should be prevented with proactive measures designed to enhance collaborative shared decision making (see Table 42.1).

B. In these days of a heightened focus on **organ systems,** numbers, monitoring, and computer-based documentation, humanizing the ICU experience—for patients, family, and staff—can be challenging. Yet it is a worthy endeavor. Burnout, as mentioned above, is a consequence of unreconciled conflict. The characteristics of burnout include a detached or dehumanizing attitude and a lack of concern for others. But the essence of ethical care involves an engaged and person-focused attitude and an abundant concern for others (patients and staff). Measures to avoid burnout and promote personalized care should be taken, such as those listed in Table 42.1.

C. Another step we have taken in our ICUs is the use of Get to Know Me posters (Fig. 42.1). These 20 × 24 inch posters in the patient's ICU rooms are filled in by the families as an opportunity for the team to get to know the patient better. The information provided by the family serves to connect the team to the (usually) voiceless patient. The interaction also helps the team develop rapport with and empathize with the family. ICU families are often under a great deal of stress—trying to maintain their home responsibilities and roles while adjusting to the ICU experience.

TABLE 42.1 Proactive Measures to Minimize Moral Distress and ICU Conflict

ICU open visitation hours
Allowing family presence during rounds
Routine proactive family meetings
Process of informed consent
Relieving patients' distressing symptoms
Sensitivity to and respect for cultural norms
Provision of spiritual support
Interdisciplinary collaborative care
Team debriefings
Ethics rounds
ICU staff meetings
Ethics consultation
Integration of palliative care principles and practices into the ICU

Get to Know Me ...

NAME: _____

I LIKE TO BE CALLED: _____
OCCUPATION: _____
IMPORTANT PEOPLE (FAMILY AND FRIENDS):
_____
_____
_____

FAVORITES
MOVIE: _____
TV SHOW: _____
BOOK: _____
MUSIC: _____
SPORT: _____
COLOR: _____
FOODS: _____
ACTIVITIES/HOBBIES: _____
QUOTE OR SAYING:
_____
_____

PETS TOO!: _____

AT HOME I USE:
☐ GLASSES   ☐ CONTACT LENSES
☐ HEARING AID   ☐ DENTURES
OTHER: _____

I UNDERSTAND INFORMATION BEST WHEN:
_____

ACHIEVEMENTS OF WHICH I AM PROUD:
_____

THINGS THAT STRESS ME OUT:
_____

THINGS THAT CHEER ME UP:
_____

OTHER THINGS I'D LIKE YOU TO KNOW ABOUT ME:
_____
_____
_____
_____

PHOTOS

FIGURE 42.1 Get to Know Me Posters. These 20 × 24 inch posters in the patient's ICU rooms are filled in by the families as an opportunity for the team to get to know the patient better.

Family members engage in multiple roles in the ICU: active presence, patient protector, facilitator, historian, coach, and caregiver. As team and family get to know each other, thus begins the process of **substituted judgment**: an aspect of shared decision making in which the surrogates speak the patient's voice.

D. Many ICUs are opening up visiting hours and allowing family to be present during ICU work rounds. Simple guidelines for making this work include inviting the family to rounds, making brief introductions, apologizing for medical jargon and offering to "translate" later, and inviting interruptions for errors; allow a short period for questions at the end of rounds and more private time later. The opportunity to observe the "work" of rounds and the transparency of communication help build trust and mutual respect. This also can increase the efficiency of communicating with families.

E. The structure and functioning of your ICU team may influence the prevalence of conflict in your ICU and how it is handled. How well do nurses, physicians, medical students, social workers, chaplains, physical and respiratory therapists, and other health professionals interact—among themselves and with families? Do you hold team debriefings after critical incidents, bad deaths, or great successes? Are work rounds interdisciplinary and collaborative? Do you hold ICU staff meetings and retreats to review educational content, your mission, and goals? Improving your ICU functioning is another means of optimizing the decision-making process that leads to optimal delivery of care.

III. TREATMENT DECISIONS

A. When there is conflict over value-laden clinical concerns, an optimal decision-making process is one that is fair, transparent, respectful, collaborative, and effective. Within some teams, there can be a diffusion of responsibility, such that the locus of decision-making authority becomes difficult to identify. In other teams, there might be a top-down authoritative approach in which some team or family members feel voiceless and powerless. Moral distress arises when persons feel powerless to alter what they perceive to be suboptimal care. And yet, regardless of the team structure, each member of the team is a moral agent and should possess some degree of moral accountability for the decisions made and actions taken. A shared decision-making paradigm locates the responsibility between the patient (or surrogate) and the clinicians, thus aiming to respect patient autonomy and the beneficent intentions of caregivers.

B. Communication is the key to the shared decision-making process. Good communication allows the clinicians to learn about the patient's values and goals and allows the patient/surrogate to learn about the clinical condition and which interventions are considered reasonable to use (after review of the patient's values and goals). The process is dynamic and allows for reassessment and adjustment of plans, on the basis of the patient's evolving condition and goals. The attending physician has the ultimate responsibility in deciding on a reasonable clinical plan.

C. Key ethical tenets come into play on a daily basis in the ICU. These include
  1. Autonomy—the right to self-govern
  2. Beneficence—the obligation to promote good and prevent/remove harm
  3. Nonmaleficence—the need to refrain from inflicting harm
  4. Justice—an allocation principle, striving for fair distribution of resources

D. Patient autonomy, the respect for an individual patient's right to make decisions about his or her own medical care, is a highly valued ethical principal in the United States. Ideally, autonomy is preserved by involving the patient in the decision-making process.

E. Informed consent preserves patient autonomy and is an ethical responsibility of the treating physician. The process of informed consent involves a dialogue between patient and health care provider(s) describing the risks/benefits of the proposed intervention as well as the pertinent alternative treatment options. Informed consent should be obtained for most procedures, therapies, and research. There are certain situations in which the informed consent process can be waived. These include emergency situations, situations in which a patient or state waiver is in place, and situations in which the patient does not have the capacity to consent (and, no surrogate is available).

F. Competent patients are able to accept and refuse medical treatments. Competence is a legal term. Individuals above the age of 18 are presumed competent unless deemed incompetent by a court previously. Decision-making capacity is a medical term. If a patient's capacity to make decisions is questioned, then a physician should evaluate the patient to determine their ability to receive and understand medical information, differentiate between options presented, and choose a course of action on the basis of the information offered.

G. In the ICU, patients often lack decision-making capacity due to illness or medication effects. In these situations a surrogate, typically a family member or health care agent, should make decisions under the principle of substituted judgment. The role of a surrogate is to make the decision that the patient would make in the given situation. This may differ from what the surrogate wants for the patient and even from what the surrogate would want for him- or herself in the same situation.

H. The patient may have prepared a document to help guide decision making in the case that the patient is unable to make decisions for him- or herself. For patients with chronic illness, discussions regarding advanced care planning should start in the outpatient setting, prior to ICU admission. This allows more time to assess the patient's understanding of their illness, clarify goals and values, and discuss reasonable clinical goals.

   1. An advanced directive is a statement specifying a patient's wishes that is designed to help guide decision making in these situations. Advance directives vary from state to state and even from institution to institution. It has been recognized that advance directives may be verbal in nature and that conversations between the patient and their loved ones may provide an acceptable framework to guide decisions.

   2. A health care proxy or durable power of attorney is a legal document prepared by the patient appointing the person they wish to make health care decisions in their place in case they are unable to make decisions themselves.

   3. A living will is a document describing therapies or interventions that the patient would wish to receive or refuse under specific circumstances. These documents often cover broad circumstances such as "persistent vegetative state" or "without meaningful recovery" and often do not apply to the nuanced situations that arise in the context of complex critical illness. Thus, these documents are often only marginally helpful and must be supplemented by communication with those close to the patient.

I. In some cases, a surrogate decision maker cannot be located for a patient. In these situations, as much information about the patient should be gathered as possible from friends, family, colleagues, primary care providers, and so forth. The patient's lifestyle and values should be taken into account to approximate a substituted judgment. In some cases, such as those where conflict has arisen regarding surrogacy, a legal guardian may be appointed to serve as a surrogate decision maker.

J. The need to perform life-saving procedures can often present suddenly in the intensive care unit, and obtaining informed consent from a surrogate may delay potential life-saving interventions. For this reason, some ICUs have implemented a **bundled** or **universal consent form**. These forms often include commonly performed procedures that may be urgent in nature such as intubation, central line placement, chest tube placement, blood transfusion, and the like.

   1. This type of bundled consent can serve as efficient way to educate patients and surrogates at the beginning of an ICU stay. It can also serve as opportunity to begin discussions regarding patient wishes and goals in the context of their current illness.

   2. However, it is possible that presenting such a complex picture early on in treatment may be overwhelming and confusing to patients and families. They may feel pressured to consent for fear that treatments will be withheld in the future.

IV. THE FAMILY MEETING

A. Family meetings are one of the most effective means to achieve shared decision making. They can also help prevent or manage conflict that arises around decision making. Think of the meeting as being like *a procedure*—with its own set of skills to master. There are organizational, communication, and emotional skills to muster in order to conduct an effective meeting. As with any procedure, preparation, performance, and follow-up are key components of the family meeting (see Table 42.2).

B. **Preparation:** Hold a premeeting staff "huddle" to assure consensus on facts; identify areas of uncertainty, conflict, or psychosocial concern; discuss agenda and goals; and identify suitable meeting facilitator, time, and location. Assure multidisciplinary staff participation (attending physician, nurse, possibly social work, chaplain, and others). Allow for adequate family/surrogate representation. Include the bedside nurse, since he or she spends the most time at the bedside and spends more time with visiting family members. He or she knows the patient's burden of care best and can communicate to family the patient's ups and downs. Since RNs

TABLE 42.2   Guide to ICU Family Meetings

1. Prepare agenda and setting
      Assure team consensus on facts
      Decide who comes to the meeting and who leads the discussion
2. Introduce participants
3. Assess patient/family understanding of the patient's prior and current circumstances and what they want to know
4. Summarize the patient's medical condition and key clinical decisions
5. What is it like for the patient now?
6. What was the patient like?
      What would the patient want in such circumstances = *substituted judgment*
7. Explore and address family fears and concerns
8. Frame recommendations
9. Plan for follow-up
10. Document meeting and communicate content to team

cover 24/7, they can provide cross-shift communication of goals of care (GOC) and treatment plans.

C. Introductions—of participants and the purpose of meeting: Invite individuals to give their name and relationship to the patient. Identify the patient's surrogate spokesperson. Politely establish a tone of courtesy and confidentiality. Clarify the broad purpose of the meeting: to identify reasonable goals and plans aligned with the patient's values, beliefs, and preferences.

D. Note, in particular, the order of steps 3 and 4 (as presented in Table 42.2): The family gets to provide their summary before the team launches into a clinical summary. This order (rather than the other way around) demonstrates respect for the patient's preferences by giving the patient/family the first opportunity to describe the situation, helps establish rapport, allows the team to learn more about the patient's illness trajectory and the family's perspectives and values, and allows the team to discern what knowledge gaps they need to address. We all have different communication styles—team and family members alike—so, listening to the family first affords insight into how *this* family communicates and their relational dynamics.

E. Steps 5, 6, and 7 deepen the opportunities to learn about *this* patient, his or her condition, and his or her preferences under such circumstances. It is the surrogate's privilege and responsibility to express the patient's voice—the patient's substituted judgment. Exploring the family's fears and concerns uncovers opportunities to manage expectations and to provide psychosocial support for realistic hopes and fears—or to provide correction for unrealistic ones.

F. After these steps have unfolded, the leading clinician can then frame recommendations (step 8) on the basis of the clinical details and the patient's values and goals. This might be introduced with the words, "In light of what we've discussed today, I recommend...." What follows is a recommendation based on the team's clinical expertise in conjunction with its understanding of the patient's goals and values. If the preceding steps have been taken, one need not ask the family to decide about *each* diagnostic or treatment option. Rather, one can propose a plan consistent with the goals and values and give family opportunity to concur with it. Recommend a treatment plan as a therapeutic time trial aimed at specific short-term goals. State how and when you will monitor success or failure of the time trial, and plan for follow-up discussions for further shared decision making. If appropriate, this might also be the point in the meeting to address code status. By this stage, the leading clinician is better equipped to make an informed recommendation of an appropriate code status.

G. Document the meeting in the record by writing a family meeting note—similar to writing a procedure note. Include who attended the meeting, what "the findings" were, what decisions and plans were made, justifications for those plans, what uncertainties or disagreements remained unreconciled, and plans for follow-up. Consider using a family meeting template to guide and document the meeting. Verbally communicate salient points to the ICU team.

H. The guidelines described above are designed to achieve shared decision making. Holding family meetings in the ICU within 72 hours of admission have been shown to increase family satisfaction, reduce the length of ICU stay, and increase the likelihood of agreement between the providers and the family about limitations of life-sustaining treatments. Family satisfaction is higher if physicians spend a smaller proportion of time

TABLE 42.3	Talking with ICU Families

Communicate regularly, using family meetings prophylactically. Involve the staff, especially the nurses. Be aware of family members who are nonparticipants.

Listen, listen for family understanding, affect, and how they make decisions. Establish trust. Acknowledge emotions. Avoid jargon. Lecture less and let the family guide you to further topics.

Provide psychosocial and spiritual support. Offer hope, not false hope. Bad news is a shock. Use support from the team. Culture and religion play key roles.

Inform family regularly about goals of care and how we know if goals are met.

Convey uncertainty; avoid false certainty. Describe treatment as a *therapeutic time trial* aimed at specific short-term goals.

Care always continues, but treatments may be withdrawn or withheld. Avoid saying we are "withdrawing care."

Don't ask the family to decide about each diagnostic or treatment option; ask them what the patient would want and allow them to concur with a plan consistent with patient values.

talking and more listening. Additional tips on talking with ICU families are provided in Table 42.3—these apply in formal family meetings and in less formal communications. Despite these efforts, uncertainty and/or conflict may arise. Redoubling communication efforts may solve the problems; sometimes, however, teams may need to seek additional help at resolving conflicts. This is covered in the section on GOC.

V. GOALS OF CARE

A. Goals of ICU therapy may vary on the basis of clinical reasonableness and patient's wishes and expectations. GOC should be discussed with the patient and/or the surrogate.

   1. For some patients, the goals are obvious, such as preventing imminent death, curing acute disease, relieving pain and suffering, and returning to their premorbid level of function. In some situations, the goal may be to delay the disease process. In others, it may be to prolong life long enough to allow the arrival of close relatives to pay last respects.

B. When discussing GOC, it is important to elicit and emphasize the patient's values.

C. After discussing the disease process and prognosis (see The Family Meeting section), the patient, a surrogate, or physician may propose a "do not resuscitate" (DNR), "do not attempt resuscitation" (DNAR), or "do not intubate" (DNI) order. The purpose of a code status is to clarify which therapies will be offered to the patient in the case of life-threatening instability. It is important to emphasize that DNR/DNAR/DNI orders do not automatically signify that a patient's condition is hopeless and to reassure that interventions to treat underlying pathology and optimize health and quality of life will continue, consistent with the patient's goals.

   1. Along these lines, it is not unusual for patients who are DNR/DNI to undergo diagnostic or therapeutic procedures. The need to reverse the DNR or DNI should be decided on a case-by-case basis. Prior to any procedure, a discussion with the patient or surrogate and providers involved is necessary. The procedure should be discussed in the context of the patient's current health status, values, and goals. For patients

undergoing elective surgical procedures requiring intubation or during which a reversible cause of cardiac arrest, unrelated to their underlying illness, may occur, it may be in line with their GOC to temporarily hold the DNR/DNI order. For severely ill patients undergoing procedures in which resuscitation would be unlikely to be effective or produce a survival consistent with their goals, they may elect to keep the DNR in place.

2. Today, patients often have multiple medical providers involved in their care and may receive treatment in multiple locations. Some states have implemented programs that provide a framework to allow patients with serious advanced illnesses to express their preferences about life-sustaining medical treatments with the purpose of relaying this information between health care providers. These are specific documents known as Physician/Medical Orders for Life-Sustaining Treatment (POLST, MOLST) or Physician Order for Scope of Treatment (POST) forms. Unlike a health care proxy or advanced directive form, these are considered to be medical order forms and are filled out by a health care professional after discussions with the patient regarding prognosis, treatments, and GOC. If a patient lacks capacity, a health care agent may sign the form on the patient's behalf. These forms can be particularly helpful in emergency situations, when the patient or health care proxy may not be immediately available to express the patient's wishes.

3. Conflict may arise when a family wishes to continue intensive interventions or "want everything done" but the medical team believes that some interventions are no longer warranted—or should not be offered. Under such circumstances, it is important to explore what is meant by the patient and family when they say they want "everything." They might not mean employ every life-prolonging intervention you can. They, like you, might want to avoid some burdensome and inefficacious treatments. Explore the nuances of their preferences and follow the steps outlined above in the section on family meetings.

4. Though there is no consensus on the precise definition of futility, clinicians often experience moral distress when they believe further intervention only serves to prolong the dying process, is ineffective, wasteful, or harmful. If open communication does not resolve the situation, then the clinician may (1) attempt to transfer the patient to another caregiver, (2) seek adjudication to replace or override the surrogate, or (3) involve institutional ethics and legal consultation to discuss limitations of life-sustaining treatment despite the wishes of the family. There might be a lower threshold to adjust a code status against family wishes than to actively withdraw life-sustaining treatments. The latter sort of decision should not be made solely by individual physicians but rather with the backing of additional critical care opinion(s), formal ethics consultation, and, preferably, with institutional policy support.

5. The institutional ethics committee is usually an interdisciplinary group of professionals trained in clinical ethics consultation. Ethics consultation offers an objective analysis of the patient's care and, drawing upon ethical principles, employs a fair process to guide the patient, clinicians, and family to a reasonable consensus or compromise. Ethics interventions have been shown to mitigate conflict and, for some, to reduce ICU length of stay, ventilator days, hospital stay, and cost (without increasing mortality).

VI. PROVIDING PALLIATIVE CARE IN THE ICU—IT'S NOT JUST FOR END-OF-LIFE

A. ICU patients are at risk for suffering a number of unpleasant sensations during routine ICU care. Their underlying illnesses and the procedures we do to diagnose and treat them can be accompanied by pain, dyspnea, anxiety, delirium, agitation, nausea, vomiting, secretions, pruritis, diarrhea, constipation, and other physical and psycho-social-spiritual discomforts. Preventing and palliating these distressing symptoms are goals shared by critical care and palliative care clinicians—whether the patient is receiving life-prolonging care or end-of-life care. Sometimes, formal palliative care consultation is warranted in the ICU, not only when patients are dying. Palliative care interventions have been shown to reduce length of stay and to improve symptom control, communication, and the quality of dying in the ICU. Social service and chaplaincy interventions can be employed as part of or separately from palliative care consultation. Patients, families, and staff are greatly supported by these services, especially under the stressful circumstances of ICU and end-of-life care.

B. General management of sedation, analgesia, and delirium is covered in Chapter 7 of this handbook. Here, we address clinical and ethical concerns related to withdrawing life-sustaining therapies from patients who are expected to die.

C. Legal and ethical opinion have established that competent individuals may refuse life-sustaining therapies, or have them withdrawn once started; they have also established that surrogates can make such decisions for patients who lack decision-making capacity. The law has evolved over time, balancing the autonomous rights of patients and the state's interest in preserving life. For surrogate decision making, states vary in their requirements of the level of evidence needed to discern the preferences of a previously competent person. So it is important to be familiar with your local legal standards.

D. Three ethical assumptions underlie the practice of forgoing life-sustaining treatment:

1. Withholding and withdrawing treatment are considered equivalent.

2. There is a difference between "killing" and "letting die."

3. One is permitted to use medications to relieve suffering at the end of life—even if side effects of those medications might hasten death—as long as the intent of using the medications is to relieve suffering. For patients who are terminally ill, risking the foreseen, but unintended, consequence of hastening death is justified under the "doctrine of double effect."

   a. Although some controversy surrounds these assumptions, they have been guiding principles for clinical practice and U.S. legal thought regarding end-of-life care.

VII. GUIDELINES FOR WITHDRAWING LIFE-SUSTAINING THERAPIES (LSTs)

A. Goals for the withdrawal of LSTs include the following:

1. Promoting comfort and respecting the wishes of the patient:

   a. Withdrawing burdensome therapies

   b. Maintaining or achieving the patient's ability to communicate, if possible

   c. Preventing or palliating distressing symptoms

2. Supporting and respecting the family

   a. Physically, emotionally, spiritually—within their cultural norms

3. Allowing death to occur

B. Your intensive focus now is the provision of comfort for this patient. All clinical **orders** should be reexamined with a goal toward palliative and comfort care. Consider consulting **palliative care**, particularly if care of

TABLE 42.4   Examples of Comfort and Palliative Measures in ICU

Continuation of general nursing care and cleanliness
Special clothing, blankets, stuffed animals
Offering of food/water to alert patients
Playing music
Nonpharmacologic sleep-promotion strategies
Control of oral secretions
Humidified air
Analgesics
Sedatives
Anticonvulsants
Antipyretics
Nonsteroidal anti-inflammatory drugs
Prophylaxis for gastrointestinal bleeding
Antiemetics

the patient will continue outside the ICU. Reassess the **equipment** in the patient's room and remove unnecessary items in order to make room for comfortable seating for family members. **Minimize monitors** (and their alarms). Therapies that increase patient comfort or relieve pain, anxiety, or agitation should be continued or added (Table 42.4). Therapies directed toward supporting physiologic homeostasis or treating the underlying disease process are no longer indicated and may be discontinued. These include many of the "routine" procedures and interventions associated with being an ICU patient (Table 42.5). The **benefit-to-burden ratio** of each intervention should be used to determine which interventions should be eliminated. The precise order of discontinuation is tailored to the patient's situation and reasonable family preferences. Most commonly, a stepwise approach is followed, with mechanical ventilation discontinued after the withdrawal of vasopressors, antibiotics, or enteral feedings.

C. **Individualized Care.** The guiding principles behind shared decision making apply in these situations: **prioritize the patient's/family's values** surrounding end-of-life practices—especially religious or spiritual and cultural—while providing situation-specific **professional advice** regarding clinical management practices. The family might not have ever experienced an ICU death. Or, perhaps they have, and it went well or went poorly. In the preparatory phases, explore the patient's/family's hopes and fears about the process. Hold a separate premeeting involving physicians,

TABLE 42.5   Examples of Routine Measures That May Be Withdrawn During the Process of Withdrawing Life-Sustaining Therapy

Frequent phlebotomy for laboratory tests
Frequent vital sign determinations
Placement of venous and arterial lines
Radiographic examinations
Aggressive chest physiotherapy and endotracheal suctioning
Debridement of wounds
Thromboembolism prophylaxis

nursing, and respiratory therapy to discuss withdrawal scenarios for *this* patient, and determine the optimal clinical options. Frame your clinical recommendations on the basis of the patient's/family's values and your clinical expertise in end-of-life care. Provide assurance of the patient's comfort throughout the process and invite family presence for as much as they feel comfortable. Assure the family that you will help them understand and cope with the end-of-life events as they unfold. Perhaps what they need most is just to hold their loved one again and prepare for a world without them.

The process of withdrawal should be clearly explained and the family educated about what to expect. For example, it is helpful to describe changes in skin color that occur, noises due to airway secretions, and the irregular breathing pattern preceding death. Explain that these changes usually are not consciously felt by the patient and that you will be vigilant to prevent or alleviate distressing symptoms. Practical wishes of the patient and family concerning the desirability of extubation can usually be accommodated. The anticipated rapidity of the dying process or realities of the patient's medical condition, however, may dictate specific choices concerning therapies to be withdrawn, the rate of withdrawal, and the ability to accommodate the requests of families. When a rapid death is anticipated, it may be impossible to accommodate requests to communicate with the patient after extubation or to hold prolonged vigils.

- **D.** Specific LSTs that may be withdrawn include the following:
  - 1. **Vasopressor and inotropic support** can be discontinued without weaning. The gradual withdrawal of circulatory support appears to offer no benefit for patient comfort.
  - 2. **Extracorporeal support therapies** are usually considered quite invasive by the patient and the family. These therapies require maintenance of vascular cannulae and the presence of additional equipment and personnel at the bedside. Intermittent extracorporeal support (e.g., intermittent hemodialysis) may simply not be restarted. Continuous renal support (e.g., continuous venovenous hemofiltration) can be discontinued. Death is usually not immediate following the discontinuation of dialysis, often occurring more than 1 week following discontinuation. Continuous circulatory support (e.g., ventricular assist, extracorporeal membrane oxygenation, intra-aortic balloon pump) can be discontinued and death anticipated soon after termination of support. Decisions regarding removal of vascular access devices not only should reflect patient comfort and family preference but also may take into account the risk of excessive bleeding due to uncorrectable coagulopathy.
  - 3. **Antibiotics and other curative pharmacotherapy.** After the decision is made to terminate LSTs, therapies directed at cure are no longer consistent with the GOC. Such therapies include cancer chemotherapy, radiation therapy, steroids, and antimicrobials—unless the treatments play a significant palliative role (such as topical antifungal agents, oral hygiene, or antibiotics aimed at treating painful lesions).
  - 4. **Supplemental oxygen.** If the avoidance of hypoxemia is no longer a therapeutic goal, supplemental oxygen may be discontinued and the patient returned to breathing room air. This is reasonable even if it is decided that mechanical ventilation will be continued. If the patient is removed from the ventilator but continues to have an artificial airway in place (e.g., endotracheal tube or tracheostomy), humidified air can be administered to avoid the irritation of drying the airway and secretions. The

continuation of supplemental oxygen often merely prolongs the dying process without providing comfort. An exception would be made for a dyspneic patient who desires to be alert for as long as possible.

5. Mechanical ventilation is the most common therapy withdrawn when LSTs are discontinued. Some physicians, however, prefer to withdraw therapies other than mechanical ventilation (such as vasopressors) with the expectation that the patient will die while still receiving mechanical ventilation. Similarly, during a prolonged illness, patients' families may have become comfortable with the surroundings of the ICU, the monitors, the artificial airway, and the mechanical ventilator. They may fear that the patient may suffer if mechanical ventilation or airway support is withdrawn, or they may believe that it is wrong to withdraw such support. Under such circumstances, it is reasonable to continue mechanical ventilation and airway support while discontinuing other LSTs. Nevertheless, mechanical ventilation does not differ morally or legally from other LSTs such as dialysis and can be discontinued if the patient or his or her proxy believes that it represents unwanted therapy.

a. Mechanical ventilation may be gradually withdrawn by decreasing the inspired oxygen to room air, decreasing positive end-expiratory pressure, and then gradually decreasing ventilatory rate. We recommend that this be done over several minutes (not hours), allowing for the titration of palliative medications. The rate of decrease is quite variable among practitioners. An overly slow "weaning" process may prolong the dying process and may provide the family with a misleading hope for survival.

b. Or, mechanical ventilation may be discontinued rapidly and humidified air administered via T-piece, or the ventilator can simply be removed from the patient and the patient extubated. Extubation may result in death more quickly compared with gradually decreasing the intensity of mechanical ventilation. It is important to anticipate, prevent, and be ready to treat dyspnea, obstruction, and air hunger.

c. The gradual and rapid techniques are each applicable in certain situations. Discuss with nursing and respiratory therapy to discern best strategy for a specific patient. The ability of the patient to maintain a patent airway, the presence of secretions, the perceptions of the patient and family, and the confounding presence of anesthetic drugs and neuromuscular blocking agents all may dictate a particular method of discontinuing mechanical ventilation. Invasive monitoring and analysis of arterial blood gas tensions or oxygen saturation are unnecessary during withdrawal of mechanical ventilation.

d. The timing of death after the withdrawal of mechanical ventilation is uncertain and depends on the etiology and severity of respiratory failure. Usually death occurs within a few hours to one day. In some studies, however, a small proportion of patients with chronic lung disease unexpectedly survived and were discharged from the hospital after withdrawal of mechanical ventilation. This observation is humbling: our prognostication is not infallible.

6. Nutrition (enteral or parenteral), fluid resuscitation, blood replacement, and intravenous (IV) hydration are considered forms of life-sustaining therapies and may be discontinued when sustaining or prolonging life is no longer the goal. Nasogastric and orogastric tubes may be removed, unless they are needed for comfort purposes. Case reports and controlled studies suggest that little, if any, discomfort

accompanies the withdrawal of enteral nutrition and IV hydration. In fact, the continuation of artificially administered fluids and nutrition can lead to edema and distressing bowel symptoms in dying persons. Nevertheless, families can be quite upset if it is perceived that their loved one is being "starved." If so, discussions would be in order about the natural slowing of metabolism during the dying process and the potential complications of artificially providing too much nutrition and hydration. A reasonable compromise might be reached, with the provision of small amounts of nutrition and hydration.

E. **Indications for Pharmacologic Intervention**
 1. **Presumption for comfort measures**. Clinicians should not withhold comfort measures for fear of hastening death. Patients who are given large doses of opioids to treat discomfort during the withdrawal of life-sustaining treatments on average live as long as patients not given opioids, suggesting that it is the underlying disease process, not the use of palliative medications, that usually determines the time of death.
 2. **Standard of care**. The administration of sedatives and analgesics during the withholding or withdrawal of life-sustaining treatments is consistent with the standard of care for critically ill patients. The majority of ICU patients do receive these medications during the withholding or withdrawal of support. Certainly, competent patients may refuse pharmacologic intervention to preserve lucidness. Drugs may not be indicated for patients who will gain no benefit (e.g., comatose patients).

F. **Specific Indications**
 1. **Pain**. The patient's report of pain or discomfort is certainly the best guide for treatment. When the patient is unable to communicate effectively, then other signs and symptoms of pain such as vocalizations, diaphoresis, agitation, tachypnea, and tachycardia may be valuable.
 2. **Air hunger/dyspnea**. Especially with the withdrawal of supplemental oxygen and mechanical ventilatory support, discomfort should be expected and anticipatory doses of anxiolytics and opioids should be administered. Additional doses should be immediately available and opioids continued as a continuous infusion. Clinicians must be immediately and continuously available to assess the patient's level of comfort and provide additional medication as necessary.
 3. **Death rattle**. Noisy, gargling breathing may occur in patients who are close to death, particularly in extubated patients. Although these sounds may be accompanied by dyspneic symptoms in the patient, they are usually more distressing to family members who are present. Treatment can include repositioning, gentle oropharyngeal suctioning, anticholinergics, and preparation and reassurance of the family.
 4. **Anxiety**. Alert patients may display varying levels of anxiety at the prospect of termination of life support. Although nonpharmacologic means of allaying anxiety can be extremely effective, sometimes patients request to be deeply sedated or unconscious prior to the discontinuation of life-sustaining therapies such as mechanical ventilation. Although death might be hastened by deep sedation, such requests can be honored.
 5. **Agitation or excessive motor activity**. Nonspecific motor activity may occur in some patients. Such activity is often interpreted as discomfort or distress by those attending the patient. It is reasonable that the level of sedation be increased in such situations. Neuromuscular blockade is never indicated because it does not treat the presumed underlying distress of the patient.

6. **Avoidance of drug withdrawal.** Often, patients are already receiving high doses of opioids or sedatives during the course of their illness and have developed drug tolerance. The patient's individual dose ranges can be used as a guide to provide increased amounts of opioids and sedatives during the discontinuation of support. Certainly, there appears to be little reason to decrease therapeutic doses of sedatives or opioids prior to the discontinuation of support for fear that the patient will not breathe adequately once the ventilator is discontinued.

VIII. PHARMACOLOGIC CHOICES (SEE CHAPTER 7)

A. **Opioids** are the first line of treatment for pain, dyspnea, or tachypnea during the discontinuation of life-sustaining measures. It is imperative that the route, dose, and schedule be individualized. IV administration is by far the most common route of administration with bolus administration providing the fastest pain relief, followed by a continuous infusion and additional bolus doses available as needed. For patients lacking adequate IV access, subcutaneous, oral, or transdermal routes of administration are options. Opioids are cardiopulmonary depressants; but these risks may be tolerated because of the proportionately desirable antidyspneic, sedative, and analgesic effects for end-of-life care (justified under principle of double effect). Gabapentin and carbamazepine are useful adjuncts for neuropathic pain.

B. **Benzodiazepines** have been the drugs of choice for the treatment of anxiety in many palliative care situations. However, because of the concern that benzodiazepines may be a risk factor for developing delirium in the ICU, critical care practice is leaning toward nonbenzodiazepines (such as propofol or dexmedetomidine) as preferable for routine sedation for mechanically ventilated adult patients. Nevertheless, in the end-of-life care setting, benzodiazepines still can play a role for their anxiolytic, hypnotic, sedative, and anticonvulsant properties. They can cause hypotension and respiratory depression, and more so when used in conjunction with opioids, but these risks are tolerable (as above).

C. **Dexmedetomidine or Haloperidol** may be indicated in the presence of delirium (acute confusional states) or agitation. These medications do not affect the respiratory drive, but dexmedetomidine can cause hypotension (hypertension with bolus administration), bradycardia, and loss of airway stability (resulting in obstruction after extubation).

D. **Propofol** is a potent hypnotic agent that can be used for sedation or for rapid induction of unconsciousness. This may be helpful for procedures and to rapidly reach a desired level of sedation. It also has helpful hypnotic, anxiolytic, antiemetic, and anticonvulsant properties, but provides no analgesia. Since dose-dependent decreases of arterial blood pressure and ventilatory drive are expected, some clinicians prefer not to use it for terminal ventilator withdrawal. The suppression of respiratory drive is enhanced by concomitant use of benzodiazepines and opioids.

E. **Barbiturates** are potent hypnotics that rapidly produce unconsciousness. Their pharmacodynamic effects are similar to those of propofol, but their pharmacokinetic profile is much less favorable. Such agents might be reserved for patients who are refractory to other, more commonly used means of sedation.

F. **Anticholinergic** medications, such as glycopyrrolate, scopolamine, ipratropium bromide, and hyoscyamine may be used to diminish copious oral and respiratory secretions that can produce death rattle. In general, atropine should be avoided because of its potential central nervous system side effects.

  G. Neuromuscular Blocking Agents are sometimes administered in the ICU to facilitate mechanical ventilation in patients with severe acute respiratory failure. The **indication for the use of neuromuscular blocking agents is lost** once the decision to forgo life-sustaining treatments is made. Neuromuscular blocking agents do not contribute to comfort of the patient and have no analgesic or sedative properties. Paralyzed patients are unable to express discomfort by attempting to communicate, move, or become tachypneic. The precise doses of opioids and anxiolytics necessary to avoid discomfort are then difficult to determine. Although it may be preferable to permit reversal of neuromuscular blockade prior to the withdrawal of mechanical ventilation, sometimes a prolonged drug effect that precludes adequate reversal or profound weakness is present. Many clinicians are uncomfortable with extubating a patient with no capability of maintaining spontaneous ventilation or a patent airway. In such cases, physicians may decide to forgo the withdrawal of mechanical ventilation or proceed only after administering high doses of sedatives and opioids to ensure the absence of patient awareness.

  H. Euthanasia is illegal in the United States. Drugs should not be administered with the sole and express purpose of causing death. Such interventions include the administration of neuromuscular blocking agents to produce apnea or the administration of potassium chloride to produce asystole.

  I. Palliative Sedation is legal in the United States and is not equivalent to active euthanasia. It is the monitored use of medications to relieve refractory and unendurable distressing symptoms. Protocols for this practice provide guidelines for the use of appropriate medications and the rationale for doing so. See, for example, Palliative Sedation Protocol of the Hospice and Palliative Care Federation of Massachusetts.

IX. MEDICAL ERRORS IN THE ICU

  A. As critically ill patients undergo more testing, monitoring, and interventions, this increases the chance for error. In fact, the rate of medical errors is higher in the ICU than in other areas of the hospital.

  B. Disclosure of medical errors should occur when harm has occurred and when it is recognized that the decision made or action taken was incorrect or that other health care providers would act differently in the same situation. Disclosure of near misses is not routinely encouraged.

  C. Open disclosure, in an empathetic, nondefensive manner, can help patients get further required treatment, facilitate financial adjustments, diminish concerns about an otherwise unexplained problem, reestablish trust, and actually strengthen doctor–patient relationship.

  D. Compassionate and sensitive disclosure may reduce the risk of malpractice litigation, whereas failure to disclose errors has been linked to increased desire to file an insurance claim.

  E. Seek advice and support from individuals in your institution skilled at disclosing medical error: there are preferred techniques for performing this difficult task.

X. SUPPORTING PROVIDERS

  A. Multiple factors in the ICU including uncertain prognosis, high incidence of conflict, and challenging end-of-life issues can result in moral distress among providers, which can lead to impairment and burnout.

    1. Impairment is the inability or pending inability of a health care provider to practice according to accepted standards as a result of substance use, abuse, or dependency.

2. It is estimated that approximately 10% to 15% of health care providers will misuse drugs or alcohol at least one time in their career. State, local, and some institutions provide impaired clinician programs for rehabilitation and treatment. Recovery rates are higher for health care professionals than for the general population and many programs assist with reentry into practice. Punitive action is rarely taken if a health care provider successfully undergoes treatment and follow-up.

3. Burnout is characterized by emotional distress, depersonalization, and sense of low personal accomplishment and is higher among ICU providers.

   a. Conflict, poor communication, work hours, work place organization, and involvement in end-of-life care are associated with increased risk of burnout. Studies have found burnout to be higher among residents, anesthesiologists, emergency medicine physicians, and oncologists. Improving overall health, increased personal support, and improving work satisfaction can help decrease burnout.

4. Ethics debriefing in the ICU can help mitigate moral distress and compassion fatigue. Such discussions can allow providers to explore alternative strategies of addressing concerns, reach a team consensus, draw from expertise of interdisciplinary team members, and help with consistent messaging to families. They can also provide awareness of moral distress and serve as educational opportunities for staff. Some ICUs schedule routine ethics rounds to discuss ethics topics, current troublesome cases, or recent past cases.

XI. SPECIAL POPULATIONS

A. **The Pediatric Patient Deserves Special Consideration**. Legally, end-of-life decisions are deferred to the parents. Ethically, however, the child may participate in these decisions, depending on his or her developmental level and decision-making capacity. If the child is too immature to participate in decisions, parents are relied on to make decisions in the child's best interest by weighing the benefit versus burden of each therapy. Pediatric intensivists must be sensitive to individual family dynamics and parenting styles when approaching end-of-life discussions for the pediatric ICU patient.

B. **Patients with Previous Disabilities**. ICUs receive some patients from both the pediatric and adult populations who have been living with previous disabilities—whether physical or cognitive. Their home caregivers usually have expertise in their home-based complex care routines. Occasionally, tensions develop between home caregivers and ICU caregivers over various elements of care or over perceptions of "quality of life." Proactive meetings among home and ICU caregivers early in the ICU course—run like the "Family Meetings" described in section IV—may help prevent or alleviate such tensions.

C. **The Chronically Critically Ill**. The term *chronically critically ill* refers to a group of patients who have survived an acute critical illness but continue to have persistent organ dysfunction requiring ongoing specialized care. Their course is usually characterized by fluctuations in care needs with slow progress and/or deterioration, which occurs over weeks to months, often interrupted by periodic acute events such as sepsis or heart failure. These patient experience frequent changes in care venue: often traveling between ICU, step down unit, short-term acute care, and long-term acute care facilities. One-year mortality is as high as 50%. In these situations, it can be difficult for patients, loved ones, and even health care providers to determine the optimum path. Continued conversations with patients and loved ones regarding prognosis, anticipated outcomes, future level of dependence, values, and goals are key since these can evolve as the state of chronic critical illness progresses. Palliative care involvement can be particularly helpful in this population.

D. Bridge to Nowhere. For some patients, a situation develops in which there is no hope for cure or improvement; yet, they seem "stranded" on a technologically complex and invasive intervention. The intervention may have been initially started as "a bridge" to some other, curative, treatment. An example of being on a "bridge to nowhere" is the continued use of ECMO for a patient who has lost candidacy for transplant or permanent ventricular assist device. In these situations, frank discussions are necessary, as well as consultations with chaplaincy, palliative care, and ethics. Before employing such therapies, clear limits should be defined.

XII. ORGAN DONATION

A. Determination of Death Using Brain Criteria. Brain death is a clinical syndrome defined as the irreversible loss of clinical function of the entire brain, including the brain stem. Prerequisites include the following:

1. Proximate cause of brain injury is known and is irreversible.
2. Exclusion of complicating medical conditions that may confound clinical assessment
3. Absence of drug intoxication or poisoning
4. Absent evidence of neuromuscular blockade
5. Core temperature greater than 36.5°C (96.8°F)
6. A period of 24 hours of observation without clinical change is necessary for comas of unknown etiology.
7. In the presence of confounding variables, brain death may be determined with the aid of ancillary testing.
   a. The three pivotal findings for brain death are **coma, absent brain stem reflexes, and apnea.**
   b. Confirmatory **ancillary tests** may be used when uncertainty about the reliability of the neurologic exam exists and apnea testing cannot be performed. In clinical practice, EEG, cerebral angiography, nuclear scan, TransCranial Doppler, CT Angiography, and MRI/MRA are currently used in adults.

B. Organ Donation after Brain Death. Patients who are declared brain dead may be considered for organ or tissue donation (with premortem patient consent or postmortem surrogate consent).

1. Due to a potential conflict of interest, conversations with the family regarding organ donation should not be conducted by the physician caring for the patient. Federal regulations require these discussions be conducted by trained personnel for the regional organ procurement agency (OPA).
2. Early contact with the OPA by ICU clinicians is critical as OPAs generally have specific guidelines regarding medications, ventilator settings, and blood work to be performed prior to organ donation.

C. Organ Donation after Cardiac Death. Critically ill patients who depend on LSTs may be considered for organ donation after cardiac death (DCD). However, the decision to withdraw LSTs must be made before—and distinct from—the discussion and decision about organ donation. In other words, LSTs are not being removed *so that* the patient can become an organ donor. Rather, a decision is made to remove unwanted, burdensome, or ineffective LSTs, and the subsequent anticipated imminent death of the patient presents an opportunity for organ donation. Only if the patient is expected to die imminently upon withdrawal of LSTs can DCD be considered.

1. DCD organ procurement is challenging and demands adherence to guiding ethical principles. The institutional guidelines for DCD organ procurement should be followed. Care for the dying patient including analgesic and amnestic medications supersedes the goal of organ procurement. The institutional policy should clearly define the following:

   a. The separation of caregiving responsibilities for the donor and for the recipient to avoid conflict of interest

   b. The physician responsible for pronouncing cardiac death is a member of the patient's care team and not a member of the transplant team.

   c. Specify if and what medications aimed at improving organ recovery may be administered before death. Permissible medications must not hasten the death of the donor.

   d. The time interval after which asystole at which death is declared (usually 2–5 minutes, to assure no autoresuscitation but to minimize ischemic damage to organs)

   e. The process for obtaining consent for and administering medications or procedures that are necessary for organ procurement, but are not otherwise of benefit to the patient (i.e., heparin administration, femoral arterial line placement, etc.)

   f. The process for allowing family presence at the time of death

   g. The time interval after which organ procurement will not be attempted in the case of unexpected patient survival after the withdrawal of life-sustaining therapies. (Time interval is 2 hours at Massachusetts General Hospital.)

XIII. ALLOCATION OF RESOURCES

A. ICU resources are not always available to persons who could benefit from them. Some patients wait in emergency departments, are triaged to other floors, or await transfer from other hospitals. Some patients might be discharged from units sooner than would be optimal for their individual benefit. Shortages of space, staff, and supplies can occur. Organs for transplant and high-tech therapies like ECMO are scarce resources. Rationing occurs. The principle of justice requires that we practice wise stewardship of resources so that they can be allocated fairly among persons. This applies across the spectrum, from chronically resource-poor settings to typically well-supplied settings facing overwhelming need, such as during pandemic flu, natural disasters, or war-torn strife.

B. Recent natural and man-made disasters (earthquakes, tsunamis, hurricanes, bombings) around the globe have inspired increased attention on the organization and functioning of medical relief efforts. This includes attention to emergency preparedness for such events or for pandemics, epidemics, and toxic exposures (influenza, Ebola, other biohazards). For example, who will get ventilators if there are not enough to go around? Who won't? Disaster teams prepare to be mobilized to distant sites, and hospitals prepare for meeting a surge in demand on resources—or, prepare to evacuate if their structure is damaged and unsafe. Strategies for resource utilization include preparation, conservation, substitution, adaptation, reuse, and reallocation. A deeper look into the practice of triage is beyond the scope of this chapter. Nevertheless, it is worth mentioning that clinicians accustomed to usual standards of care (in which they can focus on the patient in front of them) may find it ethically challenging to switch to a utilitarian goal of "the greatest good for the greatest number" if they are called upon to remove or divert a resource from the patient in front of them to another person.

C. As with other treatment decisions, optimal rationing decisions are fair, transparent, respectful, collaborative, and effective. Fairness may be the most difficult aspect to define because there are competing understandings of distributive justice (e.g., utilitarian, egalitarian, prioritarian). Some of the other aspects of decision making help attain fairness. Transparency presupposes that the decision process is explicit and open to scrutiny (and yet, intensivists' allocation of time spent with patients might involve implicit, undisclosed rationing). Being respectful includes taking into account fiduciary responsibilities and competing patient values. Collaboration insures that major decisions are not made by individuals, but, rather, at a higher-up level, in order to incorporate broader information about supply and demand, introduce objectivity and accountability, and to provide some consistency across similar situations. Effectiveness can be defined in numerous ways, including quantitatively (physiology, duration, costs) and qualitatively. Rationing is complex. So, it is right that appropriate attention be paid to allocation decisions in order to assure the best stewardship of resources and the optimal care of persons.

Selected Readings

Azoulay E, Timsit J-F, Sprung CL, et al. Prevalence and factors of intensive care unit conflicts: the conflicus study. *Am J Respir Crit Care Med* 2009;180:853–860.

Baldisseri MR. Impaired healthcare professional. *Crit Care Med* 2007;35(2 suppl):S106–S116.

Barr J, Fraser GL, Puntillo K, et al. Clinical practice guidelines for the management of pain, agitation, and delirium in adult patients in the intensive care unit. *Crit Care Med* 2013;41:263–306.

Boyle D, O'Connell D, Platt FW, et al. Disclosing errors and adverse events in the intensive care unit. *Crit Care Med* 2006;34(5):1532–1537.

Curtis JR, White DB. Practical guidance for evidence-based ICU family conferences. *Chest* 2008;134(4):835–843.

Davidson JE, Powers K, Hedayat KM, et al. Clinical practice guidelines for support of the family in the patient-centered intensive care unit: American College of Critical Care Task Force 2004–2005. *Crit Care Med* 2007;35:605–622.

Embriaco N, Papazian L, Kentish-Barnes N, et al. Burnout syndrome among critical care healthcare workers. *Anesthesiology* 2011;114(1):194–204.

Ethics in Clinical Practice Committee, Massachusetts General Hospital. Get-To-Know-Me Poster. http://www.massgeneral.org/palliativecare/assets/GetToKnowMePoster Guidelines.doc

Hamric AB, Blackhall LJ. Nurse-physician perspectives on the care of dying patients in intensive care units: collaboration, moral distress, and ethical climate. *Crit Care Med* 2007;35:422–429.

Hick JL, Hanfling D, Cantrill SV. Allocating scarce resources in disasters: emergency department principles. *Ann Emerg Med* 2012;59:177–187.

Hospice and Palliative care Federation of Massachusetts. Palliative Sedation Protocol: a report of the Standards and Best Practices Committee, Hospice and Palliative Care Federation of Massachusetts, April 2004. http://c.ymcdn.com/sites/www.hospicefed.org/resource/resmgr/hpcfm_pdf_doc/pal_sed_protocol_2004.pdf. Accessed September 6, 2014.

Hyman SA, Michaels DR, Berry JM, et al. Risk of burnout in perioperative clinicians: a survey study and literature review. *Anesthesiology* 2011;114:194–204.

Lilly CM, De Meo DL, Sonna LA, et al. An intensive communication intervention for the critically ill. *Am J Med* 2000;109:469–475.

Luce JM, White DB. A history of ethics and law in the intensive care unit. *Crit Care Clin* 2009;25:221–237.

Macintyre NR. Chronic critical illness: the growing challenge to health care. *Respir Care* 2012;57(6):1021–1027. doi:10.4187/respcare.01768.

McAdam J, Arai S, Puntillo K. Unrecognized contributions of families in the intensive care unit. *Intensive Care Med* 2008;34(6):1097–1101.

McDonagh JR, Elliott TB, Engelberg RA, et al. Family satisfaction with family conferences about end-of-life care in the intensive care unit: increased proportion of family speech is associated with increased satisfaction. *Crit Care Med* 2004;32(7):1484–1488.

Quill TE, Arnold R, Back AL. Discussing treatment preferences with patients who want "everything." *Ann Intern Med* 2009;151:345–349.

Reich DJ, Mulligan DC, Abt PL, et al. ASTS recommended practice guidelines for controlled donation after cardiac death organ procurement and transplantation. *Am J Transplant* 2009;9:2004–2011.

Santiago C1, Abdool S. Conversations about challenging end-of-life cases: ethics debriefing in the medical surgical intensive care unit. *Dynamics* 2011;22(4):26–30.

Scheunemann LP, White DB. The ethics and reality of rationing in medicine. *Chest* 2011;140(6):1625–1632.

Schultz CH, Koenig KL, Whiteside M, et al. Development of national standardized all-hazard disaster core competencies for acute care physicians, nurses, and EMS professionals. *Ann Emerg Med* 2012;59:196–208.

Shanawani H, Wenrich MD, Tonelli MR, et al. Meeting physicians' responsibilities in providing end-of-life care. *Chest* 2008;133:775–786.

Sprung CL, Zimmerman JL, Christian MD, et al. Recommendations for intensive care unit and hospital preparations for an influenza epidemic or mass disaster: summary report of the European Society of Intensive Care Medicine's Task Force for intensive care unit triage during an influenza epidemic or mass disaster. *Intensive Care Med* 2010;36:428–443.

Truog RD, Cist AFM, Brackett SE, et al. Recommendations for end-of-life care in the intensive care unit: the Ethics Committee of the Society of Critical Care Medicine. *Crit Care Med* 2001;29:2332–2348.

Truog RD, Campbell ML, Curtis JR, et al. Recommendations for end-of-life care in the intensive care unit: a consensus statement by the American Academy of Critical Care Medicine. *Crit Care Med* 2008;36:953–963.

Wilmer A, Louie K, Dodek P, et al. Incidence of medication errors and adverse drug events in the ICU: a systematic review. *Qual Saf Health Care* 2010;19(5):e7.

INDEX

Page numbers followed by *f* denotes figure; those followed by *t* denote tables